COMPREHENSIVE PERINATAL & PEDIATRIC RESPIRATORY CARE

ALWAYS: epi + fl.
↓ V-tach = defib.

When need to ID problem.
4 H's + 4 t's.

hypoxemia	tamponade
" volemia	ten. pneumo.
" thermia	toxins, poisons,
hyperkalemia	thromboembolism
hypo "	trauma
hydrogen Ions	

Jack-o-Lantern(s)?
-com

← Causes of deterior. of intub. child:
D isplacement of tube
O bstruction " "
P neumothorax
E quipment failure.

p65
FBAO _Foreign Body_
5 back blows.
Infants < 1y = chest thrust = thumbs finger.

child = abd thrust.
(heimlich)

CPR drugs
L ido
E pi
A tropine
N aloxone

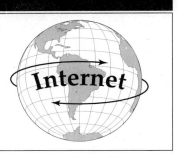

COMPREHENSIVE PERINATAL AND PEDIATRIC RESPIRATORY CARE

THIRD EDITION

Kent B. Whitaker, MEd, RRT, PA-C
Physician Assistant Program
Idaho State University
Pocatello, Idaho

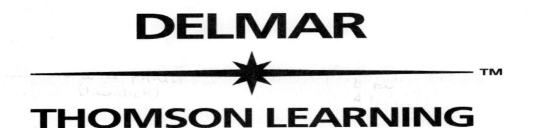

DELMAR ™

THOMSON LEARNING

Africa • Australia • Canada • Denmark • Japan • Mexico • New Zealand • Philippines
Puerto Rico • Singapore • Spain • United Kingdom • United States

NOTICE TO THE READER

Delmar Staff

Business Unit Director: William Brottmiller
Executive Acquisitions Editor: Cathy L. Esperti
Acquisitions Editor: Candice Janco
Senior Development Editor: Elisabeth F.Williams
Editorial Assistant: Maria D'Angelico
Executive Marketing Manager: Dawn F. Gerrain
Channel Manager: Tara S. Carter
Executive Production Manager: Karen Leet
Project Editor: Maureen Grealish
Production Coordinator: Nina Lontrato
Art/Design Coordinator: Jay Purcell

Library of Congress Cataloging-in-Publication Data
Whitaker, Kent B.
   Comprehensive perinatal & pediatric respiratory care / Kent B. Whitaker.—3rd ed.
     p. cm.
     Includes bibliographical references and index.
     ISBN 0-7668-1373-8 (alk. paper)
        1. Respiratory therapy for children. 2. Respiratory organs—Growth. 3. Infants (Newborn)—Diseases. 4. Neonatal intensive care. I. Title: Comprehensive perinatal and pediatric respiratory care.
     RJ434.W47 2001
     618.92'200428—dc21   2001017185

CONTENTS

PREFACE

Respiratory care practitioners working with pediatric and perinatal populations are presented with unique challenges in today's rapidly changing health care environment. Respiratory diseases represent a significant and increasing portion of pediatric and perinatal disorders. *Comprehensive Perinatal and Pediatric Respiratory Care, 3e,* has been updated and expanded to provide students with the theory and clinical expertise necessary to embark on their careers and meet these changing needs.

In this new edition, we have been grateful to the experience of a panel of subject matter experts in pediatric and perinatal respiratory care who have come together to keep the tradition of this text alive. We believe that we have responded to the market's need for more information on updated ventilators and monitors as well as new modes of ventilation. In this rapidly changing and dynamic specialty area today's special procedures quickly become tomorrow's common techniques and we have remained steadfast in our desire to provide students with information on equipment and procedures with which they will be working as they enter their careers.

We also understand that student's need their textbooks' content to correlate with information that they will find on their certification examx. To that end, we have also revised this text to correspond with the new NBRC content outline for the perinatal/pediatric specialty exam. The instructor's manual also includes a content outline of the text coded to the NBRC content outline.

In addition, we have listened to our student's needs and responded by incorporating clinical laboratories and checklists once found in a supplemental laboratory manual directly into the text. Students will now have all the necessary tools and visual aids at hand while conducting laboratory exercises. Clinical competencies are included in the text as well and allow students to assess their proficiency with specific skills.

CONTRIBUTORS

Dianne Adams, MA, RRT
Program Administrator:
Northwest New Jersey Consortium
for Respiratory Therapy Program
Saint Clare's Hospital, Dover, N.J.
Associate Professor:
County College of Morris
Randolph, New Jersey
Sussex County Community College
Newton, New Jersey

Jeff Cain, RRT
Respiratory Therapist
Department of Critical Care Support Services
C.S. Mott Children's Hospital
University of Michigan Health System
Ann Arbor, Michigan

Patricia Carroll, RRT, RN, MS
Adjunct Faculty
Respiratory Care & Allied Health
Manchester Community College
Manchester, Connecticut
Consultant and Owner, Educational Medical Consultants
Meriden, Connecticut

Gerri Davidson, RRT
Perinatal Pediatric Specialty Certified
Northeast Georgia Medical Center
Cumming, Georgia

Albert J. Heuer, MBA, RRT
Assistant Professor
School of Health Related Professions
University of Medicine and Dentistry
Scotch Plains, New Jersey

Garry Lowe, BS, RRT, RPFT
Perinatal/Pediatric Specialist
Staff Development/Stat Lab Supervisor
Respiratory Care Services
Arkansas Children's Hospital
Little Rock, Arkansas

Nancy Lowe, RRT
QI/Regulatory Affairs Coordinator
Respiratory Care Services
Arkansas Children's Hospital
Little Rock, Arkansas

Tim Opt'Holt, EdD, RRT
Professor
Cardiorespiratory Care Department
University of South Alabama
Mobile, Alabama

Kurt Riek, RRT
Respiratory Therapist
Department of Critical Care Support Services
C.S. Mott Children's Hospital
University of Michigan Health System
Ann Arbor, Michigan

Kathleen Salgado Wyka, AAS, CRT
Director Respiratory Services
Allied Health Care Services, Inc.
Orange, New Jersey

IML Contributors

Patricia Carroll, RRT, RN, MS
Adjunct Faculty
Respiratory Care & Allied Health
Manchester Community College
Manchester, Connecticut
Consultant and Owner, Educational Medical Consultants
Meriden, Connecticut

Kathleen Salgado Wyka, AAS, CRT
Director Respiratory Services
Allied Health Care Services, Inc.
Orange, New Jersey

DEVELOPMENT AND CARE OF THE FETUS: CONCEPTION TO BIRTH

CHAPTER ONE

EMBRYOLOGIC DEVELOPMENT OF THE CARDIOPULMONARY SYSTEM

OBJECTIVES

Upon completion of this chapter, the reader should be able to:

1. Describe the embryology of the morula, blastocyst, blastoderm, and trophoblast.
2. Identify the three germ layers and the body structures that evolve from each.
3. Identify the five periods of embryonic lung growth and describe the features of each period.
4. Define surface tension and describe the following:
   a. How it is developed
   b. Laplace's law
   c. Application to alveolar mechanics
5. With regard to surfactant, describe the following:
   a. Function and purpose
   b. The approximate gestational age at which immature and mature surfactant appear
   c. Components and methods to detect its presence
   d. How lung maturity is determined
6. Regarding fetal lung fluid, describe the following:
   a. Composition
   b. Function
   c. The hazards of lung fluid retention
7. Describe the embryologic development of the heart including:
   a. Development of the cardiac chambers
   b. Formation of major vessels and cardiac valves
8. With regard to fetal circulation, describe and explain:
   a. The cause of pressure differences between the right and left heart
   b. The flow of blood from the placenta, through the body and back to the placenta
   c. Each shunt that is encountered
9. Describe the location and function of the baroreceptors and chemoreceptors.
10. Describe the development of the placenta and umbilical cord and identify the major anatomical structures of each.

11. Explain the function of amniotic fluid and define the following:
    a. Polyhydramnios
    b. Oligohydramnios

KEY TERMS
---

amnion	ductus venosus	ovum
baroreceptor	ectoderm	phosphatidylglycerol
blastocyst	endoderm	phospholipid
blastoderm	fertilization	polyhydramnios
blastomere	foramen ovale	septum primum
chemoreceptor	functional residual capacity (FRC)	sinus venosus
choana	intervillous space	sphingomyelin
chorionic villi	mesoderm	surfactant
cotyledon	morula	trophoblast
dichotomy	oligohydramnios	truncus arteriosus
ductus arteriosus		

EMBRYOLOGIC DEVELOPMENT OF THE FETUS

Since we are at the beginning of a chapter that details the embryologic development of the human lung and heart, we will briefly look at the beginnings of human life. *Fertilization*, or the union of the sperm cell and the mature ovum, occurs in the outer third of the fallopian tube and begins the journey of life. From that instant on, the human body begins 40 weeks of growth and development that leads to a fully developed fetus. In the first month alone, the fetus grows in weight by nearly 3000%.

The duration of human pregnancy is referred to as either 10 lunar months of 4 weeks each, 9 calendar months in which there are 3 trimesters of 3 months each, or 40 weeks. In this text, gestational age refers to the time since conception.

Development and growth are divided into three distinct stages. The first stage is the period from conception to the completion of implantation or about 12 to 14 days. During this stage of development the developing organism is called an *ovum*. It is called an embryo during the second stage, which occurs from the end of the ovum stage to the time it measures roughly 3 cm from head to rump or around 54 to 56 days. It is during this second stage of development, that the major organ systems are developed. The embryo is extremely vulnerable to the effects of drugs, infections, and radiation. Exposure to any of these agents during this period can lead to severe congenital malformations. The name fetus is used during the third stage, from the end of the embryonic period to the end of pregnancy. The major organs have developed and now proceed to grow during this period. Because the organ systems are mostly developed, they are less susceptible to drugs, infections, and radiation. However, exposure may lead to an interruption of normal functional development of the organ systems.

Following delivery, developmental stages are identified by the following terms: Neonate is used from delivery through the first month of life, infant is used for the period from 1 month to 1 year of life, and child identifies the patient above 1 year of age.

FERTILIZATION TO IMPLANTATION

The newly fertilized ovum advances quickly through various stages of growth. Cellular division begins as the ovum travels through the fallopian tube toward the uterus. Entrance into the uterus, roughly 10 to 13 cm distance, occurs around the fourth or fifth day.

The first division or cleavage results in 2 identical cells. Further cleavage of the 2 cells results in 4 cells, 8 cells, and so forth. The cells that are produced during this rapid cleavage are called *blastomeres* and are surrounded by a transparent tissue envelope, the zona pellucida. Soon, the cells have grown substantially in number and now form a ball, called a *morula*. It is at this stage of growth that the ovum, consisting of 16 to 50 cells, enters the uterus. Fluid now begins gathering around the morula, and a cavity forms in its center. Next, fluid begins collecting in this newly formed cavity, leading to the next stage of development, the *blastocyst*. This initial fluid is a combination of uterine fluids and secretion by the cells.

The zona pellucida is now replaced by an outer layer of cells called the *trophoblast*. It is during this time that the cells begin their differentiation into their respective germ layers. As the blastocyst continues to expand, some of the cells gather toward one end forming what is known as the *blastoderm* or embryonic disc. This group of cells will become the fetus, while the trophoblast will become the placenta and its related structures.

With the loss of the zona pellucida, the trophoblast attaches itself to the lining of the uterus, the endometrium, to receive nourishment. This attachment, or implantation, normally occurs in the upper portion of the uterus. Following implantation, the blastocyst becomes completely covered by the endometrium. The trophoblast grows into the endometrial tissue, forming what will become the placenta. The various stages of development up to implantation are illustrated in Figure 1–1.

DIFFERENTIATION OF GERM LAYERS

The embryonic disc at this point includes two layers of cells, the *ectoderm* and the *endoderm*. They are named according to their location, the ectoderm being the outer and thicker layer, and the endoderm being the innermost layer. The third cell layer, known as the *mesoderm*, forms between the other two shortly thereafter (Figure 1–2). It is from these primary germ layers that all tissues, organs, and organ systems will differentiate. The structures that arise from the three primary germ layers are listed in Table 1–1.

DEVELOPMENT OF THE PULMONARY SYSTEM

The development of the pulmonary system begins soon after conception and continues well into the pediatric years. Lung development takes place in five stages, as illustrated in Figure 1–3.

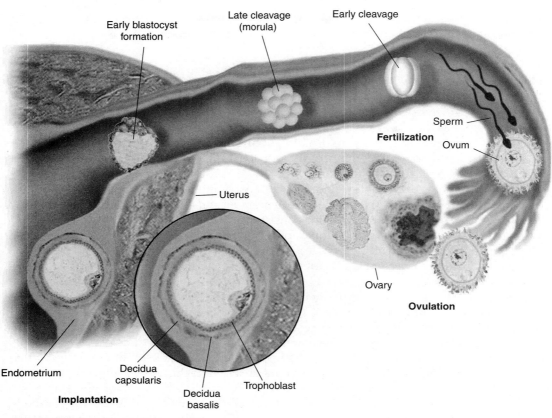

Figure 1–1 *Cellular development of the ovum.*

EMBRYONIC PERIOD

The first stage is called the embryonic period. This period of development covers the first six weeks of gestation. At roughly 21 days, the embryonic disc elongates and becomes broad at the cephalic end and narrow at the opposite end. The endoderm forms a tube-like structure, shaping the future gastrointestinal tract. The ectoderm is also developing into a cylindrical tube, forming the future central nervous system.

As the primitive gut develops, the upper portion forms the early oral and nasal openings, while the lower segment forms the pharynx and the foregut. The nasal cavities now develop from the ectoderm. The connection of the primitive mouth and the foregut, which will become the alimentary tract, occurs during the fourth gestational week.

The pharynx begins development near day 21 arising from the upper portion of the primitive foregut. A small furrow known as the laryngotracheal groove appears at the lower end of the developing pharynx.

The earliest development of the lung begins at 24 days following conception (Figure 1–3A).

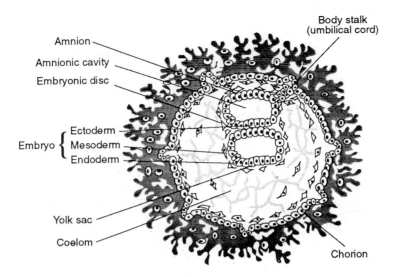

Figure 1–2 *The formation of the three germ layers.*

At this time the lung bud appears as a small pouch, arising from the laryngotracheal groove in the developing pharynx. By day 28, the small pouch has grown and now branches into the right and left lung buds. As these branches develop, they will become the right and left main stem bronchi. Both the mesoderm and the endoderm develop as the primitive airways progress in their division. The mesodermic tissue becomes the smooth muscle, connective tissue, cartilage, and blood vessels in the mature lungs.

Branching continues with lobar bronchi forming around day 31, dividing into two branches on the left bud and three branches on the right bud. The primitive mesoderm begins to differentiate into its respective muscle, tissue, and vessel formation. It is during this period that the diaphragm begins its development, becoming completely developed by the end of 7 weeks.

TABLE 1–1 Structures Arising from the Three Germ Layers

ENDODERM	MESODERM	ECTODERM
• Respiratory tract • Epithelium of the digestive tract, bladder, thyroid • Primary tissue of the liver and pancreas	• Dermis • Muscles • Bone, connetive tissue, lymphoid tissue • Reproductive organs • Cardiovascular system	• Epidermis • Hair, nails • Lens of the eye • Central and peripheral nervous system • Skin glands

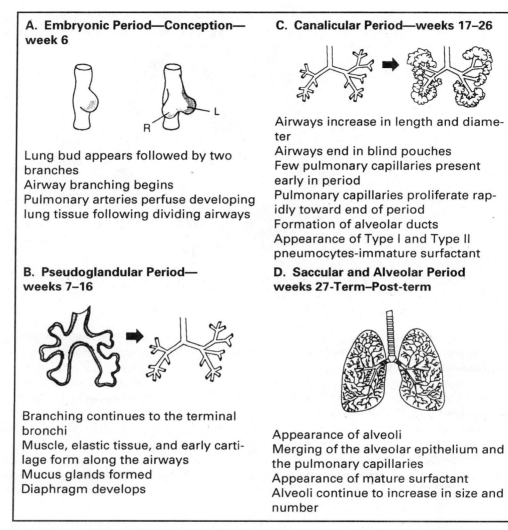

A. Embryonic Period—Conception—week 6

Lung bud appears followed by two branches
Airway branching begins
Pulmonary arteries perfuse developing lung tissue following dividing airways

B. Pseudoglandular Period—weeks 7–16

Branching continues to the terminal bronchi
Muscle, elastic tissue, and early cartilage form along the airways
Mucus glands formed
Diaphragm develops

C. Canalicular Period—weeks 17–26

Airways increase in length and diameter
Airways end in blind pouches
Few pulmonary capillaries present early in period
Pulmonary capillaries proliferate rapidly toward end of period
Formation of alveolar ducts
Appearance of Type I and Type II pneumocytes-immature surfactant

D. Saccular and Alveolar Period weeks 27-Term–Post-term

Appearance of alveoli
Merging of the alveolar epithelium and the pulmonary capillaries
Appearance of mature surfactant
Alveoli continue to increase in size and number

Figure 1–3 *Embryologic development of the lung.*

PSEUDOGLANDULAR PERIOD

The second stage is the pseudoglandular period, which covers weeks 7 to 16. This period of lung development is depicted in Figure 1–3B. By week 7 of gestation the tissue that will form the epiglottis is present. Above the epiglottal tissue, the arytenoid tissues begin developing at about the same time, eventually becoming the opening to the lower airways.

During the seventh gestational week, the membrane that separates the nasal cavity from the oropharynx disintegrates at the *choana,* opening the anterior nasal cavity to the pharynx. Failure of this membrane to disintegrate appropriately results in a blockage known as choanal atresia. This defect is discussed in more detail in Chapter 11.

Continuing at week 7 the anterior and posterior palates begin to develop, separating the oral and nasal cavities. The palates are completely developed by the end of week 12. The anterior palate eventually becomes ossified and is known as the hard palate. The posterior palate remains soft, and as such, is known as the soft palate. The area above the soft palate is the portion of the pharynx called the nasopharynx, whereas the area above the hard palate contains the nasal cavities. The vocal cords appear during week 8 as small folds of connective tissue in the larynx and are soon fully developed.

The fetal lung resembles a gland at this point in its development, thus the name pseudoglandular. Lung development during this period results in significant branching or *dichotomy.* Branching progresses from 4 generations at the beginning to 25 generations by the end of week 16, with a majority occurring between weeks 10 and 14. Segmental bronchi are present by the end of week 6, followed by the development of the subsegmental bronchi. By week 11, cartilage begins to appear in the airways and continues to form from that time. The major lobes of the lungs are identifiable by week 12.

Goblet cells, those that produce airway mucus, form in the human lung during the 13th gestational week. The mucus they produce collects in the upper portion of the cell, causing it to bulge out. This bulging causes the cell to appear as a wine glass or a goblet, hence the name. The goblet cells appear to proliferate in the larger upper airways while remaining in relatively small numbers in the small distal airways.

The bronchial glands begin development during week 13 and complete their development by week 24. Bronchial glands contain mucus-producing cells and serous cells. The bronchial gland secretions appear to contribute more to respiratory tract secretions than do the goblet cells. Ciliated cells appear sometime around week 10, and at birth are found in the airways down to the level of the terminal bronchioles. It is the cilia that move the mucus blanket up the airways, removing lung debris to the point that it can be expectorated out of the system.

CANALICULAR PERIOD

The third stage is known as the canalicular period and covers weeks 17 through 26. During the canalicular period the terminal and respiratory bronchioles continue to multiply, as shown in Figure 1–3C. It is during this period that the fetal lung undergoes a tremendous amount of vascularization. As the period advances, small outpouchings begin appearing along the walls of the respiratory bronchioles, eventually becoming the alveoli during the terminal sac period.

In these primitives alveoli, the epithelial tissue is beginning to differentiate into its two separate types. Type I will form the alveolar capillary membrane, while the Type II cells will produce pulmonary sufactant. Capillaries are present in proximity to the alveolar cavity during week 20 to 21, but it is not until week 24 to 25 that they are close enough to allow for adequate gas exchange.

SACCULAR AND ALVEOLAR PERIODS

The fourth and fifth stages are termed the saccular and alveolar periods (Figure 1–3D) covering the period from week 27 to term and into the post-term period. By week 24 to 26, the lungs have been completely formed. True alveoli, with the terminal airways called saccules, have not yet formed. True alveoli appear around weeks 32 to 34, developing from a thinning of the terminal air saccules. The number of alveoli continues to increase until the approximate age of 8 years. It is during the alveolar period that pulmonary surfactant is produced in increasing amounts by the Type II alveolar cells.

SURFACE FORCES AND THE ROLE OF SURFACTANT

At this point in development, the lung is capable of functioning as an organ of respiration. For the lung to function properly, however, strong surface forces must be overcome. An understanding of these forces and the role of surfactant in lessening their effect will now be examined.

SURFACE TENSION

Basic understanding of surface tension stems from the knowledge that similar molecules attract each other from all directions. An excellent example of this is to place a drop of water on a hard surface. The water molecules present inside the droplet attract one another from all directions, causing the water to bead. The molecules on the surface, while being drawn together and inward, are not being pulled outward by the air molecules. This causes the surface molecules to be pulled inward and together very tightly, forming a surface tension (Figure 1–4).

Surface tension is what allows a needle to float or a spider to walk across the water's surface. If you could suspend the droplet in mid-air, surface tension would cause the droplet to form a sphere. The constant inward pull of the molecules causes the droplet to retract to its smallest size. This inward pull can only be offset by an equal and opposite pressure from without.

This phenomenon of surface tension also occurs in the alveoli. Because the alveoli are largely liquid and they surround a gas, the same surface forces as described above are present in the alveoli. The surface molecules of the alveolus are attracted inward due to the lack of attraction by the gas molecules. This shrinks the alveolus to its smallest diameter.

LAPLACE'S LAW

Pierre-Simon de Laplace was a scientist who lived during the late 1700s and early 1800s. He discovered the important relationship between the internal pressure of a sphere, its radius and surface tension. According to Laplace's law, as the radius of the bubble, or in

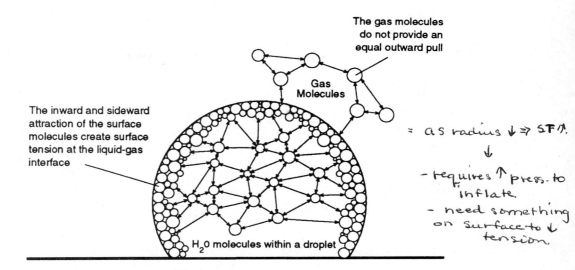

The gas molecules do not provide an equal outward pull

Gas Molecules

The inward and sideward attraction of the surface molecules create surface tension at the liquid-gas interface

= as radius ↓ ⇒ SF ↑.
↓
- requires ↑ press. to inflate.
- need something on surface to ↓ tension.

H_2O molecules within a droplet

Figure 1–4   *Surface molecules being pulled together and inward create surface tension.*

this case the alveoli, decreases, the surface tension increases (Figure 1–5). An excellent example of Laplace's law is found in a simple balloon. A new, deflated balloon requires a modest amount of pressure to begin inflation, but a balloon that is partially inflated requires much less pressure or force to inflate it further.

Applying this understanding to the alveoli, it should be clear that as the alveoli become smaller, as during exhalation, much force is required to reopen them. In this scenario, the work and energy required to inflate the lungs would quickly exhaust energy and lead to death. To overcome this collapsing force, there must be something present on the surface of the alveoli to reduce the amount of tension that develops.

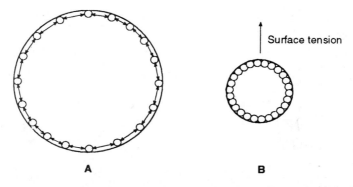

Surface tension

A

B

Figure 1–5   *As the radius decreases from A to B, the surface molecules achieve a stronger horizontal attraction, casuing an increase in surface tension.*

THE ROLE OF SURFACTANT

Surfactant is the substance found on the alveolar wall that lowers surface tension. An understanding of how surfactant lowers surface tension is given in the following example. If we were to mix a surfactant with water, the molecules of the surfactant would attract the water molecules less strongly. This would cause the molecules of surfactant to gather at the surface of the water. At the surface the weaker attractive force of the surfactant dilutes the attraction of the water molecules and thus weakens surface tension.

The physiologic importance of this is twofold. First, an alveolus that has a lower surface tension requires less counterpressure to keep it open at a smaller radius. Therefore, less musical effort is required to open and ventilate the lungs. Second, the effect of surfactant changes as the surface area of the alveoli changes. In the lung, there are many different sizes of alveoli. If surfactant does not change its influence as the alveoli change in size, then many different pressures would need to be present in the lungs to keep the different alveoli from collapsing.

Due to its unique composition and the fact that the amount remains stable in the alveoli, surfactant exerts a varying influence on the alveoli as they enlarge and shrink. As the alveoli are stretched during inspiration, the surfactant thins on the surface and tension builds. This aids in the process of passive exhalation, allowing surface tension to constrict the alveoli back down to a small size. As the alveoli become smaller, the surfactant thickens on the alveolar surface, weakening surface tension and preventing the alveoli from collapsing.

APPEARANCE AND PRODUCTION OF SURFACTANT

The first appearance of pulmonary surfactant coincides with the development of Type II pneumocytes. Surfactant is composed of *phospholipids* (mainly phosphatidylcholine [PC] and *phosphatidylglycerol* [PG]), neutral lipids, and proteins. After being produced, the surfactant is stored in the cell in what are known as lamellar inclusion bodies. The first surfactant to be produced lacks PG and is termed immature surfactant. This is first seen at 24 weeks' gestation.

During this early stage, surfactant production is easily inhibited by hypoxia, hypothermia, and acidosis. Babies born prematurely, especially those of less than 30 weeks, are extremely prone to each of these disorders. The result is a rapid deterioration in the respiratory status following delivery, commonly called respiratory distress syndrome (RDS). Mature surfactant is present around week 35, at which time PG appears.

MEASUREMENT OF FETAL SURFACTANT AND DETERMINATION OF LUNG MATURITY

From the time the immature surfactant first appears, it can be measured in a sample of amniotic fluid. Fluid produced by the lungs contributes to the amniotic fluid. Some of the surface active phospholipids excreted by the alveolar cells are carried to the amniotic fluid by the lung fluid. By withdrawing a sample of amniotic fluid and comparing the level of

PC (also called lecithin) to the level of *sphingomyelin* in the amniotic fluid, lung maturity can be predicted. Sphingomyclin is another type of phospholipid produced by the fetus that remains at a fairly stable level in the amniotic fluid throughout gestation. By comparing the levels of each in the amniotic fluid, a quick determination of fetal lung maturity is possible. This comparison is called the lecithin-to-sphingomyelin ratio (L/S ratio) (Figure 1–6).

The fetal lungs are considered mature when the L/S ratio reaches 2:1; in other words, there is twice as much lecithin as sphingomyelin. This 2:1 ratio occurs near week 35 of gestation. The achievement of the 2:1 ratio usually coincides with the onset of mature surfactant production and indicates little chance of developing in RDS.

As gestation progresses, surfactant production is enhanced. As previously mentioned, PG is produced as surfactant production reaches maturity.

This fact has led to the practice of testing amniotic fluid for the presence of PG, as well as for determining L/S ratio, as a better determinant of fetal lung maturity. The combination of L/S ratio and testing for PG is called the lung profile. Studies have demonstrated that the lung profile is a better predictor of lung maturity than either the L/S ratio or PG detection when used alone. Many factors can either delay or accelerate the production of mature surfactant. Those factors are listed in Table 1–2.

Another relatively simple method of determining lung maturity is by a test known as shake or foam test. This procedure is done by mixing amniotic fluid with ethanol. The mixture is then shaken for 15 seconds. A reading is made 15 minutes later. If there is a ring of

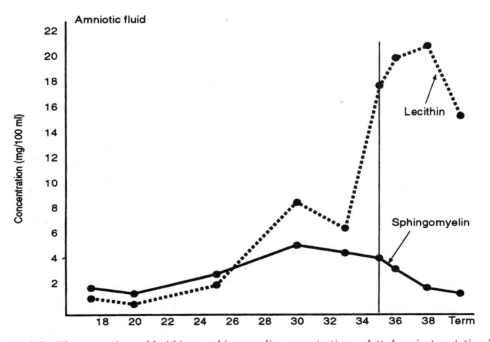

Figure 1-6 *The comparison of lecithin to sphingomyelin concentrations, plotted against gestational age. (Reprinted with permission from Gluck, L, Kulovich MV, Borer, RC, Jr., et al. Am J Obstet Gynecol. 1971; 40:440.)*

TABLE 1–2 Conditions That Delay or Accelerate Surfactant Production in the Fetus

---

Conditions that delay surfactant production:

- Acidosis
- Hypoxia
- Shock
- Overinflation
- Underinflation
- Pulmonary edema
- Mechanical ventilaiton
- Hypercapnia
- Infants of diabetic mothers classes A, B, and C
- Erythroblastosis fetalis
- The smaller of twins

Conditions that accelerate surfactant production:

- Infants of diabetic classes D, F, and R
- Maternal heroin addiciton
- Premature rupture of membranes
- Maternal hypertension
- Maternal infection
- Placental insufficiency
- Maternal administration of betamethasone or thyroid hormone
- Abruptio placentae

---

bubbles in the ethanol after 15 minutes, it shows there is enough lecithin present to create a stable foam. This technique is a fairly reliable way of determining fetal lung maturity. If foam is not present following the 15-minute period, an L/S ratio should be performed.

There are several techniques that have been successful in predicting fetal lung maturity. The concentration of lamellar bodies in the amniotic fluid has compared favorably to the lung profile in its ability to predict lung maturity. Another screening test, the amniotic fluid surfactant-albumin ratio (SAR), has been shown to be accurate in clinical studies. A third test, called the TDx-FLM assay, also can be used to predict RDS with as much reliability as the lung profile. Finally, the fluorescence polarization (FP) assay has been shown to accurately predict RDS.

Studies by Liggins and Howie that were done on fetal lung surfactant led to the discovery that lung maturation can be artificially induced.[1] These studies showed that the administration of glucocorticoids to women in premature labor increased the rate of lung maturity and decreased the rate of RDS. The limitations of this method required administration of the drug when the fetus was between weeks 27 and 34, it had to be given at least 48 hours before delivery, and delivery had to occur within 7 days of administration.

Other factors influencing lung maturation include thyroxine, thyrotropin-releasing hormone, β-adrenergic drugs, estrogen, prolactin, and epidermal growth factor.[2] In contrast to previous thinking, fetuses of preeclamptic women do not show an acceleration of lung maturation.

↑ BP @ 24w. gestation

The role of surfactant is vital. Its presence enhances capillary circulation allowing for normal ventilation/perfusion ratios. It may also offer protection to the alveolar tissues against barotrauma. Through its ability to lower surface tension and provide for stable alveoli, its presence aids in the evacuation of lung fluids.

The lack of surfactant in the lung or the deterioration of its production following birth is the leading cause of pulmonary complications in the neonate. When surfactant is not present, the lungs become stiff, noncompliant organs. Every breath requires tremendous energy, which is then quickly depicted. The unassisted neonate will soon exhaust and die from the combination of energy loss, hypoxia, and hypoventilation. It is no wonder that science has worked for so long to develop an artificial surfactant that would mimic the structure and mechanism of human surfactant. With the disruption of the normal mechanisms of surfactant production in the preemie, the administration of an artificial surfactant would result in a reduction of these lung complications. Following much trial and error, an adequate surfactant was developed. The circumstances surrounding its development and use are discussed in Chapter 17.

FETAL LUNG FLUID

The fetal lung, being a metabolically active organ and acting somewhat similar to a gland, produces and secretes its own fluid. At term, the lung is filled with about 20 to 30 ml/kg of fluid, or roughly the equivalent volume of the *functional residual capacity (FRC)*. In fetal lamb lungs, its production increases with gestation beginning at a rate of roughly 2 to 4 ml/kg/day and increasing up to 100 ml/kg/day. This fluid exits the lung through the trachea and is excreted through the mouth into the amniotic fluid. It is by this mechanism that lung surfactant can be measured in an amniotic sample.

COMPOSITION

Fetal lung fluid is of a different composition than is amniotic fluid. It has lower pH, protein, and bicarbonate, but higher concentrations of sodium and chloride. Lung fluid appears early in gestation and continues to generate until shortly before delivery, at which time production ceases.

FUNCTION

It is apparent that the lung fluid has multiple functions. One of its earliest functions is to maintain the patency of the developing airways. It also appears to play an important role in the formation, size, and shape of potential air spaces. As the lungs grow and develop, it would be difficult for them to develop their complicated structures if they were collapsed. In order for ventilation to proceed unhindered in the neonate, it is important that the lung fluid be completely evacuated from the lungs at birth. This takes place by a variety of methods. If the fetus is delivered vaginally, one third of the fluid is removed by the squeezing of the thorax as the fetus descends through the maternal pelvis. Most of the remaining lung fluid is rapidly absorbed by the pulmonary lymphatic system. This absorption takes place within a few hours following delivery.

HAZARDS OF LUNG FLUID RETENTION

It is not uncommon for neonates delivered by cesarean section to retain a larger amount of lung fluid. This is primarily due to the lack of the squeezing action on the thorax that occurs during a vaginal delivery. In these neonates, the fluid must be rapidly absorbed in order for breathing to progress. Positive pressure ventilation has been shown to distend the interstitial spaces, possibly enhancing the absorption and uptake of the fluid. Neonates who fail to remove the lung fluid adequately are prone to a syndrome known as transient tachypnea of the newborn (TTN) or RDS type II. TTN is fairly common in babies delivered by cesarean section, for reasons outlined above. TTN is discussed in more detail in Chapter 10.

DEVELOPMENT OF THE CARDIOVASCULAR SYSTEM

The importance of the heart to the growth and development of the fetus can be shown by the speed at which it develops. The heart is the first major organ to develop. This is primarily due to the tremendous growth of the fetus and its nutritional needs. Figure 1–7 illustrates the development of the heart and associated structures.

EARLY EMBRYOLOGIC DEVELOPMENT

Indistinct clumps of cells appear from the mesoderm around gestational day 21. By the end of the third week these cells have formed two tubes surrounded by a sheath of myocardial cells. The tubes begin to fuse at their center and soon form a single, continuous chamber. As early as the fourth week, the heart begins to beat. This early embryonic heart begins a twisting and folding that will eventually form the four heart chambers.

The bottom of the fetal heart begins swelling into a small cavity and contains a pair of branches known as horns. These horns are called the *sinus venosus* and will eventually become the inferior and superior vena cava and a portion of the right atrium. At the top of this small cavity, the primitive ventricle and atrium appear. A hollow tube of myocardium, the *truncus arteriosus*, grows from this primitive ventricle. The truncus arteriosus will develop into the pulmonary artery and the aorta. At this point, the heart appears as a bulging, hollow tube.

DEVELOPMENT OF THE CARDIAC CHAMBERS

The heart now begins to bend in the middle, forming itself into a rough S shape. As the heart continues its rapid growth, the sinus venosus and the atrium are pushed upward behind

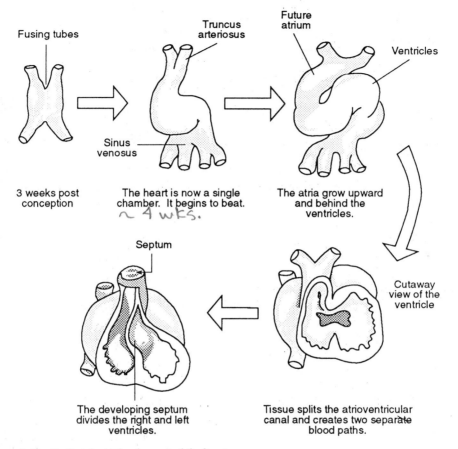

Figure 1–7 *Embryologic develpment of the heart.*

the developing ventricle. The single ventricle divides into the right and left ventricles by splitting at the center of the S. The internal chambers are identified on the outer surface by the presence of grooves, called sulci.

The blood, which began flowing around the third week, now begins a one-way flow instead of its back and forth motion. The blood enters through the sinus venosus and travels through the primitive atrium, the left and right ventricles, and out through the truncus arteriosus. By the beginning of the fifth week, the embryonic heart no longer looks like an S, but now has assumed the shape of the adult heart.

In the uppermost portion of the heart, the developing veins and arteries couple the heart to the expanding circulatory system. The single atrium divides into two separate chambers by the emergence of a tissue known as the *septum primum*. During this division, tissue growth stemming from the front and back walls of the heart form the openings between the atria and ventricles. The truncus arteriosus allows blood to exit the right ventricle and is the only outlet for blood.

FORMATION OF MAJOR VESSELS AND CARDIAC VALVES

During the sixth week the truncus is divided into two vessels by a thin tissue that spirals down the center of the truncus. These two vessels are the pulmonary artery and the aorta. This tissue continues to grow, eventually separating the right and left ventricles completely. The newly formed aorta is now the escape route for blood in the left ventricle, and the pulmonary artery provides the outlet for the right ventricle.

During this time, the valves begin to form between the atria and ventricles as well as in the root of both the pulmonary artery and aorta. In two short months, the heart has formed and begins pumping and circulating blood, a tiny replica of an adult heart.

FETAL CIRCULATION

Fetal circulation refers to the unique system of shunts and pressures that are found in the fetal circulatory system. It is important to understand and identify the flow of blood in the fetus. Of equal importance is to understand *why* the blood follows the peculiar fetal path.

The pressure found inside the fetal vasculature are the reverse of those found in the adult. Pressures in the right, or venous, system are higher than those in the left, or arterial, system. There are two reasons for this.

First, during the development of the fetus, the growing lungs provide a very high resistance to blood flow. This high resistance is secondary to pulmonary vasculature constriction caused by the low PaO_2 in the fetal blood and also by the fact that the lungs are for the most part collapsed. The collapsed lungs exert a high external force on the pulmonary vasculature, decreasing their size and increasing resistance to blood flow. The high pulmonary vascular pressures result in increased pressures in the pulmonary artery. This increases pressure in the right ventricle, right atrium, vena cava, and so forth, throughout the venous system.

The second cause of the reversal of blood pressures is the fact that the placenta offers very little resistance to blood flow. Because of the enormous amount of vasculature in the placenta, the blood flows to the placenta with relative ease. The low resistance of the placenta causes low pressures in the aorta, left ventricle, left atrium, and the entire arterial system. The combination of these two factors causes the reversal of pressures found in the fetus. With that understanding we can now look at fetal blood flow.

BLOOD FLOW AND SHUNTS IN FETAL CIRCULATION

Fetal circulation is depicted in Figure 1–8. After the fetal blood has received its oxygen and nutrients from the placenta, it collects into progressively larger and larger vessels until it

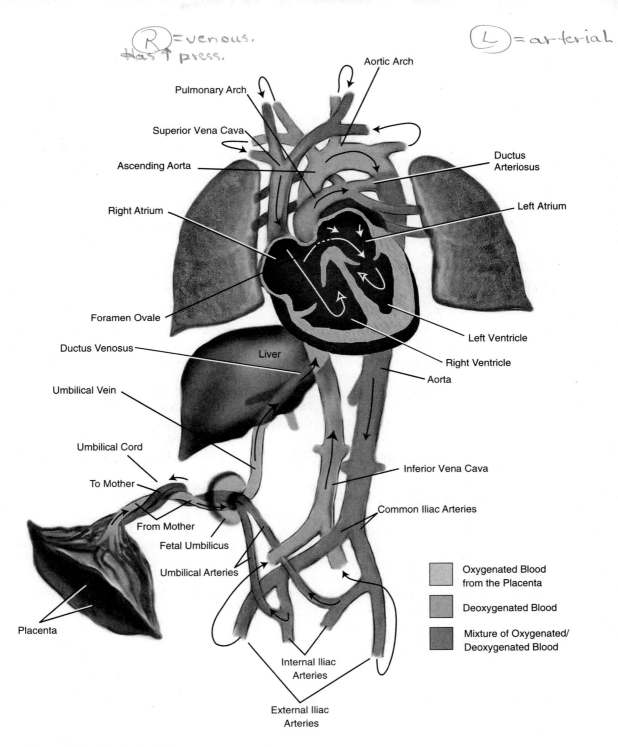

Figure 1–8 *Fetal circulation.*

arrives at the umbilical vein. The umbilical vein carries the fresh blood from the placenta through the umbilical cord and into the fetus.

Ductus Venosus.   Soon after the blood enters the abdominal cavity, the first shunt is encountered—the *ductus venosus*. Upon reaching the liver, roughly 50% of the blood flow is directed through branches of the umbilical vein into the liver. The remaining blood flow is diverted directly into the inferior vena cava through the ductus venosus. The ductus venosus is merely a continuation of the umbilical vein, which connects to the inferior vena cava.

The shunted blood mixes with blood returning from the lower extremities. This mixing causes a reduction in the total oxygen saturation of the blood. The venous blood from the extremities is true venous blood with a low oxygen content. The mixed blood continues toward the right atrium. Upon entering the right atrium, the blood mixes with the venous return of the superior vena cava. It is at this point that the second shunt is met.

Foramen Ovale.   An opening between the right and left atrium is present in the atrial septum. This opening is the second shunt, known as the *foramen ovale*. With pressures being higher in the right atrium than in the left, most of the blood in the right atrium shunts through the foramen ovale into the left atrium. On the left atrial surface of the foramen ovale is a tissue flap, which acts as a one-way valve. After birth, as pressure inside the left atrium increases and becomes greater than that in the right, the flap is held closed mechanically, preventing blood from shunting back into the right atrium.

The remaining blood, which did not pass through the foramen ovale, enters the right ventricle. Because of the anatomy of the right atrium, most of this blood comes from the superior vena cava. From the right ventricle, the blood passes through the pulmonary artery.

Ductus Arteriosus.   Upon reaching the point where the pulmonary artery branches into the lungs, the third and most familiar shunt is encountered—the *ductus arteriosus*.

The ductus arteriosus joins the pulmonary artery to the aorta. It is a short vessel with a diameter that approaches that of the pulmonary artery. Because of the high resistance in the pulmonary vasculature, most of the blood entering the pulmonary artery passes through the ductus arteriosus and enters the aorta. This leaves only 10% of the total blood supply to perfuse the lungs. The blood flow to the pulmonary system at this point serves mainly to perfuse the developing lungs.

Blood Flow Beyond the Heart.   The blood that shunts from the right to left atrium through the foramen ovale enters the left ventricle. From there it passes into the aorta, where it combines with the flow from the ductus arteriosus. As it travels through the aorta, some of the blood exits to perfuse the upper extremities, the kidneys, the gut, and other abdominal organs. Near the upper pelvic region, the aorta splits into the two common iliac arteries. The iliac arteries further divide into the external and internal iliac arteries. It is from the internal iliac arteries that the two umbilical arteries branch. Roughly 60% of the total blood flow exists the fetus through the umbilical arteries and returns to the placenta, where the cycle starts again.

THE DEVELOPMENT OF BARORECEPTORS AND CHEMORECEPTORS

BARORECEPTORS

Baroreceptors, which have the ability to detect changes in pressure, are located in the bifurcation of the carotid arteries and in the aortic arch. These receptors are actually stretch receptors and are stimulated as they are stretched or distorted in shape. Stimulation of these receptors leads to bradycardia and hypotension. Whether baroreceptors are active during fetal life or not is a subject of controversy. The progressive rise in arterial pressure during gestation, as well as the sudden increase in blood pressure and fall in heart rate that follow clamping of the cord, may show that these reflexes are present to some degree in the fetus and neonate.

CHEMORECEPTORS

Chemoreceptors, although present in the fetus, are not generally active. Immaturity of the carotid sinus synapses found in the central nervous system (CNS) may be one cause of this inactivity. Chemoreceptors are located in the carotid arteries and aorta and are called carotid and aortic bodies. Because of their sensitivity to PaO_2, $PaCO_2$, and pH, their role is in regulation of ventilation. They also have a function in the initiation of the first breath. This will be covered in Chapter 3.

DEVELOPMENT AND FUNCTION OF INTRAUTERINE STRUCTURES

These structures include the placenta, the umbilical cord, the amnion, and the amniotic fluid.

PLACENTA

During the 40 weeks of gestational development, the placenta acts as the organ of respiration for the fetus. It is through the placenta that the growing fetus receives nutrients and oxygen and rids itself of CO_2 and other wastes. Soon after the embryo implants itself in the wall of the uterus, small projections of the trophoblast begin invading the endometrium, not unlike a seed sending roots into the soil. These projections, known as *chorionic villi*, are the beginning of the placenta. The anatomy of the term placenta is illustrated in Figure 1–9.

The villi continue to branch and develop, embedding themselves deeply in the endometrium. Each villus has an outer epithelial layer and an internal connective tissue core

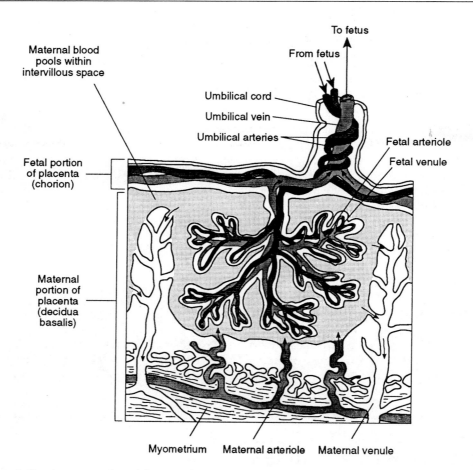

Figure 1–9 *A cutaway view of the term placenta.*

that contains the fetal vessels. As the villi continue to expand and grow, the endometrium begins eroding, creating pockets around the villi that will contain the maternal blood. These irregular spaces are known as the *intervillous spaces.*

At term, the normal placenta is round, occupies about one third of the uterine surface, and weighs around 1 pound, or 15 to 20% of the fetal weight at term. The maternal surface contains 15 to 28 segments, known as *cotyledons.* Each cotyledon contains the chorionic villus and an intervillous space.

Blood coming from the fetus follows the two umbilical arteries to the placenta, at which point they branch into smaller and smaller vessels. This branching supplies each cotyledon with a portion of the fetal blood. Upon reaching the cotyledon, the fetal blood advances throughout the branches of the chorionic villi. It is here that the exchange takes place between maternal and fetal blood. There is no contact between the two blood supplies, because they are separated by the thin epithelial layer of the villus. This allows passive exchange to proceed quite easily.

The maternal blood enters at the base of the intervillous space by way of spiral-arteries. The maternal arterial blood completely surrounds the chorionic villus, allowing a tremendous surface area for exchange. The fetal blood has high levels of CO_2 and waste materials but is low in oxygen and nutrients. In contrast, the maternal blood has high levels of oxygen and nutrients but is low in CO_2 and waste materials.

Following gradients of high to low concentrations, the fetal blood gets its needed oxygen and nutrients, while giving up the CO_2 and waste to the maternal blood. Maternal blood returns to the mother's venous system by way of venous openings in the chorionic villi, which drain into larger vessels and eventually reach the maternal vena cava.

Fetal blood, now carrying needed oxygen and nutrients, exits the villi through small veins. These veins collect the fetal blood from each cotyledon and return it to the fetus by way of the umbilical vein.

UMBILICAL CORD

The umbilical cord is the lifeline between mother and fetus. To perform this vital role, the umbilical cord has a unique makeup. A cross section of the umbilical cord (Figure 1–10) reveals three vessels surrounded by a tough, gelatinous material called Wharton's jelly. The three vessels consist of two smaller arteries and one large floppy vein. The umbilical arteries have relatively thick walls, while the vein is thin walled.

Because of the constant movement of the fetus in utero, it is possible that the umbilical cord could bend and pinch off, stopping the flow of blood to the infant. The presence of Wharton's jelly prevents this from occurring. While it is flexible enough to allow bending and movement of the cord, it is also rigid enough to prevent the cord from kinking and occluding blood flow.

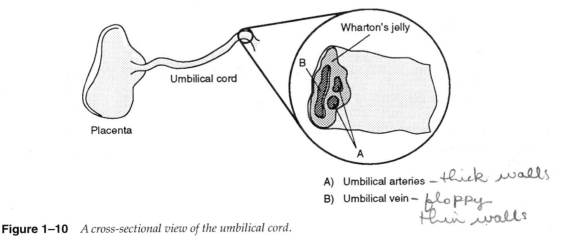

A) Umbilical arteries — *thick walls*
B) Umbilical vein — *floppy thin walls*

Figure 1–10 *A cross-sectional view of the umbilical cord.*

AMNION

The *amnion* is the sac that surrounds the growing fetus and contains the amniotic fluid. It arises from the trophoblast around the seventh gestational day. It begins as a small vesicle and develops into a sac, which covers the dorsal surface of the embryo. As gestation progresses it enlarges and surrounds the embryo.

AMNIOTIC FLUID

Fluid fills this newly developed sac, called amniotic fluid. The amniotic fluid compartment found early in pregnancy is largely made up of maternal fluids and fluid from the amniotic membrane. At the end of the 40 weeks of gestation about 1 liter of fluid is present, with a range of 500 to 1500 ml. In the last trimester alone there are increases of 30 to 40 ml per day.

Amniotic fluid is dynamic, meaning it is constantly being absorbed and replenished. There are signs that up to about 24 to 26 weeks' gestation, when keratinization of the skin occurs, the fetal skin is very permeable to amniotic fluid. Once keratinization has occurred, most of the absorption of the fluid is accomplished by fetal swallowing. The fluid is replenished by a combination of fetal urination and lung fluid. The term fetus swallows around 500 ml per day and excretes about 500 ml of hypotonic urine per day.

Polyhydramnios.   The amount of amniotic fluid present at birth is dictated by how much the fetus swallows and urinates. Abnormally large amounts of fluid, usually over 2000 ml, indicates hydramnios or *polyhydramnios*. Its presence indicates a problem with the swallowing mechanism of the fetus. Possible anomalies that may cause hydramnios include: 1) CNS malformations such as hydrocephalus, microcephaly, anencephaly, spina bifida; 2) orogastric malformations such as esophageal atresia, pyloric stenosis, cleft palate; and 3) disorders such as Down syndrome, congenital heart disease, infants of diabetic mothers, and prematurity.

The major complication for the fetus with hydramnios is the risk of premature rupture of the amniotic membranes. This condition leads to a possible prolapse of the umbilical cord and premature delivery.

Oligohydramnios.   Scant or decreased amount of amniotic fluid is known as *oligohydramnios*. Causes are usually associated with a defect in the urinary system of the fetus. Often, renal dysplasia or agenesis as well as urethral stenosis are involved. A classic example of the association between renal agenesis and oligohydramnios is Potter's syndrome. Fetal adhesion of one body part to another body part may occur if oligohydramnios develops in the first part of pregnancy. Hypoplasia of the fetal lungs is often seen in the presence of oligohydramnios.

Implications for the fetus with oligohydramnios include the risk of asphyxia secondary to compression of the umbilical cord and the danger of significant skeletal deformities.

Functions of Amniotic Fluid.   Amniotic fluid serves several important functions, outlined in Table 1–3. First, it allows the fetus to move and grow freely while within the con-

---

TABLE 1–3   Functions of Amniotic Fluid

- Protection from traumatic injury
- Thermoregulation
- Facilitation of fetal movement & prevent cord kinking

---

fines of the uterus. It offers protection to the fetus by buffering any shock or impact to the maternal abdomen. Amniotic fluid also helps in thermoregulation of the fetus. It allows the mother to go through wide changes in environmental temperature, while maintaining a fairly constant fetal temperature. During labor and delivery, the presence of amniotic fluid helps to dilate and efface the cervix. Amniotic fluid may also aid in metabolism by aiding with the water needs of the infant.

SUMMARY

The embryologic development of the fetus is an extraordinary event that begins with two cells and finishes as a fully developed child with all of the intricacies of the body systems in place. The lungs, which develop from the endoderm, begin development at 24 days with the appearance of a small outpouching on the primitive foregut. The lungs undergo five stages of growth and development, called the embryonic period, the pseudoglandular period, the canalicular period, the saccular period and finally, the alveolar period. While most lung structures are completely developed by 40 weeks, alveoli continue to increase in number for roughly the first 8 years of life.

Because the alveoli have a liquid-air interface, they are subject to surface tension which, if allowed to remain, would make normal breathing impossible. According to Laplace's law, surface tension increases as the size of the alveoli shrinks, making each successive breath more difficult, resulting in RDS. Surfactant, produced by Type II alveolar cells and stored in lamellar bodies, is secreted onto the surface of each alveoli and lowers surface tension to the point that breathing is not hindered. Fetal lung maturity can be detected by several methods, including the L/S ratio, the presence of PG in the amniotic fluid, the shake test, the concentration of lamellar bodies in amniotic fluid, the surfactant-albumin ratio, the TDx-FLM assay, and the fluorescence polarization assay. Certain drugs and hormones have been shown to influence lung maturation, including glucocorticoids, thyroxine, thyrotropin-releasing hormone, β-adrenergic drugs, estrogen, prolactin, and epidermal growth factor.

The fetal lung produces fluid throughout gestation, which helps maintain the size, shape, and patency of airways and spaces. Normally expulsed during vaginal delivery, lung fluid may be retained following cesarean section delivery and may lead to a syndrome called transient tachypnea of the newborn (TTN). Type II RDS.

The heart is the first major organ to be developed, starting to beat at roughly 4 weeks gestation. Blood flow in the fetus follows a unique series of shunts in the fetus, known as fetal circulation. The first shunt encountered is the ductus venosus, followed by the foramen ovale and finally, the ductus arteriosus. Blood flow is directed through the shunts due to a reversal of the typical pressures found in the cardiovascular system, that is, high pressure in the right heart, low pressure in the left heart.

The placenta is the fetal organ of respiration. Maternal arterial blood enters the intervillous spaces that surround the chorionic villi carrying the fetal blood. At that point, an exchange of oxygen, carbon dioxide, and nutrients takes place following concentration gradients. Blood flows from the placenta to the fetus via a large umbilical vein and is returned to the placental through two umbilical arteries.

Amniotic fluid is constantly being swallowed and absorbed and replenished through fetal urination and lung fluid. It serves several vital purposes for the developing fetus. It allows free fetal movement, protects the fetus from injury, and aids in thermoregulation. At delivery, it helps to dilate and efface the cervix. Too much amniotic fluid (polyhydramnios) or too little fluid (oligohydramnios) may indicate possible fetal anomalies and may expose the fetus to other risks.

With this brief look at fetal development, the practitioner is more able to understand the complex problems associated with premature delivery and be better able to treat these tiny patients.

References

1. Liggins CG, Howie RN. A controlled trial of antepartum glucocorticoid treatment for prevention of the respiratory distress syndrome in premature infants. *Pediatrics.* 1972;50.
2. Avery GB, Fletcher MA, MacDonald MG. *Pathophysiology and Management of the Newborn.* 5th ed. Philadelphia: JB Lippincott Co.; 1999.

Bibliography and Suggested Readings

Assali NS. *Biology of Gestation.* Vol 1, II. New York: Academic Press; 1968.
Bayer-Zwirello LA, et al. Amniotic fluid surfactant-albumin ration as a screening test for fetal lung maturity. Two years of clinical experience. *J Perinatol.* 1993;13.
Beachey W. *Respiratory Care Anatomy and Physiology, Foundations for Clinical Practice.* St. Louis: Mosby-Year Book; 1997.
Blackburn J, Loper D. *Maternal, Fetal, and Neonatal Physiology, a Clinical Perspective.* Philadelphia: WB Saunders Co; 1992.
Burton G, Hodgkin J, Ward J. *Respiratory Care: A Guide to Clinical Practice.* 4th ed. Philadelphia: Lippincott-Raven Publishers; 1997.
Chen C, et al. Clinical evaluations of the NBD-PC fluorescence polarization assay for prediction of fetal lung maturity. *Obstet Gynecol.* 1992;80.
Comroe, JH. *Physiology of Respiration.* Chicago: Year Book Medical Publishers Inc; 1965.
Cottrell GP. *Cardiopulmonary Anatomy and Physiology for Respiratory Care Practitioners.* Philadelphia: FA Davis; 2000.
Des Jardins T. *Cardiopulmonary Anatomy and Physiology.* 3rd ed. Albany, NY: Delmar Thomson Learning; 1998.
Fakhoury G, et al. Lamellar body concentrations and the prediction of fetal pulmonary maturity. *Am J Obstet Gynecol 170.* 1994;1(pt 1).

Hagen E, et al. A comparison of the accuracy of the TDx-FLM assay, lecithin-sphingomyelin ratio, and phosphatidylglycerol in the prediction of neonatal respiratory distress syndrome. *Obstet Gynecol.* 1993;82.

Harker LC, et al. Improving the prediction of surfactant deficiency in very low-birth-weight infants with respiratory distress. *J Perinatol.* 1992;12.

Herbert WN, et al. Role of the TDx-FLM assay in fetal lung maturity. *J AM Obstet Gynecol 168.* 1993;3(pt 1).

Klaus MH, Fanaroff AA. *Care of the High Risk Neonate.* 5th ed. Philadelphia: WB Saunders Co; 1999.

Larsen WJ. *Essentials of Human Embryology.* Philadelphia: Churchill Livingstone; 1998.

Lozon, MM. *Emergency Pediatric Management.* Philadelphia: WB Saunders; 2000.

Lowdermilk DL, Perry SE, Bobak IM. *Maternity Nursing.* 5th ed. St. Louis: Mosby Inc; 1999.

Schiff E, et al. Fetal lung maturity is not accelerated in preeclamptic pregnancies. *Am J Obstet Gynecol.* 1993;169.

West J. *The Essentials of Respiratory Physiology.* 6th ed. Philadelphia: Lippincott; 1999.

Posttest

1. At what stage of embryologic development does the ovum enter the uterus?
   a. zygote
   b. morula
   c. blastocyst
   d. blastoderm

2. The respiratory system arises from which of the following germ layers?
   a. endoderm
   b. mesoderm
   c. ectoderm
   d. myeloderm

3. The earliest development of the lung begins at:
   a. conception
   b. 24 days
   c. 36 days
   d. 8 weeks

4. Dichotomy of the airways occurs during which phase of lung development?
   a. embryonic
   b. pseudoglandular
   c. canalicular
   d. alveolar

5. Which of the following statements best describes surface tension?
   a. diffusion of similar molecules following concentration gradients
   b. the inward movement of surface molecules due to kinetic energy
   c. the tendency of a liquid surface to contract
   d. the attraction of surface water molecules to gas molecules

6. Which of the following, when found in amniotic fluid, is the best indicator of fetal lung maturity?
   a. PC   P.12
   b. lecithin
   c. sphingomyelin
   d. PG

7. Which of the following does not appear to accelerate fetal lung maturation?
   a. thyroxine
   b. estrogen
   c. maternal preeclampsia
   d. prolactin

8. Which of the following are true concerning lung fluid?
   I. There is approximately 20 to 30 ml/kg present at birth.
   II. At term, it is produced at a rate of 2 to 4 ml/kg/hr.
   III. It has lower pH, protein, and bicarbonate levels than amniotic fluid.
   IV. It has lower sodium and chloride concentrations than amniotic fluid.
   V. It maintains the patency of the developing airways.
   a. I, III, V
   b. II, IV, V
   c. I, II, III, V
   d. I, II, III, IV

9. Which of the following may occur following Cesarean section?
   a. RDS
   b. TTN
   c. diaphragmatic hernia
   d. aspiration pneumonia

10. The heart develops from which germ layer(s)?
   P16
   a. endoderm
   b. mesoderm
   c. ectoderm
   d. myeloderm

11. The embryologic truncus arteriosus develops into:
   I. the vena cava
   II. the pulmonary artery
   III. the atria
   IV. the aorta
   V. the right and left ventricles
   a. IV, V
   b. I, III
   c. I, II, III
   d. II, IV

12. Which of the following describes the path of blood that is shunted through the foramen ovale?
   a. from the umbilical vein to the inferior vena cava
   b. from the right to left atrium

   c. from the right to left ventricle
   d. from the iliac artery to the umbilical artery
13. The ductus arteriosus shunts blood from:
   a. the pulmonary artery to the aorta
   b. the right to left atrium
   c. the umbilical vein to the inferior vena cava
   d. the right to left ventricle
14. Which of the following statements is correct?
   a. Baroreceptors are not active during fetal life.
   b. Baroreceptors sense changes in PaO_2, pH, and $PaCO_2$.
   c. Baroreceptors are actually stretch receptors.
   d. Baroreceptors are instrumental in the initiation of the first breath.
15. In the placenta, the fetal vessels are contained in the:
   a. intervillous space
   b. cotyledon
   c. spiral arteries
   d. chorionic villi
16. Identify the umbilical vein(s) on the following diagram by circling the correct letter.

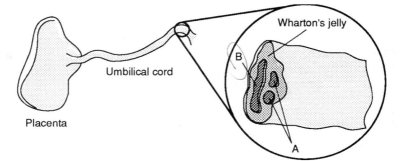

17. Polyhydramnios is defined as:
   a. an absence of amniotic fluid
   b. a decreased amount of amniotic fluid
   c. infection of the amniotic fluid
   d. an excessive amount of amniotic fluid
18. Which of the following are possible causes of polyhydramnios?
   I. hydrocephalus
   II. esophageal atresia
   III. choanal atresia
   IV. Down syndrome
   V. cleft palate
     a. II, III, IV, V
     b. I, II, IV
     c. I, II, IV, V
     d. I, II, III, IV, V

CHAPTER TWO

ASSESSMENT OF FETAL GROWTH AND DEVELOPMENT

OBJECTIVES

Upon completion of this chapter, the reader should be able to:

1. Describe at least three ways ultrasonography is used to assess fetal age.
2. Define amniocentesis and describe the role of each of the following:
   a. L/S ratio
   b. Determination of alpha-fetoprotein
   c. Bilirubin level
   d. Creatinine level
   e. Identification of meconium staining
   f. Cytologic examination of cells
3. Describe three different methods of measuring fetal heart rate.
4. Describe the cause and/or characteristics of the following:
   a. Baseline heart rate
   b. Bradycardia
   c. Tachycardia
   d. Beat-to-beat variability
   e. Accelerations
   f. Decelerations
5. Explain how fetal scalp pH is used to assess fetal asphyxia.
6. List and describe the five methods used to estimate the date of delivery.
7. Compare and contrast the contraction stress test to the nonstress test. Describe how each test is performed, and their advantages and disadvantages.
8. Describe the use of vibroacoustic stimulation, fetal movements, and amniotic fluid volume as methods of assessing fetal well-being.
9. Describe the six tests used in the biophysical profile, and how each is scored.
10. Explain the implications of meconium-stained amniotic fluid in assessing fetal status.
11. Describe chorionic villus sampling, cordocentesis, and magnetic resonance imaging in assessing fetal status.

12. Compare and contrast material estriol determination and human placental lactogen (HPL) levels as to their roles in determining fetal status.
13. Identify and list at least five factors that indicate a high-risk pregnancy.

KEY TERMS

amniocentesis

alpha-fetoprotein

anencephaly

estriol

fundus

human placental lactogen (HPL)

meconium

meningomyelocele

tocodynamometer

uteroplacental

MODALITIES TO ASSESS FETAL STATUS

Before the late 1960s and early 1970s, the attitude of the medical profession was one of "live and let die." If the infant died after birth or was born dead, there was little that could be done. The fetus was a mere unknown entity inside the mother's abdomen with little attention paid to its well-being.

As medicine advanced with new technologies and improved understanding of the unborn fetus, we entered a new era in neonatal medicine. The fetus was now being treated like a patient, and concern for its well-being began from the time of conception.

Modern technology has made it possible to monitor many aspects of the fetus. In this chapter, we will look at some of the technology now available to assess fetal status and well-being.

ULTRASONOGRAPHY

Ultrasonography has proven to be one of the more important advances in neonatal medicine. Compared to radiography, ultrasound is a relatively safe procedure and has essentially replaced it as a mode of assessment.

The modern ultrasound machine uses high-frequency sound waves to locate and visualize organs and tissues. These waves are well below the level of intensity that could damage tissues. They are transmitted from a hand-held transducer placed directly against the mother's abdomen or intravaginally through a transvaginal transducer. As the sound waves come in contact with different density tissues, some are absorbed and others are reflected to a transducer. The reflected waves are converted into a screen image, visually duplicating the targeted organ (Figure 2–1).

New high-resolution, dynamic ultrasound equipment can give the caregiver dramatic insight into fetal structures, activities, and the intrauterine environment. Modern ultrasound can give cross-sectional views of fetal organs, allowing a detailed look at possible anomalies. The development of transvaginal ultrasound has enhanced the ability to assess

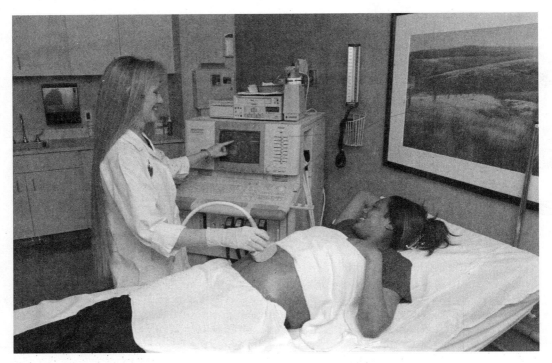

Figure 2–1 *Ultrasound examination.*

the fetus during the first trimester, when its position in the maternal pelvis make the transabdominal approach difficult.

Ultrasound has evolved from crude static displays to high-resolution, real-time B-mode displays that can show two-dimensional views and fetal/organ movement. The improved applications of ultrasound have greatly improved the ability to identify at-risk fetuses.

Ultrasound is used during pregnancy for a variety of purposes. Common usages are listed in Table 2–1.

The accurate determination of fetal age is vital in perinatal medicine in order to make clinical management decisions. This is one area in which ultrasound has made a big impact. Specific methods used to determine fetal age include crown-rump measurement (only accurate to 12 weeks' gestation), biparietal diameter (the diameter of the fetal head), abdominal circumference, and femur length. The combination of head size, abdominal circumference, and femur length can be used to estimate fetal weight. Once gestational age and weight are determined, intrauterine growth retardation (IUGR) and excessive growth (macrosomia) can be determined.

Modern ultrasound has made fetal anomalies more recognizable and manageable. Ideally, any anomaly in which there is an anatomic change in structure, or that results in a functional change in the organ or system is detectable in utero with ultrasound. The diagnostic accuracy of ultrasound in detecting anomalies increases with gestational age.[1]

TABLE 2–1   Clinical Applications of Obstetric Ultrasound

- Identification of pregnancy
- Identification of multiple fetuses
- Determiniation of appropriate fetal age, growth, and maturity
- Observance of polyhydramnios and oligohydramnios
- Detection of fetal anomalies
- Determination of placenta previa
- Identification of placental abnormalities
- Location of the placenta and fetus for amniocentesis
- Determination of fetal position
- Determination of fetal death
- Examination of fetal heart rate and respiratory effort
- Detection of incomplete miscarriages and ectopic pregnancies

---

DOPPLER ASSESSMENT OF BLOOD VELOCITIES

Doppler velocimetry is used to measure relative blood flow through umbilical, placental, and fetal vessels. While it was hoped that monitoring umbilical artery blood flow would help estimate fetal compromise, thus far it has not proven effective. Beneficial use of Doppler may be evident in predicting perinatal problems in high-risk pregnancies.[2] It is also suggested that Doppler velocimetry can decrease the number of cesarean sections, neonatal complications, and length of stay in the Neonatal Intensive Care Unit (NICU).

AMNIOCENTESIS

Amniocentesis, the obtaining of a sample of amniotic fluid, is divided into early amniocentesis (done before 15 weeks following the last menstrual period) and midtrimester amniocentesis (done during the second and third trimesters). Midtrimester amniocentesis is the most commonly performed and the oldest of all procedures for prenatal diagnosis. It is considered the "gold standard" to which other procedures are compared.[3]

Amniocentesis is performed by inserting a 3.5 to 4 inch 20 to 22 gauge needle attached to a syringe into a pocket of amniotic fluid. The position for insertion of the needle is guided by ultrasound. Once the needle is inserted, 20 to 30 ml of amniotic fluid are aspirated and placed in sterile tubes. Both the amniotic fluid and the cellular elements in the fluid are then examined.

Complications of amniocentesis include trauma, infection, and hemorrhage. Accidental puncturing of the fetus, umbilical cord, and placenta may be minor, or may lead to intrauterine hemorrhage and death. Amniocentesis is a relatively safe procedure with complication rates usually less than 1%.

Once amniotic fluid has been obtained, there are several tests for fetal well-being that can be performed on the amniotic fluid.

L/S Ratio.   Amniocentesis is used to determine lung maturity by determining L/S ratio and the presence of phosphatidylglycerol (PG). This is discussed in detail in Chapter 1.

Determination of Alpha-Fetoprotein.   Another test is the determination of alpha-fetoprotein (AFP) levels in the amniotic fluid. AFP is the main serum in the developing fetus. It normally peaks near the twelfth week of gestation and then gradually decreases. Whenever there is a break in the fetal skin, as in anencephaly or meningomyelocele (spina bifida), AFP leaks from the exposed tissues into the amniotic fluids. A high level of AFP, therefore, is a good sign of some type of neural tube defect. Acetylcholinesterase is also found in abnormally high concentrations when neural tube defects are present. In contrast, a low measurement of AFP may be useful in detecting the presence of Down syndrome in the fetus. Despite the success of AFP monitoring, Sepulveda and associates have found that high-resolution ultrasonography is more accurate in the detection of anomalies associated with elevated AFP levels.[4]

Bilirubin Level.   The level of bilirubin in amniotic fluid is an aid in detecting hemolytic diseases such as Rh incompatibility. Increases in amniotic bilirubin levels are proportional to the degree of hemolysis.

Creatinine Levels.   Creatinine levels increase in the amniotic fluid as pregnancy progresses. In the presence of normal maternal levels, amniotic creatinine levels are used to help determine fetal kidney maturity.

Identification of Meconium Staining.   Amniocentesis can detect the presence of meconium in the amniotic fluid. Normally clear, amniotic fluid becomes greenish when meconium is present. This is discussed in more detail later in this chapter.

Cytologic Examination of Cells.   The cellular elements found in amniotic fluid include cells from the skin, amnion, and tracheobronchial tree. These cells can be used to diagnose a variety of genetic and chromosomal disorders. Karyotyping of cells can be used to detect Down syndrome and other trisomy disorders.

A wide variety of disorders caused by errors in metabolism can be detected by performing biochemical and enzymatic assays on these cells.

FETAL HEART RATE (FHR) MONITORING

The average heart rate in early gestation is 140/min, dropping to an average of 120/min near term. One important factor in the management of the fetus is that the fetal heart rate (FHR) and variability (discussed later in this chapter) correlate with fetal well-being. Fetal cardiac status is measured by simple auscultation with a stethoscope, or by sophisticated electronics that are relatively simple to use.

Monitoring the heart rate of the fetus has become so common that almost every labor room has a fetal heart monitor. The major reason for this popularity is that adverse results of delivery have diminished since its advent.

FHR monitoring can identify fetal distress that may be difficult to perceive otherwise. It is well established that labor and delivery are very stressful on the infant. For this reason, FHR is usually monitored along with uterine contractions so the correlation between the two can be seen.

Because the FHR monitor shows the response of the heart to asphyxia, it is an excellent way to identify those infants who are being asphyxiated in utero.

Methods of Monitoring FHR. FHR can be monitored in one of three ways. An external abdominal transducer (Figure 2–2) can sense the movement of the fetal heart and its valves and can then determine heart rate. A second method is to place electrodes on the abdomen to pick up the electrical activity of the maternal and the fetal heart. The monitor can then electronically pick out the fetal rate and display it. By far, the most accurate method is the placement of a small spiral electrode into the fetal scalp (Figure 2–3). This requires that the

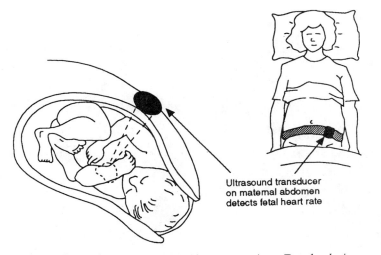

Ultrasound transducer on maternal abdomen detects fetal heart rate

Figure 2–2 *External monitoring of the fetal heart rate using a Doppler device.*

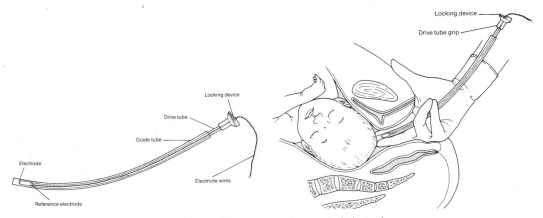

Figure 2–3 *Internal monitoring of the fetal heart rate using a spiral electrode.*

amniotic membranes be ruptured, with a small risk of infection, but the accuracy and dependability provided are unsurpassed.

Monitoring Uterine Contractions.   Uterine contractions can be monitored by one of two devices. The most commonly used device is known as a *tocodynamometer*. The tocodynamometer is strapped to the mother's abdomen at the level of the uterine fundus (Figure 2–4). As the uterus contracts, the gauge is depressed. It then transforms the degree to which it is depressed into an estimate of intensity, timing, and duration of contractions. The main drawback is its susceptibility to artifact from a variety of sources. It is also, at best, a crude estimation of intensity and does not measure actual intrauterine pressure.

A second device is the intrauterine pressure catheter. This instrument is inserted into the

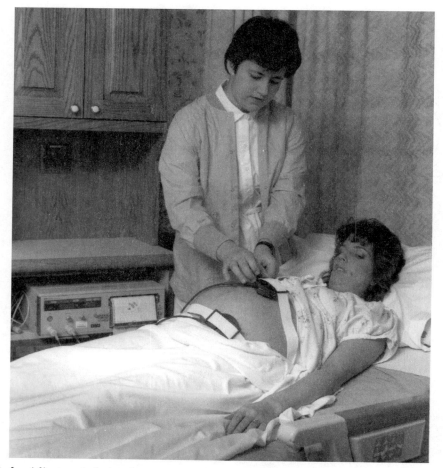

Figure 2–4   *Adjustment of a tocodynamometer to meaure uterine contractions.*

uterus through the cervix following rupture of the amniotic membranes. It can measure actual pressures in the uterus that are generated during each contraction. This device is mainly used during prolonged, difficult labors.

Determining Fetal Heart Patterns.   There are some basic patterns that are monitored with the FHR monitor. Each pattern is correlated with uterine contractions to help identify possible problems.

Baseline Heart Rate.   The first pattern is the baseline heart rate, determined by watching the rate tracing for at least 10 minutes. The normal baseline heart rate will range between 120 and 160 beats per minute (bpm). Normal fetal heart rate will vary between the high and low end, but smaller gestation fetuses will usually be closer to the high end. Although rates of 120 to 160 bpm are considered normal, each fetus must be assessed carefully. An increase or decrease in baseline heart rate of 20 to 30 bpm may be abnormal even though still within normal limits.

Variability.   When first examining the fetal heart pattern, inspect the variability of the heartbeat. A healthy, awake fetus has a constantly changing heart rate, usually between 5 and 10 bpm. The beat-to-beat variability will be reduced in the presence of CNS depression secondary to hypoxia, immaturity of the fetus, fetal sleep, or narcotic and sedative use by the mother. Samueloff and associates have indicated that variability alone cannot be used as the sole indicator of fetal well-being.[5]

Bradycardia.   A baseline heart rate of less than 100 bpm or a maintained drop of 20 bpm from the previous baseline rate is considered bradycardia. The most dangerous cause of fetal bradycardia is asphyxia. Oxygen administration to the mother may help reduce the severity of the asphyxia. Other causes of bradycardia include congenital heart block secondary to a congenital malformation, maternal systemic lupus erythematosus, administration of paracervical blocks and beta blockers to the mother, and fetal hypothermia.

Whenever fetal bradycardia is present, the primary concern should be to rule out fetal asphyxia as the cause. Fetal asphyxia can be diagnosed by the use of scalp blood pH determination, discussed later in this chapter.

Bradycardia seen during the second stage of labor is divided into end-stage and terminal bradycardia. End-stage bradycardia is accompanied by standard variability and a prior normal tracing. Normal vaginal delivery can be expected in the presence of end-stage bradycardia. In contrast, terminal bradycardia is accompanied by no variability, and delivery is performed in the quickest possible manner because it indicates fetal distress.

Tachycardia.   Tachycardia is present when the baseline is consistently above 180 bpm. The most common cause is maternal fever. Tachycardia can also be caused by fetal or maternal infection, fetal dysrhythmia, maternal dehydration, maternal anxiety, stimulation of the fetus, and asphyxia. Sympathomimetic drugs used to stop contractions, such as ritodrine, salbutamol, and terbutaline, and parasympatholytics, such as atropine, may cause fetal tachycardia when administered to the mother.

Accelerations. If FHR exceeds 160 bpm for less than 2 minutes, it is called an acceleration. Accelerations during labor are a good sign that the fetus is reacting to the contraction in a positive way.

Decelerations. If the heart rate drops below 120 bpm for less than 2 minutes, it is called a deceleration. Decelerations, in contrast to accelerations, may either be threatening or harmless, depending on their characteristics and timing. The three types of deceleration are shown in Figure 2–5.

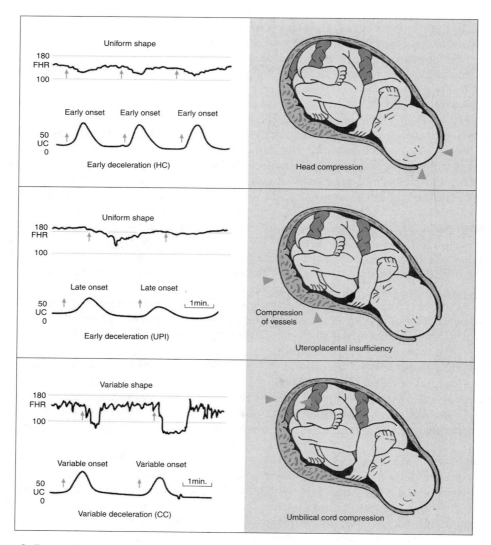

Figure 2–5 *Fetal heart rate patterns from continuous electronic fetal monitoring.*

Early or Type I decelerations closely follow uterine contractions in onset and duration. The heart rate may drop to 60 to 80 bpm during the contraction, rapidly returning to baseline following the contraction. Type I decelerations are caused by compression of the fetal head against the cervix and are benign. The bradycardia is due to a parasympathetic response and is not indicative of hypoxia.

Late or Type II decelerations do not follow uterine contractions. They occur 10 to 30 seconds following the onset of the contraction, and heart rate does not return to baseline until after the contraction is over. Even a small decease of 10 to 20 bpm from baseline is suggestive of problems. Type II decelerations are secondary to uteroplacental insufficiency during contractions, leading to fetal asphyxia.

During the contraction, the vessels of the uterus and placenta are compressed, leading to diminished transfer of oxygen from the maternal blood to the fetal blood. As the hypoxia worsens, the decelerations last longer and the beat-to-beat variability is lost. Progression of the hypoxia causes the decelerations to begin sooner and last longer, the heart rate dipping lower with each contraction.

Variable or Type III decelerations are independent of uterine contractions. They are random in their onset, duration, and severity.

Type III decelerations are usually secondary to compression of the umbilical cord, leading to hypoxia. The cord may either be wrapped around the infant's neck or be pinched between the pelvis and the presenting body part. Type III decelerations may or may not be dangerous, depending on the frequency and severity of each occurrence. Alleviation of cord compression is accomplished by turning the mother from side to side or by assuming a knee-chest position. In emergency situations, the presenting body part may be elevated to try to prevent further cord compression.

FETAL SCALP pH ASSESSMENT

The assessment of fetal scalp pH is used as a secondary tool, following FHR monitoring, in the determination of fetal well-being. It is indicated in the absence of baseline variability, late decelerations with decreasing variability, and abnormal tracings.

The acid-base balance of the fetus is determined by the viability of the placenta and its ability to exchange oxygen and carbon dioxide between maternal and fetal blood. If that exchange is disrupted, whether at the placenta or in the cord, the resultant drop in pH can be measured. The reason for the drop is twofold. First, as blood gas exchange decreases, fetal $PaCO_2$ increases, decreasing the pH. Second, in the face of hypoxia, the fetus begins to metabolize glycogen without oxygen (anaerobic metabolism), resulting in a dramatic increase in lactic acid. This metabolic acid, combined with increased $PaCO_2$, the respiratory acid, causes the pH to drop.

To get the fetal scalp blood sample, the mother is placed in the lithotomy position (Figure 2–6) and the fetal head is visualized through the cervix. This is done with a long, cone-shaped speculum or an endoscope. An incision is made with 2×1.5 mm blade and the blood sample is collected into a heparinized capillary tube. The sample should be obtained between contractions to avoid decelerations, which may cause low values. Additionally, blood flow may slow substantially during a contraction, making the obtaining of a sample more difficult.

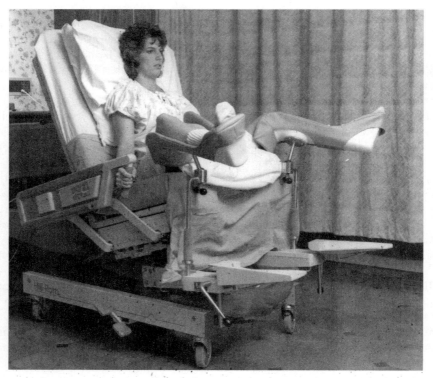

Figure 2–6 *Patient in the lithotomy position.*

Normal fetal blood pH is considered to be above 7.25. A pH of 7.2 to 7.24 shows slight asphyxia, and a pH of less than 7.2 signifies severe asphyxia. Because maternal pH can influence fetal pH, it may be necessary to determine the acid-base status of the mother concurrently.

Fetal scalp pH is useful only in the presence of abnormal FHR tracings, because a normal tracing indicates a healthy infant in most instances.

ESTIMATING THE DELIVERY DATE

The delivery date is called the estimated date of confinement (EDC) and can be calculated by a variety of methods. Although none of the methods is exact, each will help determine the time when gestation will reach 40 weeks.

NÄGELE'S RULE

Nägele's rule is the most common method of determining EDC. To determine the EDC, 3 months are subtracted from the first day of the last menstrual period. Seven days are then added to the result to determine the EDC. For example, if the first day of the last menstrual period was March 25, subtracting 3 months would arrive at December 25. Adding 7 days gives us an EDC of January 1.

The accuracy of Nägele's rule depends on a regular period of 28 days and the woman remembering her last menstrual period. The use of oral contraceptives or an irregular menstrual cycle reduces the accuracy of this method.

FUNDAL HEIGHT

The *fundus* of the uterus, which is the end opposite the cervix, can be measured on the abdominal wall as it grows with the fetus. It is fairly reliable during the first and second trimesters, but unreliable during the last trimester. To determine fundal height, a tape measure is placed on the abdomen and the distance from the symphysis pubis to the top of the fundus is measured. During the first two trimesters, gestational age correlates to this measurement in centimeters. Therefore, at 20 weeks, the fundus is roughly 20 cm above the symphysis pubis, and so forth.

QUICKENING

Quickening is the first sensation of fetal movement experienced by the mother. It generally occurs between 16 and 22 weeks, but on average occurs near week 20. Because of the large variations, quickening is at best only a very rough estimate of gestational age.

DETERMINATION OF FETAL HEARTBEAT

The fetal heartbeat can be heard as early as week 16, but is nearly always heard no later than week 20. With the use of Doppler devices, the heartbeat can be detected much earlier, possibly as early as week 8. Again, the determination of fetal heartbeat is only a rough estimation of gestational age.

BIOPHYSICAL TESTS OF FETAL WELL-BEING

With the increase in knowledge and interest in the fetus, researchers increasingly became interested in the role of the heart rate and its relationship to fetal well-being. Researchers began looking at the response of the heart to uterine contractions as a method of fetal evaluation.

THE CONTRACTION STRESS TEST

The first test using this technique was called the contraction stress chest (CST). The CST is used to determine the presence of *uteroplacental* insufficiency. One of the original forms of measuring fetal compromise, CST detects the uteroplacental insufficiency by subjecting the fetus to stress. The stress comes from an interruption of maternal blood to the intervillous spaces during contraction. A positive CST is defined as more than 50% of contractions having late FHR decelerations. With a negative CST, no decelerations are seen after any contractions. In reality most CST tests do not clearly fall into one of the above categories. For this reason, there are several other classifications that the skilled practitioner uses to interpret results, such as reactive, nonreactive, minimally reactive, and equivocal.[6]

Contraindications to the performance of the CST include placenta previa, previous vertical cesarean section, previous uterine rupture, premature labor, premature rupture of the membranes, and incompetent cervix.

A variation of the CST is the oxytocin contraction test (OCT). If spontaneous contractions are inadequate when the CST is done, the drug oxytocin is given through an intravenous line to start contractions. An alternative method is manual nipple stimulation to start contractions.

THE NONSTRESS TEST

In a healthy fetus, the heart rate increases in association with fetal body movement. Therefore, a second test was developed in which the response of fetal heart rate to fetal movements is observed. This test is called the nonstress test (NST). To classify NST results, a qualifying heart rate acceleration increases at least 15/min over baseline and lasts at least 15 seconds. A normal, reactive pattern shows at least two accelerations in conjunction with fetal movement, over a 20-minute window. A nonreactive NST occurs when the fetal heart rate does not accelerate during fetal body movement over two 20-minute periods. Some have extended the time period up to 120 minutes before declaring a nonreactive test.[7] A negative NST is often followed by a CST to evaluate the cause of the inactivity. A fetus suffering from prolonged hypoxia will have a positive CST with a negative NST. Negative CST results in the presence of a negative NST indicate the problem is one of fetal sleep or maternal narcotic or sedative ingestion.

The NST is popular mainly because it is simple to perform, is less time consuming than the CST, the patient has little discomfort, and there is little risk from induced contractions.

VIBROACOUSTIC STIMULATION

Another method of soliciting a fetal response, in addition to the NST, is by the use of vibroacoustic stimulation. In this test, a buzzer is held against the maternal abdomen. The fetal heart rate is then monitored for accelerations. The healthy fetus responds to the acoustic stimulation with an acceleration of heart rate. Failure of the heart rate to increase may indicate a compromised fetus and further evaluation should be done.

MONITORING FETAL MOVEMENT

Monitoring of fetal movement is probably the easiest means of fetal assessment. It serves as an indirect measurement of CNS integrity and function.[8] Movement can be monitored as simply as having the mother note movement, or as complex as observation with ultrasound over an extended time period. Jerky movement of the fetus has been detected as early as 7 weeks, and reaches its greatest activity between 28 and 34 weeks. Movements decrease toward term possibly due to increasing fetal size and decreasing amniotic fluid volume.

The mother first senses fetal movement sometime between 16 and 20 weeks. The test is simple in that it only requires the mother to note the number of fetal movements detected during a certain period (usually a 1-hour period). Less than 10 movements over an hour requires further testing due to the fact that fetal inactivity is associated with fetal distress and stillbirth.

ASSESSMENT OF AMNIOTIC FLUID VOLUME

It has long been appreciated that there is a link between the volume of amniotic fluid and fetal well-being. This has been demonstrated by Hadi and colleagues who indicate that adequate amniotic fluid volume relates to longer pregnancies and higher neonatal survival.[9] Amniotic fluid volume measurement may offer clues to the presence of certain anomalies such as esophageal atresia, diaphragmatic hernia, cardiac, intracranial, spinal and ventral wall defects, and urinary trace abnormalities.

THE BIOPHYSICAL PROFILE

The biophysical profile, first proposed in 1980, used information gained from five separate tests (Table 2–2). Those tests are: fetal breathing, fetal movement, fetal limb tone, the NST, and amniotic fluid volume. Each area is scored 0 or 1 depending on the finding. Vintzileos and colleagues modified the original biophysical profile by adding placental grade to the evaluation and scoring each area 0, 1, or 2 based on the finding. The biophysical profile is possibly the best overall method of fetal risk determination. Vintzileos and associates (1987)

TABLE 2–2 The Biophysical Profile

BIOPHYSICAL VARIABLE	NORMAL (2)	ABNORMAL (0)
• Fetal breathing—at least one episode of at least 30 seconds during 30-minute observation	Present	Absent
• Gross body movement—at least three body/limb movements during 30-minute observation	3 or more	2 or less
• Fetal tone—one episode of extension/flexion of limbs or trunk during 30-minute observation	Present	Absent
• Reactive NST—at least two episodes of 15 beats/min fetal heart rate accelerations during 30-minute observation	Yes	No
• Amniotic fluid volume—at least one pocket of at least 1 x 1 cm in two directions	Present	Absent

Normal Score: 8–10

found that the biophysical profile is superior to the 1- and 5-minute Apgar scores in determining fetal acidosis.[10] Figure 2–7 shows the relationship among the biophysical profile, fetal acidosis, and fetal hypoxia.

MECONIUM PRESENCE IN AMNIOTIC FLUID

Meconium is the thick, dark greenish stool found in the fetal intestine. The passage of meconium into the amniotic fluid occurs about 40% of the time in postterm fetuses of greater than 42 weeks gestation. The frequency drops to about 10% in the term infant and 3 to 5% in the preterm fetus.[11]

Meconium staining of the amniotic fluid may result from a fetal asphyxia episode, but its reliability as evidence of fetal distress is debatable. This unreliability is based on the fact that low 5-minute Apgar scores are found in only 10% of meconium-stained neonates.

The presence of meconium in the amniotic fluid is determined by amniocentesis, amnioscopy, or is visualized when the amniotic sac ruptures. One theory of asphyxia-induced meconium passage is that fetal asphyxia causes relaxation of the fetal anal sphincter and increased peristalsis of the intestine.

The most severe result of meconium release is meconium aspiration syndrome (MAS), in which meconium is aspirated into the trachea and airways. MAS and its treatment are detailed in Chapter 10.

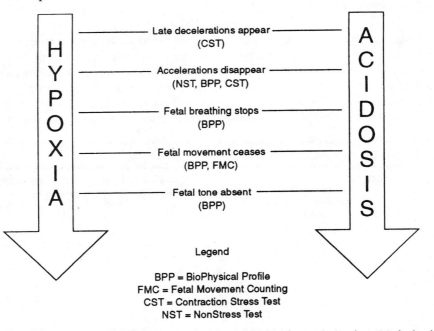

Figure 2–7 *The antepartum fetal distress cascade. (Reproduced with permission from Methods of Fetal Surveillance.* Clin Obstet Gynecol. *December 1987;30:958.*

CHORIONIC VILLUS SAMPLING

As the name implies, chorionic villus sampling is the process of removing a small sample from the chorionic villus of the placenta, which contains fetal blood and tissue. The sample is then examined for the presence of chromosomal abnormalities. Sampling can be done either transcervically, transvaginally, or transabdominally, depending on the location of the placenta. Most chorionic villus samplings are done between 9 and 12 weeks of gestation.[3] Indications for the procedure include advanced maternal age, previous child with chromosomal anomalies, or a parent carrier. It is particularly suited for DNA analysis because the amount of DNA obtained is significantly larger than that typically obtained with amniocentesis.

With the advent of high-resolution, real-time ultrasound and flexible catheters, the procedure carries a fetal loss rate of less than 1%, which is similar to that seen in amniocentesis.

CORDOCENTESIS

Cordocentesis is the in utero sampling of fetal umbilical cord blood. The base of the umbilical cord is located with ultrasound and a 22 gauge needle is inserted through the maternal abdomen into the uterus. The umbilical cord is punctured and blood samples are drawn into tuberculin syringes.

The fetal blood samples are then checked for several fetal problems, including hemoglobinopathies (e.g., sickle cell); coagulopathies (e.g., hemophilia); specific IgM antibodies to fetal infections; metabolic disorders; suspected congenital anomalies; oxygenation; and acid-base status.

This technique has evolved to be an important part of the evaluation of fetal well-being. When properly done, both fetal and maternal risk is 1% or less.[3]

BIOCHEMICAL METHODS OF ASSESSMENT

Maternal Estriol Determination. *Estriol,* a metabolite of estrogen, is secreted in high quantities by the placenta in the latter half of pregnancy. Adequate production of estriol depends on a properly functioning fetal liver and adrenal glands. Optimum levels of estriol in maternal urine require a healthy fetus, a properly functioning placenta, and a healthy mother.

With the growth and development of the fetus, the production of estriol increases. Growth retardation, fetal distress, and placental insufficiency all lead to decreased estriol production.

Estriol passes from the placenta into the maternal blood and is excreted into the mother's urine. Determinations of maternal estriol levels can be made using blood or urine samples. The mother's urine is collected over a 24-hour period and analyzed for the quantity of estriol present. Both blood and urine samples must be taken several times a week to be effective.

Fetal distress is indicated if there is a 50 to 60% decrease from the previous test, or if there is an ongoing decrease in serial values. This test is becoming unpopular owing to the high number of false-positive results, the inconvenience of 24-hour urine collection and/or weekly blood sampling, and the difficulty in outpatient management.

Human Placental Lactogen (HPL) Levels.   A second method of biochemical fetal evaluation is the determination of *human placental lactogen (HPL)* levels. Produced by the placenta and excreted into the maternal blood, HPL levels gradually increase until 37 weeks' gestation, at which point the level remains the same or decreases slightly.

Maternal serum levels are evaluated weekly, with normal ranges near term of 5.4 to 7 µg/ml. Fetal compromise may be present if HPL levels fall below 4 µg/ml after 30 weeks' gestation. As with estriol determination, HPL determination has become less popular in recent years.

MAGNETIC RESONANCE IMAGING (MRI)

The arrival of magnetic resonance imaging (MRI) has opened up new avenues not previously available. Unlike the CAT scan (computerized axial tomography), the MRI does not use radiation and therefore does not pose the risk of causing defects in the developing fetus.

MRI is especially suited for distinguishing between soft tissue structure and function. The MRI is capable of creating sagittal, axial, and coronal plane views of any part of the body. The sagittal view appears to be the most helpful in assessing fetal status in the prenatal period.

MRI imaging is indicated in those instances where ultrasonography is often insufficient, such as placental and fetal abnormalities and development of the fetal lungs and brain.

FACTORS IDENTIFYING A HIGH-RISK PREGNANCY

One of our greatest assets in caring for the sick neonate is the ability to predict those fetuses at high risk. Early in the development of perinatology it became clear that certain factors, both maternal and fetal, were present whenever a distressed infant was born. Some of these high-risk factors can be determined on the first office visit. Others appear as the pregnancy advances. Others still are only present during labor, delivery, and the postdelivery period.

Until these approaches are in common use, it is important that the neonatal practitioner have an understanding of high-risk factors. The ability to anticipate a distressed fetus will better prepare the practitioner to care for the infant. These high-risk factors are outlined in Table 2–3.

SUMMARY

Modern perinatology has evolved over the past 30 years to a complex maze of tests and procedures used to assess and treat the fetal patient. While many old techniques are

TABLE 2–3   High-Risk Pregnancy Indicating Factors

Socioeconomic Factors
1. Low income and poor housing
2. Severe social problems
3. Unwed status, especially adolescent
4. Minority Status
5. Poor nutritional status

Demographic Factors
1. Maternal age under 16
2. Obese or underweight before pregnancy
3. Height less than 5 feet
4. Familial history of inherited disorders

Medical Factors
1. Obstetric History
   a. History of infertility
   b. History of ectopic pregnancy
   c. History of miscarriage
   d. Previous multiple gestations
   e. Previous stillbirth or neonatal death
   f. Uterine/cervical abnormality
   g. High parity (many children)
   h. History of premature labor/delivery
   i. History of prolonged labor
   j. Previous cesarean delivery
   k. History of low birth weight infant
   l. Previous delivery with midforceps
   m. History of infant with malformation, birth injury, or neurologic deficit
   n. History of hydatidiform mole or carcinoma

2. Maternal Medical History
   a. Maternal cardiac disease
   b. Maternal pulmonary disease
   c. Maternal diabetes or thyroid disease
   d. History of chronic renal disease
   e. Maternal gastrointestinal disease
   f. Maternal endocrine disorders
   g. History of hypertension
   h. History of seizure disorder
   i. History of venereal and other infectious diseases
   j. Weight loss greater than 5 pounds
   k. Surgery during pregnancy
   l. Major anomalies of the reproductive tract
   m. History of mental retardation and emotional disorders

(continued)

TABLE 2–3   (continued)

---

3. Current Obstetric Status
   a. Absence of prenatal care
   b. Rh sensitization
   c. Excessively large or small fetus
   d. Premature labor
   e. Preeclampsia
   f. Multiple gestations
   g. Polyhydramnios and oligohydramnios
   h. Premature rupture of the membranes
   i. Vaginal bleeding
   j. Placenta previa
   k. Abruptio placentae
   l. Abnormal presentation
   m. Postmaturity
   n. Abnormalities in tests for fetal well-being
   o. Maternal anemia
4. Habits
   a. Smoking
   b. Regular alcohol intake
   c. Drug use and abuse

---

continually updated and improved, many new procedures and tests are developed at a staggering pace.

Of all modes used to assess the fetus, none has had more of an impact than ultrasonography. With its ability to visualize the fetus and its organs, and its relative safety, it has become a mainstay in modern perinatal medicine. Once only a guessing game, ultrasound has made the determination of fetal gestational age a nearly exact science. It is also used to detect fetal anomalies, measure amniotic fluid volume, and to safely guide the needles used for amniocentesis, chorionic villus sampling, and cordocentesis. Its cousin, Doppler velocimetry, may be helpful in predicting high-risk pregnancies.

One of the oldest methods of prenatal diagnosis is amniocentesis. Amniocentesis is useful in determining L/S ratio for lung maturity, alpha-fetoprotein levels to detect neural tube defects, bilirubin level to identify homolytic disorders, creatinine levels to determine kidney maturity, identification of meconium staining, and cell examination and karyotyping for genetic disorders.

The knowledge that fetal heart rate correlates well with fetal distress has made monitoring the fetal heart rate commonplace. When compared to uterine contractions, changes in rate and variability can be diagnostic of varying fetal distress. Bradycardia, tachycardia, and accelerations and decelerations that occur during the contraction are useful diagnostic tools.

In the absence of baseline heart rate variability, late decelerations, or abnormal tracings during labor, scalp pH assessment is useful in determining the level of asphyxia present.

Determination of the delivery date is accomplished by several methods. Nägele's rule utilizes the first day of the last menstrual period to calculate delivery date. The remaining methods—fundal height, quickening, detection of fetal heart rate, and ultrasonography—are used to assess approximate gestational age. Then, using a normal 40-week gestation, the delivery date is calculated.

The contraction stress test and the nonstress test continue to be useful in the detection of fetal compromise. Whether a test is reactive or nonreactive helps the practitioner determine the amount of stress the fetus is undergoing and whether further investigation is required. Acoustic stimulation is used to stimulate the fetus to determine if it responds appropriately. Fetal movement is relatively easy to monitor and can yield important information. Ordinarily, the mother is asked to monitor how long it takes her fetus to move 10 times. Times approaching an hour or longer require further follow-up. The amount of amniotic fluid present is diagnostic for fetal wellbeing. Normal amounts of fluid indicate less risk of early delivery and higher fetal survival.

The biophysical profile utilizes several tests in an effort to better analyze fetal wellbeing. The biophysical profile includes the nonstress test, fetal movement, breathing movements, limb tone, amniotic fluid volume, and placental grade. Each area is given a numerical rating of 0, 1, or 2, depending on the test result. The higher the score, the less chance of fetal compromise.

The presence of meconium in the amniotic fluid may be indicative of fetal asphyxia and predisposes the fetus to possible aspiration of the meconium into the trachea following delivery.

Chorionic villus sampling and cordocentesis are examples of the ability to work with the fetus while still in utero. Sampling of placental villus and fetal blood is used to detect possible genetic abnormalities, blood disorders, and acid-base imbalance.

The first step in treating a compromised fetus is predicting and anticipating those at high risk. Steps can then be taken to either prevent or minimize the effect of those risk factors. On the first visit, it is vital that a thorough history be taken to identify those patients at high risk.

It is hoped that with the basic understanding of techniques used to evaluate fetal wellness, the respiratory care practitioner can be better prepared to care for these patients.

References

1. Manning FA. Ultrasonography. In: Avery GB, Fletcher MA, MacDonald MG, eds. *Pathophysiology and Management of the Newborn.* 5th ed. Philadelphia: JB Lippincott Co; 1999.

2. Maulik D. Doppler ultrasound velocimetry for fetal surveillance. *Clin Obstet Gynecol.* 1995;38.

3. Drugan A, et al. Prenatal diagnosis: Procedures and trends. In: Avery GB, Fletcher MA, MacDonald MG, eds. *Pathophysiology and Management of the Newborn.* 5th ed. Philadelphia: JB Lippincott Co; 1999.

4. Sepulveda W, et al. Are routine alpha-fetoprotein and acetylcholinesterase determinations still necessary at second-trimester amniocentesis? Impact of high-resolution ultrasonography. *Obstet Gynecol.* 1995;85.

5. Samueloff A, et al. Is fetal heart rate variability a good predictor of fetal outcome? *Acta Obstet Gynecol Scand.* 1994;73.

6. Lagrew DC. The contraction stress test. *Clin Obstet Gynecol.* 1995;38.

7. Paul RH, Miller A. Nonstress test. *Clin Obstet Gynecol.* 1995;38.

8. Rayburn WF. Fetal movement monitoring. *Clin. Obstet Gynecol.* 1995;38.

9. Hadi HA, et al. Premature rupture of the membranes between 20 and 25 weeks' gestation: role of the amniotic fluid in perinatal outcome. *Am J Obstet Gynecol.* 1994;170.

10. Vintzileos AM, et al. The relationships among the fetal biophysical profile, umbilical cord pH, and Apgar scores. *Am J Obstet Gynecol.* 1987;157.

11. Knuppel RA, Drukker JE. *High-Risk Pregnancy: A Team Approach.* 2nd ed. Philadelphia: WB Saunders Co; 1992.

Bibliography and Suggested Readings

Avery GB, Fletcher MA, MacDonald MG. *Pathophysiology and Management of the Newborn.* 5th ed. Philadelphia: JB Lippincott Co; 1999.

Cloherty JP, Stark AR, eds. *Manual of Neonatal Care.* 4th ed. Philadelphia: Lippincott; 1998.

Cottrell GP. *Cardiopulmonary Anatomy and Physiology for Respiratory Care Practitioners.* Philadelphia: FA Davis; 2000.

Des Jardins T. *Cardiopulmonary Anatomy and Physiology.* 3rd ed. Albany, NY: Delmar Thomson Learning; 1998.

Merenstein GB, Gardner SL. *Handbook of Neonatal Intensive Care.* 4th ed. St. Louis: CV Mosby Co; 1998.

Rhoades GG, et al. The safety and efficacy of chorionic villus sampling for early prenatal diagnosis of cytogenic abnormalities. *N Engl J Med.* 1989;320.

Taussig LM, Landau LI. *Pediatric Respiratory Medicine.* St. Louis: Mosby; 1999.

Tucker SM. *Pocket Guide to Fetal Monitoring and Assessment.* 4th ed. St. Louis: Mosby; 2000.

White L. *Foundations of Nursing: Caring for the Whole Person.* Albany, NY: Delmar Thomson Learning; 2001.

Posttest

1. Assessment of the fetus in the first trimester is facilitated by which technique?
   a. high-resolution ultrasound
   b. Doppler velocimetry
   c. real-time displays
   d. transvaginal ultrasound
2. Which of the following cannot be detected by ultrasound?
   a. presence of infection
   b. position of the fetus
   c. position of the placenta
   d. volume of amniotic fluid
3. A high level of alpha-fetoprotein found during amniocentesis indicates which of the following?
   a. neural tube defect
   b. heart anomaly

   c. fetal infection

   d. Down syndrome

4. Which of the following tests done on amniotic fluid is used to help determine fetal kidney maturity?

   a. bilirubin level

   b. L/S ratio

   c. creatinine level

   d. cytologic cell examination

5. Monitoring of the fetal heart rate during labor and delivery is used to detect:

   I. uterine contractions

   II. placental insufficiency

   III. rupture of the amniotic sac

   IV. compression of the umbilical cord

   V. bradycardia secondary to a vagal stimulus

     a. I, II, III

     b. II, IV, V

     c. I, III, IV, V

     d. II, III, IV, V

6. The most accurate method of measuring fetal heart rate is:

   a. Doppler sensors

   b. stethoscope

   c. fetoscope

   d. fetal scalp electrode

7. A common cause of fetal bradycardia is:

   a. asphyxia

   b. congenital anomaly

   c. heart defect

   d. tocolytic drugs

8. Type III decelerations are caused by which of the following?

   a. uterine contractions

   b. placental insufficiency

   c. rupture of the amniotic sac

   d. compression of the umbilical cord

9. Which fetal scalp pH is the lower limit of normal?

   a. 7.30

   b. 7.25

   c. 7.20

   d. 7.15

10. A woman presents in her physician's office for an examination. The first day of her last menstrual period was October 21. Fundal height is 25 cm. Which of the following would be the estimated date of delivery?

   a. July 21

   b. July 28

   c. August 28

   d. June 21

11. What is the approximate gestational age of the fetus in question 10?
    a. 15 weeks
    b. 20 weeks
    c. 25 weeks
    d. 30 weeks
12. A fetus suffering prolonged hypoxia will demonstrate which of the following?
    a. a negative NST and positive CST
    b. a positive NST and negative CST
    c. a negative NST and negative CST
    d. a positive NST and positive CST
13. Which of the following statements are true regarding fetal movements?
    I. Fetal movements show the greatest activity between 28 and 34 weeks.
    II. Diminished fetal movements are normal early in gestation.
    III. Fetal distress and stillbirth are common findings when the fetus is inactive.
    IV. Movement has been detected as early as 7 weeks gestation.
    V. Fetal movements are very difficult to assess.
        a. I, III, V
        b. II, III,IV
        c. I, III, IV
        d. II, IV, V
14. Which of the following is not a part of the biophysical profile?
    a. nonstress test
    b. fetal movement
    c. fetal heart rate
    d. amniotic fluid volume
15. Which of the following involves removal of a fetal blood sample while still in utero?
    a. chorionic villus sampling
    b. cordocentesis
    c. amniocentesis
    d. transplacental aspiration
16. When measuring maternal estriol levels, fetal distress is indicated when:
    a. estriol is present in maternal urine
    b. estriol is absent from maternal urine
    c. levels exceed 5.4 to 7 mcg/ml
    d. estriol levels decrease 50 to 60% in maternal urine
17. Which of the following factors of maternal history places the fetus at high risk?
    I. maternal age of 37 years
    II. previous miscarriage
    III. previous premature delivery
    IV. asthma
    V. maternal obesity
        a. II, III, IV, V
        b. I, III, IV, V
        c. I, II, III, IV, V
        d. I, III, V

CHAPTER THREE

LABOR, DELIVERY, AND PHYSIOLOGIC CHANGES AFTER BIRTH

OBJECTIVES

Upon completion of this chapter, the reader should be able to:

1. List the five events that make up the birth process.
2. Compare and contrast cervical dilatation and effacement.
3. Identify the most common presentation.
4. Define station and how it is expressed.
5. Describe the sequence of events that lead to the descent and delivery of the fetus.
6. Define tocolysis and describe the various methods used to achieve tocolysis.
7. Define dystocia and describe the three etiologic factors that cause it.
8. Describe each of the following:
   a. Complete breech
   b. Incomplete or footling breech
   c. Frank breech
   d. Face presentation
   e. Transverse lie
   f. Prolapse of umbilical cord and occult cord compression
9. Identify and describe the three types of placenta previa.
10. Describe the three categories of abruptio placentae.
11. List the indications for a cesarean birth.
12. Explain why multiple gestations create high-risk pregnancies.
13. List factors that are responsible for the first breath.
14. Describe the importance of overcoming surface forces in adapting to extrauterine life.
15. Identify and describe factors that cause the change from fetal to adult circulation.

KEY TERMS
---

abruptio placentae
autosomal-recessive trait
breech
dilatation
dystocia
effacement

engagement
multigravida
occult
parturition
placenta previa

preeclampsia
primigravida
prolapse
stations
tocolysis

PARTURITION

Parturition, the process of giving birth, is a complicated occurrence that is still not fully understood. Five distinct events make up the birth process: 1) Rupture of the membranes; 2) Dilation of the cervix; 3) Contraction of the uterus; 4) Separation of the placenta; and 5) Shrinking of the uterus.

The sequence of events that starts the birth process is complicated and also poorly understood. Three primary hypotheses, however, have emerged to help explain what starts labor: 1) The withdrawal of progesterone; 2) Estrogen, causing uterine activation; and 3) Stimulation of the uterus by factors such as oxytocin and prostaglandins.[1]

We will not attempt to look at all of the complexities associated with the birth process. A basic understanding of labor and deliver is important for the practitioner and therefore we begin this chapter by examining the stages of labor and delivery.

STAGES OF NORMAL LABOR AND DELIVERY

During the latter half of the third trimester, nature begins preparing the mother and the fetus for birth. The actual date of delivery may vary 2 weeks either way from the estimated date of delivery. As the gestation nears term, the placenta begins to slow its function down and the fetus becomes more and more self-reliant in preparation for birth. An understanding of normal labor and delivery is essential to understand what causes difficult deliveries that lead to fetal demise.

Labor and delivery are broken down into three major stages, as listed in Table 3–1. A fourth stage is often listed as a recovery stage, in which the uterus shrinks and homeostasis is reestablished. The duration of each stage of labor will vary based on whether the mother is in her first pregnancy (*primigravida*) or whether she has been pregnant before (*multigravida*).

Although every stage is distinct, labor and delivery are one continuous event. False labor may be present for some time during the pregnancy. These contractions, called Braxton-Hicks, are rhythmic and fairly mild compared to true contractions.

TABLE 3–1   Stages of Labor and Delivery

STAGE	OCCURENCES	AVERAGE TIME	
		PRIMIGRAVIDA	MULTIGRAVIDA
First	Onset of regular contractions to full dilatation and effacement of the cervix	16–18 hr	7–12 hr
Second	Full dilatation and effacement of the cervix to delivery of the fetus	1 hr (can last up to 2 hr)	20 min
Third	Delivery of the fetus to delivery of the placenta	3–4 min (can last up to 45 min)	4–5 min

STAGE I OF LABOR

The first stage of labor is called stage I. It begins with the onset of the first true contraction. Actual contractions are described as coming in waves, gradually increasing in strength. The first contractions usually are 10–15 minutes apart and last 30 to 90 seconds.

Effacement and Dilatation of the Cervix.   With the onset of the first contraction, the cervix begins to stretch and widen. The stretching or thinning of the cervix is called *efface-ment*, and the widening is called *dilatation*. Effacement of the cervix is measured as a percentage. At 100% effacement, th cervix is imperceptible against the uterine wall. Dilatation is measured in centimeters (cm) as the diameter of the cervical opening. The cervix is fully dilatated at 10 cm. Effacement and dilatation are a result of the continuous pushing of the amniotic fluid and the fetus against the cervix, resulting from uterine contractions. In normal labor, the cervix primarily effaces during the early portion of stage I. Dilatation is minimal at first and then progresses rapidly toward the end of stage I, when effacement has almost completed. Effacement and dilatation of the cervix are illustrated in Figure 3–1.

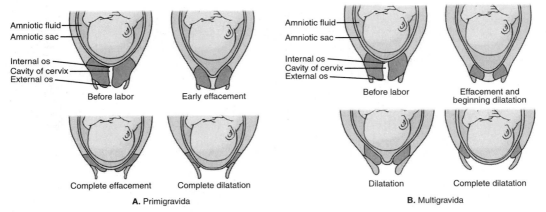

Figure 3–1   *Effacement and dilation of the cervix. A. Primigravida; B. Multigravida.*

During the initial contractions, the uterus differentiates into a thick muscular upper portion and a thin lower section. This allows the contractions to push the fetus down the birth canal.

Stage I ends when the cervix is completely dilatated and effaced. It averages between 7 and 12 hours in the multigravida, or 16 to 18 hours in the primigravida.

STAGE II OF LABOR

The second stage of labor, stage II, is the actual delivery of the fetus. The descent of the fetus through the birth canal is aided by contraction of the abdominal muscles and diaphragm by the mother. This increases intra-abdominal pressure and, along with contractions, helps push the fetus out.

Position and Engagement of the Fetus.   Ninety-five percent of all births occur with the fetus in the head-down or vertex position. Figure 3–2 shows the possible presentation in the vertex position.

As the head advances down the birth canal, it reaches different degrees of *engagement*, or *stations* (Figure 3–3). The station is the location of the head as it relates to the level of the ischial spines on the maternal pelvis. Stations are expressed in centimeters above the ischial spines as negative numbers, and below the spines as positive numbers. The head is said to be engaged in the birth canal when it reaches the spines, or a station of 0.

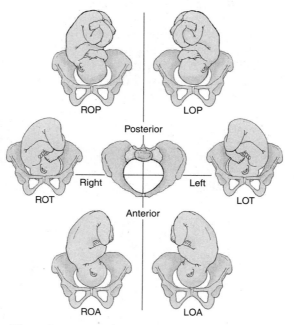

Figure 3–2   *Variations of the vertex presentation.*

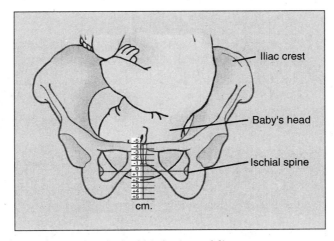

Figure 3–3 *Stages of engagement of the fetal head prior to delivery.*

Delivery of the Fetus.   As the fetus begins its descent down the birth canal, the head turns to a face-down position to accommodate passage through the pelvis (Figure 3–4). Upon delivery of the head, the fetus rotates internally to ease the passage of the shoulders through the pelvis. The upper shoulder delivers first, followed by the lower shoulder. The delivery to this point is the most time-consuming portion. Following delivery of the shoulders, the rest of the body exits quite rapidly. The umbilical cord is clamped following delivery, and the neonate begins to function outside the uterus for the first time.

The transition to the extrauterine environment is a critical time for the neonate and will be examined in more detail later in this chapter. Stage II can last from 20 minutes to 2 hours and be within normal range.

STAGE III OF LABOR

The third stage of delivery, stage III, is the expulsion of the placenta. Stage III can take 5 to 45 minutes to achieve. After the delivery of the neonate, the uterus continues to contract, tearing the placenta loose from its walls. This may be assisted by placing the neonate at the mother's breast, stimulating the secretion of oxytocin, which increases uterine contractions. Manual pressure to the abdominal wall may also help expel the placenta. Over a short time, the uterus continues to shrink and eventually returns to its original position and size.

ABNORMAL LABOR AND DELIVERY

PREMATURE LABOR AND DELIVERY

Of all the directions that neonatal research is taking, none is as important as the search for a way to prevent premature labor and delivery. There is no incubator made that can match

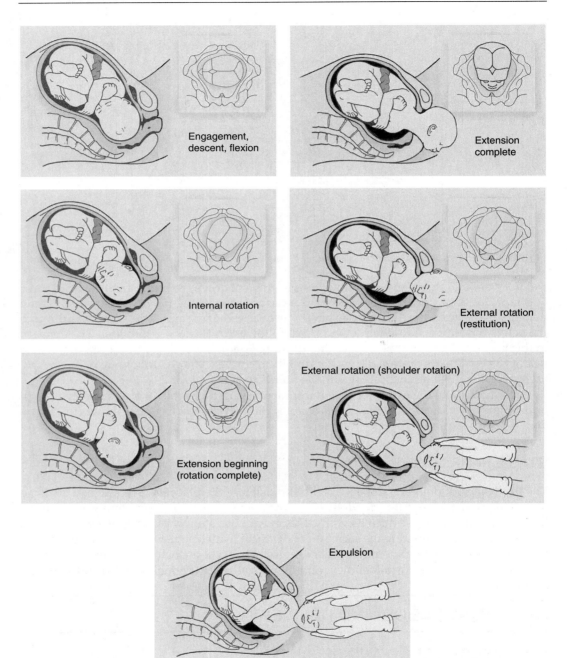

Engagement, descent, flexion

Extension complete

Internal rotation

External rotation (restitution)

Extension beginning (rotation complete)

External rotation (shoulder rotation)

Expulsion

Figure 3–4 *Normal delivery of the fetus.*

the uterus and no ventilator that can duplicate the placenta. The rate of premature labor in high-risk patients averages 40%, with a rate of premature delivery around 20%. If premature labor could be stopped, we would not have to worry about treating the many complications that result from a premature delivery.

TOCOLYSIS

The process of stopping labor is called *tocolysis*. Tocolysis is employed when premature labor threatens the premature delivery of the fetus.

Pharmacologic Tocolysis.   Many premature labors can be stopped, or at least slowed down, by the use of certain drugs. Tocolysis is often accomplished by the use of beta-sympathomimetic (adrenergic) drugs, which relax smooth muscle contractions. The common adrenergics used are terbutaline sulfate and ritodrine.

Maternal side effects of the adrenergic drugs include tachycardia, hyperglycemia, hypokalemia, anxiety, nausea, and vomiting. Fetal effects include tachycardia and hyperglycemia. Neonates may develop a rebound hypoglycemia caused by an overproduction of insulin in response to intrauterine hyperglycemia.[2] Fetuses exposed to hyperglycemia in utero often are large for their gestational age; however, the hyperglycemia seen with terbutaline use does not appear to significantly affect birthweight.[3]

Another drug in widespread use, magnesium sulfate, is an anticonvulsant drug that is successful in stopping uterine contractions. It works by decreasing muscle contractility, inhibiting uterine contractions. Neonatal effects of maternal magnesium sulfate administration may include decreased muscle tone, drowsiness, and decreased serum calcium levels.[2] Nelson and Gretcher have conducted a study indicating that the use of magnesium sulfate may protect against cerebral palsy in very low birthweight infants.[4]

With regard to their effectiveness as tocolytic agents, ritodrine and magnesium sulfate appear to be comparable according to one study by Wilkins and associates.[5] However, ritodrine seems to have more complications associated with its use. In addition to the shaking and nervousness accompanying the use of ritodrine, there is an increased incidence of maternal pulmonary edema. Blickstein and associates feel that the pulmonary edema may be secondary to an underlying cardiomyopathy, and not the drug itself.[6] Pulmonary edema, which develops in patients receiving tocolytic therapy, also appears to be associated with the presence of maternal infection.

Drugs that inhibit prostaglandin synthetase, such as indomethacin, have been used experimentally to stop prostaglandin-induced labor. Adverse fetal effects seen with indomethacin use include constriction of the ductus arteriosus, pulmonary hypertension, reduced urine production, and rarely, small bowel perforation.

Calcium channel blockers, such as nifedipine, have been shown to be effective in stopping labor. Side effects of this medication are principally seen in the mother and include nausea, flushing, headache, or dizziness. In the fetus, there is some concern that uterine and umbilical blood flow may be decreased.[7]

Indications for Tocolysis. Tocolysis is indicated when stage I labor begins prior to 37 weeks' gestation and when placenta previa is present. Preterm birth is a major cause of mortality and morbidity in the perinatal period. In one study, mortality of infants born before 37 weeks' gestation was 83%, with 66% of deaths occurring in births less than 29 weeks. Tocolysis in the 20- to 29-week gestation group is aimed at increasing survival and reducing morbidity, whereas tocolysis between 30 to 36 weeks is aimed primarily at reducing morbidity. The prediction of perinatal morbidity and identification of neonates at risk for morbidity and mortality may be aided by measuring the amniotic fluid concentration of interleukin-6.[8]

Continued research is aimed at methods of identifying those mothers at high risk of preterm birth. One such method that has shown some promise is the presence of prolactin in cervicovaginal washings.

Tocolysis should only be done when certain factors are present. These factors, described by Knuppel and Drukker are: 1) true labor must be present with at least three contractions of moderate duration and intensity in a 20-minute period; 2) the cervix cannot be dilated more than 4 cm and effaced more than 50% with intact amniotic membranes; 3) the fetus must be between 20 and 36 weeks' gestational age; 4) there should be no signs of fetal distress or disease: 5) there should be no medical or obstetric disorder that would contraindicate the continuation of labor; and 6) the mother must be willing and able to give her informed consent.[9]

Nonpharmacologic Strategies for Tocolysis. Tocolytic drugs have not proven to be effective in stopping all premature labor. This has caused research to focus on other means of preventing premature labor. Bennett and associates present four nonpharmacologic strategies that do not use tocolytic drugs. They are: 1) comprehensive, accessible family planning; 2) risk assessment and counseling before conception; 3) risk assessment for prenatal patients; and 4) patient education to identify signs of premature labor and when to seek help.[10]

DYSTOCIA (PROLONGED DIFFICULT LABOR AND DELIVERY)

Dystocia is a prolongation of labor secondary to uterine, pelvic, or fetal factors. Dystocia is present when the first and second stages of labor exceed 20 hours. Dystocia is also present when the second stage of labor exceeds 2 hours in primigravidas and 1 hour in multigravidas. Causes of dystocia are presented in Table 3–2.

TABLE 3–2 Causes of Dysocia

Uterine dysfunction (abnormal contractions of the uterus)
Abnormal fetal presentations
Excessive fetal size
Hydrocephalus
Abnormality in size or shape of birth canal

As the length of labor increases, fetal morbidity and mortality increase for three main reasons. First, the likelihood of premature separation of the placenta from the uterus is increased, causing serious fetal asphyxia. Second, compression of the umbilical cord, with subsequent fetal asphyxia, is more likely, and third, the risk of premature rupture of the amniotic sac is increased. The danger of fetal infection rises significantly if the amniotic membranes have been ruptured for more than 24 hours. We will now examine the causes of dystocia.

Dysfunction of the Uterus. A dysfunctioning uterus may contract excessively (hypertonic) or too mildly (hypotonic). When the uterus contracts hypertonically, the cervix does not dilate and efface as usual. The result may be hypoxia and asphyxia from compression of the placenta, and possibly the umbilical cord. Hypertonic contractions are the less frequent of the two varieties. Hypotonic contractions may be secondary to maternal overdosage of anesthetics or a failure of the fetus to descend normally. With hypotonic contractions, the cervix fails to dilate and efface normally, and contractions are not strong enough to expel the fetus.

Cephalopelvic Disproportion. In this abnormality, the disproportion can either be too large a fetal head or too small a maternal pelvic opening. In either case, labor is delayed by the inability of the fetus to enter and then descend the birth canal. Possible causes of a large fetal head include hydrocephaly and a growth accelerated fetus, which may occur in the presence of maternal diabetes.

Contracture of the maternal pelvis is an infrequent occurrence. It is usually a congenital problem but may be secondary to malnutrition, neoplasms, pelvic fractures, and disorders of the spine or lower extremities. Small pelvic dimensions are also seen in Asian populations and in women younger than 20 years old.[11] The pelvic opening may be diminished in either the anterior/posterior or later dimensions. Both the upper portion of the pelvic opening, the inlet, and the lower portion, the outlet, are measured. The diameter of both pelvic openings is measured by estimating the distances anteroposteriorly and transversely. This is done by manually palpating and measuring the pelvis externally.

Abnormal Presentation. Any fetal presentation other than vertex is considered abnormal (Figure 3–5). The *breech* presentation is the most common of all abnormal presentations, compromising about 3.5% of all births. Other abnormal presentations include face, brow, and shoulder or transverse lie of the fetus. Breech refers to the fetus being in a buttocks-down position.

The breech presentation is broken down into three varieties. When the feet, legs, and buttocks all present together, it is called a complete breech. An incomplete or footling breech occurs when one or both feet descend into the birth canal first. Frank breech occurs when the legs are flexed against the body, the feet being near the face, and the buttocks being the presenting part.

The primary complication of breech presentations occurs when there is a diminished pelvic size or enlarged fetal head. The problems arise after the body has been delivered and it is then discovered that the fetal head will not pass through the pelvis. At this point it is

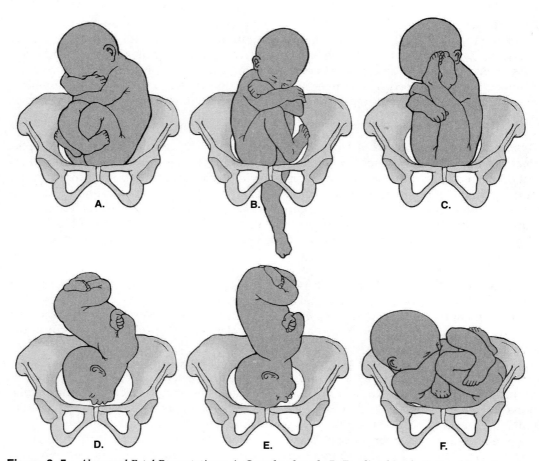

Figure 3–5 *Abnormal Fetal Presentations: A. Complete breech; B. Footling breech; C. Frank breech; D. Face; E. Brow; F. Shoulder*

too late to perform a cesarean delivery and the head must be extracted from the pelvis. This is done by manipulation and pulling on the delivered fetal body by the obstetrician. The result is often spinal cord damage and hemorrhage in the brain. Placenta previa, discussed later in this chapter, is a common cause of the breech presentation.

The fetal skull (Figure 3–6) is not a solid structure as in the adult. It is made up of several bony plates separated by what are known as sutures. In normal presentations, as the head enters the birth canal, these sutures overlap, diminishing the diameter of the fetal skull and facilitating the birth of the fetus.

In face or brow presentation the head enters the birth canal in such a way that the sutures cannot override. The result is that the head must pass through the pelvis and the birth canal at its full size. This may or may not result in prolongation of labor, depending on the size of the maternal pelvic opening. The neonate may suffer from severe facial edema follow-

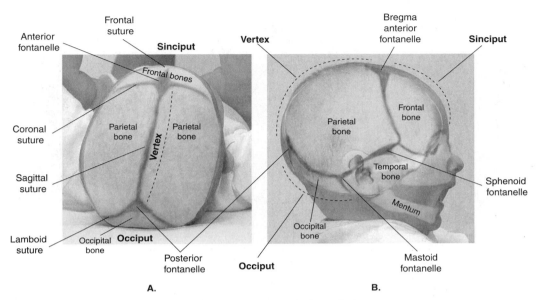

Figure 3–6 *Anatomy of the fetal skull: A Superior view; B. Lateral view.*

ing this type of delivery. Fetal mortality is increased with this type of delivery, secondary to the asphyxia frequently seen with prolonged labor.

Shoulder presentation, or transverse lie, occurs when the fetus is lying perpendicular to the birth canal. Delivery of the fetus in this state is nearly impossible and requires a great deal of manipulation to straighten the fetus. If manipulation fails, a cesarean delivery is done.

PROBLEMS ASSOCIATED WITH THE UMBILICAL CORD

Even though the Wharton's jelly, present in the umbilical cord, prevents the cord from bending to the point of occluding blood flow, it does not prevent the cord from being compressed between two body parts. This type of occlusion can occur in the uterus or in the birth canal.

Prolapse of the Umbilical Cord.   When the umbilical cord passes through the cervix into the birth canal ahead of the presenting part, it is called *prolapse* of the umbilical cord (Figure 3–7). This problem is common in breech presentations, especially footling and transverse lie, and in multiple gestations. As the fetus passes through the birth canal, the cord is easily compressed between the fetus and the maternal pelvis. Compression of the cord can also occur in the uterus and is called an *occult* prolapse.

Either of these occurrences can be dangerous to the fetus. Any interruption of blood flow through the umbilical cord leads to hypoxia, and eventual asphyxia to the fetus, and requires immediate intervention. This condition is monitored via the fetal heart monitor.

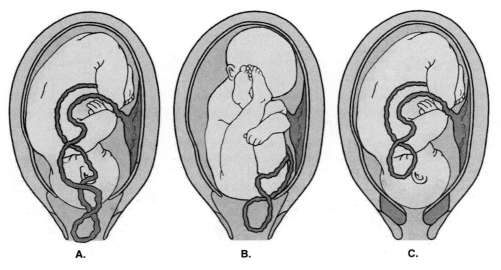

Figure 3–7   *Prolapse of the umbilical cord: A. Vertex presentation; B. Breech presentation; C. Occult prolapse*

Intrauterine cord compression can be reduced by artificially increasing the amniotic fluid volume through a process known as amnioinfusion.[12] By increasing the amniotic fluid volume, there is more room in the uterus and less chance of cord compression.

PLACENTAL ABNORMALITIES

Placenta Previa.   In most pregnancies the blastocyst attaches itself somewhere near the upper portion of the uterine cavity. When the implantation occurs in the lower portion of the uterus, it is called *placenta previa*. Three varieties of placenta previa are recognized, depending on their proximity to the cervix (Figure 3–8).

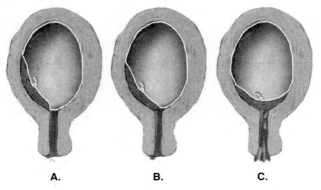

A.   B.   C.

Figure 3–8   *Placenta previa: A. Low implantation; B. Partial placenta previa; C. Total placenta previa.*

A low implantation occupies the lower portion of the uterus but does not cover the cervical opening. A partial placenta previa covers a portion of the cervical opening but does not cover it completely. Total placenta previa completely covers the opening of the cervix.

All types of placenta previa are readily diagnosed by ultrasound. It is obvious that with any type of previa, there will be varying degrees of obstruction to fetal passage. A more serious complication is the early separation of the placenta from the uterus, abruptio placentae, discussed next.

Abruptio Placentae.   Any time a normally attached placenta separates prematurely from the uterine wall, it is called *abruptio placentae.* Separation of the placenta frequently causes labor to begin. Such a pregnancy is precarious at best and requires very close monitoring by the physician. Premature labor and delivery occur more commonly with abruptio placentae. This is due to the frequent commencement of labor when the placenta separates from the uterine wall. Maternal mortality ranges from 2 to 10% in severe cases ending in fetal death. Fetal mortality approaches 50% owing to the acuteness of blood loss.

The most common cause of abruption is maternal hypertension of any origin, which includes *preeclampsia.* Maternal preeclampsia is the development of hypertension with proteinuria, edema, or both. It is of unknown etiology and usually presents after week 20 of gestation.

Additionally, abruptio placentae may be present in a other with a history of abruption, a high number of previous pregnancies, trauma, short umbilical cord, sudden uterine decompression, uterine anomalies, and compression of the inferior vena cava.

Placental separation can be partial or complete. If bleeding from the vagina is present, it is called an apparent hemorrhage. If no bleeding is evident, it is called a concealed hemorrhage. Figure 3–9 shows the different combinations of abruptio placentae that are possible. A categorization of abruptio placentae is listed in Table 3–3.

The mother and the fetus are at risk in the presence of placental abruption. Severe abruptio placentae is clinically manifested by vaginal bleeding, tetany of the uterus, tenderness of the uterus, absent fetal heart tones, and maternal hypovolemic shock. The risk to the fetus

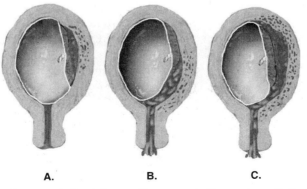

A.   **B.**   **C.**

Figure 3–9   *Abruptio placentae: A. Partial separation, concealed hemorrhage; B. Partial separation, external hemorrhage; C. Complete separation, concealed hemorrhage*

TABLE 3–3   Classification of Abruptio Placentae

Grade 0—Asymptomatic. Diagnosis is made after delivery when a small clot is found behind the placenta.
Grade 1—Vaginal bleeding. No signs of maternal shock or fetal distress. Tetany and tenderness of the uterus may be present.
Grade 2—External vaginal bleeding may or may not be present. No signs of maternal shock. Signs of fetal distress are present. Tetany and tenderness of the uterus are present.
Grade 3—External vaginal bleeding may or may not be present. Maternal shock and persistent abdominal pain are present. Fetal demise is present. Marked uterine tetany resulting in a very stiff, firm consistency. Thirty percent of cases show signs of coagulopathy.

---

is the loss of placental surface area, resulting in severe fetal hypoxia and asphyxia. Premature separation of the placenta may also lead to fetal blood loss, with subsequent anemia and shock.

Treatment of abruptio placentae includes strict management of blood volume, maintaining a hematocrit volume of 30%. This is done by the intravenous administration of blood or crystalloid solutions. The mother is instructed to lie in the lateral position to allow maximal placental circulation. Intensive monitoring of both fetus and mother is essential, and those in charge of care should prepare for emergency delivery or cesarean delivery if the signs of maternal shock or fetal distress are seen.

CESAREAN DELIVERY

Some features are delivered by way of a surgical incision through the maternal abdomen and uterus, called a cesarean delivery, or cesarean section. Cesarean deliveries are performed under anesthesia and should only be done in the presence of the following indications: prior cesarean delivery, dystocia, breech presentation, and fetal distress.[13]

Most cesarean deliveries result in a healthy neonate, but there are some possible complications. The most serious complications arise from accidental cutting of the placenta, umbilical cord, or fetus during the delivery. This can lead to serious hemorrhage and anemia. Another common complication is transient tachypnea of the newborn (TTN). This syndrome, discussed in Chapter 10, is thought to be caused by the retention of lung fluids, normally expelled as the fetus is squeezed through the birth canal.

↳ *difficult labor*

MULTIPLE GESTATIONS

Multiple gestation is the presence of twins, triplets, quadruplets, or more fetuses during the same pregnancy. The incidence of mortality is higher in multiple than in single gestations.[14] This is due in part to the high incidence of premature labor and delivery in multiple gestations. There is also an increased incidence of congenital abnormalities, growth retardation, bacterial infection, and hypoglycemia.

Several factors increase the incidence of multiple gestations. Familial inheritance predisposes the carrier female to have fraternal twins. There is a high incidence of multiple gestation among blacks, and a very low incidence in the Asian population. Multiple gestations are also more common in the older female, ages 35 to 39. The administration of clomiphene citrate (Clomid®) to induce ovulation is associated with a high incidence of multiple gestations, as is the administration of gonadotropins. It is also speculated that there is an increase in twinning following discontinuation of oral contraceptives.

Twinning is the most common type of multiple gestation, occurring in about 1 out of 99 pregnancies. Two thirds of all twins are fraternal or dizygotic and arise from the fertilization of two separate ova. Fraternal twinning is an *autosomal-recessive trait* that is carried by the daughters of mothers of twins.

The remaining one third are identical twins, originating from one ova. They are of the same sex and have an identical appearance. In contrast to fraternal twins, identical twinning is a random occurrence. Identical twins have a higher mortality rate than do fraternal twins. Whenever there is a shared placenta or umbilicus between twins, there is an increase in risk factors. One twin may receive more nutrition, or actually deplete the other twin.

For some reason, the second twin is often more compromised than the first, and it appears that female twins are healthier than male twins.

ADAPTATION TO EXTRAUTERINE LIFE

Of all the adaptations that a human undergoes throughout life, none is quite so strenuous or important as the adaptation to extrauterine life. Within a short time following birth the neonate must undergo major changes that will allow it to survive outside the uterus. The neonate must begin spontaneous ventilation and respiration. The circulatory system must change to its adult pattern, and the neonate must now provide its own energy and rid itself of wastes. The two changes that will be examined in this chapter are the establishment of breathing and the changes in the cardiovascular system.

THE FIRST BREATH

No single event is as thrilling as when a newborn takes its first breath. The breath is the sign of life, and the sound of the crying neonate is anxiously awaited by all in attendance at the delivery. What is unknown to many, however, is the magnitude of what must take place in order for the neonate to take that first breath.

Studies have shown that the fetus begins breathing movements while still in the uterus. Fetal respiratory movements have been detected as early as week 18, but most activity occurs during the last 10 weeks of gestation. These movements no doubt prepare the fetus for the time when it will be on its own.

Once the fetus has left the confines of the uterus, several events must occur to provide for an easy transition to extrauterine breathing. First, there must be something to stimulate the neonate to breathe. Factors involved in the initiation of the first breath are listed in Table 3–4.

TABLE 3–4   Initiation of the First Breath

- Asphyxia. Increased $PaCO_2$, decreased PaO_2, and pH stimulate the chemoreceptors, which then stimulate gasping.
- Recoil of the thorax. As the thorax pases through the birth canal during vaginal delivery, it is compressed. As the thorax exits the birth canal, the natural recoil of the thorax creates a negative pressure in the thoracic cavity, causing air to enter the lungs.
- Environmental changes. As the fetus passes from an environment of darkness and warmth into a bright, loud, cold environment, the abrupt change initiates a cry reflex. Additionally, tactile stimulus from handling further stimulates the cry reflex.

Factors Responsible for the First Breath.   Chemoreceptors found in the aorta and carotid arteries detect changes in PaO_2 and $PaCO_2$ levels in the blood. During the process of birth the fetus is cut off from the placenta as it descends the birth canal. As a result, fetal PaO_2 falls and $PaCO_2$ rises. These two changes stimulate the chemoreceptors, which in turn stimulate the respiratory center in the brain. The brain signals the muscles of ventilation into action. This birth asphyxia is probably the most powerful influence on stimulating the initial breath.

A second contribution to the first breath occurs during vaginal delivery. The fetal thorax is compressed as it descends through the birth canal. As it exits, the chest expands to its original size and shape. A result of this expansion is the entry of air into the lungs. Additionally, during vaginal delivery the lung fluid is expelled, creating an "empty volume" in the lungs to be filled with air upon delivery.

A third influence is the abrupt change in environment from the dark and warm uterus to the bright, cold, and noisy delivery room. These changes, combined with the physical handling of the neonate, invoke the crying reflex, which also helps stimulate the first breath.

In order for the neonate to breathe successfully, surface forces in the lung must be overcome. In the term neonate this is aided immensely by the presence of pulmonary surfactant. Surfactant greatly reduces the surface tension of the alveoli and reduces the work required of the neonate to ventilate. Chapter 1 contains a detailed discussion of pulmonary surfactant.

The initial pressure needed to overcome the surface forces of the lung has been measured and found to be as high as -100 cm H_2O. Succeeding breaths require much less negative pressure due to the establishment of the functional residual capacity (FRC). This concept is illustrated in Figure 3–10. The FRC is simply air that remains in the lung following normal exhalation.

As the alveoli are deflated following the first breath, the presence of surfactant prevents them from collapsing completely, allowing them to remain partially filled with air. With each ensuing breath a little more air remains, causing the FRC to gradually expand in the first few hours of life. The result is that each successive breath becomes less difficult and requires less energy to accomplish. Thus, the healthy neonate quickly adapts to extrauterine breathing when the lungs are mature.

THE CHANGE FROM FETAL TO ADULT CIRCULATION

Another major change that must occur in order for the newborn to successfully adapt to extrauterine life is the establishment of the adult circulatory pattern. The fetal pattern, in

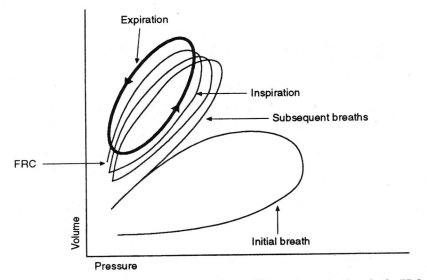

Figure 3–10 *The establishment of FRC following delivery. With each ensuing breath, the FRC gradually increases, requiring less pressure to produce larger tidal volumes.*

which the lungs are largely bypassed, cannot continue if the neonate is to survive. The actual events take place simultaneously, but each will be discussed separately here to aid understanding of what takes place. Figure 3–11 shows the change from fetal to adult circulation.

Alteration in Circulatory Pressure.   Shortly after birth, the umbilical cord is clamped. This seemingly minor occurrence causes great changes to take place in the neonatal circulation. Before clamping, the umbilicus and placenta provided a very low resistance to blood flow. Upon clamping the umbilical cord, blood flow to the placenta stops. The blood that would have gone to the placenta is now forced to perfuse the lower extremities. Being forced through a higher resistance causes the arterial blood pressure to rise. The pressure increases back up through the arterial system to the left ventricle and atrium.

As this is taking place, the neonate has begun breathing. The initiation of breathing reduces the pulmonary artery resistance, which was very high in the fetus. This reduction is accomplished by two mechanisms. First, the actual inflation of the lungs, with the resulting establishment of FRC, reduces the surrounding pressure on the pulmonary vasculature. Second, the increase in PaO_2 causes the pulmonary smooth musculature to relax from its constricted state. These two factors cause pulmonary pressures to drop, which in turn leads to a decrease in the pulmonary artery, right ventricle, and atrial pressures.

Closure of the Fetal Shunts.   The fetal cardiovascular system has now undergone a complete reversal of pressures. The left, or arterial, system has converted from low to high pressure, and the right, or venous, system has changed from high to low pressure. The left atrial pressures, now higher than right atrial, cause the tissue flap on the foramen ovale to mechanically close. Blood now flows from the right atrium to the right ventricle and no longer flows through the foramen ovale.

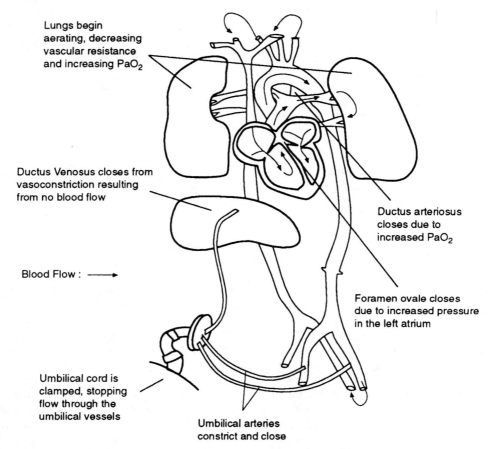

Lungs begin
aerating, decreasing
vascular resistance
and increasing PaO$_2$

Ductus Venosus closes from
vasoconstriction resulting
from no blood flow

Ductus arteriosus
closes due to
increased PaO$_2$

Blood Flow : ⟶

Foramen ovale closes
due to increased pressure
in the left atrium

Umbilical cord is
clamped, stopping
flow through the
umbilical vessels

Umbilical arteries
constrict and close

Figure 3–11 *The modifications that change fetal circulation to adult circulation.*

During the last few weeks of gestation, the smooth muscles surrounding the ductus arteriosus begin to develop. These muscles remain relaxed and open owing to the presence of specialized prostaglandins. The production of these prostaglandins is enhanced by low levels of PaO$_2$ and inhibited by high PaO$_2$ levels. As PaO$_2$ continues to increase following initiation of spontaneous breathing, the production of the ductal prostaglandins is inhibited. The absence of prostaglandins allows the smooth muscle surrounding the ductus to constrict, closing it. The closing of this shunt stops the flow of blood from the pulmonary artery to the aorta. Failure of the ductus arteriosus to close may lead to further problems, such as right-to-left shunting, left-to-right shunting, and resultant congestive heart failure. The problems confronted when the ductus fails to close are covered in detail in Chapter 12.

With the clamping of the umbilical cord, blood no longer flows through the umbilical vein or arteries. These vessels quickly constrict and eventually become supporting ligaments in the abdominal cavity. The ductus venosus constricts and becomes a ligament due to the same circumstances.

Thus the cardiopulmonary adaptation to extrauterine life is now complete. In the healthy neonate, one hardly notices that changes take place. Conversely, a failure to adapt has grave and sometimes fatal results. The cardiac and pulmonary systems are only two of many adaptations the neonate must make. It must also provide its own nutrition, fight off infection, and be kept warm. As important as each of these is, none is as important as the adaptation of the heart and lungs to the extrauterine environment.

SUMMARY

The process of human birth is a complex event that is poorly understood. Normal birth starts with the first contraction, which signals the start of stage I of labor. During this stage, the cervix effaces and dilates to accommodate the passage of the fetus. Stage II is the actual delivery of the fetus, and stage III is the expulsion of the placenta.

Many factors can lead to an abnormal labor and delivery. Of all the causes of perinatal morbidity and mortality, none is as devastating as premature labor and birth. Preventing premature labor is a major focus of perinatal medicine and is accomplished with the use of tocolytic drugs, which help slow and hopefully stop uterine contractions. Another factor resulting in abnormal labor and delivery is dystocia caused by a dysfunctioning uterus, cephalopelvic disproportion, or an abnormal fetal presentation. → *difficult labor.*

Labor and delivery can also be complicated by compression of the umbilical cord, either in utero (occult) or in the birth canal (prolapse). Complications are also seen with placental abnormalities such as placenta previa and abruptio placentae.

Approximately 25% of deliveries in the United States are done via cesarean section.[13] This mode of delivery can predispose the fetus to accidental trauma and blood loss, and TTN. Multiple gestations also have a higher incidence of mortality and can complicate the normal birthing process. → *& vag. squeeze↑ lung fluid.*

Once born, the fetus must adapt to the extrauterine environment. The stimulation of chemoreceptors, expansion of the fetal thorax, and stimulation are all factors that initiate extrauterine breathing. As the neonate continues to breathe, surface forces in the lungs are reduced by the presence of surfactant and FRC increases as compliance improves.

Another adaptation the fetus must undergo is the change from fetal to an adult circulation pattern. This occurs following a complex change of pressures between the right and left heart caused by stoppage of blood flow to the placenta and increase of blood flow to the lungs. Failure of this change to occur is called persistent fetal circulation and can lead to several neonatal problems, including shunting and heart failure.

References

1. Roberts WE, et al. Risk of preterm delivery from preterm labor in high-risk patients. *J Reprod Med.* 1995;40:95–100.

2. Merenstein GB, Gardner SL. *Handbook of Neonatal Intensive Care.* 4th ed. St. Louis: CV Mosby Co; 1998.

3. Robins GW, Blount BW, Airline A. Effective of terbutaline tocolysis on infant birth-weight. *J Fam Pract.* 1995;40:581–585.

4. Nelson KB, Grether JK. Can magnesium sulfate reduce the risk of cerebral palsy in very low birthweight infants? *Pediatrics.* 1995;95:263–269.

5. Wilkins IA, et al. Efficacy and side effects of magnesium sulfate and ritodrine as tocolytic agents. *Am J Obstet Gynecol.* 1988;159;685–689.

6. Blickstein I, et al. Ritodrine-induced pulmonary edema unmasking underlying peri-partum cardiomyopathy. *Am J Obstet Gynecol.* 1988;159:332–333.

7. Monga M, Creasy RK. Pharmacologic management of preterm labor. *Semin Perinatol.* 1995;19:84–96.

8. Yoon BH, et al. Amniotic fluid interleukin-6: a sensitive test for antenatal diagnosis of acute inflammatory lesions of preterm placenta and prediction of perinatal morbidity. *Am J Obstet Gynecol.* 1995;172:960–970.

9. Knuppel RA, Drukker JE. *High-Risk Pregnancy: A Team Approach.* 2nd ed. Philadelphia: WB Saunders Co; 1993.

10. Bennett NL, et al. New strategies for preterm labor. *Nurse Practitioner.* 1989; 14:27–28, 30, 33–34.

11. Lowdermilk DL, Perry SE, Bobak IM. *Maternity Nursing.* 5th ed. St. Louis: Mosby Inc; 1999.

12. Strong TH Jr. Amnioinfusion. *J. Reprod Med.* 1995;40:108–114.

13. Paul RH, Miller DA. Cesarian birth: how to reduce the rate. *Am J Obstet Gynecol.* 1995;172:1903–1907.

14. Gander MO, et al. The origin and outcomes of preterm twin pregnancies. *Obstet Gynecol.* 1995;85:553–557.

Bibliograhy and Suggested Readings

Avery GB, Fletcher MA, MacDonald MG. *Pathophysiology and Management of the Newborn.* 5th ed. Philadelphia: JB Lippincott Co; 1999.

Hicks GH. *Cardiopulmonary Anatomy and Physiology.* Philadelphia: WB Saunders Co; 2000.

Moore KL, Persaud TVN, Shiota K. *Color Atlas of Clinical Embryology.* 2nd ed. Philadelphia: WB Saunders Co; 2001.

Olson DM, Mijovic JE, Sadowsky DW. Control of human parturition. *Semin Perinatol.* 1995;19:52–63.

Tucker SM. *Pocket Guide to Fetal Monitoring and Assessment.* 4th ed. St. Louis: Mosby; 2000.

White L. *Foundations of Nursing: Caring for the Whole Person.* Albany, NY: Delmar Thomson Learning; 2001.

Posttest

1. Of the following, which is not part of the birth process?
   a. rupture of the membranes
   b. dilation of the cervix

    c. contraction of the uterus
    d. expulsion of the placenta
2. At a dilatation of 5 cm, the cervix is:
    a. one-quarter dilatated
    b. one-half dilatated
    c. three-quarters dilatated
    d. fully dilatated
3. The most common fetal presentation position is:
    a. occipital
    b. breech
    c. footling
    d. vertex
4. The head is said to be engaged in the birth canal when a station of _____ is reached.
    a. 0
    b. 1
    c. -1
    d. 2
5. Actual delivery of the fetus takes place during the second stage of labor and normally does not exceed:
    a. 2 hours
    b. 1 hour
    c. 30 minutes
    d. 5 minutes
6. Which of the following drugs is *not* used as a tocolytic?
    a. terbutaline
    b. beclomethasone
    c. ritodrine
    d. nifedipine
7. Dystocia could result from which of the following?
    a. breech presentation
    b. cephalopelvic disproportion
    c. uterine dysfunction
    d. all of the above.
8. Vaginal delivery of the fetus is nearly impossible in which of the following presentations?
    a. transverse lie
    b. face or brow
    c. vertex
    d. complete breech
9. A complete coverage of the cervical opening by the placenta is called:
    a. placental-cervical obstruction
    b. partial placental previa
    c. total placenta previa
    d. abruptio placentae

10. Substantial separation of the placenta from the uterus with no visible bleeding is called:
    a. partial separation
    b. complete separation
    c. apparent hemorrhage
    d. concealed hemorrhage

11. Which of the following is *not* an indication for performing a cesarean delivery?
    a. maternal fever
    b. fetal distress
    c. cephalopelvic disproportion
    d. severe maternal preeclampsia

12. Of the following, which factors explain why the mortality rate of multiple gestations is increased?
    I. an increased incidence of premature labor
    II. an increased incidence of congenital abnormalities
    III. an increased incidence of intracranial hemorrhage
    IV. an increased incidence of bacterial infections
    V. an increased incidence of hypoglycemia
        a. II, III, V
        b. I, II, IV, V
        c. I, II, III, V
        d. III, IV, V

13. The most powerful influence on the initial breath is:
    a. tactile stimulus
    b. cold stress
    c. removal of lung fluid
    d. asphyxia

14. Each breath subsequent to the first breath requires less negative pressure due to:
    a. lung fluid
    b. establishment of the FRC
    c. asphyxia
    d. decreased airway resistance

15. Clamping of the umbilical cord results in:
    a. lowering of the neonate's $PaCO_2$
    b. an improvement of oxygenation
    c. raising the neonate's arterial pressure
    d. lowering the neonate's venous pressure

16. Blood flow through the foramen ovale normally ceases when:
    a. the ductus arteriosus closes
    b. the neonate begins spontaneous breathing
    c. arterial PaO_2 rises
    d. left heart pressure exceeds right heart pressure

UNIT TWO

CARE OF THE
NEONATAL AND
PEDIATRIC PATIENT

CHAPTER FOUR

TECHNIQUES OF RESUSCITATION AND STABILIZATION

OBJECTIVES

Upon completion of this chapter, the reader should be able to:

1. List the four factors that can lead to fetal asphyxia.
2. Compare and contrast primary to secondary apnea. Describe the cardiovascular events that occur during periods of intrauterine asphyxia.
3. Discuss the effects of asphyxia on the lungs.
4. List and describe the three factors that provide proper preparation for a resuscitation.
5. Describe the ABCs of a resuscitation. Include a description of the "continuing circle" of a resuscitation.
6. Assign an appropriate Apgar score when provided with patient data.
7. Describe and discuss each step in a resuscitation as shown in Figure 4–5.
8. Describe each of the following skills as it relates to neonatal resuscitation:
   a. Thermoregulation
   b. Suctioning
   c. Positioning
   d. Tactile stimulation
   e. Evaluation of respirations
   f. Evaluation of heart rate
   g. Positive pressure ventilation
   h. Chest compressions
   i. Intubation
   j. Delivery of medications
9. List the drugs used during a resuscitation. Include correct concentrations used, dosages, and routes of administration.
10. Describe the procedure for obtaining arterial blood from the umbilical stump.
11. Discuss the indications, procedure for placement, and complications of an umbilical artery catheter.
12. Describe the sources of fetal and neonatal glucose.
13. List the serum glucose values that indicate hypoglycemia. Include a description of the clinical signs.
14. List and describe the cause of hypoglycemia, techniques used to measure glucose, and the treatment for hypoglycemia.

KEY TERMS

acrocyanosis
asphyxia
brown fat
carbonic acid
conductive
convective

erythroblastosis fetalis
evaporative
glucagon
necrotizing enterocolitis
persistent fetal circulation

primary apnea
radiant
secondary apnea
supine
Trendelenburg

OVERVIEW

For those who work with newborns, the skills and knowledge required for proper resuscitation are possibly the most important skills to possess. Every baby born is a potential resuscitation and in our society it should be expected that each newborn receive appropriate skilled care. It is to be expected that every person who practices respiratory care in a hospital setting will eventually be involved in a newborn resuscitation. For this reason, it is strongly recommended that each practitioner complete the Neonatal Resuscitation program offered jointly by the American Academy of Pediatrics and the American Heart Association. Much of the information for this chapter was obtained from that program.

WHEN TO RESUSCITATE

PRIMARY AND SECONDARY APNEA

The necessity to resuscitate a neonate is related to asphyxia, which can occur in utero during or after delivery. *Asphyxia,* which is a combination of hypoxia, hypercapnia, and acidosis, may lead to irreversible damage to the brain and other vital organs. Fetal asphyxia may be caused by any of the factors listed in Table 4–1.

First, any disorder that leads to maternal hypoxia or asphyxia will in turn lead to asphyxia in the fetus. Second, insufficient placental blood flow or a reduction in the diffusion of oxygen and carbon dioxide will lead to decreased gas transfer from the maternal to the fetal blood and vice versa. Third, occlusion or blockage of blood flow through the umbilical cord stops blood flow to the placenta and leads to asphyxia. Finally, certain fetal factors such as anemia and drug toxicity can cause fetal asphyxia.

When any of the above factors are present, the fetus initially becomes hypoxic. Because of the early development of chemoreceptors and baroreceptors in the fetal vasculature, the fetus can react to changes in blood gases while still in utero. The fetus attempts to reverse the hypoxia by beginning rapid ventilations. If the hypoxia is not corrected, the ventilatory effort ceases and the patient enters a period of apnea called *primary apnea.* At this point, the heart rate and blood pressure begin to drop.

TABLE 4–1   Causes of Fetal Asphyxia

---

1. Maternal hypoxia
   a. Low environmental oxygen
   b. Apnea associated with seizures or eclampsia
   c. Acute asthma attack
   d. Pneumonia
   e. Hypoventilation from oversedation
   f. Carbon monoxide poisoning or anemia
2. Insufficient placental blood flow
   a. Diminished blood flow to the placenta secondary to congestive heart failure
   b. Hypotension and shock
   c. Vasoconstrictive states secondary to toxemia and essential hypertension
   d. Placenta previa
   e. Abruptio placentae
3. Blockage of umbilical blood flow
   a. Prolapse of the umbilical cord
   b. Occult prolapse of the umbilical cord
   c. Nuchal cord (wrapping of the cord around the fetal neck or body)
4. Fetal disorders
   a. Hydrops fetalis (fetal cardiac failure in utero)
   b. Fetal hypotension from hemorrhage or drugs
   c. Fetal hemolytic anemia

With continued hypoxia, $PaCO_2$ rises and the pH drops, leading to asphyxia. Continuation of the asphyxia leads to a second attempt by the patient to ventilate. This time, however, the respirations are weak, gasping, and ineffective. The efforts weaken and cease, and the patient enters another stage of apnea known as *secondary apnea*. During secondary apnea, there will be no attempt to breathe again unless mechanical ventilation is started. When untreated, the heart rate and blood pressure drop until death occurs.

The return of spontaneous ventilation is a result of rapid initiation of positive-pressure ventilation (PPV) with 100% oxygen (Figure 4–1). The longer the patient has been in secondary apnea, the longer the PPV required until spontaneous breathing returns and the greater the chance of brain damage. A fetus may go through all of these stages in utero and be born in secondary apnea of unknown duration. One must therefore always assume that an apneic neonate is in secondary apnea and begin resuscitative efforts immediately. Time wasted in trying to stimulate the patient only places it at a higher risk of developing brain damage.

EFFECT OF ASPHYXIA ON THE LUNGS

As discussed in Chapter 3, the initial adaptation of the fetal lungs to the extrauterine environment requires two steps. First, the lung must rid itself of the lung fluid and become filled with air. This requires the fetus to create significant negative pressures in the thorax to over-

APNEA

Primary Apnea

When infants become asphyxiated (either in utero or after delivery), they undergo a well-defined sequence of events.

When an infant is deprived of oxygen, an initial brief period of rapid breathing occurs. If the asphyxia continues, the respiratory movements cease, the heart rate begins to fall, neuromuscular tone gradually diminishes, and the infant enters a period of apnea known as *primary* apnea. In most instances stimulation and exposure to oxygen during the period of primary apnea will induce respirations.

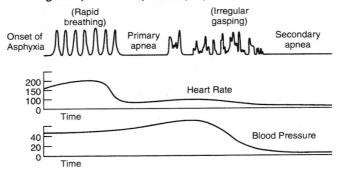

Secondary Apnea

It is important to note that gasping and muscle tone may also be depressed by drugs given to the mother.

If the asphyxia continues, the infant develops deep gasping respirations, the heart rate continues to decrease, the blood pressure begins to fall, and the infant becomes nearly flaccid. The respirations become weaker and weaker until the infant takes a last gasp and enters a period of apnea called *secondary* apnea. During secondary apnea the heart rate, blood pressure, and oxygen in the blood (Pao_2) continue to fall. The infant is now unresponsive to stimulation and will not spontaneously resume respiratory efforts. Death will occur unless resuscitation with assisted ventilation and oxygen is initiated promptly.

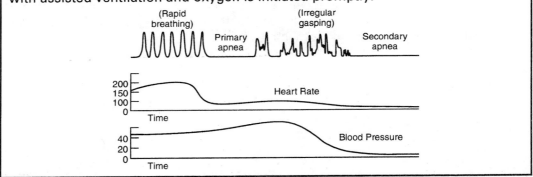

Figure 4–1 *Asphyxia induced apnea and bradycardia. (Reproduced with permission from* Textbook of Neonatal Resuscitation, *Copyright 1987, 1990, 1994, American Heart Association.)*

come the initial resistance and low compliance in the lungs. The second important step is the decrease in pulmonary vascular resistance secondary to the increasing levels of oxygen in the blood and ensuing vascular dilation.

As blood flow increases past the ventilated alveoli, PaO_2 further increases and $PaCO_2$ decreases, resulting in the eventual establishment of an adult pattern of circulation. When asphyxiation occurs, there is a disruption of one or both of these two vital steps, with the result being that the neonate does not adapt to the extrauterine environment.

The neonate who is born apneic or with shallow, ineffective respirations cannot create the necessary negative force to open the alveoli and push the lung fluid out. The presence of hypoxia, hypercarbia, and acidosis causes significant pulmonary vasoconstriction to persist in the lungs, leading to a continuation of pulmonary hypertension. Blood flow is diverted through the foramen ovale and the ductus arteriosus, completely bypassing the lungs as it did in utero. This occurrence is called *persistent fetal circulation* (PFC) and it leads to further asphyxia, because little blood is coming in contact with the ventilated alveoli.

In severe cases of asphyxia, ventilation alone does not alter blood gases because of the severity of the shunt. $PaCO_2$ remains high in the face of adequate ventilation because of the blood bypassing the lungs. In these severe cases, one resuscitative measure is to reverse the pulmonary vasoconstriction by administering sodium bicarbonate, raising the pH, and producing enough vasodilation that blood flow to the lungs increases.

It must be remembered that adequate ventilation must be maintained when bicarbonate is administered. As the bicarbonate (HCO_3) enters the bloodstream, it combines with the hydrogen ($H^{+)}$ ions to form *carbonic acid,* H_2CO_3. The carbonic acid then dissociates into water (H_2O) and carbon dioxide (CO_2), as shown in Figure 4–2. If adequate ventilation is not maintained, $PaCO_2$ builds up, worsening the acidosis.

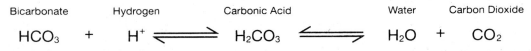

Figure 4–2 *Bicarbonate combines with hydrogen to form carbonic acid. The dissociation of carbonic acid forms water and carbon dioxide.*

PREPARATION FOR RESUSCITATION

An important determinant of a successful resuscitation is the amount of preparation that takes place before the delivery of a high-risk neonate (Table 4–2).

The first step in preparing for a resuscitation is anticipation of the depressed neonate. Anticipation involves a knowledge of the maternal history, the history of the pregnancy, and continuous monitoring of the mother and fetus during labor and delivery. Maternal history and history of the pregnancy should be examined with the high-risk factors discussed in Chapter 3 in mind.

Monitoring of the mother and fetus during labor and delivery includes maternal cardiovascular and pulmonary status and ongoing evaluation of the fetal heart rate. Proper identification and anticipation of a depressed neonate allows the team to be ready for the delivery and prepared to deal with potential problems.

TABLE 4–2   Preparation for Resuscitation

---

1. Anticipation of a high-risk delivery requires:
   a. Maternal history
   b. History of the pregnancy
   c. Continuous monitoring during labor and delivery
2. Equipment
   a. Proper equipment
   b. Variety of sizes to suit various gestational ages
   c. Checked for proper function each shift
3. Trained personnel
   a. At least one person trained in all necessary skills
   b. Must be present in the hospital to respond to unexpected high-risk deliveries

---

The second important part of the preparation is the presence of properly functioning equipment at every delivery. Equipment and supplies that should be present at each resuscitation are listed in Table 4–3. The time to discover that a resuscitation bag is not working is not after the neonate is delivered. Equipment must be checked each shift, not only for its presence, but also for proper function.

The third part of proper preparation is the presence of trained personnel who can direct the resuscitation and perform the necessary procedures. Because many asphyxiated fetuses

---

TABLE 4–3   Neonatal Resuscitation Supplies and Equipment

Suction Equipment
Bulb syringe
Mechanical suction
Suction catheters, 5F or 6F, 8F, 10F
8F feeding tube and 20-ml syringe
Meconium aspirator

Bag-and-Mask Equipment
Neonatal resuscitation bag with a pressure-release valve or pressure gauge—the bag must be capable of delivering 90% to 100% oxygen
Face masks, newborn and premature sizes (cushioned rim masks preferred)
Oral airways, newborn and premature sizes
Oxygen with flowmeter and tubing

Intubation Equipment
Laryngoscope with straight blades, No. 0 (preterm) and No. 1 (term)
Extra bulbs and batteries for laryngoscope
Endotracheal tubes, 2.5, 3.0, 3.5, 4.0 mm
Stylet
Scissors
Gloves

(continued)

TABLE 4–3   (continued)

Medications
Epinephrine 1:10,000—3-ml or 10-ml ampules
Naloxone hydrochloride 0.4 mg/ml—1-ml ampules, or 1.0 mg/ml—2-ml ampules
Volume expander, one or more of these:
  —5% Albumin-saline solution
  —Normal saline
  —Ringer's lactate
Sodium bicarbonate 4.2% (5 mEq/10 ml)—10 ml ampules
Dextrose 10%, 250 ml
Sterile water, 30 ml
Normal saline, 30 ml

Miscellaneous
Radiant warmer
Stethoscope
Cardiotachometer with ECG (oscilloscope desirable)
Adhesive tape, 1/2 or 3/4 inch
Syringes, 1, 3, 5,10, 20, 50 ml
Needles, 25, 21, 18 gauge
Alcohol sponges
Umbilical artery catheterization tray
Umbilical tape
Umbilical catheters, 3.5F, 5F
Three-way stopcocks
Feeding tube, 5F

Source: *Reproduced with permission from* Textbook of Neonatal Resuscitation. *Copyright 1987, 1990, 1994, American Heart Association.*

are born with no prior warning, it is of utmost importance that these skilled personnel be available to assist at all deliveries.

BASICS OF NEONATAL RESUSCITATION

The purpose of the resuscitation is to reverse asphyxia before irreparable damage has occurred. A successful resuscitation is divided into three steps, listed in Table 4–4, that allow the practitioner to reverse asphyxia.

Neonatal resuscitation (Figure 4–3) is a continuing cycle, which is followed until the neonate's condition is stabilized. Resuscitation begins with the evaluation of the neonate's respiratory effort. A decision is then made depending on whether the neonate has made a respiratory effort. The decision is followed by an action that will either deal with the problem, such as a lack of respiratory effort, or will advance to evaluate the next area. These three steps are continued with heart rate and color until the neonate is stabilized.

TABLE 4–4 The ABCs of Resuscitation

The steps in resuscitating newborn infants follow the well-known ABCs of resuscitation.
  A—Establish an open *airway*
  B—Initiate *breathing*
  C—Maintain *circulation*
The components of the neonatal resuscitation procedure related to the ABCs of resuscitation are
shown here.
  A— Establish an open *airway:*
    • Position the infant
    • Suction the ~~mouth, nose,~~ and in some instances the trachea   *nose then mouth*
    • If necessary, insert an ET tube to ensure an open airway
  B—Initiate *breathing:*
    • Use tactile stimulation to initiate respirations
    • Use PPV when necessary, using either
      —Bag or mask
  or
      —Bag and ET tube
  C—Maintain *circulation:*
    • Stimulate and maintain the circulation of blood with
      —Chest compressions
      —Medications

Source: *Reproduced with permission from* Textbook of Neonatal Resuscitation. *Copyright 1987, 1990, 1994,
American Heart Association.*

The actual accomplishment of this continuing cycle is discussed in detail in the following section.

STANDARD PRECAUTIONS

Whenever there is a potential for exposure to any bodily fluids or blood, a high probability during a resuscitation, the practitioner must follow standard precautions, previously known as universal precautions (Figure 4–4). It is probable that, unless one is simply observing, the baby will be handled, and the potential for a droplet of blood or fluid to hit those participating is high. Therefore, gloves, masks, and protective eye wear should be worn by all present. Additionally, a gown or apron should be worn if the possibility of blood or body fluid splashing is present.

STEPS IN A RESUSCITATION

THERMOREGULATION

The steps taken during a resuscitation are shown graphically in Figure 4–5. We will look briefly at each step separately.

The Action/Evaluation/Decision Cycle

A very important aspect of resuscitation is evaluating the infant, deciding what action to take, and then taking action. Further evaluation data is the basis for more decisions and further actions. This cycle can be represented by the following diagram.

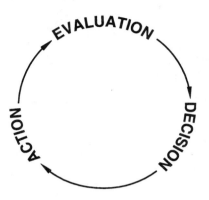

The Cycle

Efficient and effective resuscitation is brought about through a series of actions, evaluations, decisions, and further actions. As an example, at one point while you are providing tactile stimulation, you will evaluate the infant's respirations. On the basis of that evaluation, you will decide what action to take next.

Action	Evaluation	Decision	Action
	No Respirations	Need to Ventilate	Positive-Pressure Ventilation
Tactile Stimulation			
	Adequate Respirations	Make Additional Evaluation	Check Heart Rate

If your evaluation of the respirations indicates that the infant is not breathing or that the respirations are inadequate, you have the basis for deciding that the next action is to provide positive-pressure ventilation. If, on the other hand, the respirations are normal, the next action is to evaluate the infant's heart rate.

After the initiation of any action, you must evaluate its effect on the neonate and make a decision about the next step.

Figure 4–3 *The Action/Evaluation/Decision cycle. (Reproduced with permission from* Textbook of Neonatal Resuscitation. *Copyright 1987, 1990, 1994, American Heart Association.)*

STANDARD PRECAUTIONS FOR INFECTION CONTROL

Wash Hands (Plain soap)
Wash after touching **blood, body fluids, secretions, excretions,** and **contaminated items.** Wash immediately **after gloves are removed** and **between patient contacts.** Avoid transfer of microorganisms to other patients or environments.

Wear Gloves
Wear when touching **blood, body fluids, secretions, excretions,** and **contaminated items.** Put on **clean** gloves just **before touching mucous membranes** and **nonintact skin.** Change gloves between tasks and procedures on the same patient after contact with material that may contain high concentrations of microorganisms. Remove gloves promptly after use, before touching noncontaminated items and environmental surfaces, and before going to another patient, and was hands immediately to avoid transfer of microorganisms to other patients or environments.

Wear Mask and Eye Protection or Face Shield
Protect mucous membranes of the eyes, nose and mouth during procedures and patient-care activities that are likely to generate **splashes** or **sprays** of **blood, body fluids, secretions,** or **excretions.**

Wear Gown
Protect skin and prevent soiling of clothing during procedures that are likely to generate **splashes** or **sprays** of **blood, body fluids, secretions,** or **secretions.** Remove a soiled gown as promptly as possible and wash hands to avoid transfer of microorganisms to other patients or environments.

Patient-Care Equipment
Handle used patient-care equipment soiled with **blood, body fluids, secretions,** or **excretions** in a manner that prevents skin and mucous membrane exposures, contamination of clothing, and transfer of microorganisms to other patients and environments. Ensure that reusable equipment is not used for the care of another patient until it has been appropriately cleaned and reprocessed and single use items are properly discarded.

Environmental Control
Follow hospital procedures for routine care, cleaning, and disinfection of environmental surfaces, beds, bedrails, bedside equipment and other frequently touched surfaces.

Linen
Handle, transport, and process used linen soiled with **blood, body fluids, secretions,** or **excretions** in a manner that prevents exposures and contamination of clothing, and avoids transfer of microorganisms to other patients and environments.

Occupational Health and Bloodborne Pathogens
Prevent injuries when using needles, scalpels, and other sharp instruments or devices; when handling sharp instruments after procedures; when cleaning used instruments; and when disposing of used needles.

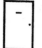

Never recap used needles using both hands or any other technique that involves directing the point of a needle toward any part of the body; rather, use either a one-handed "scoop" technique or a mechanical device designed for holding the needle sheath.

Do not remove used needles from disposable syringes by hand, and do not bend, break, or otherwise manipulate used needles by hand. Place used disposable syringes and needles, scalpel blades, and other sharp items in puncture-resistant sharps containers located as close as practical to the area in which the items were used, and place reusable syringes and needles in a puncture-resistant container for transport to the reprocessing area.

Use **resuscitation devices** as an alternative to mouth-to-mouth resuscitation.

Patient Placement
Use a **private room** for a patient who contaminates the environment or who does not (or cannot be expected to) assist in maintaining appropriate hygiene or environmental control. Consult Infection Control if a private room is not available.

This information on this sign is abbreviated from the HICPAC Recommendations for Isolation Precautions in Hospitals.

Figure 4–4   *Standard Precautions. (Courtesy of BREVIS Corporation)*

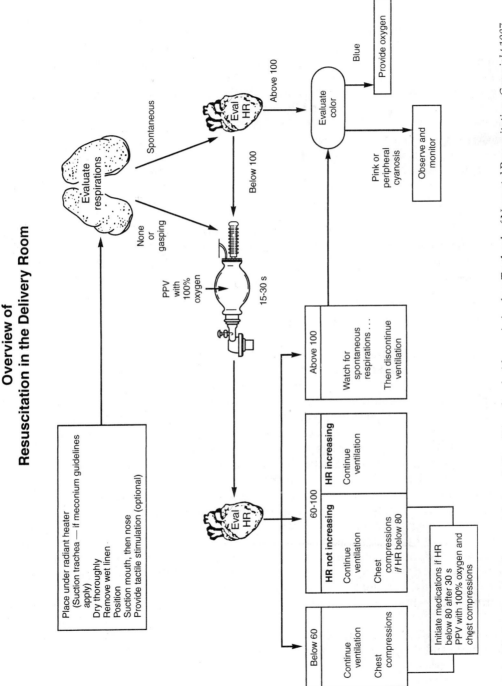

Overview of Resuscitation in the Delivery Room

Place under radiant heater
(Suction trachea — if meconium guidelines apply)
Dry thoroughly
Remove wet linen
Position
Suction mouth, then nose
Provide tactile stimulation (optional)

Evaluate respirations

Spontaneous → Eval HR

None or gasping → PPV with 100% oxygen, 15-30 s

Eval HR — Above 100 → Evaluate color

Below 100

Evaluate color — Blue → Provide oxygen

Pink or peripheral cyanosis → Observe and monitor

Eval HR

Above 100: Watch for spontaneous respirations.... Then discontinue ventilation

60-100:
HR not increasing — Continue ventilation; Chest compressions *if* HR below 80
HR increasing — Continue ventilation

Below 60: Continue ventilation; Chest compressions

Initiate medications if HR below 80 after 30 s
PPV with 100% oxygen and chest compressions

Figure 4–5 *Overview of a neonatal resuscitation. (Reproduced with permission from* Textbook of Neonatal Resuscitation. *Copyright 1987, 1990, 1994, American Heart Association.)*

The first step in resuscitating a neonate is to provide some degree of thermoregulation. The importance of this cannot be overstated. A cold neonate will not respond to resuscitative efforts as well as one whose temperature is maintained. Even though it is impractical to attempt total thermoregulation, the neonate must be protected from the most probable causes of heat loss following delivery.

Radiant heat loss is minimized by immediately placing the patient under a radiant warmer. *Conductive* loss is minimized by placing the neonate on warmed blankets, towels, or heated mattresses. Because the neonate is wet when born, it is at a high risk of *evaporative* heat loss. This is minimized by thoroughly drying the patient with a warmed towel as quickly as possible. *Convective* heat loss is a strong possibility due to the nature of the open warmer and the necessity of keeping the neonate uncovered and accessible. Convective losses can be minimized, however, by the prevention of cold drafts over the bed and keeping movement to a minimum. Once the neonate is dried, the wet towel must be removed and placed in an appropriate receptacle.

As discussed in Chapter 7, low birth weight, preterm infants are at a higher risk of heat loss. For these very small preterm infants it may be necessary to raise the temperature of the resuscitation room before delivery. Covering the patient's trunk and legs with a clear plastic sheet has also been suggested as a possibility.

MAINTENANCE OF THE AIRWAY

The next step in the resuscitation is to open the airway. This is done by positioning the neonate on its back or side in a slight *Trendelenburg* position with the neck slightly extended. Hyperextension or hypoextension of the head may result in occlusion of the airway and should be avoided. Elevating the shoulders ¾ to 1 inch with a rolled blanket or towel, as shown in Figure 4–6, helps in maintaining proper extension.

Once the proper position is achieved, the mouth is suctioned followed by suctioning of the nose. Suctioning the mouth first removes debris that could be aspirated if the patient gasps during nasal suctioning. Suctioning should be gentle and limited because stimulation of the vagal nerve in the oropharynx may induce a severe bradycardia.

If meconium is present in the amniotic fluid, further measures may be needed. Thin watery discolored amniotic fluid requires no further measures; however, the presence of thick particulate meconium in the amniotic fluid requires further attention at this time.

Upon delivery of the fetal head before the thorax is delivered, the mouth, oropharynx and laryngopharynx should be thoroughly suctioned to remove any meconium that is present. Upon delivery of the distressed neonate, the trachea is immediately intubated, suction applied to the end of the endotracheal tube, and the tube is withdrawn (Figure 4–7). Suction pressure should be set at 100 mm Hg and suction applied no more than 3 to 5 seconds.

If meconium is suctioned out of the trachea, the patient is reintubated with a new endotracheal tube and the procedure repeated until no meconium is suctioned. Blowby oxygen can be delivered to the patient to help alleviate hypoxia with PPV commencing after completion of suctioning.

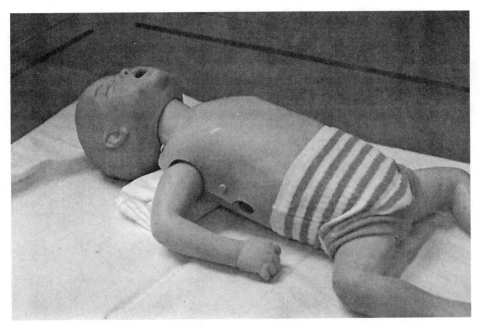

Figure 4–6 *Elevation of the shoulders to extend and open the airway.*

A significant dilemma may occur with an infant who has aspirated meconium, who is also severely depressed. The dilemma is as follows: Which is greater? 1) The risk of blowing meconium further into the lungs by providing PPV before the trachea is clear; or 2) the risk of asphyxia by not providing PPV until the trachea is clear. While the answer to this is not clear, the *Textbook of Neonatal Resuscitation* states the following: "If the baby is severely depressed, positive-pressure ventilation (PPV) may be needed even if some meconium remains in the airway."[1] Also, "In an infant with severe asphyxia, clinical judgment should be used to determine the number of reintubations. It may not be possible to clear the trachea of all meconium before initiating PPV."[1] In all cases, it is recommenced that each hospital in which resuscitation is performed establish a protocol to cover this potential problem.

EVALUATION

Respiratory Effort.   Referring to the algorithm, following the initial steps of warming, positioning, and suctioning, the patient's respiratory effort is evaluated. If the patient has gasping respirations, or is apneic, PPV may be initiated, or a very brief period of tactile stimulation may be attempted. This is done by slapping or flicking the soles of the feet and/or rubbing the patient's back. Once or twice is all that should be needed to improve the rate and depth of respirations. Blowby oxygen should be provided during the tactile stimulation. If respirations do not improve immediately, begin PPV. *Never* continue tactile

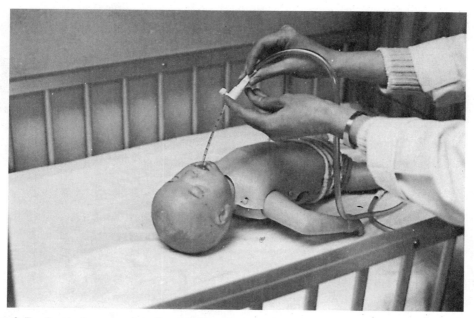

Figure 4–7 *Suctioning meconium through the endotracheal tube.*

stimulation if the patient continues gasping or is apneic. Once PPV has been initiated, or if the respiratory effort is normal, heart rate is evaluated next.

Heart Rate. The evaluation of heart rate is based on the simple determination of whether it is above or below 100 beats per minute. If below 100 bpm, PPV is initiated. If above 100 bpm, the patient's color is evaluated.

Color. The evaluation of patient color consists of determining whether the skin is blue or pink. On patients with dark complexions, color assessment may need to be done on the mucous membranes. The patient who is pink, with or without *acrocyanosis*, which is blueness of the extremities, is simply monitored and the resuscitation ends. The patient who is blue is given supplemental oxygen and gradually weaned as the body becomes pink.

Supplemental oxygen can be given via blowby through an oxygen tube or an oxygen mask. An oxygen tube, running at 5 L/min of oxygen, is initially held 1/2 inch from the nose and mouth and achieves an FiO_2 of approximately 0.8. As the skin becomes pinker, the tubing is pulled back to 1 inch from the nose and mouth and achieves approximately 0.6 FiO_2. If the patient remains pink, the tube is withdrawn to 2 inches, which is approximately 0.4 FiO_2.

From that point, the oxygen is weaned to room air and the neonate is watched for returning cyanosis. An oxygen mask with 5 L/min of oxygen flow, held firmly against the face, supplies approximately 0.6 to 0.8 FiO_2. Held loosely to the face, it provides an FiO_2 of approximately 0.4. The same procedure for weaning as with oxygen tubing is followed.

5 L 1/2" from nose = 80%.
  1 "   60%
  2 °   40%.

POSITIVE-PRESSURE VENTILATION (PPV)

Returning to the resuscitation algorithm, if PPV is indicated it must be started quickly and efficiently. PPV is indicated when the patient is apneic, gasping, or when spontaneous breathing cannot maintain the heart rate above 100 bpm.

Ventilation must always be done with an FiO_2 of 0.9 to 1.0. This is accomplished with either a flow inflating bag or a self-inflating bag. When using a self-inflating bag, a reservoir must be attached to achieve the appropriate FiO_2. Ideally, a pressure gauge is attached to the bag so inspiratory pressures can be monitored.

The mask used to cover the mouth and nose should fit the patient comfortably, as shown in Figure 4–8, without extending over the eyes or the chin. A mask that is too big or too small will make it difficult to maintain an adequate seal. Of interest to note, Paterson and associates found that the use of a laryngeal mask airway provided an effective alternative to the traditional bag-mask ventilation done during resuscitation, and may be a more easily learned skill.[2]

Before beginning PPV, the bag should be checked for proper function. This is done by turning on a flow of gas to the bag, 5 to 8 L/min, and occluding the patient connection opening. When using a flow inflating bag, the bag should inflate at this point. If it does not, there is either a leak in the bag or the flow tube is disconnected from the bag. Squeezing the bag should allow the generation of 30 to 40 cm H_2O or should open the pop-off valve if a self-inflating bag is being used.

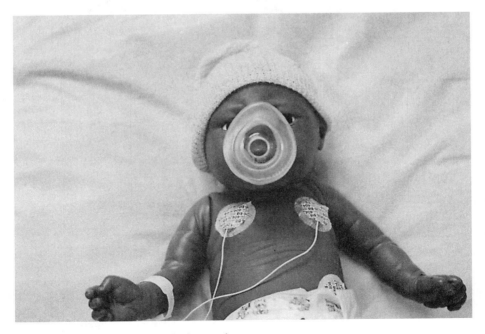

Figure 4–8 *A properly fitting resuscitation mask.*

The patient is now prepared by slightly extending the neck, being careful to avoid hyper-extension, which may close off the trachea. The mask is positioned on the patient's face and held in place by the fingers and thumb (Figure 4–9). The bag is squeezed with the finger-tips until chest expansion is observed, which may require 30 to 40 cm H_2O if it is the initial breath. Succeeding breaths will usually require 15 to 20 cm H_2O to maintain adequate chest expansion. Neonates suffering from RDS may require pressures as high as 40 cm H_2O to open the lungs. The initial rate of ventilation should be 40 to 60 breaths per minute (BPM). Ventilation is done for 15 to 30 seconds.

If PPV continues for more than 2 minutes, an orogastric tube should be inserted to alleviate gastric distension. An oral airway may also be used to maintain a patient airway when the tongue or other pharyngeal tissues are blocking the upper airway.

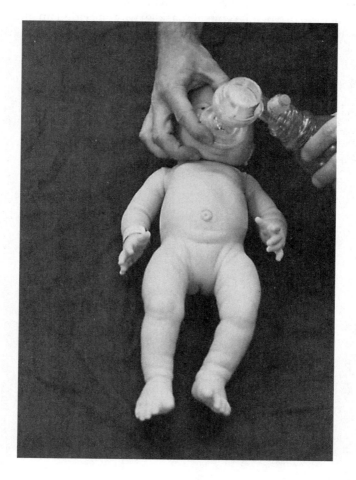

Figure 4–9 *Method of securing a resuscitation mask to the face of a neonate.*

EVALUATION OF HEART RATE (HR)

HR is evaluated after 15 to 30 seconds of ventilation, and can be determined by listening to heart sounds with a stethoscope or by grasping the umbilical stump and feeling for umbilical artery pulsations. The HR is counted for 6 seconds and multiplied by 10 to estimate the minute rate. PPV is started whenever the HR is less than 100 bpm and is continued for 15 to 30 seconds at which point the HR is reevaluated.

As the HR increases above 100 bpm, the patient is observed for the return of spontaneous respirations. PPV is continued until spontaneous respirations return, at which point it is discontinued. Following discontinuation of the PPV, the patient is stimulated and its condition closely monitored.

If the HR is between 60 and 100 bpm and increasing, following the initial 15 to 30 seconds of PPV, ventilation is continued until HR is above 100 bpm, at which point the above procedure is followed.

PPV is continued on the neonate with an HR of 60 to 100 bpm, which is not increasing. Additionally, chest compressions are started if the HR drops below 80 beats per minute.

Any neonate with an HR less than 60 bpm following 30 seconds of PPV is treated with continued PPV and initiation of chest compressions.

Any time the heart rate is less than 100 bpm and *not* increasing, check to ensure that 100% oxygen is being delivered and that chest excursion and breath sounds are adequate.

CHEST COMPRESSIONS

A persistent HR of less than 80 bpm does not provide adequate cardiac output to meet the needs of the neonate's body; therefore, chest compressions are begun. Properly performed chest compressions allow for increased blood circulation by increasing intrathoracic pressure and by compressing the heart against the spine.

Chest compressions are done by the two-finger method, which involves placing the fingertips over the lower third of the sternum, above the xiphoid process and below the nipple line (Figure 4–10). The two fingers used are the index and middle fingers, or the middle and ring fingers.

The sternum is compressed $1/2$ to $3/4$ inches at a rate of 90 per minute. Proper performance of chest compressions requires that the fingers or thumbs do not come off the thorax between compressions. Correct performance will reduce the chance of internal injuries to the neonate. The proper rate of compressions and ventilations is 3 to 1. In other words, a manual ventilation is provided after every third compression. In order to maintain a compression rate of 90/min, the three compressions and one ventilation must be given in a 2-second time period. This breaks down to 1 compression every .5 second with a 0.5-second pause for the ventilation.

Compressions are continued for 30 seconds at which point compressions and ventilations are stopped for 6 seconds to reevaluate the heart rate. This 6-second evaluation pause is repeated every 30 seconds.

Compressions are discontinued when the HR is above 80 bpm and respirations are again evaluated.

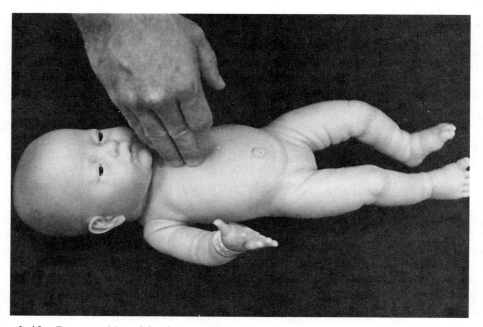

Figure 4–10 *Proper position of the chest when the two-finger method of chest compressions is used.*

INTUBATION

Intubation is indicated during a resuscitation if: 1) the bag and mask ventilation is difficult or ineffective; 2) prolonged PPV is required due to lung disease; and 3) thick meconium is present in the amniotic fluid. Intubation is also performed when a neonate is suspected of having a diaphragmatic hernia, to prevent abdominal distension.

Intubation should only be attempted by someone who is proficient in the procedure. The equipment needed for an intubation are a laryngoscope and blade with a functioning light, several endotracheal tubes of various sizes, a stylet, equipment to suction the airway, adhesive tape or other securing device, a resuscitation bag and mask with a 100% oxygen source, and lastly, an assistant. The purpose of an assistant during intubation is to help by handing equipment to the intubator, monitoring the patient during the attempt, and helping secure the tube. Continuous monitoring of the heart rate and, if possible, oxygen saturation are necessary during the intubation. The intubation should be stopped if severe bradycardia and/or desaturations occur. The patient is ventilated with 100% oxygen until the heart rate and saturations return to normal. Appropriately sized endotracheal tubes are outlined in Table 4–5.

Intubation of a term neonate will require a size 1 blade, and a size 0 blade is needed for premature patients. Straight blades are preferable in neonates and children. This is because the larynx is more superior and the epiglottis more horizontal than in adults.[3]

The endotracheal tube is prepared by placing the stylet just short of the tip of the tube to prevent trauma to the airway. This should be done with the endotracheal tube still in the

TABLE 4–5 Selecting Appropriately Sized Endotracheal Tubes

TUBE SIZE (ID MM)	WEIGHT	GESTATIONAL AGE
2.5	<1000 g	<28 weeks
3.0	1000–2000 g	28–34 weeks
3.5	2000–3000 g	34–38 weeks
4.0	>3000 g	>38 weeks

SOURCE: *Reproduced with permission from* Textbook of Neonatal Resuscitation. *Copyright 1987, 1990, 1994, American Heart Associaltion.*

protective wrapper with only the connecting adapter exposed to maintain sterility. The stylet adds extra rigidity and a fixed curvature to the endotracheal tube, facilitating the intubation.

The neonate is prepared for intubation by placing it in the *supine* position and slightly extending the neck as previously mentioned. The laryngoscope is taken in the left hand and the blade inserted into the right side of the mouth. The tong is swept to the left in a smooth motion using the left side of the blade. The blade is then lifted up and away from the roof of the mouth to visualize the glottic opening, as shown in Figure 4–11. The upper gums are *never* used as a fulcrum to pry the blade upward. At this point, it may be necessary to suction the laryngopharynx free of mucus and secretions. If the epiglottis is not visualized, withdraw the blade until the epiglottis is seen. The tip of the blade is now used to lift the epiglottis away from the glottic opening, allowing insertion of the endotracheal tube. A gentle external pressure on the trachea may help visualize the glottis.

The endotracheal tube is now inserted into the right side of the mouth and guided through the glottic opening and into the larynx. Advancement of the tube should stop when the tip is seen passing the vocal cords.

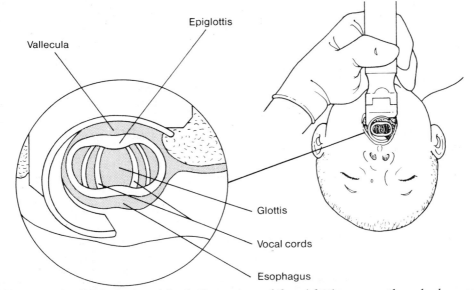

Figure 4–11 *The clinician's view of the glottic opening and the epiglottic area seen through a laryngoscope.*

Following intubation, the patient should be clinically evaluated for proper tube placement. This includes auscultation of the right and left chest, and over the stomach. The patient is also visually monitored for equal bilateral chest excursion when given a mechanical breath. When it is determined that the tube is properly positioned, it is secured with tape or other fastening device. A chest x-ray should be obtained as quickly as possible to verify proper position of the tip of the tube. The ideal placement of the tube will have its tip midway between the carina and the clavicles, as determined on the chest x-ray.

Intubation attempts should be limited to 20 seconds to minimize hypoxia. In addition, spontaneously breathing patients should be provided with blowby oxygen at 5 L/min held near the mouth and nose during the intubation. Between attempts, the patient is manually ventilated with 1.0 FiO_2 to help stabilize the PaO_2. Following verification of tube position on the x-ray, the end of the tube is cut, leaving only 4 cm outside the mouth. This helps reduce dead space and makes it easier to manage the tube.

Complications of intubation are listed in Table 4–6.

TABLE 4–6 Complications of Intubation

A number of complications can result from endotracheal intubation in neonates. An intubation procedure can produce or increase hypoxia, cause trauma to tissues, and introduce infection. However, when one is skilled in the procedure, the incidence of complications is minimized.

Study the following list; note some of the common causes of complications.

COMPLICATION	CAUSES	PREVENTIVE OR CORRECTIVE ACTIONS TO BE CONSIDERED
Hypoxia	Taking too long to intubate	Shorten intubation procedure Bag-mask ventilation with oxygen
	Incorrect placement of tube	Proper repositioning of ET tube
Bradycardia/Apnea	Hypoxia Vagal response due to the laryngoscope blade. ET tube, or suction catheter stimulating the posterior pharynx	Bag-mask, bag-ET tube ventilation with oxygen
Pneumothorax	Overventilation of one lung due to placement of tube in a main bronchus (usually the right)	Proper positioning of ET tube Appropriate ventilating pressures
Contusions or lacerations of tongue, gums, pharynx, epiglottis, trachea, vocal cords, or esophagus	Rough handling of laryngoscope or ET tube	Additional practice/skill
	Laryngoscope blade too long lor short	More appropriately sized equipment
Perforation of trachea or esophagus	Insertion of tube or stylet is too vigorous, or stylet protrudes beyond end of tube	Proper placement and curvature of stylet Gentler handling
Infection	Introduction of organisms via equipment or hands	More careful attention to clean/sterile technique

Source: *Reproduced with permission from* Textbook of Neonatal Resuscitation. *Copyright 1987, 1990, 1994, American Heart Association.*

MEDICATIONS

Several medications are used during a neonatal resuscitation, as shown in Table 4-7. These drugs are used to stimulate the heart, increase tissue perfusion, and restore acid-base balance. All resuscitation medications can be administered through a catheter inserted in the umbilical vein or artery, or a peripheral vein. Some medications can also be instilled directly into the endotracheal tube. Figure 4–12 illustrates the flowchart for the appropriate use of medications during resuscitation.

Indications for the use of medications during a resuscitation are: 1) the HR remains below 80 bpm despite PPV and chest compressions for at least 30 seconds; or 2) the HR is zero.

Epinephrine, or adrenalin, is a powerful sympathomimetic drug that increases heart rate, improves the strength of heart contractions, and causes peripheral vasoconstriction. The net effect is to increase cardiac output and increase blood flow to vital organs. Epinephrine is the first drug given when the above listed indications are met. One ml of a 1:10,000 solution is drawn up and delivered at a dosage of 0.1 to 0.3 ml/kg of body weight. Epinephrine can be delivered intravenously, or through the endotracheal tube. Either way, it should be delivered rapidly. When delivered via the endotracheal tube, the medication may be diluted with 1 to 2 ml of normal saline to aid delivery. Following delivery of the epinephrine, the heart rate should rise to 100 bpm or greater within 30 seconds. If not, epinephrine can be readministered every 3 to 5 minutes at the same dosage.

The use of volume expanders is indicated in those infants showing signs of hypovolemia. Signs include low blood pressure, pallor in the face of adequate oxygenation, heart rate above 100 with weak pulses, and failure to respond to the resuscitation. Volume expanders used in neonatal resuscitation include whole blood, 5% albumin, plasma expanders, normal saline, and Ringer's lactate. The expander is prepared by drawing 40 ml into a syringe or infusion set. The patient is then given 10 ml/kg intravenously over a 5- to 10-minute period. If the signs of hypovolemia persist, the dosage may be repeated.

In the presence of a prolonged arrest that is not responding, the patient should be given sodium bicarbonate. Sodium bicarbonate is a strong alkali that is used to buffer the metabolic acidosis that often accompanies hypoxia. Sodium bicarbonate should only be given when adequate ventilation is present. If ventilation is not adequate, as the bicarbonate combines with the hydrogen ions, their resultant carbon dioxide is not removed and builds up in the blood, worsening the acidosis. Sodium bicarbonate is prepared as either one 20 ml syringe, or two 10 ml syringes of a 4.2% solution. It is given intravenously at a dosage of 2 mEq/kg over at least a 2-minute period. The heart rate should rise to above 100 bpm within 30 seconds of delivery.

With the unfortunate widespread use and abuse of drugs, there is an ever-increasing chance that a neonate may be born under the influence of narcotics. In the presence of severe respiratory depression and a history of maternal narcotic administration within the previous 4 hours, naloxone hydrochloride (Narcan®) is indicated. Narcan® comes in concentrations of 0.4 mg/ml and 1 mg/ml and is given rapidly IV, IM, subcutaneously, or through the ET tube in a dose of 0.1 mg/kg.

TABLE 4–7   Medications for Neonatal Resuscitation

MEDICATION	CONCENTRATION TO ADMINISTER	PREPARATION	DOSAGE ROUTE*	TOTAL DOSE/INFANT			RATE/PRECAUTIONS
Epinephrine	1:10,000	1 ml	0.1–0.3 ml/kg IV or ET	**Weight** 1 kg 2 kg 3 kg 4 kg		**Total ml** 0.1–0.3 ml 0.2–0.6 ml 0.3–0.9 ml 0.4–1.2 ml	Give rapidly May dilute with normal saline to 1–2 ml if giving ET
Volume Expanders	Whole blood 5% Albumin saline Normal saline Ringer's lactate	40 ml	10 ml/kg IV	**Weight** 1 kg 2 kg 3 kg 4 kg		**Total ml** 10 ml 20 ml 30 ml 40 ml	Give over 5–10 minutes
Sodium Bicarbonate	0.5 mEq/ml (4.2% solution)	20 ml or two 10-ml prefilled syringes	2 mEq/kg IV	**Weight** 1 kg 2 kg 3 kg 4 kg	**Total Dose** 2 mEq 4 mEq 6 mEq 8 mEq	**Total ml** 4 ml 8 ml 12 ml 16 ml	Give *slowly*, over at least 2 minutes Give only if infant is being effectively ventilated
Naloxone Hydrochloride	0.4 mg/ml	1 ml	0.1 mg/kg (0.25 ml/kg) IV, ET IM, SQ	**Weight** 1 kg 2 kg 3 kg 4 kg	**Total Dose** 0.1 mg 0.2 mg 0.3 mg 0.4 mg	**Total ml** 0.25 ml 0.50 ml 0.75 ml 1.00 ml	Give rapidly IV, ET preferred IM, SQ acceptable
	1.0 mg/ml	1 ml	0.1 ml/kg (0.1 ml/kg) IV, ET IM, SQ	**Weight** 1 kg 2 kg 3 kg 4 kg	**Total Dose** 0.1 mg 0.2 mg 0.3 mg 0.4 mg	**Total ml** 0.1 ml 0.2 ml 0.3 ml 0.4 ml	
Dopamine	Weight Desired dose 6 x (kg) x (µg/kg/min) Desired fluid (ml/h)	mg of dopamine = per 100 m l of solution	Begin at 5 µg/kg/min (may increase to 20 µg/kg/min if necessary) IV	**Weight** 1 kg 2 kg 3 kg 4 kg		**Total µg/min** 5–20 mg/min 10–40 mg/min 15–60 mg/min 20–80 mg/min	Give as a continous infusion using an infusion pump Monitor heart rate and blood pressure closely Seek consultation

*IM, intramuscular; ET endotracheal; IV intravenous; SQ subcutaneous.
Source: Reproduced with permission from Textbook of Neonatal Resuscitation. Copyright 1987, 1990, 1994, American Heart Association.

Medications
Epinephrine
Volume Expander
Sodium Bicarbonate

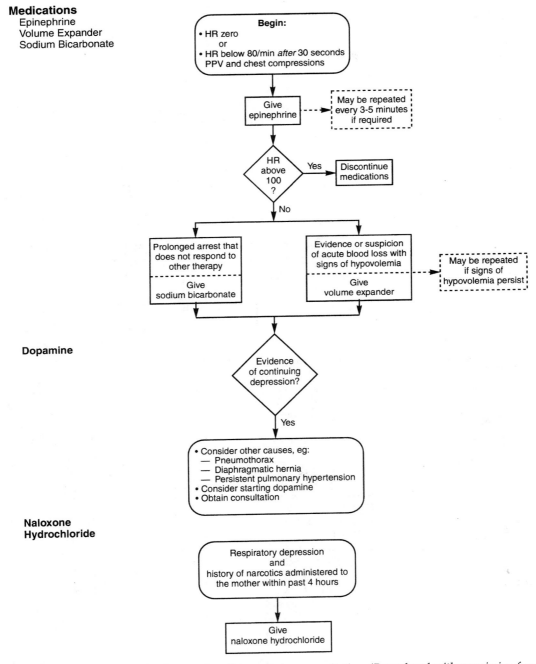

Dopamine

Naloxone Hydrochloride

Figure 4–12 *Flowchart for the use of medicines during resuscitation. (Reproduced with permission from* Textbook of Neonatal Resuscitation. *Copyright 1987, 1990, 1994, American Heart Association.)*

APGAR SCORE

The Apgar score was developed as an objective way to evaluate the condition of a neonate. The Apgar is an excellent method of assessing the effectiveness of a resuscitation, but is not to be used as a basis for making resuscitative decisions.

The five areas examined are respiratory effort, heart rate, muscle tone, reflex irritability, and color (Figure 4–13). Each area is given a score of 0, 1, or 2, depending on the response noted. The first score is assessed at 1 minute after delivery with a second evaluation performed at 5 minutes. Because the Apgar score is an objective assessment of patient status, a 5-minute score that is higher than the 1-minute score indicates the effectiveness of the resuscitation.

Apgars can be assessed every 5 minutes as needed up to 20 minutes, or when the resuscitation ends. Since the first Apgar is not given until 1 minute after birth, it cannot be used as a criterion to initiate resuscitation, but rather as an assessment of how well the neonate is responding to the resuscitation.

The 5-minute Apgar score is predictive of future impairment, with a low score being associated with a high risk of long-term damage.[4] The team can therefore use the Apgar score as an objective measurement of the response of the neonate to the resuscitation.

Apgar Scoring System

	0	1	2	1 Minute	5 Minutes
Heart Rate	None detectable	Slow irregular	Over 100		
Respiratory Effort	Apnea	Irregular shallow, gasping	Yelling, crying		
Muscle Tone	Flaccid	Some flexion of extremities	Well flexed		
Reflex	None—no response to stimulus	Grimace (withdraws)	Crying		
Color	Pale blue (shock)	Blue hands and feet, body pink (Acrocyanois)	Pink all over		

Figure 4–13 *The Apgar score.*

MANAGEMENT OF SERUM GLUCOSE

SOURCES OF FETAL AND NEONATAL GLUCOSE

During intrauterine life, the nutritional needs of the fetus are continuously supplied by the maternal circulation and regulated by the placenta. The fetus prepares for postnatal life by increasing energy stores and developing enzyme-dependent processes for rapid mobilization of stored energy. As carbohydrate stores become depleted postnatally, the neonate must develop the ability to produce hepatic glucose from alternate fuel sources. These sources, known as substrates, include ketones, glycerol, and lactate. This production is slight when compared to the major fuel sources derived from metabolism of glucose.

The rate of glucose uptake by the fetus through the placenta is directly related to the maternal blood glucose level. The glucose concentration in the fetal blood is approximately one third that in the maternal blood. Fetal stores of glycogen are present by the ninth week of gestation, and at term are approximately three times those of a healthy adult. Skeletal muscle glycogen is three to five times that of an adult, and glycogen in cardiac muscle ten times the adult.

Another energy source resides in fetal adipose tissue triglycerides that accumulate in the last trimester. These are known as *brown fat* stores. After glycogen stores are utilized, brown fat is metabolized for fuel. Brown fat is found in the scapulae, neck, axillary regions, mediastinum, and renal tissue. Due to the timing of accumulation of fat stores, neonates born prematurely are at a disadvantage, because they lack the adipose tissue stores that are used during stress.

In the immediate postnatal period the concentration of glucose in the neonate declines to approximately 50 mg/dl by 2 hours of age, but equilibrates at approximately 70 mg/dl by 72 hours after birth. The concentration may be further influenced by disturbances in extrauterine adaptations, such as hypothermia, hypovolemia, and disruptions in acid-base balance.

SERUM VALUES

Hypoglycemia has been defined as being present when whole blood glucose concentrations are less than 35 mg/dl in term neonates and less than 25 mg/dl in preterm neonates.[5] Recent studies, however, suggest that these previously held normals may require a redefinition. Changes in the feeding and care of the neonate, along with data that show higher than normal glucose levels in neonates, indicate the need for a change in the definition of hypoglycemia.

In most cases, concentrations below 45 mg/dl or greater than 125 mg/dl are abnormal after 3 days of age. Thus, any blood glucose level less than 45 mg/dl should be cause for concern and should be investigated more closely.[6]

The difficulty encountered in clinical diagnosis of hypoglycemia is the nonspecific nature of the symptoms. This is further complicated by the occurrence of symptoms at varying blood glucose levels in diverse patients.

CLINICAL SIGNS OF HYPOGLYCEMIA

Clinical signs often associated with neonatal hypoglycemia are listed in Table 4–8.

TABLE 4–8   Clinical Signs of Hypoglycemia

Tremors or jitteriness
Irritability
Exaggerated or decreased moro reflex
Apnea/tachypnea
Cyanosis
Seizures
Lethargy
Hypothermia
High-pitched or weak cry
Poor feeding
Vomiting
Cardiovascular failure and/or collapse

CAUSES OF HYPOGLYCEMIA

Hypoglycemia can result from a wide variation of pathologic conditions. A common cause of hypoglycemia is hyperinsulinism. Several causes of hyperinsulinism will be discussed.

In utero, the fetus of a diabetic mother is subjected to high levels of maternal glucose, which freely crosses the placenta. In response, the fetal pancreas secretes high levels of insulin to counter the high glucose. Following delivery the continued increased production of insulin, coupled with the loss of the maternal glucose, results in neonatal hypoglycemia. Fetuses of diabetic mothers may also have problems with *glucagon* secretion, as well as utilization of substrates such as amino acids, for the production of glucose.

Neonates suffering from *erythroblastosis fetalis,* or Rh incompatibility, demonstrate hyperinsulinism due to pancreatic islet cell hyperplasia. Hyperinsulinism may also be a problem before and during exchange transfusion in these neonates.

Insulin-producing tumors of unknown etiology are another source of hyperinsulinism. Maternal tocolytic therapy with ritodrine or terbutaline, with resultant cessation of premature labor, can additionally lead to hyperinsulinism.

Several other causes of decreased glycogen stores are listed in Table 4–9.

MEASUREMENT OF SERUM GLUCOSE

Serum glucose levels should be routinely evaluated in neonates who demonstrate risk factors for hypoglycemia. High-risk factors include infants of diabetic mothers (IDMs), Rh incompatibility, prematurity, and neonates who are small for their gestational age (SGA).

TABLE 4–9   Causes of Decreased Glycogen Stores

Prematurity
Intrauterine growth retardation (IUGR)
Starvation
Sepsis
Shock
Asphyxia
Hypothermia
Glycogen storage disease
Galactosemia
Adrenal insufficiency
Polycythemia
Congenital cardiac malformations
Iatrogenic causes (i.e., large volume and/or concentrations of glucose intravenously)

Often overlooked in the interpretation of glucose concentration are the type of sample and the method of analysis. Whole blood has a lower glucose concentration than plasma owing to the presence of red blood cells. Plasma glucose levels are therefore higher than those of whole blood by approximately 10 to 14%. Glucose levels of whole blood also vary as hematocrit values vary.

Rapid assessment of whole blood glucose can be accomplished through one of several methods. Glucose test strip methods are the most common source of assessment. Due to various problems that surround the use of test strip measurements, their use is becoming less common. Many institutions are replacing the test strips with a more accurate glucose analyzer such as those developed for home use by diabetics. Borderline blood glucose values should always be confirmed by laboratory analysis. It is important to note that blood glucose levels obtained from an umbilical artery catheter may not accurately reflect the patient's actual blood glucose. This may be secondary to contamination by dextrose containing solutions being infused through the line.[7]

TREATMENT OF HYPOGLYCEMIA

Treatment should be instituted as soon as a neonate at risk for hypoglycemia is identified. Prophylactic care includes early oral or enteral feedings, if indicated, or parenteral administration of glucose. A glucose infusion of 10% dextrose and water intravenously will provide adequate glucose for most neonates.

Treatment is started with a 200 mg/kg bolus of $D_{10}W$ given over 1 to 3 minutes. This is followed by a continuous IV infusion of 4 to 8 mg/kg/min.[5] These requirements are increased as fluid and glucose requirements change over the first few days of life. Intravenous glucose should continue until enteral feelings can be instituted.

For acute symptomatic hypoglycemia, generally 1 to 2 ml/kg of $D_{10}W$, pushed through the IV, will render the neonate normoglycemic within 1 to 2 minutes. All neonates should be monitored at least hourly until stable.

Correction of acid-base disturbances, sepsis, maintenance of normal vital signs, and attention to thermoregulation should be instituted immediately to decrease physiologic stresses and energy requirements.

OBTAINING UMBILICAL VESSEL BLOOD SAMPLES DURING RESUSCITATION

ARTERIAL SAMPLING THROUGH THE UMBILICAL STUMP

The umbilical vessels may be visualized through the Wharton's jelly of the umbilical cord. The umbilical vein is a single vessel of relatively large diameter that often appears filled with blood. The umbilical arteries are a pair of vessels of smaller diameter that usually are more opaque and whitish in appearance and appear to contain little blood.

After delivery, the umbilical arteries gradually spasm and close. Immediately after birth, however, they may be entered and an arterial sample obtained. This may be helpful in determining the neonate's status and the need for prolonged arterial access.

The cord stump should first be checked to ensure that the umbilical arteries are still pulsatile. To perform the procedure, the surface of the cord is cleaned with Betadine® and then alcohol. The umbilical cord stump is punctured with either a scalp vein needle or other small-gauged needle attached to a syringe. The needle is directed toward one of the arteries in the direction of the umbilicus, as shown in Figure 4–14.

Upon entering the artery, connect a blood gas syringe and withdraw an appropriate amount for a blood gas sample. Remove the needle from the umbilicus and tamponade the artery proximal to the site of entry.

Although blood gas samples are obtained from the umbilical arteries, the umbilical vein may also be punctured and a sample obtained. The umbilical vein carries blood returning from the fetus to the placenta and therefore reflects fetal intrapartum metabolic status.

PLACEMENT OF AN UMBILICAL ARTERY CATHETER (UAC)

Indications. An umbilical arterial catheter is indicated for use in a seriously ill neonate who may require frequent blood gas sampling, continuous arterial blood pressure monitoring, or less commonly, as a reliable route for parenteral infusions.

Procedure for Placement. The usual site for insertion of a UAC is near the umbilicus. A 5 Fr. catheter is used for neonates weighing more than 1250 g, and a 3.5 Fr. is used on neonates of less than 1250 g.

The patient is placed in a supine position and the arms and legs are restrained. Adequate control of thermoregulation, oxygenation, and ventilation must be maintained throughout the procedure.

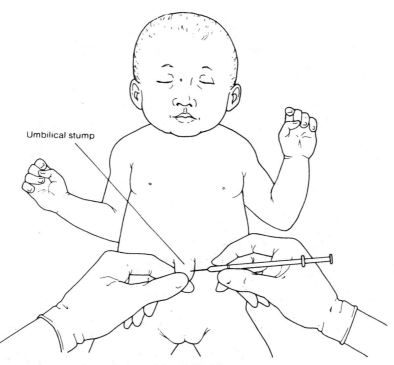

Umbilical stump

Figure 4–14 *Obtaining a blood sample from the umbilical stump.*

Sterile gloves and a gown are put on following a thorough hand washing. The catheterization tray is then opened in a sterile manner.

The cord is prepared by cleaning with povidone-iodine and then alcohol. Any excess povidone should be cleaned up to avoid skin burns in neonates of less than 1000 g. The neonate is then draped in a sterile manner, with the umbilicus showing through the drape.

Umbilical tape is next tied around the base of the cord and is used for the control of bleeding. The umbilical word is then cut 1 to 2 cm above the base. An umbilical artery is then isolated and dilated. Forceps are inserted into the artery and allowed to open, stretching the arterial wall until a catheter can be inserted.

A catheter, filled with sterile heparin flush solution, is introduced into the artery and advanced with slow, steady gentle pressure. A pulsatile blood return indicates that an umbilical artery has been cannulized. The catheter is then advanced until it is in the desired distance and an abdominal x-ray film obtained to confirm placement. Optimal placement for a low catheter is between L3–4 and at the level of T8 for a high catheter.

Complications. Thrombus formation on the catheter tip is the most common complication and may lead to a decreased circulation to one of the legs. Additional thromboembolic complications include hypertension and *necrotizing enterocolitis.*

Perforation of the vessel wall is a direct complication of the procedure. Hemorrhage from inadvertent removal of the catheter or infusion system leaks or disconnects may also occur. Vasospasm of the arterial supply to a toe, foot, or leg is often predisposed by the presence of the UAC. If wrapping the opposite leg with a warm moist diaper does not quickly relieve the vasospasm, the catheter should be removed.

SUMMARY

It is estimated that 80% of all babies born who weigh less than 1500 g will require resuscitation. Properly performed, resuscitation can make the difference between a healthy infant and a lifetime of neurologic and other problems. This chapter serves only as an overview of the steps involved in a resuscitation and should not be used as a substitute for participation in an organized neonatal resuscitation program.

Typically, the newborn who requires resuscitation has undergone a certain degree of asphyxia in utero, which leads to primary and then secondary apnea. Any infant born apneic must be assumed to be in secondary apnea and resuscitative efforts started immediately. The sooner efforts are started, the less chance of long-time sequelae from the asphyxia. The effects of asphyxia are many and include pulmonary hypertension, persistent fetal circulation, and acidosis.

A successful resuscitation begins with anticipation of the depressed neonate. This requires a knowledge of the maternal history, and a history of the labor and delivery. Also required is the ready availability of proper, functioning equipment and the presence of personnel trained in its use.

In its most basic form, neonatal resuscitation follows the time-honored ABCs: Airway, Breathing, and Circulation. Additional steps are added to meet the special needs of the newborn. Neonatal resuscitation follows a cycle in which the newborn is first evaluated regarding respirations, heart rate, and color. A decision is then made based on the evaluation, which leads to an action.

Before evaluation is performed, several steps are undertaken. These include thermoregulation, suctioning the trachea if thick meconium is present, positioning the patient to open the airway, suctioning the mouth then nose, and providing tactile stimulus if needed. The patient's respirations, heart rate, and color are then evaluated and the appropriate actions are taken as outlined on the resuscitation algorithm. The Apgar score is an excellent tool used to evaluate the overall condition of the neonate. It can also be used to assess the effectiveness of the resuscitation.

Once born, the neonate now has the responsibility to provide and maintain its own energy source—glucose. Initially, energy is derived from available glucose, stored glycogen, brown fat, and the production of glucose from ketones, glycerol, and lactate. These energy stores may be depleted more rapidly if the patient is thermally stressed, and if the work of breathing is high owing to lung disease. Ideally, the blood glucose should be kept above 35 mg/dl to prevent problems associated with hypoglycemia.

Finally, obtaining blood from the newborn is often essential during a resuscitation. In addition, the infusion of medications into the circulatory system is commonly necessary.

Blood can be drawn immediately from an umbilical artery if done before the cord vessels ligate. An umbilical artery catheter provides not only access to the arterial system for obtaining blood samples, but also for the infusion of medications.

References

1. Bloom RS, Cropley C. *Textbook of Neonatal Resuscitation.* Evanston, Ill: American Heart Association/American Academy of Pediatrics; 1994.

2. Paterson SJ, et al. Neonatal resuscitation using the laryngeal mask airway. *Anesthesiology.* 1994;80:1248–1253.

3. Finucane BT, Santora AH. *Principles of Airway Management.* Philadelphia: FA Davis Co; 1988.

4. Cloherty JP, Stark AR, eds. *Manual of Neonatal Care.* 4th ed. Philadelphia: Lippincott; 1997.

5. Merenstein GB, Gardner SL. *Handbook of Neonatal Intensive Care.* 4th ed. St. Louis: CV Mosby Co; 1998.

6. Halarnek LP, Stephenson T. Neonatal hypoglycemia, part II: pathophysiology and therapy. *Clin Pediatr.* 1998;37:11–16.

7. Butler LA, et al. Neonatal glucose determinations obtained from an umbilical artery catheter: evaluation for accuracy using an in vitro model. *Neonatal Network.* 193;12:31–35.

Bibliography and Suggested Readings

Avery GB, Fletcher MA, MacDonald MG. *Pathophysiology and Management of the Newborn.* 5th ed. Philadelphia: JB Lippincott Co; 1999.

Dantzker DR, MacIntyre NR, Bakow ED. *Comprehensive Respiratory Care.* Philadelphia: WB Saunders; 1995.

Fanaroff A, Martin R. *Neonatal Perinatal Medicine: Diseases of the Fetus and Infant.* 6th ed. St. Louis: CV Mosby Co; 1996.

Goldsmith JP, Karotkin EH. *Assisted Ventilation of the Neonate.* 3rd ed. Philadelphia: WB Saunders; 1996.

Pilbeam SP. *Mechanical Ventilation: Physiological and Clinical Applications.* 3rd ed. St. Louis: Mosby; 1998.

Taussig LM, Landau LI. *Pediatric Respiratory Medicine,* St. Louis: Mosby; 1999.

Tucker SM. *Pocket Guide to Fetal Monitoring and Assessment.* 4th ed. St. Louis: Mosby; 2000.

Posttest

1. Of the following, which does *not* cause fetal asphyxia?
    a. infection
    b. maternal asphyxia

    c. placental insufficiency

    d. occlusion of the umbilical cord

2. Which of the following is true of secondary apnea?

    a. the infant begins gasping

    b. heart rate and blood pressure rise

    c. the infant will not attempt to breathe

    d. stimulation will usually initiate breathing

3. The persistence of fetal circulation in the presence of asphyxia is secondary to:

    a. decreased cardiac output

    b. increased fluid volume

    c. arterial hypertension

    d. pulmonary hypertension

4. Equipment used for resuscitations should be checked at least:

    a. once a week

    b. every shift

    c. once a day

    d. just before use

5. During a resuscitation, which of the following are *first* evaluated?

    I. temperature

    II. patient color

    III. heart rate

    IV. respirations

    V. patient weight

      a. I, II, III

      b. II, III, IV, V

      c. II, III, IV

      d. I, II, III, IV, V

6. Assign an Apgar score to the following Caucasian infant: 2150 grams, blue dusky color all over, flaccid, HR 90, weak gasping breaths, and a weak grimace when orally suctioned.

    a. 9

    b. 6

    c. 3

    d. 1

7. Following the positioning, suctioning, stimulation, and drying of a neonate, what is the next step in a resuscitation?

    a. assess respirations

    b. assess heart rate

    c. assess color

    d. assess breath sounds

8. Which of the following would best minimize conductive heat loss in a neonate?

    a. place patient under a radiant warmer

    b. place patient on a warmed mattress

    c. dry the patient immediately

    d. blow warm air over the patient

9. Oxygen running through tubing at 5 L/min, held 2 inches from the neonate's mouth and nose, achieves what approximate FiO_2?
    a. 0.32
    b. 0.35
    c. 0.38
    d. 0.40

10. During a resuscitation, positive-pressure ventilation is indicated when:
    I. breathing effort is absent
    II. PaO_2 is less than 60 mmHg
    III. $PaCO_2$ is greater than 50 mmHg
    IV. spontaneously breathing patient's heart rate is below 100 bpm
    V. patient is blue all over
        a. I, II
        b. I, II, IV
        c. I, IV
        d. I, III, V

11. Chest compressions are started when:
    a. the heart rate is below 100 bpm
    b. the heart rate is below 80 bpm
    c. spontaneous respirations are not present
    d. cardiac arrhythmias are present

12. Which of the following factors indicate the need to intubate?
    I. prolonged positive pressure ventilation is required
    II. bag and mask ventilation is ineffective
    III. thick meconium is present
    IV. chest excursion is poor
    V. breath sounds are absent
        a. I, III, V
        b. II, III, IV
        c. I, II, III
        d. I, II, IV

13. The correct concentration and dosage of epinephrine during a resuscitation is:
    a. 1:20,000 concentration given 0.1 to 0.3 ml/kg
    b. 1:10,000 concentration given 0.3 to 0.5 ml/kg
    c. 1:10,000 concentration given 0.1 to 0.3 ml/kg
    d. 1:20,000 concentration given 0.3 to 0.5 ml/kg

14. Which of the following are complications of umbilical artery catheters?
    I. thrombus formation
    II. perforation of the vessel wall
    III. hemorrhage
    IV. pneumothorax
    V. vasospasm
        a. II, III, IV
        b. I, II, III, V
        c. II, IV, V
        d. I, II, IV, V

15. Glucose concentration in the fetus is approximately what percent of the maternal concentration?
    a. 33%
    b. 50%
    c. 75%
    d. 90%

16. A serum glucose level in premature neonates below what level indicates hypoglycemia?
    a. 100 g/dl
    b. 80 mg/dl
    c. 35 mg/dl
    d. 20 mg/dl

17. Maternal tocolytic therapy with terbutaline may lead to:
    a. decrease of maternal glucose
    b. increased fetal glucose
    c. hyperinsulinemia
    d. hypoinsulinemia

CHAPTER FIVE

ASSESSMENT OF THE NEONATAL AND PEDIATRIC PATIENT

OBJECTIVES

Upon completion of this chapter, the reader should be able to:

1. State at least 10 anatomic and physiologic differences between the infant and adult.
2. Given a patient's obstetrical history (PARA), identify the following: previous pregnancies; miscarriages; premature births; and living children.
3. Identify the physical and neurologic signs examined in the Dubowitz and the Ballard gestational age assessments.
4. Compare and contrast the Dubowitz and Ballard gestational age assessments.
5. Describe seven physical signs that are used to determine gestational age. Relate findings of each to varying gestational ages.
6. List five purposes of the neonatal physical examination.
7. Describe each of the following as it pertains to the physical examination. Include a description of the unique aspects of each examination.
   a. Quiet examination
   b. Hands-on examination
   c. Neurologic examination
8. Identify and state the 12 questions that should be evaluated during the history-taking portion of the pediatric examination.
9. List the three goals to be achieved when examining the pediatric pulmonary system. Include a description of how each goal is assessed.
10. List the four indications for performing pulmonary function tests on neonates and pediatric patients.
11. Describe the two methods used to measure compliance and resistance, and the two methods used to measure expiratory flows in the neonatal patient.
12. Briefly describe the use of helium dilution, nitrogen washout, and body plethysmography in assessing lung volumes.
13. When shown a volume-pressure loop, determine whether it is normal, or demonstrates abnormal compliance or resistance.
14. Describe the special requirements needed when assessing pulmonary function on the pediatric patient.

KEY TERMS

acrocyanosis	hyperpnea	pleural effusion
alae nasi	hypopnea	pneumotachograph
anencephaly	lanugo	purulent
caput succedaneum	methacholine	rugae
Doppler	murmur	scaphoid
fontanelle	paradoxical	thoracic gas volume
hydrocephaly	pinna	vernix

ANATOMIC AND PHYSIOLOGIC CONSIDERATIONS

Before a successful physical assessment can be performed on a neonate or pediatric patient, the practitioner must have an understanding of the anatomic and physiologic differences between adults, infants, and children.

There is tremendous variation in the anatomic and physiologic differences between the various age groups. In general, those differences are greatest during the neonatal period and become less apparent with increasing age.

CARDIOPULMONARY SYSTEM

We will begin by contrasting the differences between the cardiopulmonary systems of adults and infants.

Beginning with the upper airways, the infant tongue is proportionally larger than the adult tongue. Infants also have a large amount of lymphoid tissue in the area of the pharynx when compared to the adult. These two factors greatly increase the risk of upper airway occlusion in infants.

The epiglottis of the infant is proportionally larger, less flexible, and omega-shaped (Ω), which makes it very susceptible to trauma. The infant epiglottis also lies more horizontally than the adult.

The infant larynx lies higher in the neck in relation to the cervical spine. Additionally, the narrowest segment of the larynx is at the level of the cricoid ring. In contrast, the narrowest portion of the adult larynx is at the glottis.

All of the above factors make upper airway occlusion a greater risk in the infant than in the adult patient. Any swelling or inflammation of these structures greatly increases resistance and the patient's work of breathing.

The diameter of the trachea above the carina is roughly 4 mm at birth compared to 16 mm in the adult. The length of the trachea increases from 57 mm at birth to 120 mm in the adult.

The infant chest offers little stability because the ribs and sternum are mostly cartilage. Adequate ventilation, therefore, requires the use of the diaphragm to determine tidal volume. Any increase in minute ventilation is accomplished by increasing the respiratory rate, not the tidal volume.

Three factors are responsible for the low pulmonary reserve in infants. First, the heart is large in proportion to thoracic diameter. Thus, it imposes on the lungs and reduces the volume of gas that they can inhale. Second, as previously discussed, the thoracic cage offers little stability and makes it difficult for the patient to increase tidal volume by chest expansion. Third, proportionally large abdominal contents push up against the diaphragm, diminishing its ability to function.[1]

An additional difference in th pulmonary systems of adults and infants is the fact that infants are considered to be obligatory nose breathers. A study by Miller and coworkers demonstrated that newborns are not totally dependent on nose breathing, but do in fact mouth breathe for both spontaneous breathing and in response to natal occlusion.[2] However, because newborns breathe nasally under normal circumstances, it is important to understand the implications. Due to the small diameter of the nasal passages, any decrease in the caliber of the airway from secretions or inflammation can dramatically increase resistance to airflow and increase the work of breathing.

METABOLISM

The metabolic rate of neonates and infants is higher than in adults. The caloric requirement for neonates is approximately 100 cal/kg and decreases to 40 to 50 cal/kg in the adult.[3] The result of increased metabolism is that the neonate has a greater oxygen need proportional to body size than the adult.

Infants do not respond to medication therapy in any predictable manner, owing to differences in metabolism. Similar patients may have dramatically different reactions to the same dosage of a drug. Because of this, there are no definitive dosages or frequencies of administration established. Each time a drug is given, the dosage must be adjusted for the individual patient.

OTHER FACTORS

Neonates have a large amount of skin surface area for their body weight. An adult male has a body surface area of about 0.02 m² per kg of body weight. The term neonate has about 0.07 m²/kg, and a 28-week neonate has roughly 0.15 m²/kg.[4] This large surface area makes the neonate very prone to heat loss and resultant cold stress.

Because 80% of the neonate's total body weight is water, and that water is mainly found in the extracellular spaces, fluid balance is precarious. Overhydration and dehydration can be very difficult to avoid in the neonate.

PHYSICAL ASSESSMENT OF THE NEONATE

Following delivery and clamping of the umbilical cord, the neonate must undergo a transition from uterine life to survival outside the uterus. This initial transition is a critical time for the neonate. It is the responsibility of the practitioner to determine how well it is adapting to its new environment.

It is crucial that the practitioner be able to identify the neonate who is not adapting well. This allows the practitioner to react and treat the patient in a timely manner. The purpose of the physical assessment is just that—to determine how well the extrauterine transition is taking place.

Another important aspect of the initial assessment of the neonate is a thorough understanding of the patient's history. Of interest are those pertinent factors, which then focus the practitioner's attention on possible problems.

HISTORY

Before examining the neonatal patient, it is vital to know the important historical facts concerning the pregnancy, labor, and delivery. A basic history should also include the mother's obstetric past. The following offers a brief synopsis of a minimal history.

Obstetric History.   The practitioner should know the pregnancy history (called PARA), which is typically recorded as four numbers representing the total prior term pregnancies, premature deliveries, abortions/miscarriages, and living children. For example, a woman for whom this is the fourth pregnancy, who has had one miscarriage, one premature delivery, and two living children, would be written as PARA 3-1-1-2. The PARA can be simplified by using the mnemonic, *Texas Power And Light*, where the *T* stands for term pregnancies, *P* is for premature deliveries, *A* for abortions/miscarriages, and *L* for living children.

Pregnancy History.   The information obtained in this history is directed toward those risk factors that may have jeopardized the growing fetus. Included are exposure to teratogenic drugs, maternal drug use, and undernutrition.

Labor and Delivery History.   The history of labor can help identify a compromised fetus. It is important to obtain the following information: length of stages I and II; presentation; the use of birth assist devices; fetal heart rate—including any changes.

GESTATIONAL AGE ASSESSMENT

Until the late 1960s, the designation of prematurity, maturity, and postmaturity was based mostly on the birth weight of the neonate. A neonate of less than 2500 g was often labeled as premature. A neonate whose weight fell between 2500 and 3999 g was mature, and any weight above 4000 g was considered postmature.

These designations assumed that all fetuses grow equally in utero. In reality, each fetus grows at its own rate, some reaching 2500 g well before 40 weeks, others never reaching 2500 g even at term.

The importance of determining the neonate's actual gestational age is to allow care that focuses on the special problems of premature gestations. Assessment of gestational age, compared to birth weight, allows the neonate to be classified as growth retarded, growth accelerated, or of normal growth. This classification allows the practitioner to generate a list of potential problems and take early steps to either avoid or treat them.

Dubowitz Gestational Age Assessment. Determination of gestational age was initially a guessing game, determined from the presence or absence of certain neonatal characteristics. In 1970, a group of investigators lead by Dubowitz published several criteria to be used in assessing gestational age. The method they proposed was much more objective and reproducible than previous attempts. Using this method, the neonate's gestational age could be obtained during a routine physical examination. This scoring system is known as the Dubowitz Gestational Age Assessment, seen in Figure 5–1a–c.

The Dubowitz examines 11 physical signs and 10 neurologic signs in the newborn. These researchers found that the physical criteria are more accurate for determining gestational age than the neurologic criteria. However, when both physical and neurologic criteria are evaluated together, the assessment of gestational age is more accurate than when either criteria are evaluated alone.

Each of the areas examined is assigned a point value from 1 to 5, depending on the physical characteristic or the neurologic response of the neonate. The points are added up from each category and the resulting number corresponds to the gestational age. The Dubowitz method is usually accurate to within 2 weeks and has consistent results when used in the first 5 days of life. The Dubowitz scoring system proved to be an important step forward in neonatology. However, the need for a more rapid method became clear.

Ballard Gestational Age Assessment. In 1979, researchers presented a simplified method of assessing gestation.[5] In their studies, they found that several of the criteria used in the Dubowitz assessment were not as good at indicating gestational age as others. Their studies resulted in an examination that scores six neurologic signs and six physical signs. This system is known as the Ballard score, shown in Figure 5–2. Using the Ballard score, gestational age can be assessed from 22 to 44 weeks.

The Ballard score is comparable to the Dubowitz in reliability. The Ballard system is most reliable when the examination is done before 42 hours of life, with the ideal time being between 30 and 42 hours after delivery. With fewer categories to assess, the Ballard system takes less time to perform than the Dubowitz system. There is some question regarding the validity of shortening the Dubowitz system, because if one area is inaccurate, it has a heavier influence on the total score.

PHYSICAL EXAMINATION TO DETERMINE GESTATIONAL AGE

Physical examinations are quick, easy, and fairly reliable for determining gestational age. There will be occasions when it will be necessary to do a quick assessment of gestational age. One such time is during resuscitation.

NEUROLOGICAL CRITERIA

Neurological Sign	Score						Record Score Here
	0	1	2	3	4	5	
Posture							
Square Window							
Ankle Dorsiflexion							
Arm Recoil							
Leg Recoil							
Popliteal Angle							
Heel To Ear							
Scarf Sign							
Head Lag							
Ventral Suspension							

Total Score	Gestational Age (weeks)	Total Score	Gestational Age (weeks)	Total Score	Gestational Age (weeks)
10	27.2	30	32.5	50	37.8
12	27.8	32	33.0	52	38.3
14	28.3	34	33.6	54	38.9
16	28.8	36	34.1	56	39.4
18	29.4	38	34.6	58	39.9
20	29.9	40	35.2	60	40.4
22	30.4	42	35.7	62	41.0
24	30.9	44	36.2	64	41.5
26	31.5	46	36.7	66	42.0
28	32.0	48	37.3	68	42.6

Figure 5–1a *The Dubowitz Gestational Age Assessment.* (Reprinted with permission from Dr. V. Dubowitz.)

EXTERNAL (SUPERFICIAL) CRITERIA

EXTERNAL SIGN	SCORE					RECORD SCORE HERE
	0	1	2	3	4	
EDEMA	Obvious edema of hands and feet; pitting over tibia	No obvious edema of hands and feet; pitting over tibia	No edema			
SKIN TEXTURE	Very thin, gelatinous	Thin and smooth	Smooth, medium thickness. Rash or superficial peeling	Slight thickening. Superficial cracking and peeling, esp. hands, feet	Thick and parchment like; superficial or deep cracking	
SKIN COLOR (infant not crying)	Dark red	Uniformly pink	Pale pink; variable over body	Pale. Only pink over ears, lips, palms, or soles		
SKIN CAPACITY (Trunk)	Numerous veins and venules clearly seen, esp. over abdomen	Veins and tributaries seen	A few large vessels clearly seen over abdomen	A few large vessels seen indistinctly over abdomen	No blood vessels seen	
LANUGO (Over back)	No lanugo	Abundant; long and thick over whole back	Hair thinning, esp. over lower back	Small amount of lanugo and bald areas	At least half of back devoid of lanugo	
PLANTAR CREASES	No skin creases	Faint red marks over anterior half of sole	Definite red marks over more than anterior half; indentations over less than anterior third	Indentations over more than anterior third	Definite deep indentations over more than anterior third	

Figure 5–1b *The Dubowitz Gestational Age Assessment.* (Reprinted with permission from Dr. V. Dubowitz.)

NIPPLE FORMATION	Nipple barely visible; no areola	Nipple well-defined; areola smooth and flat; diameter < 0.75 cm	Areola stippled, edge not raised; diameter < 0.75 cm	
BREAST SIZE	No breast tissue palpable	Breast tissue on one or both side < 0.5 cm diameter	Breast tissue both sides, one or both 0.5-1.0 cm	
EAR FORM	Pinna flat and shapeless, or no incurving of edge	Incurving of part of edge of pinna	Partial incurving of whole of upper pinna	
EAR FIRMNESS	Pinna soft, easily folded, no recoil	Pinna soft, easily folded, slow recoil	Cartilage to edge of pinna, but soft in places, ready recoil	Pinna firm, cartilage to edge, instant recoil
GENITALIA MALE/FEMALE (With hips half-abducted)	Neither testi in *scrotum* Labia majora widely separated, labia minora protruding	At least one testis high in scrotum Labia majora almost cover labia minora	At least one testis fully descended. Labia majora completely cover labia minora.	

Figure 5–1b (continued)

GESTATIONAL AGE ASSESSMENT (Dubowitz)

Lily Dubowitz, M.D., D.C.H. and Victor Dubowitz, B.Sc., M.D., Ph.D., F.R.C.P., D.C.H. Department of Paediatrics and Neonatal Medicine, University of London Royal Postgraduate Medical School, Hammersmith Hospital London W 12 OHS, England

NOTES ON ASSESSMENT TECHNIQUES FOR THE NEUROLOGICAL CRITERIA

POSTURE: Observed with infant quiet and in supine position. Score 0: Arms and legs extended. 1: Beginning of flexion of hips and knees, arms extended. 2: Stronger flexion of legs, arms extended. 3: Arms slightly flexed, legs flexed and abducted. 4: Arms and legs fully flexed and hips abducted.

SQUARE WINDOW: The hand is flexed on the forearm between the thumb and index finger of the examiner. Enough gentle pressure is applied to get as full flexion as possible, and the angle between the hypothenar eminence and the ventral aspect of the forearm is measured and graded according to the diagram. (Care is taken not to rotate the infant's wrist while doing this maneuver.)

ANKLE DORSIFLEXION: The foot is dorsiflexed onto the anterior aspect of the leg, with the examiner's thumb on the sole of the baby's foot and examiner's fingers behind the baby's leg. Enough pressure is applied to get as full flexion as possible, and the angle between the dorsum of the foot and the anterior aspect of the leg is measured.

ARM RECOIL: With the infant in the supine position, the forearms are first flexed for 5 seconds, then fully extended by pulling on the hands, and finally released. The sign is fully positive if the arms return briskly to full flexion (score 2). If the arms return to incomplete flexion or the response is sluggish, it is graded as score 1. If they remain extended or are only followed by random movements, the score is 0.

LEG RECOIL: With the infant supine, the hips and knees are fully flexed for 5 seconds, then extended by traction on the feet and released. A maximal response is one of full flexion of the hips and knees (score 2). A partial flexion scores, and minimal or no movement scores 0.

POPLITEAL ANGLE: With the infant supine and the pelvis flat on the examining couch, the thigh is held in the knee-chest position by the examiner's left index finger and thumb supporting the baby's knee. The leg is then extended by gentle pressure from the examiner's right index finger behind the baby's ankle, and the poplitcal angle is measured.

HEEL-TO-EAR MANEUVER: With the baby supine, draw the baby's foot as near to the head as it will go without forcing it. Observe the distance between the foot and the head as well as the degree of extension at the knee. Grade according to the diagram. Note that the knee is left free and may draw down alongside the abdomen.

SCARF SIGN: With the baby supine, take the infant's hand and try to put it around the opposite shoulder. Assist this maneuver by lifting the elbow across the body. See how far the elbow will go across and grade according to the illustrations. Score 0: Elbow reaches opposite axillary line; 1: Elbow between the midline and opposite axillary line; 2: Elbow reaches midline; 3: Elbow will not reach midline.

HEAD LAG: With the baby lying supine, grasp the hands (or the arms, if a very small infant) and pull the baby slowly toward the sitting position. Observe the position of the head in relation to the trunk and grade accordingly. In a small infant, the head may initially be supported by one hand. Score 0: Complete lag; 1: Partial head control; 2: Able to maintain head in line with body; 3: Brings head anterior to body.

VENTRAL SUSPENSION: The infant is suspended in the prone position with the examiner's hand under the infant's chest (one hand for a small infant, two for a large infant). Observe the degree of extension of the back and the amount of flexion of the arms and legs. Also note the relationship of the head to the trunk. Grade according to the diagrams.

Reprinted by permission of Dr. L.M.S. Dubowitz, Dr. V. Dubowitz and The Journal of Pediatrics.

References: Dubowitz, L.M.S., Dubowitz, V., Goldberg, C. Clinical assessment of gestational age in the newborn infant J Pediatr 77:1 10, 1970.

Dubowitz, L.M.S., Dubowitz, V.: Gestational Age of the Newborn, Reading, Mass.: Addison-Wesley Publishing Co., 1977.

Figure 5–1c *The Dubowitz Gestational Age Assessment.* (Reprinted with permission from Dr. V. Dubowitz.)

NEWBORN MATURITY RATING & CLASSIFICATION

ESTIMATION OF GESTATIONAL AGE BY MATURITY RATING
Symbols: X - 1st Exam   O - 2nd Exam

Side 1

Gestation by Dates _____ wks

Birth Date _____ Hour _____ am/pm

APGAR _____ 1 min _____ 5 min

NEUROMUSCULAR MATURITY

	-1	0	1	2	3	4	5
Posture							
Square Window (wrist)	>90°	90°	60°	45°	30°	0°	
Arm Recoil		180°	140°-180°	110°-140°	90°-110°	<90°	
Popliteal Angle	180°	160°	140°	120°	100°	90°	<90°
Scarf Sign							
Heel to Ear							

MATURITY RATING

score	weeks
-10	20
-5	22
0	24
5	26
10	28
15	30
20	32
25	34
30	36
35	38
40	40
45	42
50	44

PHYSICAL MATURITY

Skin	sticky; friable; transparent	gelatinous; red; translucent	smooth; pink; visible veins	superficial peeling &/or rash; few veins	cracking; pale areas; rare veins	parchment; deep cracking; no vessels	leathery; cracked; wrinkled
Lanugo	none	sparse	abundant	thinning	bald areas	mostly bald	
Plantar Surface	heel-toe 40-50 mm: -1 <40 mm: -2	>50 mm; no crease	faint red marks	anterior transverse crease only	creases ant. 2/3	creases over entire sole	
Breast	imperceptible	barely perceptible	flat areola; no bud	stippled areola; 1-2 mm bud	raised areola; 3-4 mm bud	full areola; 5-10 mm bud	
Eye/Ear	lids fused loosely: -1 tightly: -2	lids open; pinna flat; stays folded	sl. curved pinna; soft; slow recoil	well-curved pinna; soft but ready recoil	formed & firm; instant recoil	thick cartilage; ear stiff	
Genitals male	scrotum flat; smooth	scrotum empty; faint rugae	testes in upper canal; rare rugae	testes descending; few rugae	testes down; good rugae	testes pendulous; deep rugae	
Genitals female	clitoris prominent; labia flat	prominent clitoris; small labia minora	prominent clitoris; enlarging minora	majora & minora equally prominent	majora large; minora small	majora cover clitoris & minora	

Scoring system: Ballard JL, Khoury JC, Wedig K, Wang L, Eilers-Walsman BL, Lipp R. New Ballard Score, expanded to include extremely premature infants. *J Pediatr.* 1991;119:417-423.

SCORING SECTION

	1st Exam=X	2nd Exam=O
Estimating Gest Age by Maturity Rating	_____ Weeks	_____ Weeks
Time of Exam	Date _____ Hour _____ am/pm	Date _____ Hour _____ am/pm
Age at Exam	_____ Hours	_____ Hours
Signature of Examiner	_____ M.D./R.N.	_____ M.D./R.N.

Provided Courtesy of

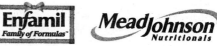

Figure 5–2 *Newborn Maturity Rating & Classification.* (Courtesy Mead Johnson Nutritionals).

A quick and fairly reliable assessment of gestational age can be made by inspecting the physical age signs, without taking the time for the neurologic examination. Using only physical signs, an assessment of gestational age can be determined in less than 1 minute by a skilled practitioner. These signs will be examined individually.

Vernix.   One of the first criteria assessed on examination of a neonate is the presence of *vernix*. Vernix is a white, cream cheese-like material that covers the fetus. It appears around 20 to 24 weeks and remains thick on the fetus until week 36, at which point it begins to disappear. It usually disappears by week 41 to 42.

Skin Maturity.   Next, the practitioner examines the neonate's skin. The appearance of the skin is an excellent indicator of gestational age. At 25 to 26 weeks, the skin is gelatinous and transparent, the blood vessels readily visible. As gestation advances, the skin becomes pink and the vessels become less and less visible. The term neonate has adult-looking skin, with many cracks and wrinkles, and no visible vessels.

Lanugo.   While examining the skin, inspect the neonate for the presence of *lanugo*. Lanugo is th fine, downy hair that covers the fetal body (Figure 5–3). It appears around week 26 and quickly covers the thorax, head, and extremities. By 28 weeks, it begins to thin and then begins to disappear around week 32. The term neonate may have lanugo on the shoulders and forehead. This is more common in neonates with dark complexions. In general, though, the lanugo has disappeared by week 40.

Ear Recoil.   Examination of the *pinna*, or the eternal portion of the ear, is helpful in determining gestational age. The cartilage in the ear is not fully present until around 34 weeks. At 25 to 26 weeks, the pinna is basically flat and will remain folded if doubled over. Cartilage first appears in the pinna around 27 to 28 weeks. At this point it has a slow recoil when folded. As each week of gestation proceeds, the pinna becomes more and more adult looking, with a rapidly increasing recoil. At term the pinna recoils instantly, similar to that of an adult.

Breast Tissue.   The breast tissue is another physical sign used to determine gestational age. At 25 to 26 weeks, the breast is barely perceptible, if at all. At 27 weeks, the breast becomes a red circle, the areola, but there is no palpable tissue behind it. The breast bud forms around week 30 and is about 1 to 2 mm in diameter. The breast bud is a firm tissue that forms behind the areola that is easily felt when palpated between the fingers. The breast continues to develop until term, at which point the bud is 5 to 10 mm in diameter, raised, and the areola is fully developed.

Genitalia.   Examination of the genitalia is very useful in assessing gestational age. At 25 to 26 weeks, the male scrotum is hardly recognizable. It has no *rugae*, and the testicles have not descended. (Rugae are the deep wrinkles in the mature scrotum.) Rugae appear and the testes begin descending around weeks 30 to 32. The scrotum continues its development until, at term, it is covered with deep rugae, and the testes have fully descended. Female genitalia undergoes very apparent changes from 24 weeks to term. At 25 to 26 weeks, the inner portion of the external genitalia, the labia minora and the clitoris, are very pronounced. As gestation advances, the outer portion, the labia majora, becomes equal in prominence. This occurs around weeks 30 to 32. The labia majora continue to grow until, at term, the clitoris and labia minora are completely covered.

Sole Creases.   Moving down to the patient's feet, next examine the creases on the sole of the foot (Figure 5–4). Deep creases of wrinkles appear on the sole of the foot beginning at the anterior end near the toes and proceeding to the heel. The creases appear as faint red lines at roughly 26 weeks. At 30 weeks, the creases have covered the anterior portion of the foot. By 34 weeks, two thirds of the sole is covered with creases. By term, the entire sole is covered by deep creases.

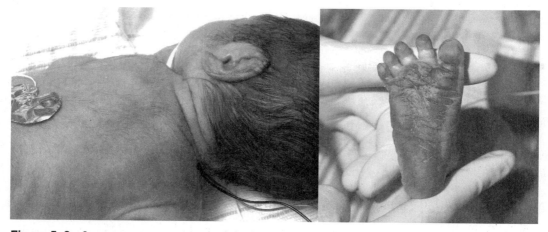

Figure 5–3 *Lanugo on a preterm neonate's back.*   **Figure 5–4** *Creases on the soles of a neonate's feet*

CLASSIFICATION OF THE NEONATE

After the gestational age of the neonate has been determined, and the weight measured, the patient can now be classified by those two factors. At any given gestational age, 80% of all neonates will weigh within a normal range. These are classified as appropriate for gestational age, or AGA. Those whose weight falls below the 10th percentile are classified small for gestational age, or SGA. Conversely, those whose weight is above the 90th percentile are classified as large for gestational age, or LGA. A typical chart used for this classifying method is shown in Figure 5–5.

PHYSICAL EXAMINATION OF THE NEONATE

There are several purposes for the physical examination of the neonate. The exam allows the practitioner to discover physical defects that may be present. These may be congenital

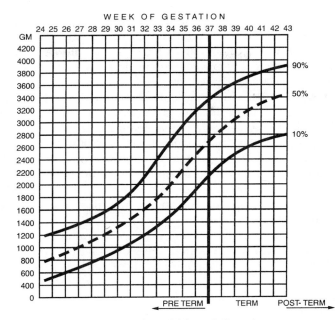

Figure 5–5 *Intrauterine Growth Curve Comparing Weight and Gestation.*

or a result of a difficult labor and delivery. If defects are discovered, the practitioner can then intervene and begin treatment.

The examination also helps to determine whether the neonate has made a successful transition to extrauterine life and the effect of the labor and delivery on the neonate. This not only includes any physical effects, but also the effect of anesthetics or analgesics on the neonate. The gestational age of the neonate is also more thoroughly assessed at this time. By completely examining the neonate, the practitioner can check for signs of infection or metabolic disease. Finally, the physical exam establishes a baseline for future comparisons.

The initial physical examination is usually done after the neonate has been stabilized and is somewhat adapted to its new environment. Of extreme importance is the maintenance of thermoregulation during the physical examination. The examination should be done in an incubator or under an open warmer to reduce heat loss.

The physical exam is usually done in two segments, a quiet observation exam followed by a hands-on exam. The quiet observation exam is necessary to observe the overall condition of the neonate in a nonstressed state, when it is not being handled or otherwise stimulated. It is difficult to assess the overall condition if the baby is upset and crying. Ideally, the patient should be nude to observe all aspects of the body. Avoid the urge to touch the patient during this part of the exam.

Quiet Examination. The first part of the quiet exam is to observe various aspects of the neonate's color. A healthy neonate with a dark complexion may be difficult to assess for oxygenation via skin color. In these neonates, it may be possible to assess the color of the mucous membranes. These membranes should be pink in a well-oxygenated patient. Those neonates with light complexions are more readily assessed for oxygenation because they will have a pinkish hue to the skin. A blue (cyanosis) or pale color of the mucosa or skin may indicate hypoxemia, and treatment with oxygen should be started immediately, followed by further assessment of respiratory status. If the exam is done in the first few hours after birth, it is likely that the body will be pink, but the feet and hands will still be blue. This is known as *acrocyanosis* and is commonly present in the first 24 hours following birth.

A yellowish hue to the skin or the eyes is secondary to jaundice. If jaundice is present, further evaluation will be necessary to determine if the jaundice is pathologic or physiologic. The differentiation of jaundice is covered in Chapter 7.

The presence of green or dark green meconium on the skin may indicate that some degree of asphyxia was present in utero. Meconium staining that was acquired in utero may only be seen if the initial examination is done before the infant is cleaned and dried. Meconium seen on the skin following cleaning and drying may be secondary to normal bowel movements and not a sign of asphyxia.

While examining the skin, assess for the presence and amount of lanugo. This is followed by a determination of skin maturity. Both of these details are an important part of the gestational age assessment, and their results should be noted accordingly.

Now focus attention on the patient's activity. Observe for symmetry of movement, good muscle tone, and normal movements of the extremities. Any asymmetry or abnormal movements may indicate fractures, paralysis, or convulsive states. A lack of good muscle tone may signify a degree of neurologic impairment. The healthy neonate will move extremities symmetrically. Asymmetry of arm or leg movements may mean a fracture or even paralysis. The movements may be jerky, but are usually short in duration.

The arm and legs will be well flexed, showing good muscle tone. The healthy neonate will usually be in the fetal position, with the legs drawn to the abdomen and arms flexed and tight to the body.

Now inspect the overall look of the patient. Start at the head and visually inspect the entire patient, taking note of any malformations or apparent anomalies. A comparison of head size to body size may help diagnose *hydrocephaly* or *anencephaly*. Abnormal bulges or bumps may be cysts or tumors that require further examination. Many congenital defects or chromosomal disorders can readily be identified by simple observation.

The last part of the quiet examination involves the observation of respiration. The respiratory rate is normally between 30 and 60 BPM. Neonates, especially those born prematurely, may have periods of apnea usually lasting 5 to 10 seconds but without cyanosis or bradycardia. This pause in breathing is called periodic breathing and is considered normal. True apnea, on the other hand, lasts longer than 15 to 20 seconds and is accompanied by cyanosis and/or bradycardia. The causes and treatments for apnea are covered in more detail in Chapter 10.

Tachypnea, or a respiratory rate above 60 BPM, could be a sign of respiratory distress and should be investigated further. Because of the relative noncompliance of the thoracic cage, newborns rely mainly on the diaphragm for their respirations. The neonate should be watched for good abdominal movement during quiet breathing. This is a sign of an intact diaphragm. Chest movement should be symmetrical during inspiration and exhalation. There should also be noticeable chest excursion during inhalation, equal on both sides.

The three cardinal signs of respiratory distress are nasal flaring, grunting, and retractions. Nasal flaring is an attempt to get more gas volume into the lungs. It is identified by a widening of the nares during inspiration, returning to normal during expiration.

The term grunting may be misleading, as the actual sound made is more of a high-pitched vocal one than a low-pitched snore. The sound is made by closing the glottis over the trachea, causing an increased lung pressure during exhalation. The positive pressure that is created helps keep the alveoli from collapsing during exhalation. The effects of respiratory distress that lead to grunting are discussed in Chapter 10.

Retractions are the inward movement of the thoracic skin surface during an inhalation. They may be mild, moderate, or severe and are found intercostally (between the ribs), above or below the sternum, or may involve the entire sternum itself. As the lung becomes less complaint with advancing respiratory distress, greater subatmospheric pressures are required in the thorax to overcome the low lung compliance. As the subatmospheric pressures become greater, the external surface of the thorax is drawn inward, creating the characteristic retractions. One good method for evaluating the degree of respiratory distress is by the Silverman-Anderson Index (Figure 5–6).

Hands-on Examination.   The final part of the physical examination is the hands-on portion. The examiner should have warm hands and a warm stethoscope. Any touching should be done gently so as not to upset the patient. A pacifier may be used to help keep the neonate quiet. As with the quiet exam, we will start at the head and work to the extremities.

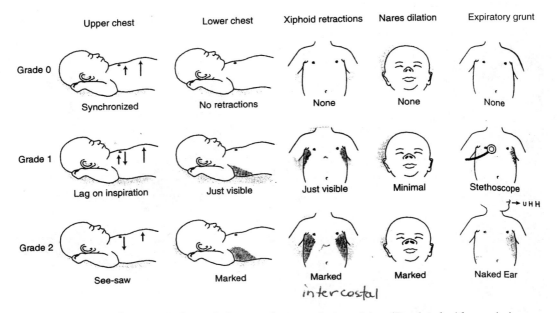

Figure 5–6   *The Silverman-Anderson Index to evaluate respiratory status. (Reprinted with permission from Silverman WA, Anderson DH Evaluation of respiratory status: Silverman and Anderson Index.* Pediatrics. *1956;17:1)*

The head should be inspected for cuts or bruises secondary to the use of forceps or other birth trauma. The head could be edematous from the pressure generated during labor. This produces what is called *caput succedaneum*. This is usually harmless and resolves in the first two days. The two soft spots, or *fontanelles,* should now be gently palpated as shown in Figure 5–7. The anterior fontanelle is diamond-shaped and usually measures 1 to 4 cm. The posterior fontanelle is triangle-shaped and is smaller than the anterior one. Both fontanelles should be firm, but soft. A bulging, tense fontanelle may signify increased intracranial pressure. Shrunken or depressed fontanelles may be secondary to dehydration.

The mouth may now be examined for the presence of clefts (openings) in the palate and any other abnormality that may hinder breathing. The ears may now be examined to determine where they fall on the gestational age assessment scale. The neck should be palpated for the presence of any cysts or tumors.

Moving to the chest, the breast tissue may now be evaluated for the gestational age assessment (Figure 5–8).

With the stethoscope, the heart is now auscultated. The normal heart rate is between 120 and 160 bpm. Heart rates below 100 bpm are considered bradycardia, and a heart rate above 160 bpm is considered tachycardia. The apical pulse, which is the point on the chest where the heart sounds are heard the loudest, is evaluated next. It is normally heard in the fifth intercostal space, midclavicularly on the left chest wall. This location, called the point of maximal impulse or intensity (PMI), is marked on the chest wall and used for future reference. Conditions that could cause the PMI to shift include pneumothorax, atelectasis, and an increase in heart size.

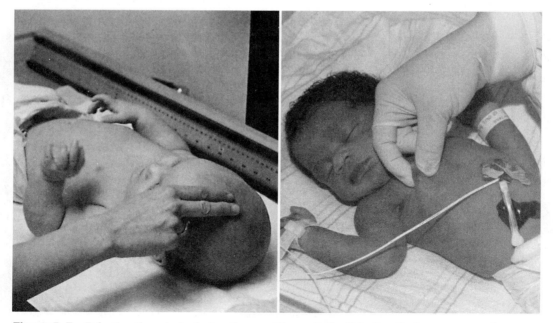

Figure 5–7 *Palpating the anterior fontanelle.*   **Figure 5–8** *Palpating the breast to assess for gestational maturity.*

The heart normally has two distinct sounds, with the first sound being slightly louder and duller than the second sound. Any sound that is heard besides the normal ones is considered to be a *murmur.* Murmurs are typically the result of turbulent blood flow in the heart. They can be caused by valvular defects, septal defects, increased blood flow, or a patent ductus arteriosus. Occasionally, the murmur of pulmonic or aortic stenosis is heard.

Systolic murmurs usually occur after the first heart sound and end before the onset of the second sound. Systolic murmurs make up most of the benign sounds, while diastolic murmurs are more indicative of heart disease. Murmurs are graded from I to IV, with I being soft and IV being loudest. Roughly 90% of murmurs in the neonatal period are benign; however, some severe heart defects may be present when no murmur is heard.

With the stethoscope on the chest, the lungs may now be evaluated (Figure 5–9). The healthy lungs will be well aerated in all segments and free of adventitious sounds. The presence of wheezes, crackles, or rhonchi should be examined further to determine their origin and to evaluate for the presence of any respiratory compromise.

Brachial pulses should now be evaluated and compared to femoral pulses (Figure 5–10). Both pulses should be equal in intensity and strength and symmetrical in rhythm. Weak pulses may indicate hypotension, diminished cardiac output, or peripheral vasoconstriction. Decreased femoral pulses in the presence of normal brachial pulses may indicate a heart anomaly such as coarctation of the aorta or patent ductus arteriosus and should be evaluated further. Conversely, bounding pulses may indicate a large right-to-left shunt through the ductus arteriosis.

Upon completion of the pulse evaluation, the blood pressure (BP) should be measured. Many factors cause neonatal BP to vary. Factors such as gestational age, weight, cuff size, and the neonate's state of alertness can all change BP readings.[6] Neonatal BP is obtained by the use of a *Doppler* device and a cuff, an electronic BP cuff, or through the umbilical artery catheter. On the small neonate, BP is best taken from the femoral artery with the cuff around the thigh.

In many instances, diastolic pressure is difficult to assess. In such cases, systolic pressure

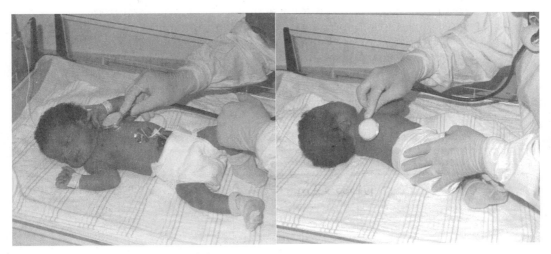

Figure 5–9 *Assessing the newborn's lungs.*

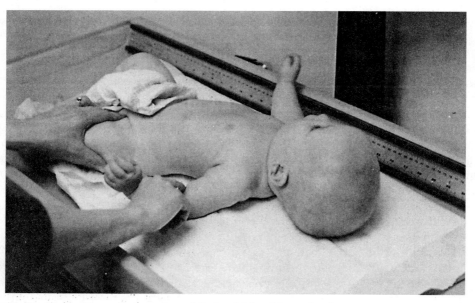

Figure 5–10 *Evaluation and comparison of the brachial and femoral pulses.*

is measured and documented. Neonatal BP begins low and increases with age and size. Normal neonatal blood pressures are listed in Table 5–1. BP continues to increase as the baby grows until it reaches its adult normal of 120/80 mm Hg.

The abdomen should now be gently palpated to check for cysts or tumors. The liver may be palpated and measured in centimeters below the right lower chest margin. The liver can normally be palpated approximately 1.5 to 2 cm below the right costal border. In right-sided heart failure, the liver is engorged with blood and may be 5 to 6 cm below the costal border.

A normal neonate will have a protruding abdomen. If the abdomen is *scaphoid* (sunken or flat), it could signify the presence of a diaphragmatic hernia.

If it is still possible, check the umbilical stump for the presence of three vessels. The presence of only two vessels is highly associated with urinary tract abnormalities.

The presence of bowel sounds should be documented with the stethoscope. The genitalia can now be examined to determine maturity. Finally, the foot can be inspected for the presence of creases.

The neonate's temperature should now be measured to assume proper thermoregula-

TABLE 5–1 Neonatal Blood Pressure Range of Normals

WEIGHT	SYSTOLIC (MM HG)	DIASTOLIC (MM HG)
750 g	34–54	14–34
1000 g	39–59	16–36
1500 g	40–61	19–39
3000 g	51–72	27–46

tion. Temperature can be assessed either rectally, aurally, or at the axilla, with the axilla being the preferred location. Axillary temperatures are reliable as indicators of thermoregulation and are within 0.10°C of rectal temperatures. Normal neonatal body temperature ranges from 36.2 to 37.3°C.

NEUROLOGIC EXAMINATION

The importance and necessity of the neurologic examination continues to be controversial. It is questionable whether the information obtained is useful for diagnosis of normal or abnormal neurologic status. Studies have shown that a fetus's neurologic system matures at a constant rate during gestation. The exam, therefore, is dependent on the degree of maturation.

Obviously, a 40-week neonate will respond differently to the neurologic exam than will a 32-week neonate. Apparent defects may be transient or permanent in nature. Until more studies are done to correlate gestational age with appropriate responses, the neurologic exam may be of limited use.

Much of the neurologic exam can be accomplished during the physical examination. The neonate's movements, crying, response to touch, and body tone are all signs that can be checked for neurologic well-being. Remaining information can be obtained by performing a series of reflex tests on the neonate.

Neonatal Reflex Tests.   To elicit the rooting reflex, gently stroke the corner of the mouth, as shown in Figure 5–11. An appropriate response is for the baby to turn its head toward the side that was stroked. The suck reflex is determined by placing a pacifier or a clean finger into the mouth. The baby should begin sucking immediately; the strength of the suck depends on how hungry the patient is. The grasp reflex is invoked by placing your index fingers into the patient's palm. The healthy neonate should immediately grasp your fingers. This is followed by placing your thumb over the fingers and gently pulling the patient to a sitting position (Figure 5–12). Be careful not to rely on the patient's grasp to be secure

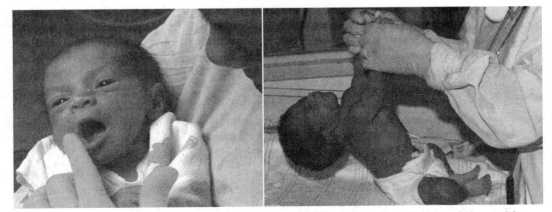

Figure 5–11 *Eliciting the rooting reflex.*   **Figure 5–12** *Lifting the patient to a sitting position using the grasp reflex.*

enough to pull him or her upright. The degree of head control can be determined with the neonate in the upright position. A healthy patient should have enough control to keep the head upright and not limply hanging down. The Moro reflex can be tested by slowly lowering the neonate back to a lying position. Just before the head touches the bed, quickly remove your fingers, allowing the patient to fall to the bed. The normal response will be an upward and outward extension of the arms and rapid flexion of the hips and knees.

If desired, the neurologic evaluation portion of the gestational age assessment can now be performed following the guidelines of the Dubowitz or Ballard systems. Findings of the neurologic examinations should be carefully evaluated because the incidence of false-positive and false-negative results is very high.

PHYSICAL ASSESSMENT OF THE PEDIATRIC PATIENT

Proper respiratory care of the pediatric patient begins with a firm understanding of the anatomic and physiologic differences between pediatric and adult patients, as discussed in the beginning of this chapter. That understanding is then used along with a physical assessment to diagnose respiratory problems and help plan a course of treatment. Certain problems and diseases are unique to pediatric patients because of these anatomic and physiologic differences.

HISTORY

Any physical examination should begin with a thorough evaluation of the patient's history. When assessing the history of the respiratory system, several questions need to be addressed. Depending on the age of the patient, questions may need to be addressed to the parents to obtain accurate information.

1. *Is the current illness an acute or chronic process?* The aim here is to determine when the symptoms appeared. Chronic problems, especially in younger patients, point to congenital problems or abnormalities. Chronic symptoms may also indicate long-term diseases such as cystic fibrosis or asthma.
2. *Are there signs of a concurrent infection?* Typical signs of infection include a fever, purulent discharges from the eyes and nose, or sputum from the lungs and swelling of the lymph nodes in the neck.
3. *If the patient has been treated for the current problem before, what was the effect of prior treatments?* This information can save a lot of time if it is known how the child has reacted to previous treatments and regimes.
4. *Have other members of the family had similar symptoms?* The presence of similar symptoms in other family members may indicate hereditary diseases such as cystic fibrosis. It may also show the presence of an infection that is being passed among family members.
5. *What is the character of the cough?* A tight, barky cough may be caused by an upper airway disease, such as croup or epiglottitis, or could indicate a foreign body obstruction. A cough may be productive or nonproductive. Expectoration does not have to

occur for the cough to be productive. A productive cough is usually defined as one in which rhonchi or crackles are heard, indicating the presence of material in the tracheobronchial tree. A dry nonproductive cough may be from an allergy, virus, or foreign body aspiration. In younger pediatric patients, a cough that is associated with swallowing suggests aspiration into the tracheobronchial tree secondary to tracheo-esophageal fistulas.

6. *What is the pattern of breathing?* Acute onset of breathing difficulty, shown by increased respiratory rate, retractions, and labored breathing, without fever, points toward an airway obstruction. If accompanied by chest pain, a pneumothorax, fractured ribs, or a *pleural effusion* may be present. Chronic patterns of labored breathing are evidence of lung or cardiac anomalies. In asthma, labored breathing may only be present during an attack.

7. *Is there a history of wheezing?* Wheezing is frequently associated with asthma. However, it can be heard whenever airway obstruction is present. It is typically loudest during expiration. Any persistent audible wheezing with an acute onset points to a foreign body lodged somewhere in the tracheobronchial tree. If the child is asthmatic, it is important to determine what medications have been given and how the asthma has reacted in past occurrences.

8. *Is cyanosis present?* Presence of cyanosis is almost always the result of some degree of hypoxemia. The exception is a cold patient, where cyanosis may be secondary to peripheral circulatory stasis, not hypoxemia. Cyanosis that persists in spite of oxygen administration signifies a right-to-left shunting of blood.

9. *Does the patient complain of chest pain?* Obviously, this will only pertain to the older pediatric patient who can verbalize. Possible causes of chest pain are many. Causes are ruled out or diagnosed by the use of a chest x-ray, location and severity of the pain, and recent history of infection or trauma. Potential sources of chest pain include the esophagus, diaphragm, chest wall, pericardium, parietal pleura, and the lung itself.

10. *What is the nature of the sputum?* When possible, a history of the color, amount, consistency, and odor of sputum will help in diagnosing lung disorders. Large amounts of thick, clear, or purulent secretions may be caused by cystic fibrosis. Foul-smelling secretions may show a lung abscess or an acute bacterial process. Blood may be present in pneumonia or bronchiectasis.

11. *What is the growth pattern of the patient?* Respiratory disease may produce failure to thrive, so called because of the failure of the patient to grow and develop normally.

12. *What is the patient's environment?* The environment includes not only the physical surroundings, but also the social and emotional characteristics of the surroundings. The presence of stressors in any of the above aspects of the environment may help diagnose the source of the respiratory problem.

EXAMINATION OF THE PEDIATRIC PULMONARY SYSTEM

When examining the pulmonary system of the pediatric patient, there are three primary goals to achieve: 1) to localize the disease, if one is present; 2) to observe for adequacy of gas exchange; and 3) to determine the nature of the patient's respirations. Each of these areas will be reviewed separately.

Localization of the Disease.   Much of the information gathered while taking the history will help in determining the location of the disease. The practitioner will then use additional information to either prove or disprove its presence. A chest x-ray is an excellent source of determining location and extent of the disease. Areas of infection or consolidation will appear as white areas on the x-ray. Air trapping, secondary to aspiration of foreign bodies or mucus plugging, will appear as a dark, hyperaerated area distal to the plugging.

Chest x-rays should never be used alone to diagnose, but only to verify what is already suspected. Thus, the practitioner should already have an idea of what the disease process is from the history and exam. The chest x-ray is then used to confirm if the disease is actually present and where it is located. Some diseases may not be detected by chest x-ray, but the information is still important in ruling out other causes of the symptoms. Chest x-rays and their interpretation are covered in more detail in Chapter 13.

Auscultating breath sounds may also be helpful in determining the location of the disease process. Figure 5–13 shows the location of the various lung segments as they relate to the exterior thorax. Breath sounds should be evaluated with an appropriately sized stethoscope, warmed before placing it on the chest. You should begin at the apices and slowly work your way down, carefully comparing similar segments in both lungs. Check for equal aeration bilaterally. The presence of adventitious sounds such as wheezes, crackles, rhonchi, or stridor in a certain segment or lobe of either lung helps localize the disease to that site.

Percussion of the chest (Figure 5–14) is another aid in assessing the location of the disease process. Involved lung areas will usually have a dull percussion note over the area of involvement. Hyperaerated areas, including pneumothoraces, will have a high-pitched, tympanic quality.

Palpating the trachea at the sternal notch (Figure 5–15) gives clues to changes in thoracic pressures. The trachea normally sits midline in the neck as it enters the thorax. The presence of atelectatic or consolidated alveoli cause the trachea to deviate toward the involved side. This deviation is the result of a slight hyperinflation of the unaffected lung and the collapse and tension of the affected lung. In the presence of a pneumothorax, or severe air trapping and hyperinflation, the trachea will deviate away from the involved lung for the same reason as mentioned above.

Assessing Adequacy of Gas Exchange.   Adequacy of gas exchange is best determined by obtaining and analyzing an arterial blood gas sample. This is covered in detail in Chapter 9. Physical signs of hypoxia include tachycardia, cyanosis, labored breathing, and a deteriorating mental state.

Signs of hypercarbia include a rapid bounding pulse, confusion or drowsiness, muscular twitching, and, in severe cases, coma. Any patient who has diminished breath sounds and any of the above symptoms should be started on oxygen therapy and a blood gas drawn immediately to evaluate the extent of hypoxia or hypercarbia.

Pulse oximeters or transcutaneous monitors are also invaluable in helping assess adequacy of gas exchange. Their use does not, however, eliminate the need to perform arterial blood gas evaluations.

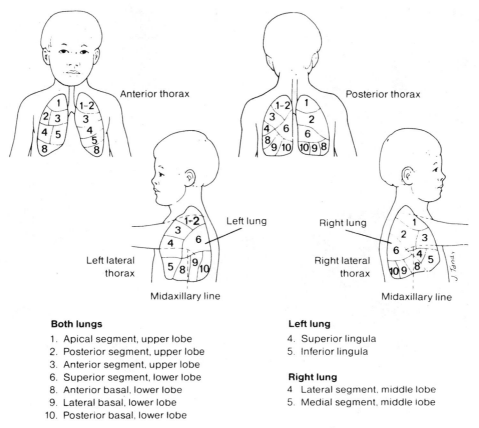

Both lungs

1. Apical segment, upper lobe
2. Posterior segment, upper lobe
3. Anterior segment, upper lobe
6. Superior segment, lower lobe
8. Anterior basal, lower lobe
9. Lateral basal, lower lobe
10. Posterior basal, lower lobe

Left lung

4. Superior lingula
5. Inferior lingula

Right lung

4 Lateral segment, middle lobe
5. Medial segment, middle lobe

Figure 5–13 *The lung segments and their relationship to the exterior thorax.*

Determining the Nature of Respirations. The last part of the physical examination of the pulmonary system involves determining the nature of the patient's respirations. This includes evaluating the rate, depth, rhythm, and ease of breathing.

Rate. The respiratory rate is a good indicator of distress. An elevated rate is usually secondary to decreased lung and chest wall compliance. The difficulty is in determining what is a normal respiratory rate for the pediatric patient. The normal respiratory rate falls rapidly during the first years of life, leveling off during late adolescence and early adulthood. The respiratory rate is often higher when the patient is awake and slows during sleep. After age 1, any resting quiet respiratory rate above 40 should be investigated further. As the child reaches 5 years and above, a resting rate above 35 is suspect and should be followed up to assess its cause.

Depth. The depth of ventilation may be difficult to assess. Extremes are easily detected, but assessment between the two extremes requires much practice and observation. The

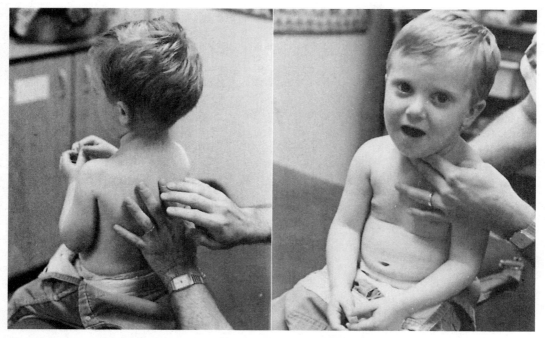

Figure 5–14 *Percussion of the thorax to assess the location of consolidation or other lung processes.*

Figure 5–15 *Palpating the sternal notch to assess the position of the trachea.*

normal breath should have some chest expansion accompanied by abdominal movement. As the breaths becomes more and more shallow, the chest and abdominal movements decline. An overly deep breath, called *hyperpnea,* is found in patients with metabolic acidosis, fever, severe anemia, and in deadspace-producing diseases. Too shallow breathing, called *hypopnea,* results from metabolic alkalosis, paralysis of the diaphragm, or central nervous system disorders.

Rhythm.   The last area of assessment is the rhythm of breathing. Normal quiet breathing is regular, interrupted only by an occasional sigh. Any apnea or irregular rhythm in the breathing witnessed in the pediatric patient is abnormal and should be investigated further. Either of these abnormalities could be associated with neurologic problems such as hypoxic-ischemic insults.

Ease of Breathing.   The effort of breathing is divided into two categories: labored and normal breathing. The presence of labored breathing, indicated by retractions, may be a sign of airway obstruction. Retractions may occur intercostally, substernally or suprasternally, and subclavicularly or supraclavicularly. As the airway obstruction worsens, retractions increase in severity. Flaring of the *alae nasi,* the external opening of the nose, is also a sign of labored breathing.

NEONATAL AND PEDIATRIC PULMONARY FUNCTION TESTING (PFT)

The purpose of testing pulmonary function in neonatal and pediatric patients is to identify those patients at risk for pulmonary problems, diagnose the dysfunction, and aid in selection of treatments aimed at improving the dysfunction, and/or reducing acute and long-term complications.[7]

With the advent of computers, the performance of PFTs on neonates has become available to most NICUs. PFTs are used to reduce the risks associated with mechanical ventilation, while optimizing the patient/ventilator interaction. Technology has also produced airway connectors that have acceptable amounts of deadspace—a problem that severely limited PFTs on neonates before this development.

Pulmonary function values vary over a wide range of ages and sizes. Differences in anatomy and physiology between adults and infants must also be considered when pulmonary tests are being performed. An additional concern that could potentially lead to inaccurate results is the lack of patient cooperation and inability to comprehend and follow commands, which is often seen in pediatric patients.

INDICATIONS FOR PULMONARY FUNCTION TESTS

There are four main indications to the performance of PFTs on neonates and pediatric patients. They are: 1) Diagnosis of lung disorders; 2) Follow the natural history of lung diseases and/or lung growth; 3) Evaluation of therapeutic responses; and 4) Prediction of subsequent dysfunction.[8]

CONTRAINDICATIONS FOR PULMONARY FUNCTION TESTS

The *AARC Clinical Practice Guideline* identifies three contraindications and four relative contraindications that should be evaluated before performing PFTs on neonates or pediatrics. These contraindications are: 1) Active pulmonary bleeding; 2) Open chest wound; and 3) Untreated pneumothorax. Relative contraindications include: 1) The risk of interrupted ventilation outweighs the benefit of the PFTs; 2) Sedating the patient may cause untoward clinical events in the presence of some conditions (central hypoventilation, central nervous system depression, obstructive sleep apnea, severe obesity, esophagitis or gastritis, and hepatic or renal dysfunction); 3) The level of patient sedation/paralysis is inadequate; and 4) The patient is uncooperative or combative.[8]

PULMONARY FUNCTION TESTS ON NEONATES

The ability to measure pulmonary compliance, resistance, and flow rates in the neonatal patient allows the practitioner to maximize the benefit of therapeutic treatments. Following trends in compliance allows the practitioner to optimize ventilator settings and avoid unnecessarily high pressure or rates.

Changes in resistance and flow can indicate bronchospasm or other obstructions that can then be treated. A gradual decreasing trend in values may help in the diagnosis and treatment of bronchopulmonary dysplasia.

The major disadvantage of performing pulmonary function tests on neonates is the inability of the patient to follow commands. The tests must be done using invasive measurements and often require sedating the patient, which may further compromise the results. Either of the mentioned techniques can be performed on intubated or nonintubated patients.

The basic pulmonary function test requires the measurement of airflow and transpulmonary pressure, which is the difference between the pressure in the pleural space and that at the mouth. Several parameters can then be measured (frequency, tidal volume, and minute volume) or calculated (compliance, resistance, and work of breathing). We will now examine how compliance, resistance, and work of breathing are determined.

Measurement of Compliance and Resistance.   The "Classic method." The first necessary measurement to calculate compliance and resistance is airflow, obtained by placing a *pneumotachograph* inline with an endotracheal tube (ETT) or a face mask. The second measurement, transpulmonary pressure, is obtained by measuring the difference between mouth and pleural pressures. Mouth pressure is simply obtained by placing a pressure monitor inline to the face mask or ETT and pleural pressure is assessed by placing a catheter into the distal esophagus and measuring the pressure at the tip.[9]

A disadvantage with this testing is that accurate results are only obtained if the measured esophageal pressure actually represents an average pleural pressure. To measure lung compliance, three factors must be measured. The tidal volume is measured by the use of a pneumotachograph attached to a face mask. The proximal airway pressure is measured through a port, also attached to the face mask. Pleural pressure is estimated by the esophageal catheter. Measuring the proximal and pleural pressure at the same point during a breath allows for the determination of transpulmonary pressure. This is obtained by subtracting the pleural from the proximal pressure. Dividing the transpulmonary pressure into the patient's tidal volume results in the compliance of the lug.

It is apparent that an inaccurate pleural pressure reading will result in an inaccurate compliance measurement. There are several factors that could result in the esophageal pressure differing from pleural pressure. Cardiac artifact from a misplaced catheter could alter pressure readings. To avoid this problem, the catheter should be placed in the lower third of the esophagus. *Paradoxical* movement of the chest wall during ventilation causes different pleural pressures at any given tidal volume within the thorax. This paradoxical movement is caused by the horizontal position of the ribs and the lack of mineralization of the bony ribs, both giving rise to a very compliant chest wall. During REM sleep, the activity of the intercostal muscles changes, causing increased distortion of the rib cage and making the measurement of pleural pressures difficult.

In any of these situations, no clinically consistent pleural pressure exists and neither compliance nor resistance can be accurately measured.

Occlusion Techniques to Measure Compliance and Resistance. Another method of determining lung compliance in the neonate is to measure alveolar pressure at a known lung volume. Alveolar pressure can be obtained by occluding the airway following an inspiration and measuring the pressure generated in the airway while the respiratory muscles are relaxed. This can be accomplished by the use of the face mask and pneumotachograph. A measured tidal volume is then delivered to the patient. Exhalation is prevented by occluding the expiratory valve on the mask. The pressure is measured through the mask by a manometer once a plateau has been achieved. Exhalation is then allowed to occur and compliance is calculated by dividing the plateau pressure into the tidal volume. To be accurate, the occlusion time must be short enough so a spontaneous respiratory effort does not occur.

This technique is not without problems. First, a true pressure plateau must be reached at the mouth to ensure relaxation of the respiratory muscles. A struggling patient will not allow for accurate results. Second, in the diseased lung, diverse regional lung time constants may not allow for equilibration of pressures within the lung during the short time between occlusion of the airway and the onset of a spontaneous breath. This problem can be somewhat lessened by occluding the airway at several points before end inspiration, and averaging the compliances found at each point.

Measuring Work of Breathing. Work of breathing reflects the amount of energy required by the lungs to overcome airway resistance. It is usually calculated by the computer as the area inside a pressure-volume loop that the patient creates. Pressure-volume loops are explained later in this chapter. As pulmonary mechanics worsen (resistance increases or compliance decreases), the amount of work increases and the neonate must expend more energy to maintain ventilation.

Measurement of Expiratory Flows. On the adult, forced expiratory flow are easily measured by instructing the patient to blow forcefully into the measuring device. It is obvious that this technique is not possible on the neonatal patient. Two methods are employed to measure forced expiratory flows. The first method is to physically squeeze the thorax to force exhalation.

Studies by England have shown that the external pressure needed to provide the desired results varies from patient to patient and is lower in patients with lung disease than in normal patients.[10] Thus, the use of a standard pressure to squeeze the chest of all patients will not result in accurate measurements.

The second method of measuring expiratory flows is to apply a suction to the airway and measure the flows generated. With either described method, it is possible that the application of an external pressure, or the negative pressure applied to the airway, may alter the mechanical characteristics of the airway and give erroneous results.[10]

Measurement of Lung Volumes
Functional Residual Capacity (FRC). There are three basic methods used to measure the FRC of an infant: helium dilution, nitrogen washout, and body plethysmography. We will briefly examine each technique.

Helium dilution involves the closed-system rebreathing of a gas with a known helium volume and concentration. This technique, because of its effectiveness and simpleness, is probably the best method for use with neonates. Nitrogen washout is an open-system circuit in which the infant breathes 100% oxygen while the exhaled volume and concentration of nitrogen are analyzed. Both methods involve the placement of a mask over the mouth and nose, or attachment of the circuit to the endotracheal tube on intubated patients. Calculation of FRC is then done following prescribed equations. These techniques are only totally reliable in patients with good gas distribution and minimal small airway disease.[11]

In contrast to the preceding techniques, body plethysmography is able to measure all of the thoracic gas volume, regardless of disease or distribution. To perform a measurement of *thoracic gas volume* (TGV) using plethysmography, the infant is placed in the body box and the airway is occluded at end expiration. As the infant attempts to inhale, the chest expands and produces an increase in volume in the plethysmograph. The change in volume is measured by a change in pressure in the plethysmograph. Mouth pressure is also measured with a differential pressure transducer. By applying Boyle's law, $P \times V - P' \times V'$, the TGV can then be calculated by the following equation[11]:

$$TGV = (\text{barometric pressure} - \text{water vapor pressure}) \times V/P - \text{deadspace}$$

where V/P = exchange in volume divided by the change in pressure. The amount of trapped gas in the thorax can be determined by subtracting the FRC from the TGV.

A relatively old technique, impedance plethysmography, is based on the concept that chest wall motion changes the impedance between two electrodes, which can then be converted to volume measurement. New research is using this concept and its possible use in neonates with a technique called respiratory inductive plethysmography.[12] As this procedure is perfected, it may prove to be an acceptable alternative to traditional methods of performing pulmonary functions.

Crying Vital Capacity. The crying vital capacity has been advocated as an alternative to assess lung volume when FRC or TGV determinations are difficult.[11] To assess the crying vital capacity, tidal volume is measured while the patient is crying. This may be useful in evaluating the course of RDS and other diseases that alter the FRC.

PULMONARY FUNCTION PROFILE

This data of lung volumes and pulmonary pressures provided by the PFT computer are used to create a profile of the patient's pulmonary function status using a volume-pressure loop and a flow-volume loop. To obtain a volume-pressure loop, volume measurements are plotted on the vertical line and pressure on the horizontal. A normal volume-pressure loop is shown in Figure 5–16. The compliance of the lung is indicated by connecting points of no airflow on the loop and examining the slope of the line, as shown in Figure 5–16. Changes in lung compliance are seen by a change in the slope of the line, as seen in Figure 5–17. Conversely, changes in airway resistance are seen as an increase or decrease in the area of the loop, as shown in Figure 5–18.

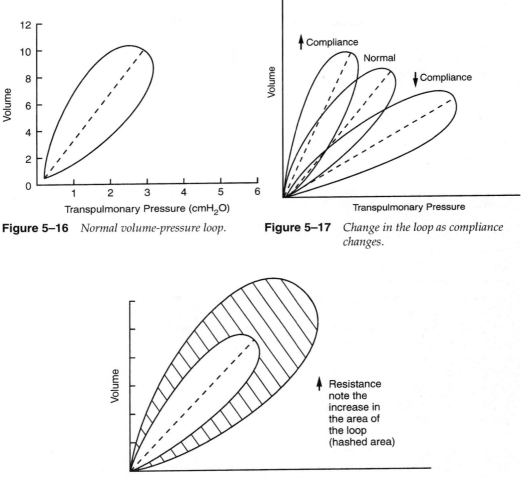

Figure 5–16 *Normal volume-pressure loop.*

Figure 5–17 *Change in the loop as compliance changes.*

Figure 5–18 *Change in the loop as resistance changes.*

Another useful comparison is the relationship between tidal volume and airflow, called a flow-volume loop. The flow-volume loop, shown in Figure 5–19, detects abnormalities in the airways. In a patient with increased airway resistance, the loop narrows as shown in Figure 5–20.

To complete the profile, the calculated FRC is added to the above information. As an example, in the face of decreased compliance knowing whether the FRC is normal or decreased can help the practitioner narrow the possible causes between RDS (decreased FRC) and pneumonia (normal FRC).[13]

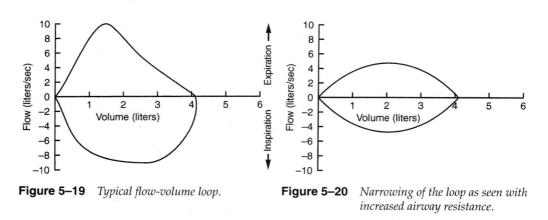

Figure 5–19 *Typical flow-volume loop.*   **Figure 5–20** *Narrowing of the loop as seen with increased airway resistance.*

PULMONARY FUNCTION TESTS ON PEDIATRIC PATIENTS

Pulmonary function tests done on pediatric patients yield a wealth of information. Measurement of expiratory flow curves is helpful in the diagnosis of early obstructive disease. For example, the flow measurements at small lung volumes (V_{max} 25) may be decreased before a decrease in spirometer values is seen.[14]

Provocation of bronchospasm is possible in many childhood asthmatics by having them exercise, especially in cool air. Bronchospasm may also be provoked with the use of antigens and *methacholine* aerosolization. The benefit of these types of pulmonary function tests is to determine the cause and extent of childhood asthma.

The diagnosis and progression of cystic fibrosis is aided by the close following of FVC and FEV_1. Less than expected increases in both values as the child grows is typical of obstructive disease.

Pulmonary function tests are helpful in following the patient with bronchopulmonary dysplasia (BPD) following hospital discharge. The patient is tested over time to evaluate the status of the lung disease. Future problems with exercise intolerance or bronchospastic disease may be avoided in these patients. Pulmonary function testing can also help differentiate between the deconditioned patient and those with bronchospastic disease as causes of exercise intolerance.

The performance of pulmonary function tests on pediatric patients, including those in their teens, is mainly dependent on the cooperation and maturity of the subject. Age is not always predictive of patient maturity. For example, two 5-year-old patients may be opposite in their ability to follow commands and cooperate and so will have vastly different results.

Assuming that the patient is cooperative and able to follow commands, the performance of pulmonary function tests on pediatric patients is basically the same as on adults. There are, however, a few special requirements that must be considered.

Accuracy of Equipment.   Although the equipment is not different from that used for adults, it should be accurate at low volumes and flows. Desired accuracy should be ±3% of the reading, or 30 ml, whichever is greater, for volumes. Accuracy for flows should be ±5% or 0.1 liter per second, whichever is greater.[14]

Practitioner Training. It is important that the person performing the test understand children. They must have a high level of patience to teach the patient the proper techniques. The person and the environment must be friendly so the patient will be at ease and not be frightened.

Interpretation of Results. Before any attempt is made to interpret results, the patient effort must be verified as being acceptable. There should be no artifacts from coughing, slow onset, or early termination of the maneuver. To be considered acceptable, the patient should produce three forced vital capacity maneuvers that are within 10% of the best effort.[14] Comparison of measured values must also be made to suitable pediatric references and standards and not to regressed adult values.

Determination of Total Lung Volume. Where there is no evidence of severe airway obstruction, nitrogen washout and helium dilution are generally reliable for the determination of total lung capacity and residual volume. A body plethysmograph may also be used, but may not be tolerated as well by the patient. Young patients may not be able to tolerate the confining nature of the plethysmograph, making accurate measurements difficult.

DLCO Tests. The diffusing capacity of carbon monoxide (DLCO) is rarely done on the pediatric patient for three main reasons: 1) smaller lung volumes necessitate smaller washout volumes when obtaining helium and carbon monoxide plateau concentrations; 2) it is difficult to get a 10-second breath hold from the patient; and 3) there is a low incidence of interstitial lung disease in the pediatric group.[14]

Arterial Blood Gas Analysis. Finally in the pediatric patient where pulmonary function measurements are not possible, an arterial blood gas may be helpful in diagnosing respiratory symptoms. In many lung diseases, the arterial PaO_2 and $PaCO_2$ will change before changes in lung function are noted.

SUMMARY

Assessment of the neonatal and pediatric patient requires the practitioner to first understand the differences—both anatomic and physiologic—in comparison to the adult patient. Differences in the cardiopulmonary system make these patients more prone to airway occlusion, trauma, and afford them less pulmonary reserve. Understanding the difference in metabolism is vital before treating with medications and when considering caloric intake.

Assessment of the neonate is divided into history, physical examination, and neurologic examination, and serves several purposes. First, it allows the practitioner to evaluate how well the patient is adapting to the extrauterine environment. Second, it allows for the identification of anomalies that may be present. Third, it allows for the determination of gestational age and establishing whether the neonate is appropriately grown for its gestational age.

The chapter also focuses on evaluation of the cardiopulmonary system of the pediatric patient. A series of questions are presented, which will help the practitioner focus attention on pertinent details that will aid in diagnosis and treatment. Physical examination of the same system allows the practitioner to identify physical findings that support or rule out possible diagnoses determined from the history.

Pulmonary function testing, previously relegated to research laboratories, has now become available for use in the neonatal population with relative ease of use and safety, thanks to computer and microchip technology. Testing on neonates can identify existing lung problems and monitor the efficacy of treatment. It can also be used to improve the patient/ventilator system by allowing the practitioner to fine tune parameters to best meet the patient's needs. PFTs done in the pediatric population are usually well tolerated, but rely on patient cooperation to obtain accurate results.

References

1. Shapiro BA, et al. *Clinical Application of Respiratory Care.* 4th ed. St. Louis: Mosby-Year Book; 1991.

2. Miller MJ, et al. Oral breathing in newborn infants. *J Pediatr.* 1985;107:465–469.

3. Whaley LF, Wong DL. *Essentials of Pediatric Nursing.* 5th ed. St. Louis: CV Mosby Co; 1996.

4. Wilkins RL, et al. *Clinical Assessment in Respiratory Care.* 4th ed. CV Mosby Co; 2000.

5. Ballard JL, et al. A simplified score for assessment of fetal maturation of newly born infants. *J Pediatr.* 1979;95:769–774.

6. Merenstein GB, Gardner SL. *Handbook of Neonatal Care.* 4th ed. St. Louis: Mosby Co; 1997.

7. Greenspan JS, Abbasi S, Bhutani V. Sequential changes in pulmonary mechanics in the very low birth weight (≤ 1000 grams) infant. *J Pediatr.* 1988;113:732–737.

8. AARC Clinical Practice Guideline. Infant/toddler pulmonary function tests. *Resp Care.* 1995;40:761–768.

9. Cullen JA, et al. Pulmonary function testing in the critically ill neonate, part II: methodology. *Neonatal Network.* 1994;13:7–13.

10. England SJ. Current techniques for assessing pulmonary function in the newborn and infant: advantages and limitations. *Pediatr Pulmonol.* 1988;4:48–53

11. Thibeault DW, Gregory GA. *Neonatal Pulmonary Care.* Norwalk, Conn.: Appleton-Century-Crofts; 1986.

12. Alderson SH, Warren RH. Respiratory inductive plethysmography: application in infants. *Resp Care.* 1995;40:114–120.

13. Greenspan JS, et al. Pulmonary function testing in the critically ill neonate, part I: an overview. *Neonatal Network.* 1994;13:9–15.

14. Eisenberg JD, Wall MA. Pulmonary function testing in children. *Clin Chest Med.* 1987;8:661–667.

Bibliography and Suggested Readings

Avery GB, Fletcher MA, MacDonald MG. *Pathophysiology and Management of the Newborn.* 5th ed. Philadelphia: JB Lippincott Co; 1999.

Beachey W. *Respiratory Care Anatomy and Physiology.* St. Louis: Mosby; 1997.

Bing DR, Porter SL. Pulmonary function testing in infants. In: Barnhart SL, Czervinske MP, eds. *Perinatal and Pediatric Respiratory Care.* Philadelphia: WB Saunders Co; 1995.

Cloherty JP, Stark AR, eds. *Manual of Neonatal Care.* 4th ed. Philadelphia: Lippincott: 1997.

DesJardins T. *Cardiopulmonary Anatomy and Physiology.* 3rd ed. Albany, NY: Delmar Thomson Learning; 1998.

Goldsmith JP, Karotkin EH. *Assisted Ventilation of the Neonate.* 3rd ed. Philadelphia: WB Saunders Co; 1996.

Harwood R. *Exam Reviews and Study Guide for Perinatal/Pediatric Respiratory Care.* Philadelphia: FA Davis; 1999.

Lynam LE, Algren S. Pulmonary function testing: a tool for managing the mechanically ventilated patient. *Neonatal Network.* 1993;12:61–64.

Pilbeam SP. *Mechanical Ventilation: Physiological and Clinical Applications.* 3rd ed. St. Louis: Mosby; 1998.

Taussig LM, Landau LI. *Pediatric Respiratory Medicine.* St. Louis: Mosby; 1999.

White L. *Foundations of Nursing: Caring for the Whole Person.* Albany, NY: Delmar Thomson Leaning; 2001.

Wong DL. *Whaley & Wong's Nursing Care of Infants and Children.* 6th ed. St. Louis: Mosby; 1999.

Posttest

1. Which of the following are true regarding the anatomic and physiologic differences between adults and infants?
    I. infants have a proportionally larger tongue.
    II. infants have a proportionally larger epiglottis
    III. infants have a proportionally larger body surface area
    IV. the infant trachea is only a third the diameter of the adult's
    V. infants have a higher oxygen consumption
        a. I, II, III, IV
        b. I, II, IV, V
        c. I, III, V
        d. I, II, III, IV, V

2. While reviewing a patient's chart before her delivery, you note the previous history shows PARA 3-1-0-2. Which of the following is TRUE?
    a. the patient has had 1 miscariage
    b. one previous birth is not living
    c. this is her third pregnancy
    d. there have been no premature deliveries

3. Identify which of the following are included in the Ballard gestational age assessment.
   I. ear recoil
   II. presence of edema
   III. sole creases
   IV. skin appearance
   V. presence of lanugo
      a. I, III, IV, V
      b. I, II, III, IV
      c. II, III, IV
      d. I, III, V

4. Upon examination of a newborn, you find thick vernix covering the infant, gelatinous translucent skin, thick lanugo over the body, faint red lines on the soles of the feet, flat areola with no bud, slow ear recoil, a male genitalia that shows no scrotal rugae or testicular descent. The proximate gestational age of this infant is:
   a. 35–37 weeks
   b. 32–34 weeks
   c. 29–31 weeks
   d. 26–28 weeks

5. Which of the following are done during the quiet examination?
   I. assess skin color
   II. palpate the fontanelles
   III. assess patient movement
   IV. overall visual inspection
   V. auscultation of breath sounds
      a. II, II, V
      b. I, II,IV
      c. I, III, IV
      d. III, IV, V

6. Increased intracranial pressure is indicated when:
   a. the fontanelles are bulging or tense
   b. the infant has an abnormal cry
   c. the pulse is bounding and asynchronous
   d. a caput succedaneum is present

7. A pediatric patient presents with a history of a dry, nonproductive cough. You would suspect which of the following?
   a. cystic fibrosis
   b. asthma
   c. foreign body aspiration
   d. myasthenia gravis

8. When assessing a pediatric patient, you discover that the patient has a rapid bounding pulse, confusion, and muscular twitching. Which of the following is suspected?
    a. hypoxia
    b. hypokalemia
    c. hypercarbia
    d. hypocarbia

9. Which of the following is NOT an indication to performing PFTs on a neonate or pediatric patient?
    a. assess the extent of a pneumothorax
    b. diagnose lung disorders
    c. evaluate therapeutic response
    d. predict the risk of pulmonary dysfunction

10. Of the following, which may result in inaccurate pleural pressure readings when an esophageal balloon is used?
    I. increased airway resistance
    II. cardiac artifact
    III. paradoxical chest movement
    IV. REM sleep
    V. presence of infection
        a. I, II, III
        b. II, IV, V
        c. I, III, V
        d. II, III, IV

11. Body plethysmography uses which of the following gas laws to measure thoracic gas volume?

    a. $\dfrac{P}{T} = \dfrac{P'}{T'}$

    b. $\dfrac{V}{T} = \dfrac{V'}{T'}$

    c. $\dfrac{V \times P}{T} = \dfrac{V' \times P'}{T'}$

    d. $P \times V = P' \times V'$

12. This volume-pressure loop shows which of the following?

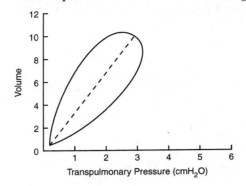

a. decreased compliance
b. increased airway resistance
c. tracheal stenosis
d. normal findings

13. An accurate pulmonary function study done on a pediatric patient is mainly dependent on:
a. cooperation and maturity of the patient
b. the availability of pediatric pulmonary function equipment
c. the disease state of the infant
d. the ability of the practitioner

CHAPTER SIX

RESPIRATORY CARE PROCEDURES

OBJECTIVES

Upon completion of this chapter, the reader should be able to:

1. List the indications for airway clearance.
2. List the contraindications of airway clearance therapy.
3. Briefly describe each of the following airway clearance techniques:
   a. Positive expiratory pressure (PEP)
   b. Forced exhalation technique (FET)
   c. Autogenic drainage
   d. High-frequency chest compression
   e. Flutter valve therapy
4. Describe the procedure for performing CPT including:
   a. Auscultation
   b. Postural drainage
   c. Percussion
   d. Vibration
   e. Removal of secretions
5. Discuss the following as they apply to aerosol delivery:
   a. Particle amount
   b. Particle size
   c. Particle characteristics
   d. Airway anatomy
   e. Ventilatory pattern
6. Discuss the advantages and disadvantages of each of the following:
   a. Small volume nebulizer (SVN)
   b. Metered dose inhaler (MDI)
   c. Dry powder inhaler (DPI)
7. List the indications for aerosolized drug therapy.
8. Describe the equipment used to deliver aerosolized medications. Compare and contrast updraft nebulizers to mainstream nebulizers.
9. Discuss the procedure for placement of a medication nebulizer inline to a ventilator circuit.

10. List and describe the hazards of aerosolized medications.
11. Explain the techniques used to prevent ventilator malfunction when aerosolizing ribavirin into a ventilator circuit.
12. Describe the indications for and hazards of suctioning and the equipment used. Review alterations in the procedure when the patient's clinical signs indicate.
13. Discuss the indications for and hazards of oxygen therapy.
14. Describe, for each of the following, its role in oxygen delivery:
    a. Oxygen blenders and flowmeters
    b. Oxygen analyzers
15. Compare and contrast bubble and wick humidifiers.
16. Describe the indications, hazards, and approximate FiO_2 for each of the following:
    a. Oxygen hood
    b. Oxygen cannula
    c. Simple oxygen mask
    d. Nonrebreathing mask
    e. Venturi mask
    f. Tent
    g. Incubator
    h. Resuscitation bags

KEY TERMS

Bourdon gauge	lavage	rhonchus
crackle	mainstream nebulizer	Thorpe tube
emesis	nosocomial	Trendelenburg
epistaxis	reconcentration	updraft nebulizer
hydrophobic	reflux	wheeze
hydroscopic		

AIRWAY CLEARANCE

One of the most widely studied aspects of respiratory care is that of airway clearance. Procedures and techniques have changed fairly dramatically from the early days where patients were hung over the edge of the bed and pounded on.

Normally, airway clearance relies on effective mucociliary action and an effective cough. Assistance in airway clearing becomes important when either of these two mechanisms become dysfunctional and result in mucus retention. As mucus increases in the airways, obstruction occurs and leads to air trapping, atelectasis, ineffective gas exchange, inflammation, and infection.

The traditional treatment for increased mucus retention is chest physiotherapy, which consists of postural drainage, percussion, and drainage. Several new techniques are being investigated and used in a effort to increase airway clearance. These new procedures are called airway clearance techniques, or ACTs.

INDICATIONS

The need for airway clearance is based on careful assessment of the patient's pulmonary status. Indications are not specific to any age group but apply to any patient meeting the criteria. Indications are listed in Table 6–1.

The indications for airway clearance can be effectively divided into four general categories: conditions that result in increased retention of secretions; diseases that produce excessive secretions; aspiration; and prophylaxis.

The premature neonate is prone to atelectasis secondary to a lack of pulmonary surfactant present with RDS. If severe enough, atelectasis can lead to large areas of shunting with worsening arterial blood gases. Airway clearance is used not only to help prevent atelectasis, but to help reinflate those areas that are atelectatic. Another complication of RDS is damage to lung tissues from ventilator pressures, oxygen and lack of surfactant, leading to BPD. The damaged alveolar and airway tissues secrete a larger amount of fluids and mucus into the airways, increasing the chance of occlusion and atelectasis. Efficient removal of these secretions during the course of the disease may help in preventing complications such as infection, air trapping, and barotrauma.

Airway clearance is especially needful in the neonatal patient because of the small diameter of the airways. Any accumulation of secretions can lead to severe imbalances in ventilation/perfusion ratios. Once intubated, the airway diameter is reduced even further by the endotracheal tube. Once intubated, the airway diameter is reduced even further by the endotracheal tube. Occlusion of the tube with secretions results in increased airway resistance and subsequent increases in ventilatory pressures. Intubation disrupts the normal cough mechanism, making mechanical removal of secretions necessary.

Postoperatively, or posttrauma, the patient may be unable or unwilling to cough because of the pain involved. The cough mechanism may also be limited by paralytic or neuromuscular diseases. In either case, the lack of effective coughing allows secretions to build

---

TABLE 6–1   Indications for Airway Clearance

Retained Secretions	*Excessive Secretions*	*Aspiration*
Atelectasis	Cystic Fibrosis	Meconium
RDS	Pneumonia	Foreign body
BPD	Asthma	
Intubation	Bronchitis	*Prophylaxis*
Ineffective cough mechanism	Bronchiectasis	Postextubation
Pain		
Paralysis		
Neuromuscular diseases		
Ciliary dyskinesia		

in the airways. Finally, the inability of the cilia to beat in a coordinated fashion (dyskinesia) or total paralysis of the cilia, prevent the secretions from being moved up the airways to be removed.

There are several disease processes that cause the lungs to secrete an increased amount of mucus into the airways. With some diseases, such as cystic fibrosis, abnormally thick mucus makes removal even harder. Other diseases include pneumonia, asthma, bronchitis, and bronchiectasis.

Any aspiration, whether it be of meconium in a newborn, or a foreign body, should benefit from the use of airway clearance techniques.

Following extubation, several days may be required before the patient is able to produce an effective cough. During this time, assistance with airway clearance is prophylactic in preventing the buildup of secretions.

CONTRAINDICATIONS AND HAZARDS

Airway clearance therapy is not without detrimental side effects. Contraindications of treatment and postural drainage are listed in Table 6–2.

Hypoxemia that may occur during the treatment and the ensuing tracheal suctioning of the infant is a significant hazard. Hypoxemia is frequently associated with patient agitation and tracheal suctioning.

Treatment should be stopped in patients who require more than a 0.25 increase in FiO_2 to maintain an adequate PaO_2. The use of transcutaneous monitors and pulse oximeters can help reduce hypoxemic episodes during CPT and tracheal suctioning. By watching the infant's PaO_2 or saturation during the procedure, the practitioner can increase FiO_2 levels in response to patient hypoxemia.

Airway clearance often requires various movements of the patient. Water that has condensed in the tubing must be removed before the start of the treatment to prevent draining the water into the patients airway.

Another hazard involves the use of postural drainage positions. The possibility of emesis and possible aspiration of feedings is of great concern. Placing the baby in a head-down position (*Trendelenburg*), especially following a feeding, and then percussing the infant,

---

TABLE 6–2   Contraindications of Airway Clearance Therapy

Pulmonary hemorrhage
Excessive agitation or hypoxemia during treatment
Feedings within the previous 45 minutes to 1 hour
History of reflux
Neonates of less than 1200 g birth weight or less than 32 weeks' gestation
History of intraventricular hemorrhage of greater than grade I, or less than 7 days postbleed
Untreated pneumothorax
Congestive heart failure

---

greatly increases the chance of *emesis* and potential aspiration. To prevent this, treatment should never be done within an hour following feedings. It is best done 15 to 20 minutes before feedings, when the chance of emesis is minimal. Postural drainage should never be done on patients with a history of *reflux*. If treatment is to be done, it should be performed with the infant in an upright position.

Postural drainage increases the intracranial pressure (ICP) when the patient is placed in the Trendelenburg position. The increase in ICP predisposes the early gestation baby to intraventricular hemorrhage (IVH). Studies have shown that infants of less than 1500 g are at a high risk for IVH.[1] It is therefore recommended that neonates of less than 1500 g not be placed in the Trendelenburg position because of the risk.

An additional concern involving preemies of less than 1200 g is the integrity of the skin. Percussion on these patients may cause skin damage that leads to edema, excoriations, and bruising.

TECHNIQUES

This discussion will begin with a look at several new airway clearance techniques and end with a review of traditional chest physiotherapy.

Positive Expiratory Pressure (PEP). PEP therapy is relatively new to the United States and Canada. It was developed in Denmark and is now extensively used in that country. PEP therapy is done using a flow resistor, mask or mouthpiece, through which the patient breathes in and out. As the patient exhales, a positive pressure is created in the airways. The pressure is monitored and adjusted, with pressures being either low (15 to 30 cm H_2O) or high (60 to 80 cm H_2O).

This inspiration/expiration is done 10 to 20 times, and is followed by a forced exhalation technique (discussed next). These two techniques are repeated until secretions are expelled. The concept behind PEP therapy is to increase the transmural pressure of the airways and cause dilatation. Airway dilatation then allows gas to pass any obstruction and reach collapsed lung units. Allowing the gas to enter into previously occluded areas may improve oxygenation and ventilation and additionally improve the mobilization of secretions toward the larger, central airways.

Forced Exhalation Technique (FET). FET is used as an adjunct to use with other secretion removal techniques. FET is a way of modifying a patient's cough to avoid airway closure secondary to airway instability. It is performed by having the patient inhale slowly and then "huffing" forcefully 2 to 3 times. FET differs from a cough in that the glottis remains open during the "huff." FET combined with controlled breathing exercises is termed the active cycle of breathing (ACB) and consists of interspersing the FET with deep relaxed breaths. These relaxing breaths use diaphragmatic excursion to enhance lung volumes and promote an effective cough.[2] ACB is followed by a forceful cough to remove loosened secretions.

Autogenic Drainage.   Autogenic drainage is a technique in which the patient breathes at three different lung levels. In the first phase, the patient inhales a normal tidal volume and exhales midway into the expiratory reserve volume (ERV). This maneuver allows mucus lining the airways to loosen. At the next level, the patient inhales slightly above normal tidal volume and again exhales to mid-ERV. This allows for collection of the mucus from the periphery to the mid-central airways. For the third level, the patient inhales to near vital capacity and then exhales to the beginning of ERV. This maneuver is similar to a FET and allows removal of the secretions.

A distinct advantage to autogenic drainage is that it requires no equipment and can be done in any location and at any time. One disadvantage is that it may be difficult for the patient to properly learn and perform the technique.

High-Frequency Chest Compression.   The concept of this therapy is that by applying high-frequency oscillations to the chest wall, the vibrations are transferred to the airways. This results in improved gas liquid interface and improved mucus clearing. Presently, this therapy is provided by way of an inflatable jacket that is worn by the patient. The jacket is inflated and deflated extremely rapidly by a pump attached to it, resulting in the high-frequency oscillations.

Flutter Valve Therapy.   This device combines PEP therapy with high-frequency oscillations applied to the airways. It is done by having the patient exhale into the flutter device. During the exhalation, the valve creates 10 to 20 H_2O of pressure and a ball flutters in the pipe, causing the oscillations that are transmitted to the airways.

Traditional Chest Physiotherapy.   The traditional method of performing chest physiotherapy consists of five techniques: auscultation; postural drainage; percussion; vibration; and removal of secretions.

Auscultation.   Auscultation involves listening to the sounds being produced in the lungs during the ventilatory cycle. The practitioner listens for sounds that may indicate the presence of airway secretions and/or reduced ventilation to a certain lung segment. Although the terminology for defining breath sounds is diverse, the definitions set forth by the American Thoracic Society (ATS) and the American College of Chest Physicians (ACCP) should be used. They recommend that a high-pitched continuous sound be called a *wheeze,* a continuous low-pitched sound be called *rhonchus,* and the term *crackle* for discontinuous sounds.[3] The presence of coarse crackles or rhonchus usually indicate the presence of airway secretions.

Postural Drainage.   Having auscultated the lung fields, the practitioner determines the proper position for the patient to best facilitate drainage of the affected area. The patient is positioned in such a way that gravity is used to drain the site. This requires an understanding of the anatomy of the airways on the part of the practitioner. Figure 6–1 illustrates the relationship of the segmental airways to the exterior thorax. The various positions used to drain each lung segment are illustrated in Figure 6–2.

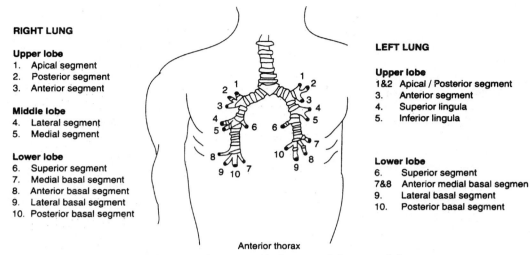

RIGHT LUNG

Upper lobe
1. Apical segment
2. Posterior segment
3. Anterior segment

Middle lobe
4. Lateral segment
5. Medial segment

Lower lobe
6. Superior segment
7. Medial basal segment
8. Anterior basal segment
9. Lateral basal segment
10. Posterior basal segment

LEFT LUNG

Upper lobe
1&2 Apical / Posterior segment
3. Anterior segment
4. Superior lingula
5. Inferior lingula

Lower lobe
6. Superior segment
7&8 Anterior medial basal segmen
9. Lateral basal segment
10. Posterior basal segment

Anterior thorax

Figure 6–1 *The relationship between the segmental airways and the external thorax.*

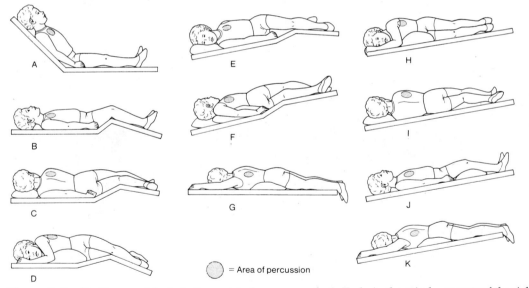

= Area of percussion

Figure 6–2 *Positions used to drain the various lung segments. A. To drain the apical segments of the right and left upper lobes—torso elevated 30°. B. Drainage of the anterior segments of the right and left upper lobes—patient supine. C. Drainage of the posterior segment of the right upper lobe—patient prone, right side elevated 45°. D. Drainage of the posterior segment of the left upper lobe—head elevated 15°, left side elevated 45°. E. Drainage of the left lingular segment—head down 15°, patient lies on right hip, shoulders turned to lie flat on bed. F. Drainage of the right middle lobe—head down 15°, right side elevated 45°. G. Drainage of the apical segments of both lower lobes—patient prone. H. Drainage of the lateral basal segment of the left lower lobe—head down 39° left side elevated 45°. I. Drainage of the lateral basal segment of the right lower lobe—head down 30° right side elevated 45°. J. Drainage of the anterior basal segment of both lower lobes—head down 30° patient supine. K. Drainage of the posterior basal segments of both lower lobes—head down 30° patient prone.*

The patient should be left in the position, and the thorax should be percussed or vibrated for 2 to 5 minutes. If postural drainage is to be done alone, as in those patients who cannot tolerate percussion or vibration, the patient should remain in the position for 15 to 20 minutes.

Percussion. Percussion is the rhythmic clapping on the thorax over the affected lung area to loosen secretions. Percussion on larger patients is done with the hands or with a mechanical percussor. The small size of the neonatal thorax prevents the use of hands for percussion and thus, percussion is usually done with the aid of special devices. These devices may be obtained commercially or can be made from resuscitation masks, as shown in Figure 6–3.

These cups are held between the fingers and percussion is achieved by the rhythmic up and down motion of the practitioner's hand. A variation of the cup held in the fingers is the rubber cup attached to a plastic wand, shown in Figure 6–4. The plastic wand is held between the thumb and index finger and percussion is done by a rhythmic movement of the wrist, similar to playing a drug. On the preemie, percussion may not be possible because of the fragility of the patient.

For larger patients, there are several commercially available mechanical percussion devices. These devices may be powered by compressed gas or electricity. One such pneumatic percussor is shown in Figure 6–5.

Percussion is done with enough force to produce a "popping" sound, but lightly enough to avoid trauma. Patients with BPD may have fragile bones and require special care when being percussed. Percussion is done over the rib cage to avoid damage to the liver or other abdominal organs. A light covering on the skin will reduce the chance of brushing and make the procedure more tolerable for the patient. Each area is percussed for 1 to 5 minutes as indicated.

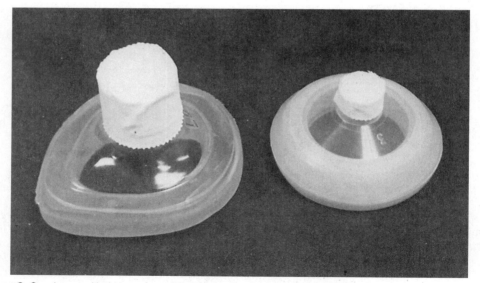

Figure 6–3 *A resuscitation mask modified to use for chest physiotherapy.*

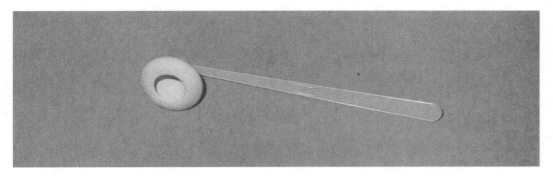

Figure 6–4 *A neonatal percussor.*

Vibration. Vibration differs from percussion in that it is a rapid, constant motion, rather than the rhythmic clapping. Vibration is used to help loosen secretions in the airways and aid their mobilization. Vibration can be done with the fingertips by placing them on the thorax and rapidly vibrating them. An easier method is to use a commercially available vibrator, designed to be used on small neonates, shown in Figure 6–6.

Vibration is best done during expiration to allow gas flows to aid the movement of the secretions. As with percussion, care must be exercised when the vibration is done to ensure toleration by the patient.

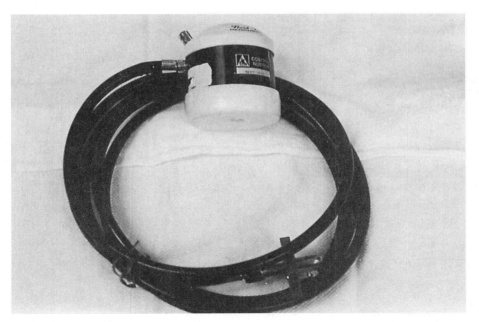

Figure 6–5 *A commercial percussor.*

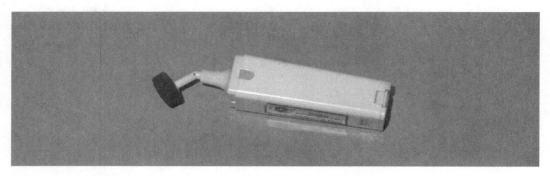

Figure 6–6 *A neonatal vibrator.*

Removal of Secretions. At the completion of the postural drainage, percussion, and vibration, the patient is prepared for the removal of secretions. Older pediatric patients should be instructed to use FET.

Younger patients may need to be suctioned both orally and nasally. To avoid bradycardia secondary to hypoxemia, which may accompany suctioning, the nonintubated patient should be hyperoxygenated before performing the suctioning. This can be done via blowby from the resuscitation bag, or by increasing the FiO_2 to the oxygen delivery device being used. The procedure for suctioning is covered later in this chapter.

AEROSOLIZED DRUG THERAPY

Aerosolized medications can be delivered by one of several methods: the small volume nebulizer (SVN), which is run by a compressed gas source; large volume nebulizer (LVN), also powered by compressed gas (both the SVN and LVN are jet nebulizers); the metered dose inhaler (MDI), powered by compressed gas; and the dry powder inhaler (DPI) in which the patient's inspiratory effort powers the delivery of medication.

The goal of treatment with aerosolized medications is to delivery an adequate amount of medicine to the desired sites in the pulmonary tree with a minimum of side effects. This being the case, an effective treatment depends on four factors: 1) The size and amount of particles produced; 2) The characteristics of the particles; 3) The anatomy of the airways; and 4) The patient's ventilatory pattern. Unfortunately, of these four, none can be altered by the practitioner. Understanding the ideal situation for each factor can aid the practitioner in modifying the therapy and instructing the patient when possible to best provide therapy.

PARTICLE AMOUNT AND SIZE

Particle amount and size is dependent on the type of nebulizer used. Jet nebulizers are easy to use and in common use in many NICUs; however, one drawback is that particle size varies tremendously among nebulizers. When run continuously, much of the medication is lost during expiration, thus reducing the amount of drug available to the lungs. This can be reduced slightly with the addition of a reservoir that collects some of the aerosol produced during exhalation and makes it available on the next inspiration.

PARTICLE CHARACTERISTICS

The major characteristic of aerosol particles that affects deposition is its ability to take on additional water. This is called *hydroscopic* growth. These aerosols grow larger when added to an environment of high humidity, which makes them more likely to deposit higher in the airway. Other characteristics that determine aerosol deposition include the concentration and viscosity of the drug and the velocity at which it is delivered. More drug is delivered when the volume of diluent is increased.[4]

Studies have demonstrated that the lung deposition of aerosolized drugs delivered to intubated infants is only about one-twentieth of that in nonintubated adults and about one-tenth that of intubated adults. The implication is that higher dosages are needed when delivering aerosolized drugs to an intubated infant in order to achieve a dose equivalent to that received by nonintubated patients.

ANATOMY OF THE AIRWAYS

In general, the narrower the airway, the more deposition of drug. This is important in the neonatal and pediatric populations because their airways are narrow to begin with. Add to that the effect of bronchoconstriction, secretions and endotracheal tube, and the amount of drug reaching the terminal airways and alveoli is probably negligible.

VENTILATOR PATTERN

Aerosol delivery is best enhanced when laminar inspiratory flow is obtained followed by a brief pause. For the patient, this requires a slow deep breath followed by an inspiratory pause. The timing of the aerosol is also important. Ideally, aerosol should be available from the onset of inspiration. This does not present a problem with continuous jet nebulization, but can pose a problem when an MDI is used. If not activated at the proper time, the amount of delivered medication can drastically change. When giving an aerosol to a mechanically ventilated patient, it may aid aerosol deposition by lengthening inspiratory time, reducing flow rate and adding a short inspiratory pause at the end of inspiration.

Aerosolized drug delivery has limited use in the NICU setting. One reason for this limited usage is due to the unknown drug effects and dosages on the neonate. With improved drugs and increased experience, however, aerosolized drugs are being used to a greater extent as part of the care of the premature infant.

In the case of the pediatric patient, aerosolized drugs have long been used in the treatment of several respiratory-related disorders. A problem exists regarding which is the best and most effective way to deliver the medication. An effective aerosol treatment requires a cooperative patient who can follow verbal commands. Unfortunately, very few infant and pediatric patients are cooperative enough to hold a mouth piece or allow the practitioner to hold a mask over the mouth and nose.

SVN

The main advantage to the use of SVN therapy is that it requires little patient coordination. This makes it useful in very young patients. SVN therapy is also advantageous in acute distress or in the presence of reduced inspiratory flows and volumes. The use of SVNs allows modification of drug concentration and additionally allows the aerosolization of almost any liquid drug. Finally, SVNs are effective with minimal breath holding, which may be difficult for younger patients.

Major disadvantages to SVN therapy are: it is relatively expensive; it is less easily transported; both cleaning and preparation are required; the dose delivery is inefficient; it delivers a cold, wet spray when used with a mask or blowby; and it provides a medium for bacteria to grow. When used inline with a ventilator, jet nebulizers have additional drawbacks. The high humidity of the inspired gas may aid in the hydroscopic growth of the particle, resulting in deposition in the circuit or upper airway, again reducing the amount of drug delivered.

LVN therapy is used when it is desirous to deliver a medication over a long period of time. Continuous nebulizer therapy is used to treat acute recalcitrant asthma in which a SVN does not deliver enough medication to have an effect.

MDI

The advantages to the use of MDIs are that they are very portable, they provide efficient drug delivery, and they require a very short preparation and delivery time. An advantage to the use of MDIs inline with a ventilator is the resistance of the particles to hydroscopic growth due to accompanying surfactants.[5]

Disadvantages include: the difficulty of coordinating the breath and delivery of the drug; fixed drug concentrations; limited choice of drugs; possible reaction to the propellants used; the possibility of oropharyngeal impaction; and the possibility of aspiration of a foreign body. The use of spacers reduces the necessity of hand-breath coordination, and reduces the chance of oropharyngeal impaction. With regard to use with neonates, there is substantial concern about the chemicals and gases used in the delivery of MDI medications. Their effect on neonates is unknown. Because of this, the American Association for Respiratory Care and the American Respiratory Care Foundation issued a statement indicating that due to the danger of hypoxia when the propellant gas of the MDI mixes with the patient's tidal volume, patients being ventilated at tidal volumes less than 100 ml should not receive inline MDI therapy.[6]

DPI

The advantages to using DPI devices include those mentioned with MDI devices; in addition, limited hand-breath coordination is needed, no propellants are used, and the drug doses are easily counted. Disadvantages to using DPI devices include: a limited number of drugs available; possible irritation of the airway from the dry powder; possible reaction to the carrier; it requires high inspiratory flowrates; it requires loading before use; and it is less useful in the presence of acute obstruction.

INDICATIONS

Most aerosolized drugs fall into one of three categories: bronchodilators, mucolytics, and steroids. For a bronchodilator to be indicated, some degree of bronchoconstriction should be present. On the premature infant and the pediatric patient, this may be manifest by decreased breath sounds, decreased chest expansion, presence of wheezes and retractions, increased respiratory rate, nasal flaring, grunting, increasing ventilatory pressures, increasing FiO_2 requirements, and an increasing $PaCO_2$.

Depending on the age and maturity of the pediatric patient, bronchoconstriction may also be verified by the results of pulmonary function studies. A decreased vital capacity and peak expiratory flow will help to diagnose bronchoconstriction.

The indication for the use of an aerosolized mucolytic is the presence of thick secretions that are difficult for the patient to expel. It is sometimes difficult to detect the difference between the presence of thick, copious secretions and bronchospasm. The patient may or may not have loud rhonchi when auscultated. The patient may also show the same signs as the patient with bronchoconstriction. As mucus fills the airways, the effect is the same as a narrowing of the lumen, thus the similarity of signs.

Inhaled steroids are indicated when an inflammatory pulmonary process is present, such as BPD or asthma. While the exact mechanism of action is not known, steroids are thought to have antivasopressin effects, enhance surfactant production and β-adrenergic receptor function, stimulate antioxidant production, and improve pulmonary microcirculation.[5]

A patient who shows any of the above signs is a candidate for aerosolized drug therapy. Once the treatment has been started, the practitioner must evaluate the effectiveness of the treatment and watch carefully for any complications. The use of these drugs, their dosage, and hazards is covered in detail in Chapter 8. Effectiveness of the treatment in the neonatal patient is indicated by improved breath sounds, increased chest expansion, and decreased signs of work of breathing.

EQUIPMENT

Most SNVs will work equally well using a mouthpiece, mask, or attached inline to a ventilator circuit. The most common nebulizer in use is the *updraft* type, which is used mainly in the vertical position. A tee piece is attached to the top of the nebulizer. The mouthpiece is inserted into one end of the tee piece, and a short length of aerosol tubing is placed on the opposite end of the tee to act as a reservoir. One study showed that the use of an expiratory reservoir significantly increased the amount of inhaled medication compared to the absence of a reservoir.[7]

For patients who require a mask, the setup is the same except that the mask is placed where the mouthpiece would be (Figure 6–7). Another possible use is to insert the top of the nebulizer into the bottom opening of an aerosol mask and either hold the mask over the mouth and nose or use the elastic strap to secure the mask to the patient's face (Figure 6–8).

One of the drawbacks of the updraft nebulizer is that it must be in a vertical position to nebulize properly. Fortunately, some of the newer nebulizers are designed to nebulize in a vertical or horizontal position. An updraft nebulizer can be used equally well in a pediatric ventilator circuit or a neonatal circuit. Adapters must be used to join the nebulizer to the circuit (Figure 6–9).

A less common type of SVN that is well adapted for use in the ventilator circuit is the *mainstream nebulizer* (Figure 6–10). The mainstream nebulizer has an advantage in that it does not require additional tubing to adapt it to the circuit. It is designed to be used in the horizontal position, which helps tremendously when being used inside an incubator.

Use of an MDI requires an actuator device that triggers the canister and diverts the aerosol horizontally. To avoid the hazard of misaiming the device or holding it too close or distant, it is generally recommended that the MDI be used with a spacer device. The spacer

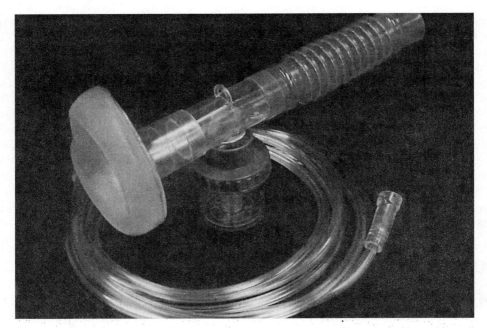

Figure 6–7 *Replacing the nebulizer mouthpiece with a mask. Used on patients who are unable to use a mouthpiece.*

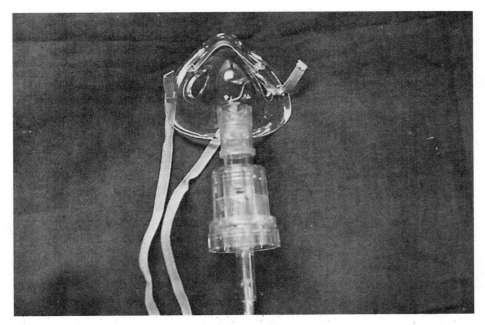

Figure 6–8   *An aerosol mask to deliver an aerosolized medication.*

is usually a chamber into which the medication is ejected, allowing the patient to then inhale the medication with less coordination needed. Adapters also exist, which are placed inline with a ventilator circuit, allowing the MDI to be discharged directly into the circuit.

DPI therapy uses a special apparatus that dispenses the medication from a capsule or a blister packet as the patient inhales. Currently, there is no mechanism for using DPI therapy on patients being mechanically ventilated.

Considerations for Use on Intubated Patients.   One of the biggest hazards associated with the use of aerosol delivery inline to the ventilator circuit is the potential increase in tidal volumes and peak pressures during ventilation. The problem is due to the necessity of providing 6 to 8 L/min of flow to properly nebulize the medication. Salyer and associates' recommended solution is to place the nebulizer at the humidifier outlet and nebulize during exhalation.[8] This allows the aerosol to fill the inspiratory limb of the circuit to be delivered to the patient with the next breath.

Another possible alternative is to reduce the ventilator gas flow proportionally to the flow being used to power the nebulizer. In addition to helping reduce tidal volumes and pressures, this may help prevent a buildup of inadvertent positive and expiratory pressure (PEEP) and the resultant increase in mean airway pressure. The additional flow added by a small volume nebulizer is usually not enough to affect flow patterns in larger circuits such as those used in pediatric patients, and, subsequently, does not need compensation.

When an SVN is to be used inline with a ventilator circuit, the cool gas of the nebulizer mixing with the warm gas of the humidifier leads to condensation. This may cause the

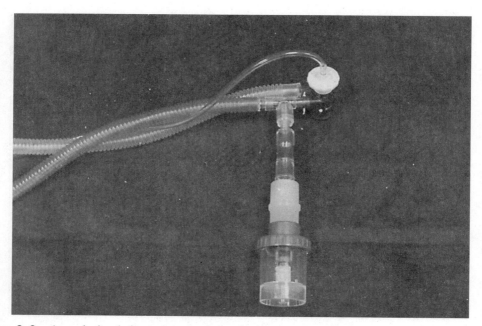

Figure 6–9   *An updraft nebulizer adapted to be used inline to a ventilator circuit.*

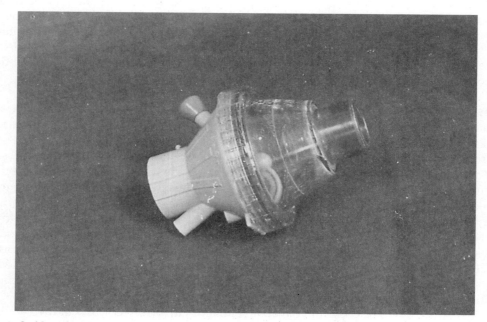

Figure 6–10   *The Bird Micronebulizer, supplied as a mainstream nebulizer.*

RESPIRATORY CARE PROCEDURES • 163

medication to rain out in the tubing and not reach the patient. For this reason, it may be more effective to either bypass or turn off the humidifier during the treatment. Upon completion of the treatment, the humidifier should be promptly connected or turned back on.

If the humidifier is to be left on, the following concerns should be noted. Certain ventilator circuits have a distal temperature probe to measure gas temperature as it enters the patient. In these instances the nebulizer should be placed distally to the probe. A nebulizer that is placed proximally to the probe will cool the gas and cause the humidifier to intensify its heat output. When the nebulizer is removed, the gas temperature could potentially burn the patient's airways. By placing the nebulizer after the probe, the humidifier continues to maintain the proper heat output.

HAZARDS AND COMPLICATIONS

Although aerosol therapy is a relatively safe procedure, there are certain conditions, described below in Table 6–3, that could be hazardous to the patient and require the attention of the practitioner.

Infection. Hospital acquired *nosocomial* pneumonias are frequently linked to the use of contaminated nebulizers. Contaminated nebulizers can carry bacteria-laden aerosol into the sterile environment of the lungs. Nosocomial pneumonia can occur from the use of contaminated multiuse medication vials, or from Legionella-contaminated tap water used to clean the nebulizer. Recommendations from the Centers for Disease Control and Prevention (CDC) for the prevention of nosocomial pneumonia include disinfecting and rinsing the nebulizer with sterile water following each treatment, or airdrying the nebulizer. Nebulizers must be replaced between patients with sterile ones and the practitioner must ensure that only sterile fluids, dispensed aseptically, be used in the nebulizer.

TABLE 6–3   Hazards Associated with SVN Therapy

Nosocomial infection
Medication side effects
Drug reconcentration
Ventilator malfunction
Excessive noise

Medication Side Effects. As mentioned, specific drugs and their particular side effects are covered in Chapter 8. However, there are some conditions unique to the use of medication nebulizers that will be discussed here.

The nature of bronchodilators causes them to affect not only the smooth muscle of the airways but also stimulate the heart and the smooth muscle of the vasculature. Early bronchodilators had very potent effects in all three areas. In contrast, modern bronchodilators minimally stimulate the heart and vessels while having a strong effect on the smooth muscle.

Reaction to drugs varies depending on the size and maturation of each patient. For this reason, the practitioner must watch the patient for changes in the cardiovascular system, muscle tremors, and nervousness. Nebulized mucolytics, especially acetylcysteine (Mucomyst), may cause bronchospasm in certain patient groups, particularly asthmatics. Because of this side effect, acetylcysteine is given with a bronchodilator.

Drug Reconcentration. Another potential hazard exists in the form of *reconcentration* of the nebulized drug. As the drug is nebulized, larger droplets return to the fluid reservoir. As the fluid reservoir gets lower, the concentration of the drug in the solution increases. Thus, toward the end of the treatment, the drug is in a higher concentration and could potentially produce more side effects.

Other Hazards. It is possible that depositing medication on the ventilator expiratory valve may cause it to stick, resulting in hazardous PEEPs and inspiratory times. This problem can be minimized by placing a filter into the expiratory tubing to prevent the aerosolized medication from reaching the valve. Some nebulizers create a high level of noise that could potentially be harmful to the small preemie. To avoid problems with noise when used with that patient group, the nebulizer should be placed in the ventilator circuit outside the incubator.

SMALL PARTICLE AEROSOL GENERATORS (SPAG)

The SPAG unit shown in Figure 6–11 is a unique device designed and intended for the administration of the drug ribavirin to treat respiratory syncytial virus. No other medication should be delivered through the SPAG unit and conversely, ribavirin should not be delivered through any other device. The administration of ribavirin, along with hazards and precautions, are covered in Chapter 8.

As mentioned, the SPAG unit is unique in its operation (Figure 6–11). Ribavirin is reconstituted in a large reservoir within the SPAG unit. Compressed gas enters the unit into a pressure regulator and is reduced to a working pressure of 26 psi. The gas is then fed to two separate flowmeters. One flowmeter supplies a gas flow to the nebulizer inside the reservoir. The nebulized particles exit the top of the reservoir and are met by flow from the other flowmeter. Together, the two flows enter a drying chamber. Inside the drying chamber, the nebulized particles undergo evaporation and are significantly reduced in size to between 1.2 and 1.4 microns. The particles then exit the drying chamber and are delivered to the patient. Ribavirin from the SPAG unit can be delivered to a mask, hood, tent, or ventilator circuit.

Because ribavirin can precipitate and accumulate on the walls of the ventilator tubing and the endotracheal tube, extreme care must be taken when administering the drug with mechanical ventilation. It is recommended that it only be used in this fashion by those who are familiar with this mode of delivery and with the ventilator. Several procedures have been shown to reduce risk associated with administering ribavirin via a ventilator. Suctioning of the ETT tube should be done very 1 to 2 hours and close monitoring of pressures

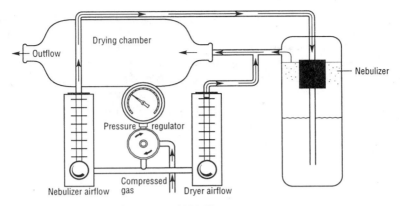

Figure 6–11 *Small particle aerosol generator (SPAG).*

done every 2 to 4 hours. The use of a heated wire circuit may also reduce precipitation of the drug. One-way valves are used to prevent the drug from entering the humidifier or ventilator, and to prevent ventilator flow from entering the SPAG unit. The use of disposable exhalation valves, which are changed out every 4 hours, reduces the risk of clogging and excessive pressures. The flow of ribavirin from the expiratory circuit to the environment is slowed by the placement of bacteria filters in the expiratory circuit.

SUCTIONING

Many patients present with factors that promote the retention of airway secretions. The intubated patient has a decreased ability to remove airway secretions spontaneously and must be aided by the practitioner. Secretions that block the airway increase resistance and subsequently increase work of breathing. As airway resistance increases, airflow is diminished and ventilation decreases.

Proper suctioning must be done in a manner that does not compromise the clinical status of the patient or the sterility of the airways.

INDICATIONS

Oral, nasal, and tracheal suctioning should be done when indicated. The basic indication for suctioning is the need to remove secretions. The secretions may be located in the trachea, pharynx, mouth, or nose. Intubated patients may require frequent suctioning of the endotracheal tube (ETT) to preserve its patency.

Suctioning through the ETT should be performed on an as-needed basis, ranging from every hour to every 4 to 6 hours depending on the amount and consistency of pulmonary secretions. Clinically the patient may show worsening chest excursion, and on auscultation, coarse crackles and rhonchi may be heard. Often the mucus is seen in the ETT. These signs all indicate the need for tracheal suctioning. Suctioning should be done following a CPT treatment to remove any secretions that may have been lodged and to prevent their aspiration back into the trachea.

Suctioning of the nose, nasopharynx, mouth, and oropharynx is indicated to provide hygiene to the intubated patient. On the nonintubated patient the same areas are suctioned to provide hygiene, as well as prevent aspiration of secretions and maintain the airway patent. Oral and nasal suctioning can also be done to stimulate a cough.

Due to its effect on the patient's ventilatory status, suctioning should be done at least 20 minutes before a blood gas sample. Tracheal suctioning is additionally indicated when a sputum culture or Gram stain is requested.

EQUIPMENT

The equipment needed to perform suctioning is listed in Table 6–4. Due to the fact that bradycardia and hypoxemia often accompany suctioning, monitors that measure the heart rate and oxygen levels of the infant should be used. These monitors must be easily visualized by the person performing the suctioning.

A stethoscope is necessary to access breath sounds before and after the suctioning. Noting the change in breath sounds indicates the effectiveness of the procedure.

A resuscitation bag and mask must be readily available at the bedside. In the event of a prolonged bradycardia that does not respond to stimulus, or in the case of an accidental extubation, a properly functioning resuscitation bag is life-saving. The FiO_2 delivered to the bag should be set 0.10 above the current FiO_2 before beginning the procedure. In the case of prolonged bradycardia, the FiO_2 should be increased to 1.0 while bagging the patient.

When suctioning the ETT there should be sterile saline available to *lavage* the airway. The neonatal patient will require only a few drops, whereas the larger pediatric patient may require several milliliters of solution. In either instance, there should be enough saline available to provide adequate lavage.

If the patient is to be suctioned nasally, the use of a water-soluble jelly will facilitate the passage of the catheter into the nares. The jelly should be opened and then squeezed onto a sterile field placed nearby. The sterile catheter is then drawn through the jelly before inserting it into the patient's nares. If an assistant is present, he or she may place the jelly directly onto the catheter, being careful not to contaminate it.

TABLE 6–4 Equipment Needed to Suction

Cardiac, oxygen saturation, and/or transcutaneous monitors
Stethoscope
Resuscitation bag and mask with oxygen source and pressure manometer
Sterile saline for lavage
Sterile suction catheter kit with gloves (appropriately sized)
Suction regulator set at appropriate suction level
Water-soluble jelly as needed

A suction regulator set at −50 to −80 mm Hg for neonates and −80 to −100mm Hg for pediatric patients and an appropriate collection canister are both required before suctioning.

The suction tubing that connects the catheter to the canister should be long enough to allow the procedure without pulling or kinking. The end of the tubing should be placed at a site that allows an easy connection to the suction catheter without breaking sterility.

The last piece of equipment is a suction catheter of the proper size. Table 6–5 shows the proper sizes for suction catheters used on neonates. The kit should contain at least one sterile glove, a sterile suction catheter, and a sterile water basin.

An alternative method of suctioning is the use of inline suction devices, which incorporate a suction catheter covered by a protective sheath and a patient connection "T-piece." The advantage to these types of suction devices is the ability to suction the patient without disconnecting the ventilator, less risk of contamination, and less overall cost (Figure 6–12).

PROCEDURE

It is recommended that suctioning always be done with two people: one to perform the suctioning procedure, the other to monitor the patient and provide support as needed.

The first task in preparing the airway for suctioning is the preparation of the equipment. Select the appropriately sized suction catheter, using Table 6–5 as a guide.

The technique of inserting the suction catheter into the ETT until resistance is felt may lead to trauma of the tracheal mucosa. To avoid possible injury, the suction catheter should be inserted only to the tip of the ETT.

The proper catheter insertion distance is determined by noting the cm mark on the exterior ETT, which corresponds to the level of the adapter (Figure 6–13). The adapter length, which is approximately 4 cm, is added to the cm mark on the ETT. This represents the distance from the tip of the ETT to the opening of the adapter and can then be used to determine the appropriate depth of catheter insertion. Once the insertion distance is determined, it should be noted and placed on a card near the patient's bedside to allow for consistency when suctioning.

TABLE 6–5   Selecting Suction Catheter Sizes

Intubated patients:	
Endotracheal Tube (mm I.D.)	*Suction Catheter (French)*
2.5	5,6
3.0	5,6–8
3.5	8–10
4.0	8–10
Nonintubated patients:	
Age	*Suction Catheter (French)*
Preemie	5,6
Term newborn	5,6–8
Newborn to 6 months	8–10

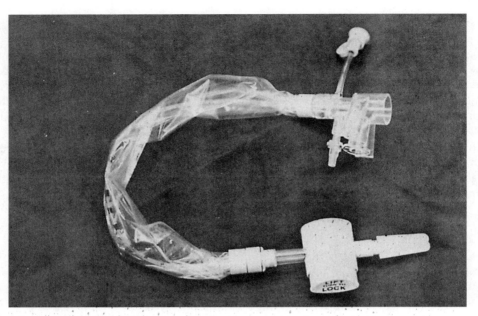

Figure 6–12 *A closed suction device.*

The vacuum pressure is now adjusted by occluding the opening of the suction tubing and adjusting the vacuum to the previously mentioned settings.

After washing the hands, the lungs are auscultated to assess the presence of mucus in the airways and to serve as a guide to determine the adequacy of the suctioning. Before suctioning, the patient should be hyperoxygenated for 1 minute with an FiO_2 0.10 to 0.15 higher than is currently being used. When a manual resuscitation bag is used, it is important to have a pressure manometer inline.

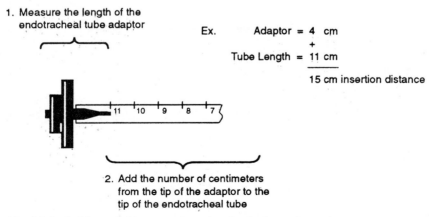

1. Measure the length of the endotracheal tube adaptor

   Ex.   Adaptor = 4 cm
                              +
        Tube Length = 11 cm
        _____
        15 cm insertion distance

2. Add the number of centimeters from the tip of the adaptor to the tip of the endotracheal tube

Figure 6–13 *Method of determining proper insertion depth of a suction catheter.*

After aseptically opening the package and donning the gloves, the catheter is removed from its protective package. When the patient is inside an incubator, the catheter should be wrapped around the hand or inside the clenched hand to protect it from being contaminated as the hand is inserted into the porthole.

If the patient is to be lavaged, a few drops of sterile saline are instilled into ETT followed by two to three mechanical breaths. The suction catheter is now inserted into the ETT to the predetermined distance, suction applied, and the catheter rotated and withdrawn. The entire suctioning procedure should not take more than 10 seconds, with a maximum of 5 seconds with suction applied. The procedure is repeated as needed until the secretions have been removed. Careful monitoring of the vital signs will help prevent hypoxemia and bradycardia.

HAZARDS

Hazards associated with suctioning are listed in Table 6–6. The major hazard related to tracheal suctioning is bradycardia. Bradycardia is defined as a heart rate below 100 bpm. In the neonate, a heart rate below 100 bpm indicates lack of proper oxygenation and a decrease in cardiac output secondary to decreased contractility of the myocardium. It is therefore a serious hazard that requires rapid care by the practitioner.

Bradycardia can be induced by way of two mechanisms. First, stimulation of the vagus nerve located in the trachea or in the oropharynx and nasopharynx can cause bradycardia. Vagal stimulation may be lessened by limiting the time that the suction catheter is in the trachea or pharynx. Insertion and removal of the suction catheter should last no longer than 10 seconds. It may be less hazardous to the patient to perform repeated, short-duration suctioning rather than one or two prolonged procedures.

A second mechanism of bradycardia is hypoxia brought on by the tracheal suctioning. Hypoxia-induced bradycardia can be lessened by hyperoxygenating the infant before performing the procedure and by limiting the application of suction to 5 seconds.

As with many procedures done on neonates, suctioning produces a significant amount of stress to the patient. In addition to bradycardia and hypoxemia, suctioning causes an increase in the amount of arousal, stressful facial expressions, and an increase in autonomic activity. The effect of this psychological stress is not fully understood, but certainly is not helpful to the patient's well-being. One study has shown that the use of music and vibroacoustic therapy may help reduce the agitation associated with suctioning.[9]

TABLE 6–6 Hazards of Suctioning

---

1. Bradycardia
   a. Vagal Response
   b. Hypoxemia-induced
2. Hypoxemia
3. Mucosal damage
4. Atelectasis
5. Airway contamination
6. Accidental extubation

Other potential hazards of suctioning include mucosal damage, atelectasis, airway contamination, and extubation. Mucosal damage may aid mucus plugging in the distal airways, leading to V/Q mismatches and worsening patient status, and may also lead to tissue swelling and edema, increasing resistance in the airway. Damage to the mucosa is reduced by regulating the insertion distance of the suction catheter as mentioned above.

OXYGEN THERAPY

Oxygen may be the most misunderstood drug in use today. Oxygen, in the eyes of many, is a wonder drug that can cure many problems. The purpose of this section is to look at oxygen as a drug that must be used with as much prudence as any other drug. Oxygen has side effects and complications that may further injure the lungs of the compromised patient. This section discusses those complications as well as the many methods and devices used to deliver oxygen to neonatal and pediatric patients.

INDICATIONS

The main indication for the administration of oxygen is the presence of hypoxemia in the patient. Hypoxemia is defined as a level of oxygen in the blood that is less than normal. Acceptable room air arterial PaO_2 for a neonate ranges from 40 to 70 mm Hg, whereas in the older pediatric patient a PaO_2 of less than 80 mm Hg (55 mm Hg at 5000 ft.) is considered hypoxic.

The diagnosis of hypoxemia is made by one of several methods. Actual measurement of the oxygen present in the arterial blood by arterial blood gas analysis is the most reliable source for determining hypoxemia. Transcutaneous monitoring and pulse oximetry offer rapid, noninvasive alternatives to diagnose the presence of hypoxemia. The methods of obtaining and interpreting blood gas results is covered in more detail in Chapter 9.

The average arterial PaO_2 at sea level of the normal term infant at birth is only 16 mm Hg, increasing to 51 mm Hg at 20 minutes and nearing 75 mm Hg 5 hours after birth. In contrast, the average arterial PaO_2 in the normal preemie at 3 to 5 hours after delivery is 60 mm Hg, increasing to 73 mm Hg after 24 hours.

Hypoxemia may be suspected when the patient shows signs of respiratory distress. Those signs include retractions, expiratory grunting, nasal flaring, and cyanosis. A word of caution regarding the assessment of cyanosis: The skin will not appear cyanotic until 5 g of hemoglobin become desaturated. If the patient has a low hemoglobin, there may be a significant level of hypoxemia present with no sign of cyanosis.

HAZARDS

The hazards associated with the use of oxygen are listed in Table 6–7. There is a strong correlation between high levels of arterial oxygen, and the development of retinopathy of pre-

TABLE 6–7 Hazards of Oxygen Use

Retinopathy of prematurity
Oxygen toxicity leading to bronchopulmonary dysplasia
Cerebral vasoconstriction
Fire hazard

maturity (ROP). Even though oxygen levels are not the only factor, it is still suspected as playing a major role in its development. Chapter 10 discusses the development of ROP in more detail.

The toxic effects of oxygen are seen in the development of bronchopulmonary dysplasia (BPD). High levels of oxygen administered over a prolonged period may cause a breakdown and destruction of alveolar tissues, leading to a loss of surface area for gas exchange. High levels of oxygen also cause a constriction of the cerebral vasculature, possibly reducing much-needed blood flow to a developing brain. On the other end of the spectrum, if too little oxygen is delivered, the patient may continue to suffer the effects of hypoxemia.

With these hazards in mind, the goal of oxygen therapy is to maintain a PaO_2 that is high enough to avoid the dangers of hypoxemia, but also low enough to avoid complications such as ROP, BPD, and oxygen toxicity. Arterial PaO_2 of 50 to 70 mm Hg are recommended to meet this criterion.

Another hazard that must be considered is the fire danger associated with oxygen use. Oxygen is not an explosive gas; however, it intensifies combustion to the point that a small spark or flame may instantly become an inferno. Instruction must be given to those who may work with or visit the patient that no type of flame of spark may be used in the presence of an oxygen-enriched environment. In all cases, whenever oxygen is in use, precautionary signs advising of the danger of combustion must be placed at the bedside and at the entrance to the room.

EQUIPMENT

We begin this section on oxygen equipment by examining those points that are common to all oxygen administration, expanding to common devices used to deliver the oxygen to the patient.

Oxygen Blenders and Flowmeters.   The oxygen blender, shown in Figure 6–14 is the usual starting point for the administration of various concentrations of oxygen. The blender is first connected to a 50 psi source of oxygen and air. The gases go through a series of regulators to lower the pressure to a workable level and then are mixed to achieve the desired concentration of gas.

The desired concentration is determined by the practitioner, who selects the FiO_2 on the blender via a rotating dial. Any concentration of oxygen from 0.21 to 1.0 is possible. The blended gas is then passed to the exterior of the device, where a flowmeter is used to direct the proper flow of gas to the patient.

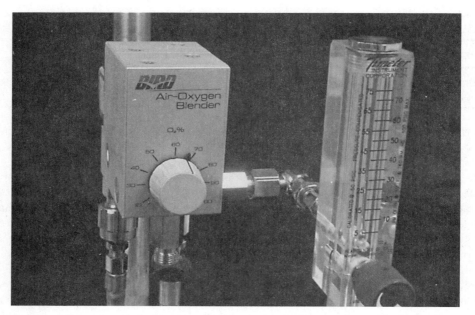

Figure 6–14 *A flowmeter attached to an oxygen blender for the delivery of a specific O_2 concentration.*

Flowmeters come in two varieties. The less accurate of the two uses a curved copper tube that measures flow as a byproduct of pressure. This device is called a *Bourdon gauge* and is usually found on cylinder regulators. Figure 6–15 shows a Bourdon gauge. The more accurate flowmeter is the *Thorpe tube,* depicted in Figure 6–16, which uses a ball or pin inside a calibrated tube to measure flow. On either type, gas flow is measured in liters per minute on a calibrated scale located on the flowmeter. A flowmeter can also be used to administer 1.00 oxygen directly from the 50 psi source to the patient.

Oxygen Analyzers. Although most oxygen blenders indicate an approximate FiO_2 on the mixture dial, few will be entirely accurate. If a precise oxygen percentage is desired, it is essential that an oxygen analyzer be placed in the system to monitor delivered oxygen percent. The only precaution is to place the analyzer in the system proximal to the humidifier, because the wet gas may cause erroneous readings. The analyzer should be calibrated to room air and 1.00 oxygen to ensure accuracy before being placed in the system. Thereafter, a calibration should be done at least every 8 hours, and possibly every 4 hours to ensure accuracy and prevent drifting.

Humidifiers. After leaving the blender and before reaching the patient, the gas should pass through a humidification device. Gases are stored in a dry state and therefore require the addition of humidity before being administered to a patient. This is especially true of the intubated patient whose normal humidification mechanism is being bypassed. Low flows of oxygen delivered via a cannula may not require humidification on older patients,

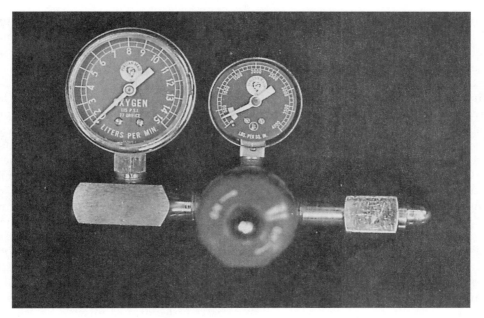

Figure 6–15 *A Bourdon gauge used to measure gas flows.*

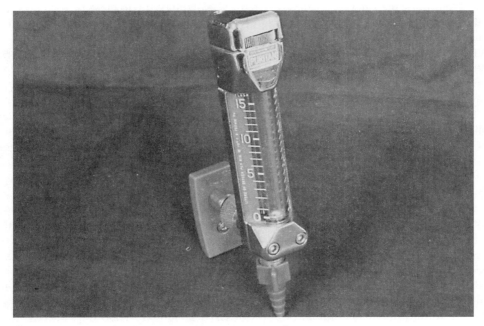

Figure 6–16 *A Thorpe tube flowmeter used to measure gas flows.*

because normal airway mechanisms provide adequate moisture to the gas. Younger patients may require humidification even at low flows due to smaller tidal volume to weight ratios and gas to tissue surface areas. The addition of humidity at high flows helps prevent drying of the airways, which leads to impairment of mucus cleaning, potential infection, and atelectasis.

Humidification devices fall into two classes: low flow and high flow. Low flow humidity systems are usually designed for flows of 10 L/min or less. A low flow system supplies a relatively small amount of humidity and does not heat the gas. These devices are classified as bubble or diffuser humidifiers. This type of humidifier allows the gas to bubble up through a reservoir of sterile water. The gas picks up water molecules as it rises to the surface. Oxygen cannulas and simple masks are examples of modalities that use the bubble humidifier.

High flow systems, usually having flows greater than 10 L/min, are designed to provide a fully saturated gas at a desired temperature. Warmed, fully saturated gas delivery is essential for intubated patients for reasons previously mentioned. A warm, humid gas can also be invaluable in preventing evaporative heat loss in the small neonate. Varieties of this type of humidifier include large volume jet nebulizers, advanced bubble humidifiers, and passover humidifiers.

Large volume jet nebulizers produce an aerosol by using Bernoulli's principle, which lowers the lateral pressure around the jet that draws water up a capillary tube. When the water reaches the jet, the gas breaks it up into an aerosol, which is then carried with the gas to the patient. A heater is either attached to a steel plate at the bottom of the reservoir, or placed around the nebulizer orifice. Caution must be exercised when gas flow is interrupted through the nebulizer not to allow the water in the reservoir to overheat. Most jet nebulizers have a built-in air entrainment port, which allows various FiO_2 to be achieved.

When using a jet nebulizer, it is important that the total flow meets or exceeds the patient's inspiratory flow. This is ensured by a continual stream of aerosol exiting the exhalation posts during inspiration.

Passover humidifiers use either a heated water-saturated wick or a heated chamber covered by a *hydrophobic* material (Figure 6–17). The wick is a material that absorbs water by capillary action. A heater surrounds the wick, and as it heats, the water evaporates. The source gas is then passed through the humidifier, over the wick where it picks up the heated water vapor, and out to the patient. The hydrophobic material used in the other variety of humidifier allows the heated water vapor to pass through, but not the actual liquid water. The water is fed to the top of the heater surface underneath the hydrophobic material where it is rapidly heated and evaporated.

As the warmed humidified gas passes through the tubing that carries it to the patient, the cooler air surrounding the tubing cools the gas. This results in a rain-out or condensation of the molecular water on the walls of the tubing. This could pose a potential danger if the accumulated water were allowed to drain toward the infant. To prevent this, some type of collection device should be placed in the tubing at the lowest point between the humidifier and the patient.

Certain humidifiers resist the rain-out problem by placing a heated wire into the tubing. The wire keeps the gas at the desired temperature as it travels through the tubing, thus

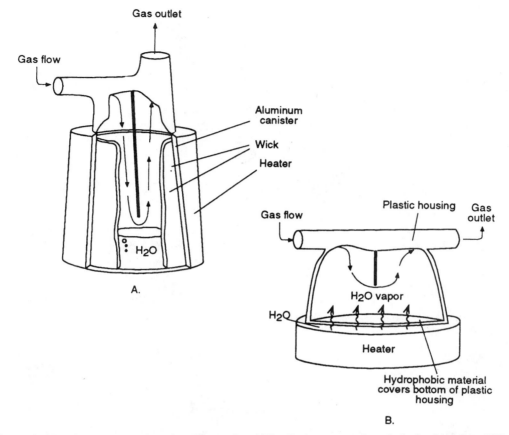

Figure 6–17   *A. A cutaway view of a wick-type humidifier. B. A cutaway view of a hydrophobic humidifier.*

greatly reducing rain-out. These devices (Figure 6–18) are most commonly found on venti-lator circuits. When this type is used, the gas temperature is measured as it exits the humid-ifier and again at the patient connection. By keeping the distal gas temperature warmer than the humidifier temperature, the patient is given a more consistent humidity and tempera-ture of gas, with less rain-out.

Oxygen Hood.   An oxygen hood is a clear, plastic hood that fits over the infant's head, shown in Figure 6–19. It provides an oxygen-enriched environment for the patient with rel-ative ease and comfort. Oxygen hoods are generally used with FiO_2 of less than 0.50. A patient requiring more than 0.50 oxygen can be managed in a hood; however, it becomes difficult to maintain consistent concentrations above that level. This is due in part to the large neck opening and the less-than-tight seal around the edges of the hood, allowing ambient gas to dilute the hood gas.

An infant requiring high levels of oxygen should be closely assessed for signs of respi-ratory distress or other problems. An increasing FiO_2 requirement is frequently the result

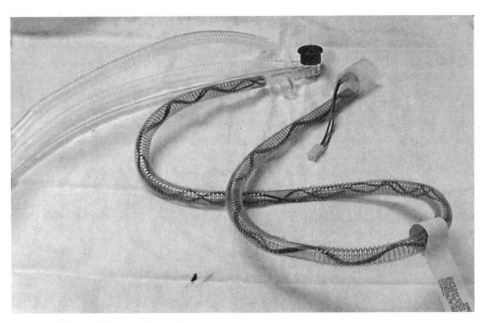

Figure 6–18   *A heated wire ventilator circuit.*

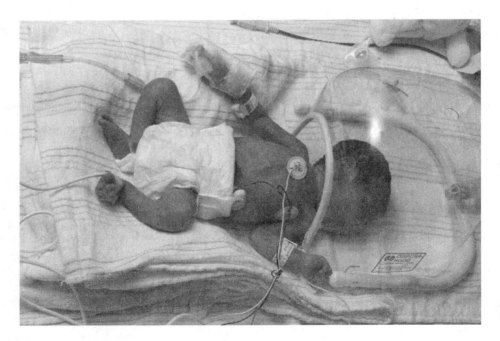

Figure 6–19   *An oxygen hood used to deliver oxygen.*

of worsening respiratory status and may require more intensive measures than an oxygen hood can provide. Due to the layering effect of the oxygen in the hood, the FiO_2 should be monitored at the level of the patient's face to ensure accurate readings.

There are some hazards associated with the use of an oxygen hood that pose potential problems. If too low a gas flow is used, there is a chance of CO_2 retention in the hood. According to Gale and associates, a flow of more than 7 L/min should be used to avoid this problem.[10] Although unlikely, it is also possible for the infant's breathing to become hampered by the face being pressed against the wall of the hood, or the neck opening being too tight and occluding the airway. High or low gas temperatures blown into the hood may cause the infant to overheat or become chilled. This could make thermoregulation of the patient difficult to maintain. To avoid thermoregulatory problems, gas temperatures should be maintained at temperatures equal to that within the incubator.

Oxygen Cannulas and Masks. Oxygen cannulas are used on those patients with chronic oxygen need. Chronic oxygen use is often associated with bronchopulmonary dysplasia (BPD). Cannulas can also be used as a tool to wean the patient from an oxygen hood, gradually weaning the patient to room air. Flows used on the neonatal patient are usually less than 1 L/min. Flows greater than 4 L/min may lead to nasal mucosal drying and *epistaxis* and should be used cautiously. Although the exact FiO_2 delivered via a cannula depends on the patient's age, size, tidal volume, and respiratory rate, it can be estimated. At 0.25 L/min, the FiO_2 will range from 24 to 27%. At 0.50 L/min, approximate FiO_2 is 26 to 32%, and at 1 L/min, the FiO_2 is roughly 30 to 35%.

Neonatal and pediatric cannulas are available from various manufacturers. The pediatric-sized prongs are shorter in length and smaller in diameter than their adult counterparts, due to the smaller size of the pediatric patient. The neonatal cannula has prongs that are even shorter and smaller, accommodating the even smaller neonatal nose and face. An option for the smaller patients is to cut off the prongs and position the resultant hole below the nasal openings (Figure 6–20).

The combination of small size and constant movement may make it difficult to keep the cannula in place. On such difficult patients, it may be helpful to tape the cannula to the face. This is best done with a tape designed to cover IV sites. These tapes have good holding capabilities and can be used for fairly long periods without causing skin breakdowns.

Oxygen masks provide higher percentages of oxygen than cannulas but are used infrequently because they are not tolerated as well by the small patient. Oxygen masks come in assorted designs, each devised for specific oxygen requirements. When used on a neonate, a simple oxygen mask will provide 60 to 80% FiO_2 at 5 L/min when tight against the face. A loosely placed mask provides about 40% FiO_2 at 5 L/min. On the older pediatric patient, liter flows of 6 to 8 L/min provide a range of 35 to 45%, depending on the size and age of the patient.

Nonbreathing masks are similar in design to the simple mask except for the addition of a reservoir bag to the bottom of the mask. There are also rubber flaps over the exhalation ports that allow exhaled gas to exit the mask, but prevent entrainment of room air. This type of mask (Figure 6–21), if functioning properly, can provide 70 to 100% FiO_2 at flows of 6 to 15 L/min.

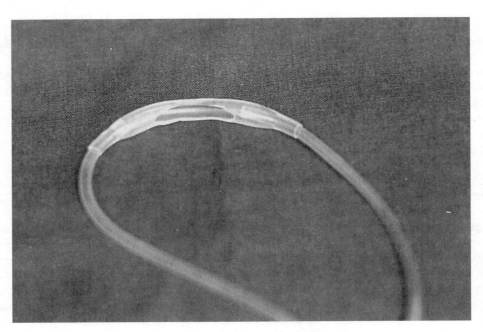

Figure 6–20 *A nasal cannula with the prongs removed for use on preemies.*

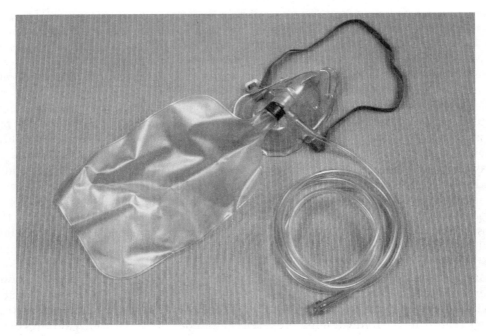

Figure 6–21 *A nonrebreathing oxygen mask.*

Venturi masks (Figure 6–22) use various sized openings on a Venturi device to entrain room air and achieve precise oxygen concentrations in the mask. Common oxygen concentrations available with Venturi masks are 24, 28, 31, 35, 40, and 50%. To achieve the desired FiO_2, it is important to use the proper oxygen liter flow for the particular Venturi device. Total flow entering the mask is a combination of the oxygen flow and the entrained flow of room air. At a concentration of 24%, the entrainment ratio is 20:1. At an oxygen flow of 4 L/min the total flow to the mask is 84 L/min. At a 50% concentration, the ratio is 1.75:1. With an oxygen flow of 12 L/min total flow to the mask is 33 L/min.

Hazards present with the use of any oxygen mask include possible aspiration in vomiting patients, skin necrosis from a tight mask, low FiO_2 if the mask is loose, and CO_2 retention in the presence of low oxygen flows. Whenever a mask is used, it must have an oxygen flow sufficient to flush out the patient's exhaled gases and prevent rebreathing CO_2. To avoid this problem, flows should not be set below 5 L/min. The exception to this is when masks are used on neonatal patients. In these circumstances, lower flows may be used because of the smaller tidal volumes.

Tents. Tents are plastic enclosures that cover the entire patient. Figure 6–23 illustrates one variety of tent. Tents come in various sizes to accommodate a variety of patient sizes. Tents most commonly provide an oxygen-enriched, cool mist to the patient environment for the treatment of croup or other types of upper airway swelling. The internal environment of

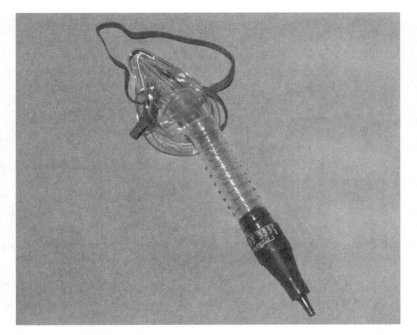

Figure 6–22   *A Venturi-type oxygen mask.*

the tent is cooled from 5 to 10°C below ambient temperature by the effects of evaporation or the use of a refrigeration unit. Due to the large size of the tent and the layering effect of the oxygen, FiO_2 should be monitored near the patient's face to ensure accurate measurement. The tent is usually supported by some type of external or internal framework.

There are several hazards associated with tent use. High-output nebulizers can create a fog inside the tent that makes it difficult to observe the patient. In severe cases of airway obstruction, it is vital to monitor the patient closely and watch for signs of distress. The presence of a thick mist may hamper this effort.

Because of its oxygen-enriched environment, a tent has a higher fire danger. All those working with tents, including parents and the patient, must be familiar with the dangers of flames or sparks in this environment. The patient should not be given toys that create sparks to avoid any possible problems.

Another possible hazard is that the high degree of moisture in the environment could potentially overhydrate the neonatal patient through the respiratory tract. Close monitoring for signs of overhydration should be observed in these patients.

Finally, although extremely unlikely, it is possible that the patient could become asphyxiated by an accidental lodging of the head between the mattress and the tent, or by a collapse of the tent onto the patient. These hazards can be greatly lessened with proper instruction and observation.

Incubators.   Incubators provide a temperature-controlled and relatively quiet environment for the neonatal patient. Figure 6–24 illustrates an incubator. It is possible to provide

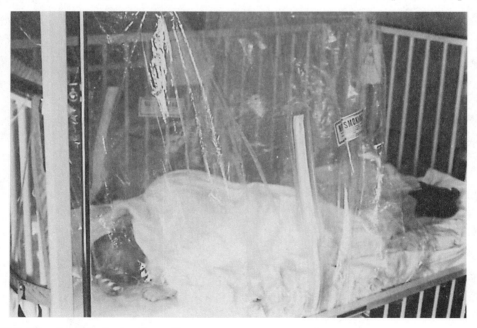

Figure 6–23   *A mist tent set up in a crib.*

the patient's oxygen needs directly into the incubator. Blended, warmed, and humidified oxygen can be blown into the incubator to achieve the desired FiO_2. Due to the previously mentioned effect of oxygen layering, the FiO_2 should be measured near the patient's face.

Most incubators allow the direct flow of oxygen into the incubator through a venturi located on its side. The concentration of oxygen delivered depends on the liter flow of oxygen into the venturi.

The main problem encountered with this type of oxygen delivery is that the constant opening of the doors and portholes and the relatively large size of the incubator make it very difficult to maintain a consistent FiO_2. Ideally, if the patient requires an FiO_2 of higher than 0.25, it may be more easily managed with an oxygen hood.

Resuscitation Bag.   Oxygen delivery via a resuscitation bag is not considered to be a normal route of delivery, but is more commonly used during emergencies or other short-term applications (Figure 6–25). Two types of bags are now in use: self-inflating and flow-inflating.

Self-inflating bags are designed to reinflate following decompression. The gas delivered to the patient is entrained into the bag on each reinflation. With a proper reservoir attached

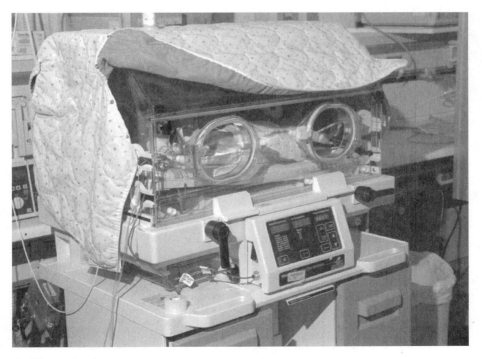

Figure 6–24   *An incubator.*

and sufficient oxygen flow, most self-inflating bags can achieve FiO_2 of between 0.80 and 1.00. Without a reservoir, or with inadequate flow rates, the FiO_2 is unpredictable and not appropriate for most situations.

Flow-rating bags, on the other hand, have the advantage of providing the percentage of oxygen that is used to power them. FiO_2 of 1.0 can be achieved simply by using pure oxygen to inflate the bag. Flow rates are adjusted to allow reinflation of the bag between breaths. Faster rates require higher flows, whereas in the self-inflating bag, the reinflation time remains constant regardless of rate.

Oxygen may be delivered either by blowby or by the use of a pressure mask over the mouth and nose. Use of a resuscitation bag on a neonate or pediatric patient requires that a method of measuring inflating pressures be present.

Modern neonatal resuscitation bags have two ports, usually found on the patient elbow attachment, as seen in Figure 6–26. As indicated by the manufacturer, one port is for the entrainment of oxygen and the other for connection to a pressure manometer. When used on an intubated patient, it may be preferable to entrain the oxygen into the port that is distal to the patient connection. This will prevent a retardation of exhalation caused by the direct flow of gas onto the end of the ETT. The alternate port should be attached to an accurate pressure manometer to monitor ventilatory pressures, avoiding potential barotrauma while bagging. Ideally, a pressure manometer should also be used on a self-inflating bag for the same reasons.

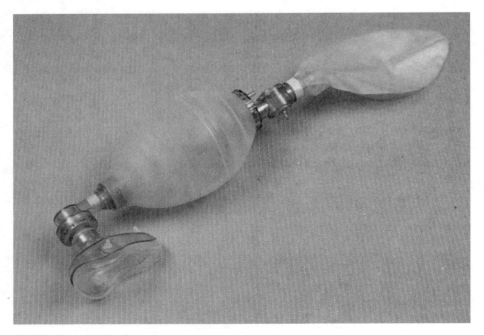

Figure 6–25 *Resuscitation bag.*

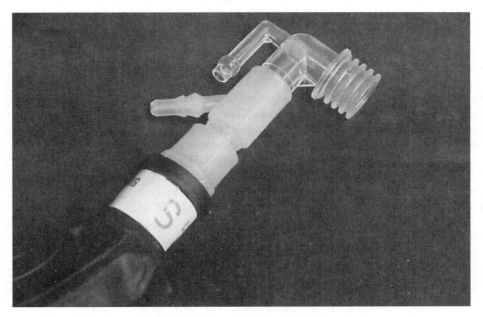

Figure 6–26 *Ports found on the elbow of some neonatal resuscitation bags.*

Pressure masks come in a variety of sizes and shapes. The ideal mask should form a tight seal around the patient's mouth and nose, and not cover the eyes if possible. The seal should be able to be maintained with minimally applied pressure.

SUMMARY

When respiratory care first evolved, technicians were called on to bring oxygen tanks to the various floors. They then began setting up the oxygen tanks in the rooms and attaching the patients to masks and cannulas. As technologies in respiratory care evolved and the understanding of the pulmonary system increased, the respiratory technician was the natural person to fill the new niche created. From simple beginnings, respiratory care has evolved into a highly technical and skilled profession with therapies, treatments, and procedures improving year by year. This chapter is a basic look at the traditional therapies and treatments done by the respiratory care practitioner.

One of the staples of respiratory care through the years is that of chest physiotherapy, or CPT. New techniques have evolved to augment traditional CPT, which includes vibration, percussion, postural drainage, and removal of secretions. These new procedures include forced exhalation technique (FET); active cycle of breathing (ACB); positive expiratory pressure (PEP); autogenic drainage (AD); high-frequency chest compression (HFCC); flutter valve applications; and exercise.

Another traditional treatment modality used in respiratory therapy is the delivery of aerosolized medications. While the small volume nebulizer remains the most common method of delivery, newer delivery techniques such as metered dose inhalers and dry powder inhalers are increasing in popularity.

Studies have fond MDIs to be as effective in aerosol delivery as the SVN, while being easier to administer, with less hazards and complications. A special nebulizer, the SPAG unit, is used exclusively to administer the antiviral drug ribavirin.

Suctioning the patient's airway is a job that is frequently handed to the respiratory care practitioner. If done improperly, suctioning may lead to hypoxemia, bradycardia, and tracheal damage; therefore, the performance of suctioning must follow a strict guideline of proper timing, use of the proper size catheter, insertion to the proper depth, and for the proper time interval. Although following these guidelines does not guarantee an absence of side effects, they can at least be minimized.

The administration of oxygen is probably one of the most common procedures done on patients in the hospital. Neonates and pediatric patients are no exception. Oxygen is delivered via any one of several methods and appliances, depending on the amount of oxygen and humidity needed by the patient.

References

1. Avery GB, Fletcher MA, MacDonald MG. *Pathophysiology and Management of the Newborn*. 5th ed. Philadelphia: JB Lippincott Co; 1999.

2. Lewis R. Chest physical therapy. In: Barnhard SL, Czervinske MP, eds. *Perinatal and Pediatric Respiratory Care*. Philadelphia: WB Saunders Co; 1995.

3. Ward JJ. Lung sounds: easy to hear, hard to describe [editorial]. *Resp Care*. 1989; 34(1):17–19.

4. Fink JB, Jue PK. Humidity and aerosol therapy for pediatrics. In: Barnhart SL, Czervinske MP, eds. *Perinatal and Pediatric Respiratory Care*. Philadelphia: WB Saunders Co; 1995.

5. Southgate WM. Aerosolized pharmacotherapy in the neonate. *Neonatal Network*. 1995;14:29–36.

6. Aerosol Consensus Statement. *Chest*. 1991;100:1006–1009.

7. Pisut FM. Comparison of medication delivery by T-nebulizer with inspiratory and expiratory reservoir. *Resp Care*. 1989;34:985–988.

8. Salyer JW, et al. The effect of continuous in-line nebulization on tidal volume during ventilation of an infant lung model [abstract]. *Resp Care*. 1990;35:1121.

9. Burke M, et al. Music therapy following suctioning: four case studies. *Neonatal Network*. 1995;14:41–49.

10. Gale R, et al. Accumulation of carbon dioxide in oxygen hoods, infant cots and incubators. *Pediatrics*. 1977;60:454.

Bibliography and Suggested Readings

Aloan CA. *Respiratory Care of the Newborn: A Clinical Manual*. 2nd ed. Philadelphia: JB Lippincott Co; 1997.

Andersen JB, Falk M. Chest physiotherapy in the pediatric age group. *Resp Care.* 1991;36:546–554.

Barnhart SL, Czervinske MP. *Perinatal and Pediatric Respiratory Care.* Philadelphia: WB Saunders Co; 1995.

Bloom RS, Cropley C. *Textbook of Neonatal Resuscitation.* Dallas: American Heart Association/American Academy of Pediatrics; 1994.

Burton GG, et al. *Respiratory Care, a Guide to Clinical Practice,* 4th ed. Philadelphia: JB Lippincott Co; 1997.

Dantzker DR, MacIntyre NR, Bakow ED. *Comprehensive Respiratory Care.* Philadelphia: WB Saunders Co; 1995.

Goldsmith JP, Karotkin EH. *Assisted Ventilation of the Neonate.* 3rd ed. Philadelphia: WB Saunders Co; 1996.

Hardy KA. A review of airway clearance: new techniques, indications, and recommendations. *Resp Care.* 1994;39:440–452.

Hierholzer WJ, chairman. Guideline for prevention of nosocomial pneumonia: Centers for Disease Control and Prevention. *Resp Care.* 1994;39:1191–1236.

Kacmarek RM. Ribavirin and pentamidine aerosols: caregiver beware [editorial]. *Resp Care.* 1990;35:1034–1035.

Kacmarek RM, et al. *Current Respiratory Care.* Burlington, Vt: BC Decker Inc; 1988.

McPherson SP. *Respiratory Therapy Equipment.* 6th ed. St. Louis: CV Mosby Co; 1999.

Pilbeam SP. *Mechanical Ventilation: Physiological and Clinical Applications.* St. Louis: Mosby; 1998.

Shapiro BA, Peruzzi WT, Kozlowski-Templin R. *Clinical Application of Blood Gases.* 5th ed. St. Louis: Mosby; 1994.

Taussig LM, Landau LI. *Pediatric Respiratory Medicine.* St. Louis: Mosby; 1999.

Tucker SM. *Pocket Guide to Fetal Monitoring and Assessment.* 4th ed. St. Louis: Mosby; 2000.

Posttest

1. Of the following, which are indicates for CPT?
   I. asthma
   II. atelectasis
   III. cystic fibrosis
   IV. prolonged bed rest
   V. ventilator care
     a. I, III, IV
     b. II, III, IV
     c. I, II, IV, V
     d. I, II, III, IV, V

2. To ensure maximum effectiveness, PEP should be followed by what technique?
     a. FET
     b. autogenic drainage
     c. high-frequency chest compressions
     d. CPT with postural drainage

3. Which of the following is not part of traditional CPT?
   a. postural drainage
   b. percussion
   c. hyperoxygenation
   d. removal of secretions

4. Which of the following modalities to administer aerosolized medication requires the least amount of patient coordination?
   a. MDI alone
   b. MDI with a spacer
   c. SVN
   d. DPI

5. Of the following, which are indications for aerosolized medication therapy?
   I. wheezing
   II. retractions
   III. increased respiratory rate
   IV. increased peak expiratory flow
   V. increasing FiO_2 requirements
      a. I, III, IV, V
      b. II, IV
      c. II, III, V
      d. II, III, V

6. One advantage to the mainstream nebulizer is that:
   a. it is less expensive
   b. it can be used horizontally
   c. it produces smaller particle size
   d. it can be reused

7. Placement of a medication nebulizer in the ventilator circuit between the humidifier and the distal temperature probe may cause:
   a. overheating of the circuit when the nebulizer is removed
   b. malfunction of the nebulizer
   c. overhydration of the infant
   d. contamination of the ventilator circuit

8. Which of the following would be considered hazards of aerosol drug therapy?
   I. infection
   II. medication side effects
   III. drug reconcentration
   IV. overhydration
   V. intraventricular hemorrhage
      a. I, II, III, IV
      b. III, IV, V
      c. II, III, IV
      d. I, II, IV, V

9. Which of the following is not a disadvantage of MDI therapy?
   a. fixed drug concentrations

b. not indicated in patients younger than 12 years

c. possible reaction to the propellants

d. possible oropharyngeal impaction

10. The *greatest* hazard associated with the aerosolization of ribavirin into a ventilator circuit is:

   a. medication may not reach the patient

   b. precipitation and accumulation of the drug on vent tubing and ETT

   c. malfunction of the oxygen analyzer

   d. patient may receive a lethal dose of the medication

11. While suctioning the endotracheal tube following a CPT treatment, the patient becomes bradycardic. Which of the following should the respiratory care practitioner do?

   a. continue the procedure, but shorten the duration of suctioning

   b. stop the procedure and order a stat chest x-ray

   c. when done, select a larger catheter and use less negative pressure

   d. stop the procedure, hyperoxygenate the patient, and shorten the duration of suction with subsequent attempts.

12. The main indication for oxygen administration is:

   a. increasing altitude

   b. barotrauma

   c. hypoxemia

   d. hyperventilation

13. Which of the following is true regarding gaseous oxygen?

   a. it supports and intensifies combustion

   b. it causes spontaneous combustion in plastics

   c. it is the sole causative factor in the development of ROP

   d. its atmospheric concentration is higher at sea level.

14. The type of flowmeter often found on cylinder regulators is the:

   a. Thorpe tube

   b. Bourdon gauge

   c. dual reducing valve

   d. Wilkinson tube

15. A bubble humidifier is best used with what type of oxygen administration device?

   a. ventilator

   b. head box

   c. cannula

   d. incubator

16. A physician orders a pediatric patient to be on an FiO_2 of 0.35. Which of the following devices would best deliver the ordered FiO_2?

   a. cannula at 3 L/min

   b. simple mask at 6 L/min

   c. nonrebreathing mask

   d. Venturi mask

CHAPTER SEVEN

GENERAL CONSIDERATIONS OF CONTINUING CARE

OBJECTIVES

Upon the completion of this chapter, the reader should be able to:

1. Discuss the physiology of thermoregulation, including a description of the thermoneutral zone and nonshivering thermogenesis.
2. Define the internal thermal gradient (ITG) and describe the reasons why a preemie has a decreased ability to maintain its ITG.
3. Describe each of the following as it relates to the external thermal gradient (ETG). Include examples for each type of heat loss and a description of how each method of heat loss may be prevented or reduced in the nursery.
   a. Radiant
   b. Conductive
   c. Convective
   d. Evaporative
4. Describe how a neonate reacts to cold stress and to hyperthermia.
5. Discuss thermoregulation of the neonate in the delivery room and nursery to include methods of heat loss prevention.
6. Compare and contrast incubators and open warmers, focusing on the advantages, disadvantages, and thermoregulation in each.
7. Explain the physiologic effects of overstimulation of the premature neonate.
8. Identify and describe those factors involved in behavioral-based care.
9. Describe the use of environmental controls and parental involvement in reducing overstimulation and increasing more normal interactions and relationships.
10. Describe the physiologic factors that make the skin of the preemie more susceptible to trauma.
11. Discuss those factors that will reduce skin trauma on the neonate.
12. Describe the distribution of body water and its solutes. Compare and contrast the percentage of extracellular fluid and intracellular fluid between the preemie and the term neonate.
13. Describe the balance principle as it pertains to fluid and electrolyte balance. Identify the components of intake and output.

14. Identify and describe the three methods of determining fluid deficit. Estimate the degree of deficit when given patient clinical data.
15. Identify at least five factors that influence insensible water loss. Calculate the approximate insensible water loss when given the necessary information.
16. Describe the functions of sodium, potassium, calcium, magnesium, chloride, and phosphate in the neonate.
17. Relate the causes of hyponatremia, hypernatremia, hypokalemia, hyperkalemia, hypocalcemia, hypercalcemia, hypomagnesemia, and hypermagnesemia.
18. Describe how electrolytes are maintained and the importance of monitoring electrolytes.
19. With regard to jaundice, describe the following:
    a. Physiology
    b. Causes
    c. Pathologic jaundice
    d. Complications
    e. Treatment
20. Describe the clinical signs and treatment of necrotizing enterocolitis.

KEY TERMS

anaerobic	gastroschisis	myelomeningocele
brown fat	guaiac	omphalocele
conjugated	hydrops fetalis	parenteral
Crigler-Najjar syndrome	hypersosmolar	servo-controlled
encephalocele	hypotonia	sodium-potassium exchange resin
enteral	kernicterus	stratum corneum
galactosemia	Lucey-Driscol syndrome	turgor

THERMOREGULATION

Homeostatic thermoregulation can best be defined as the maintenance of equality between heat dissipation and heat production by the body. Normal thermoregulatory mechanisms maintain a balance of heat production and heat loss to maintain a core temperature of 37°C. Thermoregulation is one of the most important aspects in the care of the neonate. The human neonate is extremely vulnerable to cold stress and its complications at birth.

Heat balance must be considered in all aspects of the care of the neonate and must be constantly monitored and evaluated. Human neonates have the ability to maintain fairly stable core temperatures when placed in a proper environmental temperature.

After delivery, an environmental temperature should be maintained that falls within the thermoneutral zone. The thermoneutral zone is that temperature range in which the metabolic rate is at a minimum and, thus, oxygen consumption is at its lowest. When this temperature is achieved, the neonate is thermally balanced with its environment, neither gain-ing nor losing heat. There is no exact environmental temperature at which all neonates will achieve thermoneutrality. This is due to the diversity of metabolic rate, gestational age, and weight. Current recommendations are to maintain an environmental temperature that achieves a rectal temperature of 36.5 to 37.5°C and an abdominal skin temperature of 36 to 36.5°C.

In the adult, heat can be produced by metabolic and physical activity (shivering). The newborn, however, has a diminished shivering response and relies entirely on the metabolism of brown fat for heat production. Around gestational weeks 26 to 30, the first *brown fat* cells appear. The cells enlarge in size and number as the pregnancy advances. The fetus stores the brown fat around the great vessels, kidneys, scapulas, axilla, and the nape of the neck. Brown fat is highly vascularized and innervated by neurons from the sympathetic system.

In the presence of cold stress, the neonate responds by increasing stimulation of the sympathetic nervous system. Increased stimulation causes an increase in the amount of norepinephrine released. Norepinephrine is released from the nerve endings in the sympathetic system. Increased levels of norepinephrine activate lipase, which breaks the brown fat into free fatty acids. These acids are then hydrolyzed into glycerol and nonesterified fatty acids. The oxidation of the nonesterified fatty acids produces heat, which then increases the baby's temperature. This breakdown of brown fat with the subsequent production of heat is called nonshivering thermogenesis.

THE PHYSIOLOGY OF HEAT LOSS

Heat loss from the core of the body in the environment follows two gradients (Figure 7–1).

Internal Thermal Gradient. The internal thermal gradient (ITG) is the temperature difference between the warm body core and the cooler skin. The ITG is regulated by many factors. Among these are the metabolic rate, the amount of subcutaneous fat present, the amount of surface area available for dissipation of heat, and the distance from the body core to the skin surface.

A premature neonate has a diminished ability to maintain the ITG for several reasons. Neonates have a large amount of skin surface area in relation to body weight. This results in a large area for heat to dissipate. The premature neonate has a relatively thin layer of skin and decreased amounts of subcutaneous and brown fat. Consequently, it has less insulation to prevent heat loss. Additionally, the brown fat stores deplete rapidly, resulting in a loss of the ability to generate heat through nonshivering thermogenesis.

Another factor is that the preemie is often unable to take in enough calories to maintain the level of nutrients for heat production. The metabolic response of the preemie to cold is impaired by hypoxemia. This presents a problem because most premature neonates suffer some degree of pulmonary problem leading to hypoxemia. Frequent handling, which is often required in the care of the preemie, disposes the patient to the cold environment outside the incubator.

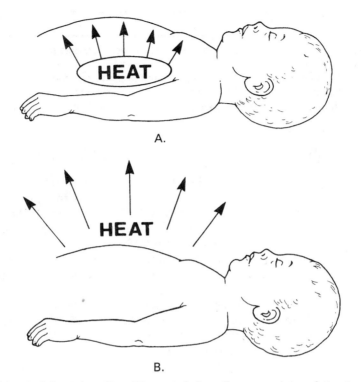

Figure 7–1 *A. The internal thermal gradient. Heat travels from the warmer internal structures to the cooler skin. B. The external thermal gradient. Heat travels from the skin to the cooler environment.*

External Thermal Gradient. The temperature difference between the skin and the environment is called the external thermal gradient (ETG). The ETG is determined by environmental factors that are controllable by the practitioner. There are four factors that determine heat loss through the ETG, listed in Table 7–1 and described below.

Radiant heat loss is the dissipation of heat from the neonate to cooler objects that surround the patient but are not in direct contact. The cooler objects are not limited to those within the incubator, but may be in the same room, or even outdoors if a window is nearby. The radiation of the sun's heat is an example of radiant heat.

Conduction is the transfer of heat from the body to a cooler surface on which the neonate is lying. The colder the surface, the more heat is lost. Conduction of heat can also occur in reverse if the surface is warmer than the skin.

Convection is the loss of heat from the skin to moving air. The velocity and the temperature of the air determine the amount of heat lost. Convection is the principle behind wind chill factors, which make temperatures colder in a wind.

As water changes states from a liquid to a gas, heat is released. This is called evaporation. Evaporative loss occurs as insensible (from the skin and respiratory tract), and sensible (sweating from the skin).

TABLE 7–1   Methods of Heat Loss

- Radiant—the dissipation of heat from the neonate to cooler objects surrounding but not touching the neonate.
- Conductive—the transfer of heat from the neonate to a cooler surface in contact with the neonate.
- Convective—the loss of heat from the neonate to air current passing over the neonate.
- Evaporative—the loss of heat that accompanies the evaporation of water from the surface of the neonate's skin.

COLD STRESS: RESPONSE AND COMPLICATIONS

Thermoreceptors located in the skin detect changes in environmental temperature. Receptors located in the face are the most sensitive and respond the quickest. A cold stress, or hypothermia, is any lowering of the thermoneutral temperature. It should be remembered that the adult thermoneutral zone is far below that of the newborn. A cold environmental temperature for the neonate may be uncomfortably warm or even hot to the adult.

Cold stress can be initiated by the opening of incubator doors or cold gas blowing onto the neonate from a resuscitation bag. It may also be triggered by placing the neonate on a cold scale or countertop.

The initial response to hypothermia is peripheral vasoconstriction. This results in a shunt of the blood away from the skin, helping to maintain the ITG. Peripheral vasoconstriction, however, leads to *anaerobic* metabolism and metabolic acidosis. The presence of acidosis may lead to pulmonary vasoconstriction with worsening hypoxemia and acidosis. Hypoxemia acts to further restrict the neonate's response to the cold stress and worsens the acidosis. Simultaneously, the hypothermia triggers nonshivering thermogenesis, which boosts heat output. With the increased metabolism of brown fat, glucose levels begin to fall, potentially leading to hypoglycemia.

The combination of peripheral vasoconstriction and brown fat metabolism causes the neonate's body temperature to remain homeostatic for a time. If the stress is corrected quickly, the patient may suffer no permanent effects. A continued cold stress, however, may lead to the deterioration of the patient condition and possibly death. A neonate who is being continually cold stressed may maintain normal body temperature, but at the expense of critical calories needed for growth.

RESPONSE TO HYPERTHERMIA

Hyperthermia, as opposed to hypothermia, is temperature that is above normal. The effects of hyperthermia can be as severe as those associated with hypothermia. The initial response of the neonate is a vasodilation of the peripheral vessels to help dissipate heat. This is followed by an increase in metabolism and oxygen consumption. Hyperthermia may result from infection, dehydration, improperly functioning incubators, radiant warmers, humidifiers, and phototherapy lights.

Continuous monitoring of patient and environmental temperature is essential to avoid hyperthermia from malfunctioning equipment.

THERMOREGULATION IN THE DELIVERY ROOM

The goal of thermoregulation in the delivery room is to maintain an environmental temperature such that the neonate's core temperature remains in the normal range of 36.5 to 37.5°C. To achieve this goal, all avenues of heat loss must be minimized or eliminated.

Prevention of Evaporative Loss. The neonate is at the highest risk of heat loss shortly after delivery. Every newborn should immediately be completely dried with a prewarmed towel or blanket. The head and face are particularly important. This drying helps reduce evaporative heat losses.

Prevention of Radiant Loss. The neonate should then be wrapped in a warm blanket and immediately placed beneath a radiant heater for resuscitation or examinations. A cap or other covering should be placed on the head as shown in Figure 7–2. Due to a tremendous amount of heat loss from the head, placement of a cap greatly reduces heat loss.

Prevention of Convective and Conductive Loss. The small preemie is more easily thermoregulated if placed on a warming mattress. The neonate should be kept covered as much as possible while on the open warmer to avoid convective losses. As quickly as possible, the neonate should be placed in a prewarmed incubator. The longer the patient is left out in the open, the greater the chance of hypothermia.

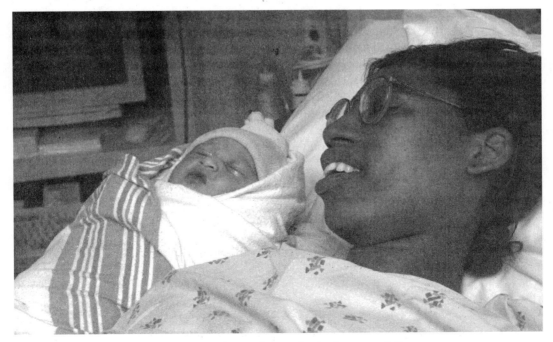

Figure 7–2 *Placement of a cap on a newborn to help maintain thermoregulation*

THERMOREGULATION IN THE NURSERY

Incubators and Thermoregulation. Once in the incubator, several precautions can be taken to avoid unnecessary heat loss. Skin temperature should be maintained at 36.5°C by a *servo-controlled* incubator. As previously discussed, at a skin temperature of 36 to 36.5°C, metabolism is at its lowest point. The servo-control uses the skin temperature to increase or decrease the heat output of the incubator into the environment. The operator designates a set point for skin temperature. If skin temperature falls below the set point, the incubator warms the environmental temperature until skin temperature rises above the set point. At that point, the heater returns to its normal output.

Modern incubators also monitor the environmental temperature and maintain it at neu-trothermal ranges. When using a servo-control, it is vital that the skin probe be securely attached to the neonate. Hyperthermia could occur if the skin probe becomes loose.

Radiant heat losses can be lessened by several methods. Modern incubators incorporate an inner plastic wall on the interior of the incubator (Figure 7–3). This inner wall is warmed to the incubator's environmental temperature and thus reduces the amount of heat that is radiated by the baby to the external wall of the incubator. Aluminum foil can also be used to line the interior of the incubator (Figure 7–4) to reflect radiant heat back toward the patient. Radiant losses can also be lessened if the incubator is kept away from air condi-tioner ducts and windows, which cool the external wall.

Conductive losses can be minimized by using warming mattresses or other warming devices under the patient.

A common cause of convective heat loss in the incubator is resuscitation bag that is left on, blowing cold gas over the patient's head. If the resuscitation bag is to be left on, it should be positioned so it does not blow on the patient.

Evaporative heat loss can be controlled by creating a "swamp" environment around the patient. This is done by directing warmed and humidified gas into the incubator.

Thermoregulation in Open Warmers. Radiant heat loss is difficult to manage in the open warmer. Placing a shield over the neonate reduces the amount of radiant loss, but it also reduces access to the infant. Reduction of patient access takes away a major advantage of using an open warmer.

Evaporative heat loss in the open warmer can be minimized by providing a closed envi-ronment around the patient and creating a "swamp" as described above.

Convective heat loss is lessened by keeping the neonate out of areas of air movement. Convective losses are most profound in open warmers, where it may be necessary to cover the patient with plastic or a shield to protect it from air currents. Shields and plastic sheets can also be used in the incubator to protect the small preemie from convective and radiant losses.

Conductive heat loss can be lessened by not placing the neonate on cold surfaces or allowing cold items to come in contact with the skin. In the open warmer, the patient should be placed on blankets that insulate the neonate from the cold mattress. A common source of conductive heat loss is weighing the neonate. The procedure of weighing requires that the patient be placed directly on the scale with only a paper covering. Weights should be

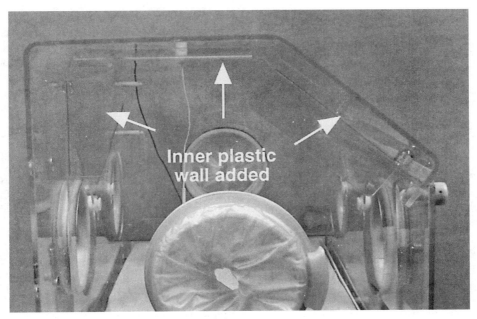

Figure 7–3 *The addition of an inner wall to the incubator to reduce radiant heat loss to the cooler incubator wall*

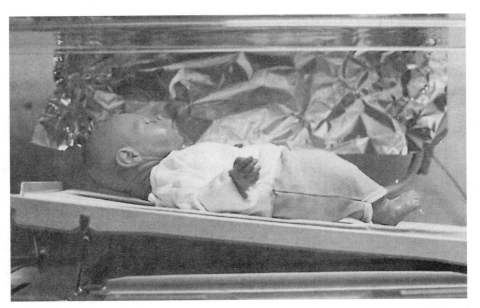

Figure 7–4 *A sheet of aluminum foil lining the incubator. The foil reflects back heat toward the patient, reducing radiant heat loss.*

done as quickly as possible to reduce conductive losses. An alternative method is to keep the patient covered while weighing, removing the coverings after the patient is returned to the incubator, and weighing the coverings alone. The weight of the coverings is then subtracted to arrive at the weight of the patient.

INCUBATORS VERSUS OPEN WARMERS

The perfect device to maintain thermoregulation in the neonate has yet to be developed. Modern incubators and open warmers each serve a distinct purpose.

Open Warmers. The primary advantage of the open warmer (Figure 7–5) is access to the patient. This is critical during times of resuscitation or other emergencies where several people must have access to the patient. Disadvantages include difficulty in thermal management and the inability to control the environment.

Incubators. One advantage to the use of an incubator is that it provides a controlled environment that allows for better thermal management. The closed environment may also serve as a barrier to excessive handling of the patient by nursery personnel. The incubator also provides a somewhat quieter environment than the open warmer. The major disadvantage to an incubator is in patient access. During an emergency, it may be necessary to remove the neonate from the incubator to allow adequate access for procedures.

DEVELOPMENTAL NEEDS OF THE HIGH-RISK NEONATE

Much discussion and research has occurred over the past decade surrounding the developmental needs of high-risk neonates. Before the 1980s, the NICU was viewed as a sensory deficient environment. Many believed that hospitalized neonates needed considerable stimulation to overcome their functional disabilities. It was also believed that normal functioning would occur more quickly if aggressive development therapies were used.

More recently, concerns have centered around the impact of the environment on the developing nervous system of the neonate. There exists significant clinical evidence that the environment as well as treatment protocols affect the systemic and cerebral circulation, as well as oxygenation. These studies have revealed a possible causal relation between NICU caregiving protocols and physiologic stress. More recent studies have demonstrated that care must be individualized to the patient, because no two neonates respond to environmental stimulation the same way. It has been recommended that each infant be individually assessed and a specific care plan started.[1]

PHYSIOLOGIC CONSIDERATIONS

The nervous system of a neonate is anatomically immature. The chemical and physiologic function of the nervous system is primitive when compared to the adult. Additionally, the

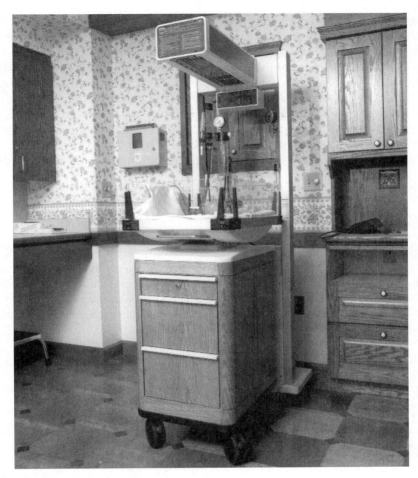

Figure 7–5 *An open warmer.*

cerebral hemispheres show poor distinction between gray and white matter. Most neuronal cells, which conduct nerve impulses, are present at birth but are immature in their function. In the premature neonate, there is little nerve myelination and the synaptic junctions are at an early stage of formation. It appears that neurologic function in a neonate is largely controlled at the brain stem and spinal cord level, and that existing brain functions are hyperreactive.

THE EFFECTS OF OVERSTIMULATION

Immature or stressed neonates have limited energy and can be exhausted by excessive stimulation. With the increased survival rate of premature neonates, the risk for developmental handicaps and morbidity in the presence of overstimulation is increased. Studies have shown that the preterm neonate finds itself in a "mismatch" between brain expectancy and environmental input leading to a form of self-analgesia.[2] It has been theorized that the NICU environment may interfere with both the maturation and the organization of the neonate's central nervous system. Furthermore, it is felt that another imbalance exists in that hearing and vision receive overwhelming overload, while tactile and vestibular needs are not met. A study by Zahr and Balian demonstrated significant changes in both behavioral and physiologic responses to typical nursing interventions and NICU noises.[3]

The importance for the practitioner then is to reduce the amount of visual and acoustic stimulation in the NICU. Early intervention can reduce long-term disability in this patient group.

BEHAVIORAL-BASED CARE

Behavioral-based care is founded on the concept that care is provided to the neonate based on observed behaviors that indicate times of nonstress. The positive effects of intervention may be diminished if stimuli is offered at inappropriate times. It is therefore important to correlate interventions with times of nonstress. The approach then is to develop a plan of behaviorally supported care for each at-risk neonate. The timing of patient stimulation should be based on several factors, as listed in Table 7–2.

TABLE 7–2   The Timing of Patient Stimulation

Sleep/wake state
Activity level
Approachability
Oxygenation status

Neonates should not be stimulated while they are asleep. Sleeping patients should not be disturbed, to allow a conservation of energy and to prevent a negative response by the neonate. Stimulation should be avoided when behavioral stress cues (such as gaze aversion, facial grimaces, hiccoughs, and irritability) and physiologic cues (cyanosis, hypoxemia) are present.

Neonates should be handled only when behavioral and physiologic signs dictate. The timing of interventions is an important key to an effective, safe interaction. Clustering of caregiving and procedures should be minimized to allow adequate recovery time between treatments and to decrease the chance of overstimulation. Nonemergency procedures should be postponed or delayed if possible.

The practitioner should ensure that oxygenation is adequate before and during interventions. If oxygen saturations decrease during intervention, it should be stopped and then restarted when saturation is acceptable. The neonate should be turned and positioned only as necessary. The neonate's response to procedures, especially if stressful, should be monitored for a minimum of 5 minutes following completion. One method that has shown promise in reducing the stress of minor pain and stress-inducing procedures is facilitated tucking. This is done by holding the patient's extremities flexed and close to the body.

ENVIRONMENTAL CONTROLS

Environmental controls to decrease excess stimulation should be instituted in the NICU whenever possible. These include scheduled periods without intervention or "quiet time." The patient should not be disturbed during this time, except in an emergency. Care should be taken to avoid loud noises and bright lighting. The importance of reduced lighting is detailed in a study that showed a significance in oxygen saturation in neonates who were subjected to increasing light brightness. Both workers and parents should avoid loud laughing and talking at the bedside. Attention to details such as the quiet closing of garbage can lids and incubator portholes makes a tremendous difference. Critically ill neonates should be placed in a bedspace where traffic and noise level are minimal.

One method that has been shown to decrease the noise level in the incubator is to cover it with a custom-made blanket.[4] This method is not without its critics, however. They point out that covering the incubator does not allow for visualization of the patient. Thus, serious problems such as extubation, kinking of the endotracheal tube, IV problems, or loss of an umbilical artery catheter may go unnoticed until serious complications have occurred.[5]

PARENTAL INVOLVEMENT

Efforts to involve the parents in the care of their neonate should begin as soon as possible. Parents should be taught ways in which they can help in the care of their newborn. Being a part of the team not only helps the parents overcome feelings of helplessness, but also helps bond the infant-parent relationship. A strong relationship between the neonate and the parents is an accurate predictor of good future cognitive function in the neonate.

One tool, kangaroo care, is beneficial for both the infant and parent. Kangaroo care involves placing the infant upright on the parent's chest for skin-to-skin contact (Figure 7–6). Kangaroo care has been shown to help parents overcome the feelings of separation with their infant. For the infant, it has been shown to reduce the amount of time in active states and to promote deep sleep.[6]

SKIN CARE OF THE PREMATURE NEONATE

Of special concern when working with premature neonates is the care and protection of the skin. Understanding several factors relative to fetal skin development will aid in good skin care.

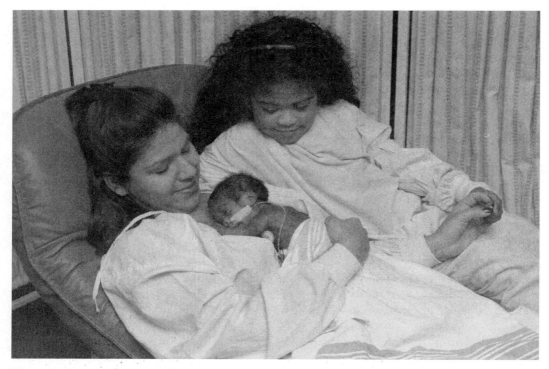

Figure 7–6 *Kangaroo care for a premature infant.*

PHYSIOLOGIC FACTORS

The skin of the premature neonate is very permeable to anything placed on it. Toxic substances used on adult skin for protection or to remove adhesive tape absorb very readily into the preemie's skin, creating the potential for systemic effects.

Another factor is a diminished cohesion between the surface epidermis and the underlying dermis. The bond between an adhesive tape and the epidermis may be stronger than the epidermal/dermal bond. The result is potential epidermal stripping when removing the tape.

The skin of the preemie is additionally sensitive because the *stratum corneum* layer is extremely thin. This is the top layer of the epidermis, which serves as the main barrier against microorganisms. Tape removal could very easily result in the removal of the stratum corneum.

Intensive care medicine requires that many monitors and other devices be taped to the skin of the neonate. These include temperature probes, umbilical artery catheters, endotracheal tubes, transcutaneous monitors, and pulse oximeters. Conventional-medical tapes are traditionally used to secure these devices. Many times, barriers such as tincture of benzoin are sprayed or painted onto the skin to enhance adhesion of the tape. Because of the above mentioned problems with the skin of these patients, severe damage may occur to the skin when these tapes are removed.

SKIN CARE RECOMMENDATIONS

With the above information in mind, some practical applications can be implemented to reduce damage to the skin of the preemie. Only mild soaps should be used when cleaning the skin. These soaps are best applied with a cotton ball to avoid abrading the skin.

Many spray-on skin barriers are plastic polymers, which may absorb into the skin and lead to systemic toxicity. Traditional adhesive removal swabs are saturated with a solvent that is readily absorbed through the premature patient's skin. There are adhesive removal swabs currently available that use citrus oils that are nontoxic to dissolve the adhesive barrier. These would be the preferred adhesive removers to use on the preemie.

One recent study examined the use of pectin-based adhesives. Pectin-based adhesives are used to secure ostomy bags to the abdomen. The study looked at the use of the barrier between the skin and the tape to lessen epidermal damage and at the same time allow adequate adhesion of the device to the skin. The results of this study show that pectin-based adhesive should be used between the skin and tape whenever the taping of equipment to the skin is necessary.[7]

Monitors such as transcutaneous monitors (TCMs) or pulse oximeters must be next to the skin to perform functionally. On the premature patient, both devices may be held in place with Coban-type wraps or fabric straps using a Velcro closure (Figure 7–7). Coban is a stretchable bandage material that sticks to itself but does not stick to skin.

A final recommendation is the use of transparent IV site dressing covers to protect areas of skin excoriation or breakdown. This will protect the injured area from further damage and allow the skin to heal.

FLUID AND ELECTROLYTE BALANCE

Water is the major component of both the fetus and the newborn. Other compounds are dissociated, transported, dissolved, or transported in water. These compounds may also undergo chemical reactions within water and contribute to cellular and body functions. Compounds that dissolve in water and separate into charged particles (ions) capable of conducting an electric current are called electrolytes. Electrolytes are essential for cellular and organ functions and to maintain fluid and acid-base balance.

Fetal fluid and electrolyte status is regulated by both maternal and fetal mechanisms. Maternal disorders of fluid and electrolyte balance, diseases that affect uterine perfusion, and maternal IV therapy during labor may create a fluid and electrolyte imbalance in the neonate at birth. Most fetuses, however, are born in reasonable fluid balance for their gestation.

After birth, changes in fluid and electrolyte balance must occur, which are dependent on gestational age. The neonate's own regulatory mechanisms, combined with the interventions of the caretakers, unite to achieve fluid and electrolyte balance. Abnormalities in fluid

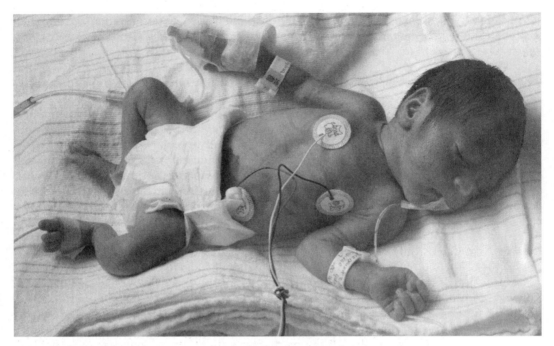

Figure 7–7 *A pulse oximeter strapped to the foot of a premature infant.*

and electrolyte balance occur with certain disease states. These diseases include respiratory disorders, asphyxia, congenital heart disease, *hydrops fetalis*, sepsis, renal disorders, urinary tract anomalies, endocrine disorders, and decreased skin integrity.

DISTRIBUTION OF BODY WATER

Total body water (TBW) decreases from a high of 95% of body weight at 13 to 14 weeks to approximately 78% of body weight at term. TBW is the total of extracellular fluid (ECF) and intracellular fluid (ICF). ECF is further divided into two compartments: interstitial fluid (ISF), which bathes many of the cells of the body, and intravascular fluid, which is the plasma volume (PV).

As gestation increases, and continuing postnatally, ECF decreases while ICF increases. ECF is greater in volume than ICF prenatally, but at about 3 months of age ICF volume passes and exceeds ECF. At term, ECF is roughly 45% of body weight, whereas ICF is 33% of body weight. This progression is shown in Figure 7–8. Postnatal changes in ECF are the most dramatic occurrence in the fluid and electrolyte adaptation of the neonate.

During the first days after birth most neonates experience a decrease in TBW caused by a reduction in ECF. The ECF volume shrinks secondary to a loss of water and ECF electrolytes. This results in a 5 to 15% decrease in weight from birth weight. During these first few days, several periods of diuresis may occur, resulting in full-term neonates losing about 5 to 10% of their birth weight in water, and premature neonates about 5 to 15% of their birth weight.

The timing of this reduction in ECF is altered in certain disease states, most notably in those associated with respiratory distress. An improvement in the respiratory status often follows the onset of diuresis. An exception to this is respiratory distress syndrome (RDS), where induced diuresis is not followed by the same degree of improvement. Excess fluid and/or water intake during the first few days expands the ECF and may delay patient improvement or cause deterioration in cardiopulmonary status.

DISTRIBUTION OF SOLUTES

The total body solute composition changes as gestational age advances. The total amount of sodium and chloride per kg/weight decreases with increasing gestational age. These changes are a result of the decrease in ECF. Total body potassium content per kg/weight remains relatively constant throughout gestation.

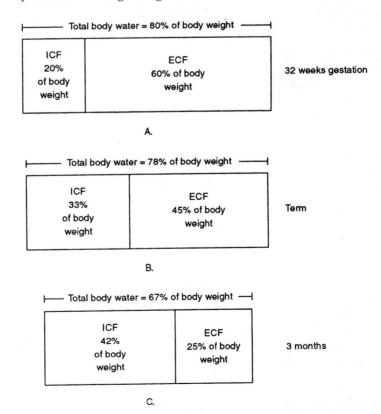

Figure 7–8 *The comparison of ECF to ICF: A. a 32–week preemie; B. a term neonate; and C. a 3-month-old infant*

The main electrolytes of the ECF are sodium and chloride. The minor electrolytes are potassium, calcium, magnesium, bicarbonate, and protein. Plasma and interstitial fluid are similar in composition, with the exception that plasma has a higher amount of protein.

The major electrolytes of ICF are potassium, magnesium, and phosphate, with sodium and bicarbonate being present in much smaller quantities than in ECF. Postnatally, the distribution of the electrolytes reflects the changes in body fluid distribution. For example, as ECF volume decreases with increasing postnatal age, total body sodium and chloride content per kg/weight continue to decrease. During the first weeks after birth, ICF electrolyte content per kg/weight remains relatively unchanged.

Postnatally, the intake of the neonate will influence the establishing of electrolyte homeostasis. Most important in this regard is sodium intake. Excess sodium intake delays contraction of the ECF in the early neonatal period. This is particularly true when combined with excess water intake.

Because sodium is mainly found in the ECF and water remains with the sodium, excess sodium prevents the reduction of the ECF and may even cause it to increase. The excess volume in the ECF may worsen and/or delay improvement in cardiorespiratory disorders. The premature neonate is especially vulnerable to this because of renal immaturity.

BALANCE PRINCIPLE

Like other organisms, the neonate's body water composition is determined by input minus output. When the input equals the patient's output, it is said to meet the neonates' maintenance requirements. In this situation, the fluid, electrolyte, and nutritional requirements are the same as the losses. There will therefore be no weight gain or loss when input and output are balanced.

When intake and output are not equal, this balance is upset. When the intake of a given component exceeds its output, the neonate is said to be in positive balance with regard to that component. Conversely, when output is more than intake, there is a negative balance for that component.

Adequate growth requires that intake exceed output in the proper proportions. Weight gain is not synonymous with growth. As discussed previously excess water and/or sodium intake, or the inability to excrete water and/or sodium, may result in overexpansion of the ECF. Under these circumstances there is a weight gain but no growth of new issues. Similarly, weight loss may reflect water or sodium losses in excess of intake, rather than inadequate nutrition.

In the first few days of life, there normally exists a negative balance for most components. The negative balance of sodium and water during this period results in the reduction of the ECF. With growth, there is a positive sodium and water balance, although the increase in ECF is proportionately less than the increase in the rest of the body.

COMPONENTS OF INTAKE AND OUTPUT

Water and electrolyte intake for the newborn consists of that contained in feedings, IV fluid, medications, and transfusions. Patients on mechanical ventilators may even absorb water through the lungs from the humidity provided. The normal newborn regulates the intake of these, along with other nutrients.

In the case of the sick newborn, intake is generally controlled by the physician in amount and composition. Output of fluid and electrolytes occurs chiefly through the urine. Additional output occurs with stool, skin, and respiratory losses. Abnormal losses of fluid and electrolytes occur with diarrhea, emesis, nasogastric tube drainage, thoracotomy tube losses, damaged skin, and other factors that increase insensible water loss.

Urine losses primarily affect sodium and water balance. With diarrhea, bicarbonate loss may become significant. Gastric secretions contain considerable amounts of hydrogen, chloride, potassium, and sodium ions. Emesis and nasogastric tube drainage may therefore lead to a negative balance for these electrolytes in addition to the water loss. Thoracotomy tube drainage is similar to plasma in composition and results in a loss of ECF, including proteins.

ESTIMATING FLUID DEFICIT

Fluid deficits may vary from minimal, with no apparent clinical consequences, to profound, with the clinical picture of hypovolemic shock. Assessing the patient for fluid deficit and estimating the amount requires looking at three categories of data: 1) history; 2) physical exam; and 3) laboratory values.

Historical information that is useful in assessing hydration is available from the nursing flow sheets and nurses' notes. A review of intake versus output may show whether intake and output have been deficient or excessive in relation to each other. Urine output may be diminished in the presence of advanced fluid deficit. Recent weight changes should be reviewed and the current percent of birth weight noted, because these can provide an estimate of the volume of fluid deficit.

A comparison of the weight change to the difference in intake and output will help determine if the weight change is expected. In addition, the patient must be assessed as to whether the weight change was beneficial. For example, in the first days of life when the ECF is reduced, a weight loss is expected and may bring about a clinical improvement. However, if the patient has lost more than expected and shows signs of hypovolemia or dehydration, a fluid deficit may exist. Vital signs may reveal a low or decreasing blood pressure, tachycardia, or increasing baseline heart rate.

Reviewing the amount of blood that has been withdrawn may indicate a compromise of the vascular volume. This occurs when about 10% of the baby's blood volume has been withdrawn over a short period.

Signs of dehydration or hypovolemia may be present on physical exam. Examination of the skin and head is most helpful when assessing for fluid deficit. The perfusion of the skin is decreased with larger fluid deficits, and decreased skin *turgor* may be present. Decreased turgor is manifested by skin that, when grasped and raised between two fingers, slowly returns to its previous position. Decreased turgor is difficult to assess in the premature neonate because of less subcutaneous fat.

The presence of edema may indicate that total body water is adequate, but does not rule out hypovolemia. In the presence of edema, the fluid deficit may be a deficit in vascular fluid. Examination of the head can show a sunken anterior fontanelle with increased over-lapping of sutures in the presence of fluid deficit. Overlapping of sutures is not abnormal in newborns; therefore, changes from previous examinations are important.

Mucous membranes may also be noted to be dry. With increasing fluid deficits, the hematocrit, serum sodium, blood urea nitrogen (BUN), and serum protein tend to increase. Without these data, fluid deficits may be roughly approximated in the manner described in Table 7–3, providing the neonate has normal serum sodium values. Serial weights and observation of vital signs should follow efforts to replace fluid deficits. Reassessment of the deficit can then determine the adequacy of therapy and if modifications need to be made.

TABLE 7–3   Estimation of Fluid Deficit in the Patient with Normal Sodium Levels

---

- 5% Dehydration—oliguria, dry mucous membranes, slightly sunken anterior fontanelle
- 10% Dehydration—signs of 5% dehydration plus: decreased skin turgor, decreased perfusion, sunken eyes, definite sunken anterior fontanelle
- 15% Dehydration—signs of 10% dehydration plus: signs of shock (tachycardia, hypotension, decreased pulses, poor perfusion), altered sensorium

---

INSENSIBLE WATER LOSS (IWL)

Insensible water loss is water lost by evaporation from the skin and respiratory tract. This evaporative loss is proportional to the surface area of the skin and mucosa and is greatly influenced by the type of environment the patient is in—in particular, the relative humidity of that environment.[8] Other factors that influence IWL include temperature and skin integrity. Table 7–4 lists those factors that increase IWL.

IWL may be estimated by subtracting the patient's output from the input, and then subtracting the change in weight from the result [IWL = Intake – Output – (change in weight)]. This method is helpful in estimating IWL over several days, which is then used to estimate the patient's fluid needs. The instruments used to measure intake, output, and weight present enough inaccuracy to make this only an approximation. Also, the output includes measurable fluid losses only and therefore does not include water lost in stools. There are several clinical factors that influence IWL.

TABLE 7–4   Factors That Increase Insensible Water Loss

Early gestational age
Respiratory distress
Environmental temperature above the neutrothermal zone
Elevated body temperature
Skin breakdown and excoriations
Congenital skin defects (neural tube disorders)
Radiant warmer
Phototherapy
Increased motor activity and crying

Level of Maturity. Mature babies have increased skin thickness and, therefore, less evaporative loss per equivalent surface area. In contrast, premature neonates have greater evaporative losses due to decreased skin thickness.

Size. Larger babies will have a greater surface area from which to have evaporative loss, resulting in a higher absolute IWL. Smaller babies, particularly those who are small for gestational age, will have higher surface area-to-body weight ratios. They will, therefore, have higher per kilogram IWL.

Respiratory Distress. Increased gas movement through the respiratory tract will increase the amount of IWL from the airways.

Humidity. Increased ambient or inspired humidity will decrease IWL from the skin and respiratory tracts, respectively. This is most important in very small babies with decreased skin thickness.

Temperature. Increased environmental or body temperature increases IWL.

Skin Breakdown or Injury. Even the skin of premature baby prevents some evaporative loss, and any break in skin integrity increases IWL. Similarly, lesions such as *omphalocele, gastroschisis, myelomeningocele,* or *encephalocele,* which are not covered with skin lead to increased evaporative loss. This is not only because of a poorer barrier to evaporation, but also due to the increased surface area from which evaporation can occur. Occlusive dressings decrease this source of evaporative loss.

Radiant Warmers and Phototherapy Lights. Radiant heat increases evaporative losses, and air currents that are common in open warmers further increase IWL. Humidity under an open warmer depends on room humidity, unless a heat shield is used over the baby and humidity is added under the heat shield. Radiant heat from phototherapy lights increases evaporative water loss.

Heat Shields. Heat shields made of plastic may be placed over the baby to decrease radiant heat loss from the baby. This decreases the evaporative loss.

Motor Activity. Very active babies will have an increased IWL, whereas inactive babies will tend to have a lower IWL.

FUNCTIONS OF ELECTROLYTES

Differences in electrolyte concentrations across cell membranes create an electric charge necessary for many cellular functions. For example, neuronal transmission and contraction of smooth, skeletal, and heart muscle all require such electrolytic gradients.

Sodium. Sodium is important in the regulation of water balance and the distribution of water in body components by virtue of its osmotic activity. It is also necessary for muscular and neuronal function.

Potassium. Potassium is one of the main constituents of ICF. It plays an important role in acid-base balance. With increased hydrogen ion concentration in the blood, hydrogen ion diffuses into cells and potassium diffuses out, providing quick buffering of an acidosis.

Calcium. Calcium plays an important role in the clotting mechanism and is integral in muscular and heart function. It is also the major mineral deposited in bone.

Magnesium. Magnesium is also deposited in bone and is also necessary for many enzyme functions and calcium regulation.

Chloride. Chloride is a major anion providing electrical neutrality and is important in acid-base balance.

Phosphate. Phosphate is an essential component in energy metabolism and bone deposition.

ELECTROLYTE DISORDERS

Table 7–5 summarizes the types and causes of electrolyte disorders that can occur in the neonate.

Hyponatremia. Hyponatremia, a decrease in body sodium, may be caused by inadequate sodium intake, excess sodium loss due to renal immaturity or diuretics, or dilutional from excess body water. In the first two instances, total body sodium content is decreased and treatment is directed toward increasing sodium intake. With dilutional hyponatremeia, the total body sodium content may actually be increased. Its treatment consists of eliminating the excess total body water and with it the excess sodium.

Hypernatremia. Hypernatremia, an excess of body sodium, is generally due to a loss of body water in excess of sodium. It is usually due to insensible water losses not replaced adequately with IV fluids or feedings. Treatment involves replacing the water deficit. Caution is required when replacing the water, because with severe degrees of hypernatremia, the baby may become *hyperosmolar*. Replacement of the water deficit will lead to water entering all cells. Seizures may result if water enters brain cells too rapidly.

Hypokalemia. Hypokalemia, an inadequate amount of potassium, may be caused by several factors. Those factors include inadequate potassium administration, diuretic therapy, and gastric losses. Hypokalemia may also occur during the high output phase of acute renal failure. Treatment consists of increasing the potassium supplement to the patient.

Hyperkalemia. Hyperkalemia, an excess of body potassium, is caused by either excess potassium administration or acute renal failure. Treatment for mild-degree hyperkalemia involves restricting the patient's potassium intake. For severe hyperkalemia, treatment with sodium bicarbonate, calcium, insulin-glucose infusions, *sodium-potassium exchange resin*, or dialysis may be necessary.

Hypocalcemia. Hypocalcemia, a deficit of body calcium, is classified according to the timing of its onset. Early onset hypocalcemia begins in the first 3 days of life. It may be caused by maternal factors such as hyperparathyroidism, pregnancy-induced hypertension, or diabetes mellitus. It may also be caused by certain neonatal conditions such as asphyxia, cesarean delivery, or prematurity and its complications. Late onset hypocalcemia begins after 3 days of age. Causes include phototherapy, furosemide therapy, renal disease, intravenous lipid infusions, and ingestion of a formula with a suboptimal calcium-to-phosphorus ratio.

The clinical presentation of both forms can include jitteriness, irritability, apnea, and seizures. Treatment is the administration of calcium.

TABLE 7–5 Types and Causes of Electrolyte Disorders in the Neonate

DISORDER	DEFINITION	CAUSES
Hyponatremia	Decrease in body sodium	Inadequate sodium intake, excess loss secondary to diuretics or renal immaturity, excess body water
Hypernatremia	Excessive body sodium	Loss of body water in excess of sodium
Hypokalemia	Deficit in body potassium	Inadequate potassium administration, diuretic therapy, gastric losses, high output renal failure
Hyperkalemia	Excessive body potassium	Excessive administration of potassium, acute renal failure
Hypocalcemia	Decreased body calcium	Early Onset: Maternal factors: hyperparathyroidism, pregnancy induced hypertension, diabetes mellitus Neonatal factors: asphyxia, cesarean delivery, prematurity Late Onset: phototherapy, furosemide therapy, renal disease, intravenous lipid infusions, ingestion of formula with suboptimal calcium to phosphorus ratio
Hypercalcemia	Excessive body calcium	Excess IV calcium administration, maternal and neonatal factors
Hypomagnesemia	Deficit of body magnesium	Associated with hypocalcemia
Hypermagnesemia	Excessive body magnesium	Maternal magnesium sulfate therapy during labor, administration of magnesium containing antacid to the neonate

Hypercalcemia. Hypercalcemia, an excess of body calcium, is much less common than hypocalcemia. It is frequently caused by excess IV calcium administration, but may also be caused by maternal hypoparathyroidism or neonatal diseases beyond the scope of this text.

Hypomagnesemia. Hypomagnesemia, an insufficient amount of magnesium, is most frequently associated with hypocalcemia and may present with the same clinical signs.

Hypermagnesemia. Hypermagnesemia, or excess amounts of magnesium, is usually secondary to maternal magnesium sulfate therapy during labor, but may also occur after administration of an antacid containing magnesium to the neonate. The patient presents with *hypotonia*, lethargy, and may be apneic. Treatment includes ventilatory support and correction of acid-base and other electrolyte abnormalities.

MAINTENANCE OF ELECTROLYTES

The ingredients of intravenous fluids may be adjusted in response to the needs of the patient. Intravenous fluids may be used as a supplement to *enteral* feedings or may be the total *parenteral* nutrition. Enteral feedings of standard formulas or human milk meet the electrolyte requirements of most full-term newborns. For those babies with other requirements, there are special formulas designed to provide more or less sodium, or more calcium and phosphorus.

MONITORING OF FLUID AND ELECTROLYTES

When total parenteral nutrition is being provided the neonate, frequent monitoring of electrolytes is required. Sodium, potassium, chloride, calcium, and possibly phosphate are particularly important and must be monitored until a stable growth rate has been achieved. As feedings are started, continued monitoring is necessary to ensure that the neonate can meet electrolyte requirements as the intravenous portion is tapered. Once full feedings have been achieved, monitoring is not necessary unless there has been a persistent abnormality or signs of possible electrolyte disturbance.

Patients on diuretic therapy, particularly furosemide, need routine monitoring of electrolytes and acid-base status. Replacement therapy to correct chloride and phosphate deficiency is important in these patients and will help diagnose and treat metabolic alkalosis.

NEONATAL JAUNDICE

Jaundice is the yellowish-orange skin color that accompanies increased levels of bilirubin in the blood, called hyperbilirubinemia. Most bilirubin comes from the breakdown of old erythrocytes into its constituent parts. The globin portion is reused as a protein elsewhere in the body. The heme, which is the iron portion of the red blood cell, is the source of the bilirubin. Bilirubin is a waste product that is normally eliminated from the body through the intestinal tract or the kidneys.

Jaundice is common in neonates, occurring in 25 to 50% of all term neonates, with a higher percentage in preemies. It is important to distinguish between physiologic jaundice, which is normal, and patholigic jaundice, which is abnormal.

Typically, bilirubin is measured by taking a blood sample from the neonate and determining the plasma concentration. A noninvasive jaundice meter that can detect plasma bilirubin transcutaneously has recently been produced. One drawback is the influence of skin color on the readings. To offset this, a standardization curve was developed, which improves the predictive value of the readings.[9]

PHYSIOLOGY

Bilirubin is normally handled by the body in the following manner. Upon the destruction of the red blood cell, enzymes reduce the hemoglobin and produce bilirubin and carbon monoxide. The bilirubin at this point is called unconjugated, or indirect-reacting. It is released into the plasma, where it is bound to the protein albumin, which carries it in the blood to the liver. In this form, the unconjugated bilirubin is not water soluble, but is very soluble in fatty tissues, especially brain tissue. In the liver, the bilirubin is released from the albumin. The bilirubin then undergoes a series of reactions with a glucuronide radical, glucuronyl transferase, and the resultant bilirubin becomes combined, or *conjugated*, to the glucuronide and now is water soluble.

The conjugated bilirubin, also called direct-reacting or direct bilirubin, is passed into the intestine through the biliary tree. Direct bilirubin that enters the bloodstream may also be excreted by the kidneys. Of interest to note is that the process of conjugation requires oxygen and glucose to be present. Therefore, lack of either may contribute to hyperbilirubinemia.

Although hyperbilirubinemia is present to some degree in all neonates, jaundice does not appear until bilirubin levels exceed 4 to 6 mg/dl.

CAUSES OF JAUNDICE

Most neonatal jaundice falls into the category of physiologic jaundice. There are several causes of neonatal jaundice.

Neonates have a large amount of bilirubin production in the first days of life. This is due in part to a higher percentage of erythrocytes in the neonate, and the fact that the erythrocytes have a shorter life span (70 to 90 days) than in adults. Therefore, as these cells break down, they release large amounts of bilirubin into the system. There is also a significant amount of reabsorption of bilirubin from the intestine.

These two factors greatly increase the amount of bilirubin present in the neonatal blood. The neonatal liver is unable to conjugate all the excess bilirubin, which further increases the amount of serum bilirubin.

Certain blood disorders cause jaundice in newborns. Maternofetal blood incompatibility, either Rh or ABO, is a frequent cause of jaundice. Premature black neonates are especially prone to a deficiency of the enzyme G-6-PD, which disrupts erythrocyte metabolism and leads to hemolysis. Abnormal erythrocyte contours also make them vulnerable to hemolysis. Hemolysis may occur when excess doses of vitamin K_3 are given, especially in the presence of G-6-PD deficiency.

Jaundice may result from hemorrhages in the fetal body. The hemorrhage may be in the skin, brain, or may be internal. A lack of the enzyme glucuronyl transferase, a major enzyme in the conjugation of bilirubin, has been linked to neonatal jaundice. Two syndromes, *Crigler-Najjar* and *Lucey-Driscol*, are associated with this disorder.

Bacterial and viral infections may impair liver function and lead to hyperbilirubinemia. Septic infections may also cause hemolysis of erythrocytes.

Several other factors are associated with jaundice. Infants of diabetic mothers have a high incidence of jaundice. The exact mechanism is unknown; however, it is believed that the frequency of prematurity and RDS in these patients are factors. Jaundice is often seen in breast-fed neonates. It is thought that substances in breast milk inhibit the activity of glucuronyl transferase in the liver.

Jaundice is also seen in the presence of *galactosemia* and hypothyroidism. The administration of maternal drugs, especially oxytocin to induce labor, has been shown to increase neonatal bilirubin levels. Jaundice is often seen in neonates who are fed soon after delivery, possibly caused by immaturity of the hepatic system.

An uncommon but very serious disorder causing jaundice is biliary atresia. Although the exact cause is unknown, it has been seen with congenital rubella infections. Atresia of the biliary tree obstructs the outflow of bile, which is a major vehicle for ridding the body of bilirubin. It is seen mostly in term neonates and in females twice as often as in males.

PATHOLOGIC JAUNDICE

Pathologic jaundice can be determined by using the following criteria: 1) jaundice appears within the first 24 hours following birth; 2) serum unconjugated (indirect) bilirubin levels exceed 13 mg/dl in term neonates and 15 mg/dl in premature neonates; 3) indirect levels rise more than 5mg/dl in a 24-hour period; 4) direct (conjugated) bilirubin levels exceed 1.5 mg/dl; and 5) the jaundice persists beyond 7 days in term neonates and beyond 14 days in the preemie.[10]

COMPLICATIONS AND TREATMENT

The most serious complication of hyperbilirubinemia is *kernicterus* (bilirubin encephalopathy). Because of the high affinity for fat that unconjugated bilirubin possesses, in high levels it crosses the blood-brain barrier and attaches itself to the brain cells. This leads to neurologic deficits, including locomotor dysfunction, cerebral palsy, and hearing impairment.

The exact level of bilirubin that will produce kernicterus is unknown. Levels as low as 3.3 mg/dl have been reported to have caused kernicterus. Levels of 20 mg/dl for term neonates and 15 mg/dl for preemies are often listed as upper limits, with treatment beginning at levels of 10 mg/dl. It is important to treat hyperbilirubinemia quickly and efficiently because of this unknown association between bilirubin levels and kernicterus. Table 7–6 illustrates guidelines for the management of hyperbilirubinemia.

Treatment must begin with the determination of whether the jaundice is physiologic or pathologic. Pathologic symptoms must be further investigated as to their cause. The most common method of treatment for moderate levels of hyperbilirubin is the use of phototherapy lights. The most effective light is in the blue spectrum. The blue light causes the bilirubin to decompose by photooxidation forming water-soluble bilirubin products that are then excreted by the kidneys and through the bile. Phototherapy lights increase insensible water loss, so care must be taken to counteract the loss.

New methods of phototherapy involve the use of fiberoptics. The infant is covered in a blanket in which fiberoptic fibers have been placed. The light is then able to reach a larger area of the patient's skin while reducing the effects of IWL. These devices have been shown to be superior to traditional phototherapy in recent studies.[11, 12]

High levels of hyperbilirubinemia are treated by exchange transfusion in an attempt to rid the neonatal body of factors causing hemolysis. The indications for exchange transfusion are listed in Table 7–7. Exchange transfusions usually involve a two-volume exchange. The patients blood volume is estimated by weight, which approximates 80 ml/kg. The procedure is performed by withdrawing 5 to 20 ml of blood, depending on the weight of the patient, from the catheter. The same amount of fresh blood is then replaced to the patient. This is done until all of the fresh blood is gone. Two-volume exchange transfusions remove and replace about 87% of the patient's blood volume.

Other treatments include the administration of phenobarbital and albumin. Phenobarbital induces microsomal enzymes and increases bilirubin conjugation and excretion. It has numerous side effects, however, and so must be used cautiously. The administration of albumin increases the capacity of the blood to transport unconjugated bilirubin to the liver.

TABLE 7–6   Management of Hyperbilirubinemia

INDIRECT BILIRUBIN LEVEL	TREATMENT
<5	None
5–9	Phototherapy, if caused by hemolysis
10–14	Exchange transfusion if levels occur within first 24 hours. Phototherapy if patient is less than 2500 g.
15–19	Exchange transfusion if levels occur within first 48 hours. Possible exchange on patients less than 2500 g with levels occurring after 48 hours. Phototherapy on patients greater than 2500 g with levels occurring after 48 hours.
>20	Exchange transfusion

Source: Cloherty JP, Stark A. R., eds. Manual of Neonatal Care. *4th ed. Philadelphia: J. B. Lippincott; 1997.*

TABLE 7–7   Indications for Exchange Transfusion

• Correction of severe anemia
• Treatment of hemolytic disease by removing antibody-coated red blood cells
• Removal of excessive amounts of unconjugated bilirubin

NECROTIZING ENTEROCOLITIS (NEC)

NEC is an idiopathic disorder characterized by ischemia and necrosis of the intestine. In its mildest form, abdominal distention is present. At its worst, perforation of the intestine occurs, leading to sepsis and eventually death. Risk factors include prematurity, asphyxia, and formula feeding.[13]

ETIOLOGY

The cause of NEC is known to be multifactorial, but three main factors are seen as key etiological factors: 1) mucosal wall injury; 2) bacterial invasion into the damaged intestinal wall; and 3) formula in the intestine.[14] Injury to the intestinal mucosa may be secondary to ischemia and/or decreased blood flow to the gut. Maternal cocaine abuse has also been implicated. Factors leading to ischemia and decreased blood flow are listed in Table 7–8.

The next step in the onset of NEC is the invasion of bacteria into the damaged intestinal tissue. Following mucosal wall injury, the intestine loses its defense against bacterial invasion. Once the bacteria have invaded the intestinal tissue, necrosis and the formation of gas in the intestinal wall, called pneumatosis intestinalis, occurs. Pneumatosis intestinalis is visible on x-ray, as shown in Figure 7–9. In some cases , the bacterial invasion is unrelenting and leads to the passage of bacteria into the circulation, causing sepsis, or perforation of the intestine, allowing bacteria into the abdominal cavity, causing profuse peritonitis.

TABLE 7–8   Factors Leading to Ischemia and Decreased Blood Flow

INJURY	POSSIBLE CAUSES
Ischemia	RDS
	Apgar scores <5
	Abruptio placentae
	Apnea
	Hypertonic oral medicines
	Bowel obstruction
Decreased blood flow	PDA with left to right shunting
	Exchange transfusion
	Umbilical artery catheter
	Polycythemia
	Shock

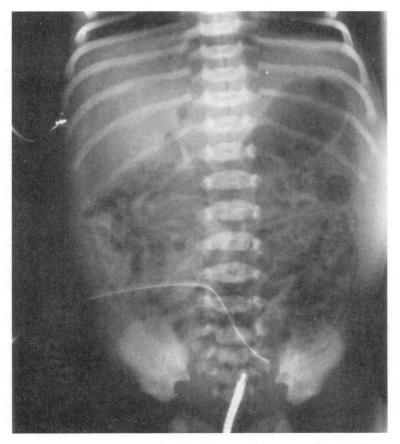

Figure 7–9 *Gas bubble seen in the intestinal wall with necrotizing enterocolitis (NEC)*

The final factor, formula feeding, is seen in 95% of infants with NEC.[14] It is theorized that formula may interfere with intestinal blood flow, contribute to mucosal damage, and provide the substrate for the intestinal bacteria. In contrast to formula, human breast milk may enhance gastrointestinal function and has been shown to be protective against NEC.[15]

CLINICAL SIGNS AND TREATMENT

The first confirmatory sign that will be seen in the presence of NEC is guaiac-positive stools, which is the presence of blood in the stools. The invasion of the bacteria results in bleeding, which may not be visible in the stool. It is therefore important to perform a *guaiac* check on each stool to determine if blood is present. Abdominal distention becomes apparent as the disease advances by increasing abdominal girth measurements. The patient may have bile residuals and bile-tainted emesis. Feedings may be poorly tolerated, demonstrated by increased residuals and frequent emesis. Lastly, the patient may show general signs of sepsis, which are lethargy and increased FiO_2 requirements.

The best treatment of NEC is avoidance of factors that lead to its presence. Good hand washing is mandatory when treating all neonates, especially those with suspected NEC. Oral feedings are stopped immediately and nasogastric suctioning started to empty the stomach of bile residuals. Feeding is started via hyperalimentation through an IV, and antibiotics, such as ampicillin and gentamicin, are administered. Abdominal x-rays are done frequently for follow-up and to rule out intestinal perforation. The FiO_2 is also increased to raise arterial PaO_2 levels and aid in mucosal regeneration. Studies have indicated that nitric oxide maintains the integrity of gastric mucosa. Because of this, it has been suggested that a potential treatment for NEC is L-arginine, a nitric oxide substrate. In a piglet study, a continuous infusion of L-arginine was show to markedly reduce intestinal injury.[16]

The presence of gastrointestinal perforation or full-thickness necrosis requires surgical resection of the affected area.

SUMMARY

This chapter focuses on several aspects of continuing care that are important for the practitioner to have an understanding. Thermoregulation is of utmost importance in the ongoing care of a neonate, as well as older patients. A patient who is not thermoregulated will waste energy and reserves in an attempt to stay warm. Ideally, the thermoneutral temperature should be maintained as much of the time as possible. The thermoneutral temperature varies from patient to patient. It is the environmental temperature that maintains a rectal temperature of 36.5 to 37.5°C, or an abdominal skin temperature of 36.0 to 36.5°C.

Heat loss occurs by one of four mechanisms: 1) radiant—the dissipation of heat from the patient to cooler surroundings not in direct contact; 2) conduction—the transfer of heat to cooler surfaces in contact with the patient; 3) convection—the loss of heat from the body to air moving across the skin; and 4) evaporation—the heat lost when water is changed to a gas. An understanding of these four mechanisms allows the practitioner to take precautions in preventing unnecessary heat loss.

Another very important consideration in the care of the premature infant is control of the NICU environment in order to meet the developmental needs of the patient. The premature infant is developmentally immature, both physiologically and neurologically, and excessive stimulation in either area can have serious consequences. Interventions such as planning procedures during times of nonstress, keeping the lights and sound levels low, facilitated tucking, and kangaroo care have all been shown to reduce the amount of stimulation the infant receives.

As an organ system, the skin of a preemie is also immature and very susceptible to injury. Additionally, absorption through the skin is enhanced, and use of solvents or polymers on the skin may lead to toxicity. Skin injury can be reduced by using a pectin-based adhesive between the skin and tape. The pectin-based adhesive allows the skin to grow and develop while protecting it from the trauma associated with tape removal. Monitors can be applied using Velcro closures, or Coban tape, which do not stick to the skin.

One of the most difficult components in the care of a premature neonate is fluid and electrolyte balance. Because a preemie's body weight is mostly water, and a majority of the body water is extracellular, fluid balance can be difficult to achieve. Because of their effect on the lungs and compliance, a basic understanding of fluid balance and the major ions and their function helps the practitioner involved in respiratory care. Additionally, an understanding of insensible water loss and those mechanisms that increase it, aids the practitioner in helping control fluid balance.

Jaundice is a common occurrence in newborns. While it is common, it is important to distinguish normal physiologic jaundice from pathologic jaundice. Hyperbilirubinemia can lead to severe neurologic complications, called kernicterus. Knowing the normal mechanisms of bilirubin production as well as when and how to treat, can prevent kernicterus from occurring.

Finally, necrotizing enterocolitis is a serious gastrointestinal disorder that every practitioner working with neonates needs to be aware of. The importance of good hand washing cannot be emphasized enough in helping prevent this disease. Rapid and effective identification of the disease may prevent serious complications such as sepsis and peritonitis. Assurance of adequate oxygenation may also help prevent the disease, or slow its progression.

References

1. Shogan, MG, Schumann, LL The effect of environmental lighting on the oxygen saturation of preterm infants in the NICU. *Neonatal Network*. 1993; 12:7–13.

2. Gorski, PA, et al. Handling preterm infants in hospitals: stimulating controversy about timing stimulation. In: *Infant Stimulation*. Skillman, NJ: Johnson and Johnson; 1987.

3. Zahr, LK, Balian, S Responses of premature infants to routine nursing interventions and noise in the NICU. *Nurs Res*. 1995; 44:179–185.

4. Saunders, AN Practice applications of research. Incubator noise: a method to decrease decibels. *Pediatr Nurs*. 1995; 21:265–268.

5. Treas, LS Incubator covers: health or hazard? *Neonatal Network*. 1993; 12:50–51.

6. Ludington-Hoe, SM, et al. Kangaroo care: research results, and practice implications and guidelines. *Neonatal Network*. 1994; 13:19–27.

7. Dollison, EJ, Beckstrand, J Adhesive tape vs. pectin-based barrier use in preterm infants. *Neonatal Network*. 1995; 14:35–39.

8. Horns, KM Physiologic and methodologic issues: neonatal insensible water loss. *Neonatal Network*. 1994; 13:83–86.

9. Linder, N. Noninvasive determination of neonatal hyperbilirubinemia: standardization for variation in skin color. *Am J Perinatol*. 1994; 11:223–225.

10. Avery, GD, Fletcher, MA, MacDonald, MC *Pathophysiology and Management of the Newborn*. 5th ed. Philadelphia: JB. Lipponcott Co.; 1999.

11. Garg, AK, et al. A controlled trial of high-intensity double-surface phototherapy on a fluid bed versus conventional phototherapy in neonatal jaundice. *Pediatrics*. 1995; 95:914–916.

12. Tan, KL Comparison of the efficacy of fiberoptic and conventional phototherapy for neonatal hyperbilirubinemia. *J Pediatr*. 1994; 125:607–612.

13. Caplan, MS, et al. Role of asphyxia and feeding in a neonatal rat model of necrotizing enterocolitis. *Pediatr Pathol.* 1994; 14:1017–1028.

14. Parker, LA Necrotizing enterocolitis. *Neonatal Network.* 1995; 14:17–26.

15. Schanler, RJ Suitability of human milk for the low-birthweight infant. *Clin Perinat.* 1995; 22:207–222.

16. Di-Lorenzo, M, et al. Use of L-arginine in the treatment of experimental necrotizing enterocolitis. *J Pediatr Surg.* 1995; 30:235–240.

Bibliography and Suggested Readings

Cloherty, JP, Star, AR, eds. *Manual of Neonatal Care.* 4th ed. Philadelphia: Lippincott; 1997.

Corff, KE. An effective comfort measure for minor pain and stress in preterm infants: facilitated tucking [abstract]. *Neonatal Network.* 1993; 12:74.

D'Apolito, K Hats used to maintain body temperature. *Neonatal Network.* 1994; 13:93–94.

Klaus, MH, Fanaroff, MB *Care of the High-Risk Neonate.* 5th ed. Philadelphia: WB Saunders Co.; 1999.

Merenstein, GB, Gardner, SL *Handbook of Neonatal Intensive Care.* 4th ed. St. Louis: CV Mosby Co.; 1998.

Patten, BM *Human Embryology.* 2nd ed. New York: The Blakiston Co. Inc.; 1953.

Thomas, K Thermoregulation in neonates. *Neonatal Network.* 1994; 13:15–22.

White-Traut, RC, et al. Environmental influences on the developing premature infant: theroretical issues and applications to practice. *J Obstet Gynecol Neonatal Nurs.* 1994; 23:393–401.

Wong, DL *Whaley & Wong's Nursing Care of Infants and Children.* 6th ed. St. Louis: Mosby; 1999.

Posttest

1. Oxygen consumption is lowest in the neonate at which of the following skin temperature ranges (°C)?
    a. 35.5–36.0
    b. 36.0–36.5
    c. 36.5–37.0
    d. 37.0–37.5

2. Which of the following are involved in nonshivering thermogenesis?
    I. guanosine
    II. norepinephrine
    III. acidase
    IV. lipase
    V. nonesterified fatty acids
        a. I, III, V
        b. II, IV, V

   c. II, III, V

   d. II, III, IV

3. Premature newborns have a decreased ability to maintain body heat. Which of the following are reasons for that decreased ability?

   I. large body surface area

   II. increased amount of subcutaneous fat

   III. thin skin layer

   IV. preemies have a lower thermoneutral environmental temperature

   V. reduced ability to intake calories

     a. I, II, III, V

     b. I, III, V

     c. II, IV, V

     d. I, III, IV, V

4. A small preemie is placed on a warming mattress inside an incubator lined with aluminum foil. The environmental temperature is maintained at 33°C. Flow to the resuscitation bag is turned on inside the incubator with the flow of gas passing over the infant's head. This baby is at risk of losing heat through which of the following methods?

     a. convective

     b. conductive

     c. evaporative

     d. radiant

5. The initial response of a neonate to cold stress is:

     a. acidosis

     b. shivering

     c. decreased metabolism

     d. peripheral vasoconstriction

6. Radiant heat loss following delivery can be minimized by which of the following?

   I. complete drying of the neonate

   II. wrapping patient in a warm blanket

   III. placing a cap on the patient's head

   IV. placing the patient on a warming mattress

     a. I, III

     b. II, IV

     c. II, III

     d. I, II, III, IV

7. Which of the following is an advantage to using an open warmer?

     a. ease of patient access

     b. less chance of conductive heat loss

     c. better thermoregulation

     d. ability to control the environment

8. A baby who is being overstimulated may show which of the following signs?

     a. shaking

     b. seizures

    c. hiccoughs

    d. hyperventilation

9. An important part of environmental control is:

    a. active stimulation of the infant

    b. quiet times

    c. music played inside the incubator

    d. alternating bright and dim lights to simulate day and night

10. Which of the following are skin care recommendations for premature neonates?

    I. use spray-on skin barriers to protect the skin

    II. use solvent-based adhesive removers to remove tape

    III. use pectin-based adhesives between the skin and tape

    IV. use Coban wraps to hold TCMs on the skin

    V. cover the skin with benzoin before applying tape

        a. II, IV

        b. I, III, IV

        c. III, IV, V

        d. III, IV

11. Which of the following may cause abnormalities of fluid and electrolyte balance in neonates?

    I. maternal IV therapy

    II. asphyxia

    III. cold stress

    IV. sepsis

    V. endocrine disorders

        a. I, III, IV

        b. II, IV, V

        c. I, II, IV, V

        d. I, II, IV

12. The percentage of ICF that comprises TBW passes and exceeds the percentage of ECF at what approximate age?

    a. 10 days

    b. 3 months

    c. 18 months

    d. 3 years

13. Excessive intake of sodium in the postnatal period would lead to:

    a. delayed contraction of the ECF

    b. enhanced contraction of the ECF

    c. delayed contraction of the ICF

    d. hypothermia and acidosis

14. Sodium and water balance are primarily affected by:

    a. oral intake

    b. the presence of diuretics

    c. urine losses

    d. insensible water loss

15. Which of the following would indicate a fluid deficit in a neonate?
    I. decreased skin turgor
    II. increased skin turgor
    III. sunken anterior fontanelle
    IV. decreased tear production
    V. increase in suture overlap
        a. I, III, V
        b. II, IV, V
        c. II, III, IV
        d. I, II, III, IV, V
16. Which of the following would most greatly increase insensible water loss?
    a. increased gestational age
    b. neonates who are large for their gestational age
    c. the presence of RDS
    d. the use of heat shields
17. A patient with a diminished clotting mechanism would possibly have an imbalance in which electrolyte?
    a. sodium
    b. calcium
    c. potassium
    d. phosphate
18. A neonate appears clinically with jitters, irritability, apnea, and seizures. The probable cause is:
    a. hyponatremia
    b. hypokalemia
    c. hypomagnesemia
    d. hypocalcemia
19. A term neonate has an indirect bilirubin level of 5 mg/dl. The following day, the level has risen to 9 mg/dl. You would:
    a. do nothing, this is normal
    b. start phototherapy
    c. administer albumen
    d. suggest another sample be analyzed
20. The initial sign of NEC is:
    a. feeding intolerance
    b. increased abdominal girth
    c. bile residuals
    d. guaiac-positive stools

CHAPTER EIGHT

PHARMACOLOGY IN NEONATAL AND PEDIATRIC RESPIRATORY CARE

OBJECTIVES

Upon completion of this chapter, the reader should be able to:

1. List and discuss the physiologic factors and mechanisms of drug transfer across the placenta.
2. Define a teratogenic substance and describe its actions on the fetus.
3. Discuss each of the following as it relates to neonatal and pediatric pharmacokinetics. Include a description of the routes of absorption and the methods of distribution.
   a. Absorption
   b. Distribution
   c. Metabolism
   d. Excretion
4. Briefly describe how antibiotics work against bacteria, fungi, and viruses.
5. List the nine categories of antibiotics and at least one antibiotic from each category.
6. For each of the following cardiovascular conditions, describe at least one drug that is used in its treatment:
   a. Congestive heart failure
   b. Closure of the ductus arteriosus
   c. Pulmonary hypertension
   d. Hypotension
   e. Edema
7. List at least one drug from each of the following categories of respiratory medications. For each drug listed, describe briefly its indications and dosage:
   a. Sympathomimetic
   b. Parasympatholytic
   c. Steroid
   d. Antiviral
8. Describe at least one drug from each of the following categories. Include the indications and adverse effects:
   a. Anticonvulsant
   b. Steroid

      c. Sedative
      d. Paralytic
   9. Describe the effects of maternal drug abuse on the fetus.

KEY TERMS

active transport	facilitated diffusion	pseudocholinesterase
anuria	hydrolysis	reduction
beta-lactam	ototoxic	simple diffusion
conjugation	oxidation	teratogen
dyscrasias	pharmacokinetic	ultrafiltration
extravasation	pheochromocytoma	

INTRODUCTION

The study of pharmacology in the neonatal and pediatric populations is a complicated, intricate, and challenging subject. Therapeutic actions and adverse effects of many drugs may be quite different in neonates, infants, or older children than in adults. This is due to continuous changes that occur as the child develops, with respect to growth, and the associated pharmacodynamic responses.

Only 25% of all U.S. Food and Drug Administration (FDA) approved drugs are labeled as safe and effective in children. The available data for the remaining 75% of drugs are inadequate to allow for FDA approval in the pediatric population.

This chapter outlines many of the complicated and challenging factors associated with drug therapy in the neonatal and pediatric populations as well as defining therapeutic parameters for many of the drugs used in the treatment of neonates.

As technology improves, new medicines are constantly being added to the assortment used in neonatal and pediatric care. For this reason, it is impossible to provide an updated list of all drugs currently being used. It is strongly recommended that the practitioner have at her/his disposal a current neonatal/pediatric pharmacologic manual for the latest information on drugs, dosages, and their uses.

PLACENTAL DRUG TRANSFER

Soranus of Ephesus during the second century A.D., wrote: "Even if a woman transgresses some or all of the rules mentioned (i.e., administration of drugs, sternutatives, pungent substances, and drunkenness, especially during the first trimester) and yet miscarriage of the fetus does not take place, let no one assume that the fetus has not been injured at all. For it has been harmed: it is weakened, becomes retarded in growth, less well nourished, and in general, more easily injured and susceptible to harmful agents; it becomes misshapen and of ignoble soul."[1] This shows an early understanding of the effects of maternal drug use on the fetus. This chapter begins by examining those factors that determine the effects of drugs on the fetus.

PHYSIOLOGIC FACTORS

Several factors should be kept in mind when considering the effects of drugs on the fetus. The extent to which drugs cross the placenta from the mother to the fetus varies, but many drugs reach concentrations in the fetus of 50 to 100% of the levels in maternal blood. The total amount of blood protein is less in the fetus and often results in more free drug, especially for drugs that are highly protein bound in the maternal blood.

MECHANISMS OF PLACENTAL DRUG TRANSFER

The major mechanisms by which drugs cross the placenta are: *ultrafiltration, simple diffusion, facilitated diffusion, active transport,* and breaks in the placental villi. Drug transfer across the placenta is determined by the concentration difference across the placenta, the lipid solubility of the drug, the degree of ionization of the drug, and the molecular weight of the drug. Figure 8–1 outlines the process of drug transfer across the placenta.

EFFECTS ON THE FETUS

Many drugs have been known to cause physical and/or mental developmental abnormalities in the embryo or fetus. These are known as *teratogens* or teratogenic substances.

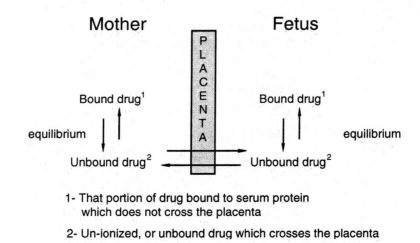

1- That portion of drug bound to serum protein which does not cross the placenta

2- Un-ionized, or unbound drug which crosses the placenta

Figure 8–1 *Drug transfer across the placenta.*

Teratogens may cause spontaneous abortion, congenital malformations, intrauterine growth retardation, mental retardation, and carcinogenesis. The effects of teratogens are dependent on several factors. Those factors include the dose of drug that actually reaches the embryo or fetus, the length of exposure to the teratogen, the gestational age of the fetus at the time of exposure, and other drugs concurrently being taken by the mother.

Generally, the first trimester of pregnancy is the most critical time for teratogens to have an effect; however, drugs may also have teratogenic effects during the second and third trimesters.

Drugs may have an adverse effect on labor and delivery if taken late in pregnancy. Additionally, the neonate is exposed to the drug, which could lead to prolonged exposure and toxicity.

NEONATAL AND PEDIATRIC PHARMACOKINETICS

Pharmacokinetics is a general term for the process by which drugs enter the body (absorption), are distributed throughout the system (distribution), are changed or altered from the original compound (metabolism), and eventually leave the body (excretion). This section will describe this process, with emphasis on the neonatal and pediatric populations.

ABSORPTION

A drug may enter the system through a variety of mechanisms: through the gastrointestinal tract, intramuscularly, by topical absorption through the skin and respiratory tract, and through direct intravenous administration.

Gastrointestinal Tract. The absorption of drugs from the gastrointestinal (GI) tract is often regulated by pH-dependent diffusion and gastric emptying time.

At birth, gastric pH is between 6 and 8 but falls to a pH of 1 to 3 in the first 24 hours after birth. This decrease is not present in premature neonates because of an immature acid-secreting mechanism. The pH then returns close to neutral, and there is no further acid secretion until the 10th and 15th day after birth. Normal adult values for GI acidity are reached by about 2 years of age. The difference in pH of the stomach for the neonate may affect the normal absorption of both basic and acidic drugs such as penicillins, phenobarbital, and phenytoin.

Gastric emptying time in the newborn infant may be as long as 6 to 8 hours and does not approach the adult values until 6 months of age. Many factors can influence the gastric emptying time, including gestational maturity, postnatal age, and type of oral feeding (human milk or formula), and unpredictable peristalsis in the newborn.

Intramuscular Administration. The intramuscular absorption rate of drugs in the newborn is altered owing to many factors. Factors include variability in the blood flow to various muscles, a decrease in muscular contractions, and the low muscle mass in the neonate.

Skin. The absorption of drugs through the skin of the newborn is greatly increased. Newborns generally have thin, well-hydrated skin, which allows for increased permeability and therefore an enhanced drug absorption.

Respiratory Tract. The combination of extensive vascularization, large surface area, and thin tissue separating the airway lumen and blood vasculature makes the respiratory tract ideally suited for absorption of drugs. Although most drugs administered to the respiratory tract have a topical effect, certain drugs used during resuscitation are purposely instilled into the lungs to achieve rapid systemic absorption. Drugs that may be given this route include epinephrine and Narcan.

Intravenous Administration. Intravenous administration of drugs bypasses all of the previously described complications of drug absorption due to the drug being readily available in predictable amounts within the system. The effective dose of a drug can therefore be more accurately calculated.

DISTRIBUTION

Following the absorption or injection of a drug into the bloodstream, it is distributed into interstitial, cellular, and extracellular fluids. The rate and extent of distribution are dependent on the physical and chemical properties of the drug.

Lipid-Soluble Drugs. In general, lipid-soluble drugs that readily cross cell membranes are distributed throughout all fluid areas. Lipid-soluble drugs are distributed very rapidly into the heart, brain, liver, kidney, and other highly vascularized tissues and more slowly into muscle tissue and fat cells. Drugs that are less lipid soluble and that do not readily cross cell membranes may gather in tissues at higher concentrations than in plasma.

Many drugs are bound to plasma proteins (mostly plasma albumin), and their protein binding ability influences their activity throughout the system. Lipid-soluble drugs generally have a high affinity to be protein bound. Often, more than 90% of a lipid-soluble drug will be bound to plasma proteins. This leaves only 10% of unbound or free drug available to cross cell membranes and exhibit its maximal pharmacologic activity.

Binding to Serum Proteins. Many drug interactions and toxicity reactions occur when drugs compete for binding to serum proteins, thus increasing the unbound portion of one or more of the drugs being administered. Several factors can significantly reduce the plasma protein binding of many drugs in the premature and full-term newborn. These include a reduced plasma protein concentration, a lower binding capacity of fetal serum albumin, a lower blood pH, and increased level of unconjugated bilirubin competing with the drug-binding sites. These are all factors to consider when calculating drug dosages for premature infants.

Volume of Distribution. Another area for consideration when calculating dosages in premature infants is the volume of distribution. The volume of distribution is a proportional factor that relates the amount of drug in the body to the plasma concentration. The volume of distribution of many drugs in infants is different from adults for two main reasons. First, neonates have a decreased plasma protein binding capacity, and second, neonates have an increased extracellular fluid volume per kilogram of body weight. Extracellular fluid areas include the gastrointestinal tract, the cerebrospinal fluid, aqueous humor, endolymph fluid, and joint fluids.

Extracellular fluid volume decreases from 50% of body weight in premature infants to 35% in 4- to 6-month-old infants, to 25% in 1-year-olds, and to 20% in adults. Total body water decreases from 86% in premature infants to 70% in full-term infants. This implies that the loading dose (on a mg/kg basis) of a water-soluble drug would decrease as the infant's age and weight increased.

METABOLISM

Metabolism is the changing or alteration of the drug to a different form, either active or inactive, as the next step in the pharmacokinetic process. The primary site within the system where drug metabolism takes place is the liver; however, drug metabolism is also accomplished in other areas such as the plasma, kidney, and the gastrointestinal tract.

The liver produces many enzymes that aid the metabolism of drugs. In the premature and newborn infant, the ability of the liver enzyme system to mediate the metabolism of drugs is greatly reduced.

There are basically four types of drug metabolizing biochemical reactions that take place in the liver: *conjugation, oxidation, reduction,* and *hydrolysis.* The premature infant generally has a decreased ability for drug metabolism by all of these mechanisms, which is one of the factors that causes an increased half-life of the drug or drugs being administered. Half-life is the amount of time required to reduce a drug level to one half its initial value.

Several drugs, such as phenobarbital, have the effect of increasing the enzymatic activity of the liver. Exposure to these drugs may require the dosages of other drugs to be reevaluated.

EXCRETION

Because most drugs are poorly metabolized in the premature infant, the excretion of a drug is the most important factor in the termination of a drug's effects. Drugs can be eliminated from the body through various routes, including the kidneys (primary site of elimination), via biliary and fecal excretion, and through other body fluids such as sweat and saliva.

The renal function, both glomerular filtration rate and tubular secretion, in premature and full-term infants is not completely developed at the time of birth. The renal function of infants does not achieve the same level as in adults until the child is between 6 months and 1 year of age. The creatinine clearance, as a measure of renal function, of full-term infants is generally 20 ml/min and increases to 60 ml/min by one month of age. In contrast, the creatinine clearance of premature infants (less than 34 weeks' gestation) is 16 ml/min and only increases to 40 ml/min by one month of age.

Drugs that are not extensively metabolized and are primarily excreted through the kidneys are therefore eliminated more slowly in premature infants and dosage adjustments must be made. Drugs that rely on the glomerular filtration rate (GFR) for their effect (i.e., diuretics) may have to be increased due to the reduction in GFR.

MEDICATIONS

The study of pharmacology could be a lifetime study, especially when one considers that there are several thousand drugs available for use. To list each drug used in the neonatal/pediatric population could fill an entire volume. The approach to pharmacology in this chapter is to give the reader a general overview of therapeutics in the neonatal and pediatric populations. Antibiotic therapy makes up a large portion of therapeutics and therefore is treated differently than the other medications. An overview of antibiotic therapeutics is given, with the specific medications discussed in their groups so the reader can appreciate the role of antibiotics in the care of infants and children. Because they represent a smaller portion of drugs used, the other medications discussed are considered individually.

ANTIBIOTICS

A wealth of antibiotics are available for treating a variety of infections, and each year many new antibiotics become available. Therapeutics with antibiotics is a science in and of itself. Since the discovery of penicillin many years ago, antibiotic therapy has become complex and spread out with numerous drugs falling under various categories of drugs. Before using an antibiotic, there are three basic principles that must be observed: 1) Unless the situation is life-threatening, identify the infective organism whenever possible. Identification of the organism allows the practitioner to use the appropriate antibiotic for which the organism is susceptible; 2) Always consider the pharmacologic and toxicologic aspects of the drug before it is started; 3) The response of the patient to the drug is extremely variable in the infant and pediatric population.

Groups of antibiotics include the penicillins, cephalosporins, aminoglycosides, macrolides, quinolones, tetracyclines, sulfonamides, antifungals, and antivirals.

Penicillins

Mode of Action. Penicillins are *beta-lactam* antibiotics. The term beta-lactam refers to the chemical structure of the drug. The cell wall of the bacteria has several layers. The beta-lactam drugs penetrate the outer membrane through small canals in structures called porins. At the level of the cytoplasmic membrane, enzymes that are sensitive to the beta-lactams, called penicillin binding proteins (PBPs), are found. When the drug attaches to the PBPs, two processes kill the bacterial cell.

First, the attachment of the drug causes an interference in cell wall synthesis, and second, the cell releases an enzyme that is autolytic and lyses the cell.

Classification and Uses. There are four classifications of penicillins available.

Natural Penicillins. The natural penicillins include penicillin G, which is combined with benzathine to provide a slow release of the drug. Penicillin G is used for gram-positive bacteria such as streptococci, and gram-negative coverage for pneumococci, *Haemophilus influenzae,* and gonococci. The second is penicillin V, which is acid-resistant and better tolerates oral administration. It has the same coverage as penicillin G, but is thought to be less active against gram-negative bacteria.

Penicillinase-Resistant Penicillins. In an attempt to survive, some bacteria have developed the ability to produce an enzyme that inactivates the beta-lactam drugs. This enzyme is called penicillinase, or beta-lactamase. Several of the penicillin drugs are resistant to this enzyme and are effective against those bacteria that produce it. There are numerous reports, however, of bacteria, especially staphylococcus, that have become resistant to these antibiotics. *Staphylococcus aureus,* which has become resistant to methicillin, is called methicillin resistant *Staphylococcus aureus,* or MRSA. Reports of resistance to this antibiotic have been documented. Any drug that is said to be effective against staphylococcus should be understood to not include MRSA.

The penicillinase-resistant group includes methicillin, nafcillin, cloxacillin, dicloxacillin, and oxacillin. These drugs are used almost exclusively to treat resistant strains of staphylococcus.

Aminopenicillins. The aminopenicillins include ampicillin and amoxicillin. These drugs are used to treat gram-positive bacteria (except *S. aureus*), and gram-negatives such as *Shigella, H. influenzae, Salmonella, Proteus mirabilis,* and *Escherichia coli.* For use with bacteria that are producing beta-lactamase, ampicillin is combined with sulbactam, and amoxicillin is combined with clavulanic acid. These two chemicals inhibit beta-lactamase and prevent the drug from being inactivated by the enzyme.

Antipseudomonal Penicillins. The drugs in this category have been chemically altered to make them more useful against difficult bacteria such as pseudomonas. These drugs include azlocillin, mezlocillin, piperacillin, ticarcillin, and carbenicillin. For use with beta-lactamase producing bacteria, clavulanic acid is combined with ticarcillin and another anti-beta-lactamase drug, tazobactam, is combined with piperacillin. The addition of these chemicals makes the drugs useful against staphylococcus, enterococcus, and *Bacteroides fragilis.*

Cephalosporins
Mode of Action. The cephalosporins are similar to the penicillins chemically in that they also have a beta-lactam ring and thus act on the bacteria in the same manner as the penicillins. Cephalosporins are often used in patients who are allergic to the penicillins. Their chemical structure makes them less susceptible to bacteria that produce beta-lactamase. The cephalosporins have been developed in generations, with each successive generation of drugs becoming broader spectrum.

First-Generation Cephalosporins. This group of drugs is most active against gram-positive bacteria such as staphylococcus and streptococcus, and moderately active against gram-negative bacteria, such as *E. Coli, Klebsiella,* and *Proteus.* These drugs are often used in surgical prophylaxis, especially before orthopedic and cardiovascular surgeries. Drugs in this category include cephalexin, cephalothin, cefadroxil, cephradine, cephapirin, and cefazolin.

Second-Generation Cephalosporins. The second generation of cephalosporins is more potent than first generations against gram-negative bacteria, while maintaining good gram-positive activity. Second-generation cephalosporins are often used to treat community acquired pneumonias. Penetration of the CNS is probably limited in these drugs. Drugs include cefaclor, cefamandole, cefoxitin, cefuroxime, cefonicid, ceforanide, cefmetazole, cefotetan, cefprozil, cefpodoxime, and loracarbef.

Third-Generation Cephalosporins. These antibiotics possess the broadest spectrum and have the most potent activity against the gram-negative bacteria. Third-generation cephalosporins are further divided into those with pseudomonal activity and those without. The antipseudomonal drugs include ceftazidime and cefoperazone. Those without pseudomonal activity include cefotaxime, ceftizoxime, cefriaxone, and cefixime.

Other Beta-Lactam Drugs. Two other drug categories are included with the beta-lactams, which are not penicillins or cephalosporins. Because of their broad activity, they are often humorously referred to as the "Gorillacillins." These drugs are the monobactams, and the carbapenems, each only having one drug currently. The monobactam drug, aztreonam, is effective against aminoglycoside- and cephalosporin-resistant gram-negative organisms. Its spectrum of activity is the same as the aminoglycosides, without the nephrotoxic and *ototoxic* side effects. The carbapenem, imipenem, is a synthetic agent that has broad-spectrum activity against gram-positive and gram-negative bacteria; it is also used to treat MRSA where it is resistant to vancomycin.

Aminoglycosides. The aminoglycosides include gentamicin, kanamycin, neomycin, spectinomycin, streptomycin, amikacin, netilmicin, and tobramycin.

Mode of Action. While not entirely understood, it is believed that the aminoglycosides inhibit bacterial protein synthesis by irreversibly binding the ribosomal subunits, thus "freezing" the elongation process.

Uses. The aminoglycosides are considered the cornerstone of gram-negative bacterial infections. Aminoglycosides are often used in combination with other antibiotics to reduce the potential for resistance and to enhance the bacteriocidal activity. Uses include the treatment for gram-negative sepsis or bacteremia, pneumonias, and enterococcal infections.

Hazards. The use of aminoglycosides has been associated with renal toxicity. Normally, pediatric and neonatal patients are at a low risk for renal toxicity. Another potential hazard is that of ototoxicity, which affects hearing and balance. Although the mechanism is not totally understood, it is thought that the risk is associated to the dose and duration of the drug.

Macrolides. Drugs currently available in the macrolide group include erythromycin, clar-ithromycin, and azithromycin. Erythromycin is the prototype drug, while clarithromycin and azithromycin are newer generation drugs.

Mode of Action. The macrolides are similar to the aminoglycosides in that they bind to the ribosomal subunit of the bacteria. An important difference is that the bind is reversible, making them bacteriostatic instead of bacteriocidal.

Uses. The macrolides have both gram-positive and gram-negative coverage. Organisms susceptible to macrolides include streptococcus and staphylococcus, *H. influenzae, Neisseria gonorrhoeae, N. catarrhalis, Legionella, Mycoplasma pneumoniae, Chlamydia pneumoniae* and *C. trachomatis, Mycobacterium*, and *Toxoplasma gondii.*

Hazards. The major hazard associated with the macrolides is the inhibition of hepatic metabolism of certain drugs resulting in elevated serum concentrations and potential toxicities. These drugs include theophylline, carbamazepine, astemizole, terfenadine, and cisapride.

Quinolones. This class of drug, also called 4-fluoroquinolones, includes ciprofloxacin, ofloxacin, lomefloxacin, norfloxacin, and enoxacin.

Mode of Action. The quinolones inhibit DNA gyrase, the enzyme that nicks strands of DNA to promote the twisting or untwisting of the DNA strand, and then reseals the nicks. By inhibiting this enzyme, DNA replication is inhibited and the bacteria are effectively eliminated.

Uses. In general, the quinolones are not used as first line agents. They are effective against staphylococcus, but have poor activity against streptococcus and because of this are generally not recommended for gram-positive infections. Gram-negative acitivity include *E. coli, Klebsiella, P. mirabilis, Morganella,* and *Pseudomonas* (if used combined with an aminoglycoside).

Hazards. Quinolones inhibit hepatic enzymes and can cause increased serum levels, and possible toxicity in drugs that are hepatically metabolized. The quinolones are also extensively excreted renally and the dose should be adjusted in patients with renal problems.

Tetracyclines and Chloramphenicol. Drugs in this category include tetracycline, chlortetracycline, oxytetracycline, demeclocycline, doxycycline, minocycline, methacycline, and chloramphenicol.

Mode of Action. The tetracyclines and chloramphenicol prevent protein synthesis at the level of the binding of transfer RNA/amino acid complexes to the ribosomes. This action disables the bacteria's ability to reproduce and therefore makes tetracyclines bacteriostatic.

Uses. All tetracyclines are active against most gram-positive cocci, and against many gram-negative bacilli. Mycoplasma and Chlamydia are also inhibited. The tetracyclines are often used as a substitute for patients who cannot tolerate, or are allergic to erythromycin. Chloramphenicol is the drug of choice to treat typhoid fever. It is also used to treat *H. influenzae, N. meningitidis*, and *S. pneumoniae* and is bactericidal against these organisms. Because choloramphenicol penetrates well into the eye and brain, it is effective at treating susceptible infections in those organs.

Hazards. Tetracyclines should not be used in patients younger than 8 years old due to the fact that they can permanently stain the teeth. Hazards with choloramphenicol include: aplastic anemia, which has a low incidence but high mortality; dose-related bone marrow depression; and "gray baby syndrome," which is manifest as circulatory collapse in premature infants and neonates with doses in excess of 50 mg/kg/day or serum levels >20–25 mcg/ml.

Sulfonamides and Trimethoprim. The sulfonamide, sulfamethoxazole, is given with trimethoprim, providing a raised activity level and widened spectrum of activity than when used alone. Other sulfonamides include sulfisoxazole, sulfadiazine, sulfamethizole, sulfadoxine, and sulfasalazine.

Mode of Action. In order for a bacterium to reproduce, para-aminobenzoic acid (PABA) must be converted to folic acid. The steps in formation are first PABA, then dihydrofolate, tetrahydrofolate, and finally, folic acid. The sulfonamide drugs prevent the conversion of PABA to dihydrofolate, and trimethoprim prevents the conversion of dihydrofolate to tetrahydrofolate. The two, therefore, work synergistically to stop bacterial reproduction.

Uses. The sulfonamides are used to treat various gram-positive and some gram-negative infections, such as *E. coli, Klebsiella, Proteus, Shigella, Xanthomonas maltophilia*, and *Nocardia*. Trimethoprim has activity against many gram-positive cocci, and most gram-negative rods.

Hazards. Sulfonamides have been associated with acute hemolytic anemia, aplastic anemia, agranulocytosis, thrombocytopenia, and leukopenia. The sulfonamides also have a higher than normal rate of hypersensitivity reactions. Because a large percentage of trimethoprim is eliminated by the kidneys, the dosage must be closely monitored in patients with renal insufficiency.

Antifungals. Fungal infections are commonly seen as an opportunistic skin infection, often occurring in areas that are warm and moist. These infections are usually treated with topical antifungals, but may require oral therapy if severe. Fungal infections of the blood and CNS carry a high risk of mortality and morbidity and must be treated aggressively with oral antifungal agents. The oral antifungals include amphotericin B, nystatin, flucytosine, ketoconazole, miconazole, griseofulvin, fluconazole, and intraconazole.

Mode of Action. Most of the antifungals work by inhibiting enzymes in the cell membrane and binding membrane sterols, making them more permeable.

Uses. Antifungals vary greatly in their ability to treat infections and it is necessary to identify the organism before treating, to ensure coverage. In general, the antifungals are used to treat *Aspergillus, Candida, Blastomyces, Coccidioides, Cryptococci, Histoplasma, Leishmania,* and *Sporotrichum.*

Hazards. One of the most common side effects seen with IV antifungals, especially amphotericin B, is the so-called "shake and bake" syndrome, consisting of chills, fever, headache, myalgias, hypotension, nausea, and vomiting. Chronic use of oral antifungals can lead to nephrotoxicity, thrombophlebitis, and anemia.

Antivirals. Common antivirals include amantadine, rimantadine, acyclovir, famcyclovir, valacyclovir, vidarabine, zidovudine, ganciclovir, didanosine, and zalcitabine. Ribavirin, an aerosolized antiviral agent, is discussed in more detail below.

Mode of Action. In order to understand how antivirals work, it is useful to review how viruses reproduce. When a virus attaches itself to a cell, it injects an enzyme messenger into the cell, which forces the cell to replicate the DNA of the virus. Chemically, the antiviral drug is similar to the amino acid thymidine. As the antiviral drug is placed in the DNA chain in place of the thymidine, further attachment of amino acids is blocked and thus the reproduction of the virus is stopped. It is for this reason that antiviral drugs are referred to as chain terminators.

Uses. Most of the antiviral drugs are used to treat HIV related illness. Other indications are herpes simplex infections, cytomegalovirus retinitis, varicella zoster, and influenza virus infections.

Hazards. Each antiviral drug has its own side effects and hazards and many are dose related. Mild effects may include nausea and vomiting. More advanced hazards include phlebitis, CNS toxicity, depressed bone marrow function, convulsions, pancreatitis, and peripheral neuropathy.

Ribavirin. Ribavirin is a broad-spectrum antiviral drug that is specifically used in the neonatal population for the treatment of bronchiolitis caused by respiratory syncytial virus (RSV). Ribavirin is delivered via a unique device called the Small Particle Aerosol Generator (SPAG 2). The use of this device is covered in Chapter 6.

Ribavirin comes as 6 grams of a sterile powder that is reconstituted by adding 50 to 100 ml of sterile water with no additives. This solution is then transferred to a sterile 500 ml flask in the SPAG-2 unit and further diluted with sterile water to a volume of 300 ml. This final concentration contains 20 mg of drug per ml. With this concentration, the SPAG-2 unit delivers a mist of approximately 190 mg of ribavirin per liter. The dose delivered to the respiratory tract can then be estimated by using the equation in Table 8–1.

The dose and administration of ribavirin for the treatment of RSV is the same for ventilated and nonventilated patients. Treatment to ventilated patients is covered in Chapter 6. The mist from the SPAG-2 unit is delivered to the patient via a hood, tent, or mask. When

TABLE 8–1   Estimating Ribavirin Delivery

TOTAL DOSE = MV x DOI x 0.19 x 0.7

MV	=	Minute Volume (liters)
DOI	=	Duration of inhalation (minutes)
0.19	=	Concentration of ribavirin delivered
0.7	=	Fraction of inhaled dose deposited in the respiratory tract

given via a hood or tent, the aerosol is delivered at a rate of 15 lpm, and at 12 lpm when delivered to a mask. The patient receives the aerosol continuously for 12 to 18 hours daily for 3 to 7 days. The exact length of treatment is determined individually for each patient and is based on the severity of illness, age of the patient, and the presence of underlying diseases.

Environmental Exposure Concerns. Evidence from animal studies shows a potential for teratogencity with exposure to ribavirin. Additionally, no established data defining safe levels of exposure have been produced. Until studies show that exposure does not provide a risk, health care providers and visitors must protect themselves, and be protected from exposure to ribavirin. This is true especially for those females who are pregnant, or trying to become pregnant. The most frequent adverse effects reported are eye irritation, headache, nasal and throat irritation, pharyngitis, nausea, dizziness, fatigue, and rash.

The amount of environmental exposure varies tremendously depending on the method of delivery, length of exposure, number of patients being treated in a room, size of the room, room ventilation, administration schedules, and the integrity of the SPAG-2 unit. To minimize environmental exposure, several precautionary measures have been devised. When a tent or hood are used, an outer hood or cover can be placed over the primary hood or tent. A vacuum tube is then placed in the space between the outer and inner covers. The idea behind this procedure is that any excess ribavirin delivered to the inner hood or tent, will escape to the space between the two covers. It is then evacuated through the vacuum tube to the outside, or through filters that remove the ribavirin. Other measures include requiring all who enter the room to wear gowns, gloves, goggles, and masks. Surgical masks do not filter the ribavirin. This makes the use of special, small particulate filter masks necessary. Except when immediate care is required, the SPAG-2 unit should be shut off remotely, 10 to 15 minutes before entering the room. It is also recommended that ribavirin only be delivered in isolation rooms that are under negative pressure, have adequate air exchange, and vent to the outside.

Other Antibiotics. Several other antibiotics exist that are not generally categorized. These include clinadamycin, lincomycin, vancomycin, and metronidazole. Clindamycin and lincomycin are limited for use with anaerobic infections and severe gram-positive infections. The primary use of vancomycin is in the treatment of MRSA, enterococci, and *Clostridia*. Metronidazole is very active against gram-negative anaerobes, amoebae, and *Trichomonas*.

CARDIOVASCULAR MEDICATIONS

Adenosine
Indications. Adenosine is indicated for the acute treatment of sustained paroxysmal supraventricular tachycardia (SVT).

Dosages. The starting dose for adenosine is 50 mcg/kg given intravenously rapidly over 1 to 2 seconds. The dose is then increased 50 mcg/kg every 2 minutes until sinus rhythm returns, for a total of 250 mcg/kg.

Effects. Adenosine is the active metabolite of adenosine triphosphate (ATP). Its action consists of depressing sinus node automaticity and AV conduction. Response is expected within 2 minutes of the dose.

Adverse Effects and Precautions. The most common adverse effects are flushing, irritability, and dyspnea, which normally resolve within 1 minute. Transient arrhythmias have been known to develop between the termination of SVT and normal sinus rhythm. Thirty percent of patients treated have a recurrence of SVT.

Atropine
Indications. Atropine is used in the reversal of severe sinus bradycardia, especially in the presence of parasympathetic influences (drugs, carotid sinus reflex).

Dosages. Atropine is given at a dosage of 0.01 to 0.03 mg/kg intravenously over a 1-minute period. It can also be given via the endotracheal tube at 2 to 3 times the intravenous dose, followed immediately by 1 ml of normal saline (NS).

Effects. Atropine is an anticholinergic drug. As such, it blocks the parasympathetic receptors, thus reducing the stimulation of the parasympathetic branch that is causing bradycardia.

Adverse Effects and Precautions. Cardiac arrhythmias have been reported, often during the first 2 minutes following administration. Because of its effects on the gastrointestinal tract, abdominal distention, and esophageal reflux may be increased.

Epinephrine
Indications. Epinephrine is used during resuscitation for the treatment of acute cardiovascular collapse. It may also be used as a short-term treatment for cardiac failure that is resistant to other drugs. Additionally, it is used subcutaneously in the treatment of acute bronchospasm.

Dosages. For bradycardia and hypotension, epinephrine is given 0.1 to 0.3 ml/kg of a 1:10,000 concentration.

Effects. As a powerful sympathomimetic agent, epinephrine causes an increase in the rate and force of heart contractions, dilation of the bronchial smooth muscles, and constriction of the peripheral vasculature.

Adverse Effects and Precautions. Arrhythmias such as premature ventricular contractions and ventricular tachycardia may be seen. The vasoconstrictive effect may lead to renal vascular ischemia.

Digoxin (Lanoxin®)

Indications. Digoxin is indicated for use in atrial fibrillation, atrial flutter, paroxysmal atrial tachycardia (PAT), cardiogenic shock, and all degrees of congestive heart failure (CHF). congestive heart failure is the primary indication for use in neonates.

Dosages. An initial loading dose of digoxin (known as digitalization) is required to provide peak concentrations in the affected tissues and should be dosed as shown in Table 8–2.

The maintenance dose of digoxin is 20 to 30% of the digitalizing dose per day divided into two doses given every 12 hours. For example, the loading dose for a 2-kg preterm infant should be 30 to 50 mcg with a maintenance dose of 3 to 7.5 mcg administered every 12 hours. The relative dose of digoxin in infants is higher than in adults. This is due to a decreased digoxin receptor binding affinity in the neonatal myocardium. Digoxin can be administered orally, intravenously, or intramuscularly.

Effects. The effect of digoxin involves both a direct action on cardiac muscle and the specialized conduction system and indirect action on the cardiovascular system, which is mediated by the autonomic nervous system. The indirect actions effectively depress the sinoatrial (SA) node and prolong conduction to the atrioventricular (AV) node. Direct actions include increasing the force of myocardial systolic contraction, increasing the refractory period of the AV node, and increasing the total peripheral resistance.

Contraindications. Digoxin is contraindicated in patients with ventricular fibrillation, ventricular tachycardia, or who are hypersensitive to the drug.

Adverse Effects and Precautions. Common adverse effects include vomiting, anorexia, bradycardia, and arrhythmias. These adverse effects relate to the narrow range of therapeutic and toxic concentrations that occur within the body, and close monitoring of cardiac function and blood levels for the drug should be performed.

TABLE 8–2   Initial Loading Dose for Digoxin

Preterm Infants: 15–25 mcg/kg
Full-term Infants: 20–30 mcg/kg
1–24 months: 30–50 mcg/kg

Indomethacin Sodium Trihydrate (Indocin® IV)

Indications. Indomethacin is indicated to close a hemodynamically significant patent ductus arteriosus (PDA). Clinical factors used to decide on its use include patient weights between 500 and 1750 g and a persistent PDA following 48 hours of fluid restriction, diuretics, digoxin, and respiratory support. Clinically, a hemodynamically significant PDA is identified by the presence of the following: respiratory distress, continuous murmur, hyperactive precordium, and cardiomegaly.

Dosages. Indomethacin is administered to neonates in three doses given at 12- to 24-hour intervals by the intravenous route only. Table 8–3 shows the recommended dosages by age.

If closure or significant reduction of the ductus arteriosus occurs after 48 hours or more from completion of the first course of therapy, no further doses are necessary. If the ductus arteriosus reopens, a second course of one to three doses may be given as described in Table 8–3.

Contraindications. Indomethacin is contraindicated in infants who have proven or suspected untreated infections, bleeding (particularly intracranial hemorrhage or gastrointestinal (GI) bleeding), thrombocytopenia, coagulation defects, or significant renal function impairment.

Adverse Effects. Major adverse effects experienced with the use of indomethacin include bleeding and coagulation problems, renal dysfunction characterized by decreased urinary output and elevated serum creatinine, and GI bleeding. Apnea has been reported following administration of indomethacin. However, a causal relationship to indomethacin therapy has not been established.

Precautions. The use of indomethacin may conceal the signs and symptoms of infection. The drug should be stopped if clinical signs and symptoms of liver disease develop. The drug may be very irritating and should be administered carefully to avoid *extravasation* into the tissue.

Alprostadil-Prostaglandin E₁ (Prostin® VR Pediatric)

Indications. Alprostadil is indicated to maintain the patency of the ductus arteriosus until corrective surgery can be performed. It is used in neonates with congenital heart defects who depend on the patent ductus for survival.

TABLE 8–3 Recommended Dosage of Indomethacin

AGE AT FIRST DOSE	DOSAGE (MG/KG)		
	1st	2nd	3rd
Less than 48 hours	0.2	0.1	0.1
2–7 days	0.2	0.2	0.2
Greater than 7 days	0.2	0.25	0.25

Dosages. Alprostadil is administered by continuous intravenous infusion into a large vein or through an umbilical artery catheter. The infusion should be started at a rate of 0.1 mcg/kg/min until an adequate therapeutic response is seen. The response is an increased PaO_2 for infants with restricted pulmonary blood flow or increased systemic blood pressure and blood pH in infants with restricted systemic blood flow. The rate of infusion should be reduced to as low a level as possible and still maintain an adequate response.

Effects. Alprostadil causes vasodilation, inhibits platelet aggregation, and relaxes smooth muscle of the ductus arteriosus. Infants with an initially low PaO_2 value (less than 40 mm Hg) appear to have a greater increase in blood oxygenation than those with PaO_2 values greater than 40 mm Hg.

Contraindications. There are no known contraindications to the use of alprostadil.

Adverse Effects. Fever, seizures, flushing, bradycardia, hypotension, apnea, and diarrhea are several of the major adverse effects seen with alprostadil use.

Precautions. Alprostadil should be infused for the shortest length of time in the lowest dose possible to produce positive effects. Use cautiously in infants with bleeding tendencies due to the drug's inhibition of platelet aggregation. Alprostadil should not be used in patients with respiratory distress syndrome. Routine or constant monitoring of arterial pressure, blood oxygenation, systemic blood pressure, and blood pH should be performed.

Dopamine HCl (Intropin®)

Indications. Dopamine is indicated for the correction of hemodynamic imbalances present in the shock syndrome due to decreased cardiac function in congestive heart failure, trauma, endotoxic septicemia, renal failure, and myocardial infarction.

Dosages. Dopamine is administered by continuous intravenous infusion only at a rate of 2 to 20 mcg/kg/min and titrated according to the patient's response.

Effects. Dopamine is a catecholamine that is naturally occurring within the body. Its effects are seen both directly on alpha and beta-1 receptors as well as indirectly by releasing norepinephrine throughout the system. Beta-1 effects cause an increase in cardiac output through positive inotropic effects on the myocardium. Dopamine dilates the renal vasculature and causes an increase in glomerular filtration rate, renal blood flow, and sodium excretion. In low doses, cardiac stimulation and renal vascular dilation occur, and in larger doses, the alpha-adrenergic effect of vasoconstriction occurs.

Contraindications. Contraindications are *pheochromocytoma* (a type of chronic hypertension) tachyarrhythmias, or ventricular fibrillation.

Adverse Effects. The most common adverse effects encountered with the use of dopamine are ectopic heartbeats, tachycardia, hypotension, vasoconstriction, and vomiting.

Precautions. Dopamine should be used in conjunction with blood, plasma, and fluid replacement. Routine and/or constant monitoring of blood pressure, pulse pressure, and urine output should be performed. If extravasation occurs, phentolamine (Regitine®) should be administered throughout the area of extravasation.

Dobutamine (Dobutrex®)

Indications. Dobutamine is indicated for short-term treatment to increase cardiac output due to decreased contractility from organic heart disease or cardiac surgical procedures.

Dosages. Dobutamine is administered by continuous intravenous infusion only at a rate of 2.5 to 10 mcg/kg/min and titrated according to the patient's response. The maximum recommended infusion rate is 40 mcg/kg/min.

Effects. Dobutamine is a drug chemically related to dopamine with most of its effects exhibited on the beta-1 receptors. Dobutamine has very little effect on the alpha receptors and does not cause the release of norepinephrine, nor does it have any effect on the renal vasculature.

Contraindications. Dopamine is contraindicated in patients with idiopathic hypertrophic subaortic stenosis (IHSS).

Adverse Effects. There are several dose-related adverse effects, including increased heart rate, increased blood pressure, and increased ventricular ectopic activity. Infusions continuing longer than 72 hours have not been associated with more adverse effects than shorter-duration infusions with the exception that tolerance to the drug has been reported with infusions lasting longer than 3 days.

Precautions. The use of dobutamine should be in concert with blood, plasma, and fluid replacement. Continuous monitoring of ECG and blood pressure should be performed.

Tolazoline (Priscoline®)

Indications. Tolazoline is indicated for the treatment of persistent pulmonary hypertension of the newborn. Treatment should only be started when arterial oxygenation cannot be maintained by oxygen and/or mechanical ventilation.

Dosages. Tolazoline is given as an initial dose of 1 to mg/kg, followed by an infusion of 1 to 2 mg/kg per hour. The response to the drug usually occurs within 30 minutes of administration.

Effects. Tolazoline has a direct effect on blood vasculature, causing vasodilation. It has additional stimulatory effects on the heart and gastrointestinal tract. Tolazoline reduces pulmonary artery pressure by reducing vascular resistance.

Contraindications. The only contraindication is a hypersensitivity to the drug.

Adverse Effects. Adverse reactions following the administration of tolazoline have been observed; however, their frequency of occurrence is not documented. Adverse effects include hypotension, tachycardia, arrhythmias, nausea, vomiting, diarrhea, pulmonary and gastrointestinal hemorrhage, skin flushing, thrombocytopenia, and edema.

Precautions. In the presence of acidosis, the effects of tolazoline on the pulmonary vasculature may be decreased.

DIURETICS

The class of drugs termed diuretics encompasses a wide variety of agents including carbonic anhydrase inhibitors, thiazides, loop diuretics, potassium-sparing diuretics, and osmotic diuretics. The use of carbonic anhydrase inhibitors, osmotic diuretics, thiazides, and potassium-sparing diuretics in neonates is very limited. Even though thiazides are the most common diuretic in use today, they are not as effective as the loop diuretics (that is, furosemide) in the neonate due to immature renal tubular function, and a lesser glomerular filtration rate, compared with children and adults.

Acetazolamide (Diamox®)
Indications. The diuretic acetazolamide is often used in conjunction with furosemide to slow the progression of hydrocephalus in patients who are not candidates for surgery.

Dosages. The initial dose is 5 mg/kg every 6 hours, injected slowly intravenously (IV) or orally (PO). The dosage is increased to 25 mg/kg as tolerated.

Effects. Acetazolamide works by inhibiting carbonic anhydrase in the renal tubules. The result is sodium and bicarbonate remain in the tubule and an alkaline diuresis occurs. Acetazolamide also decreases the rate of cerebral spinal fluid (CSF) formation and inhibits seizure activity.

Adverse Effects and Precautions. Premature infants are at risk of developing metabolic acidosis, which may be severe even in low doses. Hypokalemia is also a possibility.

Bumetanide (Bumex®)
Indications. Bumetanide is a diuretic used in patients with congestive heart failure, renal insufficiency, or edema that is refractory to furosemide.

Dosages. The dosage of bumetanide is 0.015 to 0.3 mg/kg per dose, given once every 24 hours.

Effects. Bumetanide is a loop diuretic and is 40 times more potent than furosemide. It also decreases CSF production by a weak carbonic anhydrase inhibition.

Adverse Effects and Precautions. Imbalances in water and electrolytes are frequently seen. In particular, hyponatremia, hypokalemia, and hypochloremic alkalosis are seen. This drug is also potentially ototoxic, but not to the degree of furosemide.

Chlorothiazide (Diuril®)
Indications. Chlorothiazide is a diuretic used to treat mild to moderate edema and hypertension. It may be used in conjunction with furosemide or spironolactone. It has been shown to improve pulmonary function in patients with BPD.

Dosages. Chlorothiazide is dosed at 10 to 20 mg/kg every 12 hours. It can be given intravenously or orally.

Effects. Chlorothiazide's diuretic action is a result of inhibition of sodium reabsorption in the distal nephron. This causes an increase in sodium loss and with it, an increase in water loss.

Adverse Effects and Precautions. The most commonly seen adverse effects are hypokalemia and other electrolyte abnormalities. Hyperglycemia and hyperuricemia are also seen.

Furosemide (Lasix®)
Indications. Furosemide is indicated for the treatment of fluid overload, symptomatic patent ductus arteriosus, hypertension, and pulmonary interstitial edema.

Dosages. Furosemide may be administered orally, intravenously, or intramuscularly. The recommended oral dose is 2 to 6 mg/kg administered every 8 to 12 hours. The recommended intravenous or intramuscular dose is 1 mg/kg initially followed by 2 mg/kg no sooner than 2 hours after the initial dose. An intravenous or intramuscular dose of 1 mg/kg/day to a maximum of 6 mg/kg/day divided every 4 to 12 hours is recommended.

Effects. Furosemide inhibits the reabsorption of electrolytes (specifically sodium and chloride) in the proximal and distal tubules and in the loop of Henle. Diuresis from furosemide results in enhanced excretion of multiple electrolytes. Furosemide also has some renal vasodilator effects by decreasing renal vascular resistance and increasing renal blood flow, causing an increase in glomerular filtration rate.

Contraindications. Furosemide is contraindicated in patients with *anuria*, a cessation of urine output, or who are hypersensitive to the drug.

Adverse Effects. Fluid and electrolyte imbalances are the most common and important adverse effects and should be monitored carefully, especially in the neonate. Electrolyte imbalances (particularly hypokalemia and hypochloremia) may lead to metabolic alkalosis, and potassium supplementation may be necessary in the neonate during furosemide therapy. Other adverse effects include reversible or permanent hearing impairment (usually caused by rapid intravenous administration of too high a dose), dizziness, anorexia, blood *dyscrasias* (abnormal blood or bone marrow condition), and hyperglycemia and glycosuira.

Precautions. Observation for signs of hypovolemia and electrolyte imbalances should be carefully monitored. Periodic urine and blood glucose monitoring should be performed.

Spironolactone (Aldactone®)

Indications. Spironolactone is used in combination with other diuretics in the treatment of congestive heart failure and BPD.

Dosages. Spironolactone is dosed 1 to 3 mg/kg every 24 hours orally.

Effects. Spironolactone is a competitive antagonist of mineralocorticoids (aldosterone). It increases the excretion of calcium, magnesium, sodium, and chloride, and decreases the excretion of potassium. The effects are usually not seen before 2 to 3 days after starting therapy.

Adverse Effects and Precautions. The most common adverse effects are rashes, vomiting, diarrhea, and headaches. There is also a dose-dependent androgenic effect in females.

RESPIRATORY DRUGS

The medications given for the respiratory system are those that cause a relaxation of the bronchial smooth muscles leading to bronchodilation. These drugs are given to the patient aerosolized in a small volume nebulizer or through the intravenous line. We will first examine the aerosolized drugs, and then turn our attention to the bronchodilators administered intravenously.

Aerosolized Drugs. The aerosolized bronchodilators, as with other drugs given to neonates, are not specifically approved for use in neonates, so extreme care and caution must be used when administering these drugs. This category of drugs is divided into four groups: sympathomimetics, parasympatholytics, corticosteroids, and other drugs. We will examine the drugs that fall in each group.

Sympathomimetics. Sympathomimetics are also called beta adrenergics. The name adrenergic comes from their ability to act like adrenalin on the beta sites and cause smooth muscle relaxation. At the effector site, which, in this case, is the bronchial smooth muscle cell, the stimulation of the beta site results in the stimulation of adenyl cyclase, which, in turn, catalyzes the formation of cyclic 3′,5′ adenosine monophosphate (cAMP) from adenosine triphosphate (ATP). This series of reactions is illustrated in Figure 8–2. The presence of cAMP causes the smooth muscle to relax, leading to bronchodilation. cAMP is inactivated by the enzyme phosphodiesterase into AMP, losing the bronchodilatory effect. Stimulation of the bronchial smooth muscle beta site, whether by the sympathetic system or by a sympathomimetic drug, increases the level of 3′,5′ AMP and causes dilation.

All sympathomimetic drugs share the same indication for use, that is, the prevention and treatment of reversible bronchospasm. They also share common adverse reactions and interactions. Adverse reactions include tremors, nervousness, dizziness, insomnia, head-

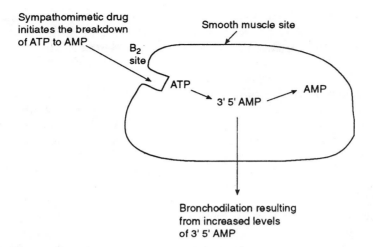

Figure 8–2 *Sympathetic reactions leading to bronchodilation.*

ache, tachycardia, palpitations, hypertension, nausea, and vomiting. The adverse reactions are often secondary to the inherent stimulation of the beta-1 cardiac sites and may also be due to a slight degree of alpha-site stimulation.

A drug interaction common with all sympathomimetics occurs when they are used in combination with propranolol or other beta blockers. Beta-blocking drugs may inhibit the bronchodilatory effect of the sympathomimetic drug, and care must be exercised when used together. A common, potentially dangerous effect of sympathomimetics is a paradoxical bronchospasm that may occur following abuse of the drug.

Albuterol (Proventil®)
Concentration and Dosage. Albuterol comes in a 20-ml vial at a concentration of 5 mg/ml, or 0.5% solution. It is also supplied in unit dose, 3 ml of a 0.083% solution, which is 2.5 mg of albuterol, mixed in 2.5 ml normal saline. When given via a small volume nebulizer, the dosage for the patient 13 and older is 0.5 ml of the 0.5% solution, mixed with 2.5 ml of normal saline. This results in a total dosage of 2.5 mg of albuterol per treatment, given 4 times a day. The dosage of aerosolized albuterol given to children of less than 13 years should be examined on an individual basis, with the dosage titrated as needed.

Metaproterenol Sulfate (Alupent®, Metraprel®)
Concentration and Dosage. Metaproterenol for inhalation comes in a solution with a concentration of 5%. Normal dosage for inhalation is 0.3 ml of a 5% solution diluted with 2.5 ml normal saline. Again, when used with smaller patients, the dosage is titrated according to size and age.

Terbutaline Sulfate (Brethine®, Bricanyl®, Brethaire®)
Concentration and Dosage. Terbutaline comes in a concentration of 1 mg/ml, or a 0.1% solution. It is designed to be given subcutaneously at a dosage of 0.01 mg/kg, but can also

be aerosolized for inhalation. The dosage for that route has not been established and must be determined by the physician on an individual basis. Terbutaline is also available as a metered dose inhaler (MDI), giving a dose of 0.2 mg/puff. In tablet form, terbutaline comes in 2.5- and 5-mg sizes.

Racemic epinephrine (Micronephrine®, Vaponephrine®)

Concentration and Dosage. Racemic epinephrine is supplied for inhalation as a 2.25% solution. The normal dosage is 0.5 ml of solution, diluted with 2.5 to 3 ml of normal saline or sterile water. In addition to being used to treat bronchospasm, racemic epinephrine is indicated for use with upper airway edema producing disease, such as croup. The stimulation of the alpha sites, on the laryngeal blood vasculature, results in vasoconstriction, with a reduction of edema and swelling.

Parasympatholytics. The action of the parasympathetic system in bronchospasm (Figure 8–3) is opposite that of the sympathetic system. When the parasympathetic system is stimulated, acetylcholine is released at the cholinergic receptor site and stimulates the production of guanyl cyclase. Guanyl cyclase is the enzyme that converts guanosine triphosphate (GTP) to cyclic 3.5 guanosine monophosphate (cGMP). The action of cGMP causes smooth muscle contraction and also enhances the release of mediators from the mast cell.

The action of the parasympatholytic drugs is to block the cholinergic receptor site to acetylcholine, thus stopping the formation of cGMP and reducing the bronchospasm. Drugs that exert this effect are called cholinergic blockers or parasympatholytic drugs. Due to the slow nature of the parasympathetic system, these drugs are of no value during an acute attack, but are used as prophylaxis to bronchospasm.

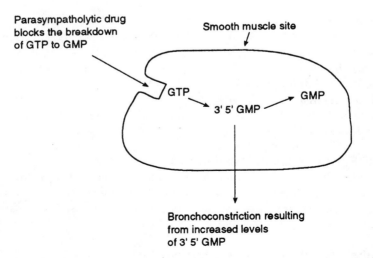

Figure 8–3 *Parasympathetic reactions which cause bronchoconstriction.*

Atropine

Concentration. Atropine comes in ampules in a concentration of 1 mg/0.5 ml, which results in a 0.2% solution. It is also available as 2.5 mg/0.5 ml, resulting in a 0.5% solution.

Dosage. The recommended dosage for a child is 0.05 mg/kg given 3 to 4 times per day.

Side Effects. Side effects of atropine include dry mouth, blurred vision, and palpitations. Atropine also has a drying effect on secretions. This may pose problems in the patient with thick, viscous secretions.

Ipratropium bromide (Atrovent®). Chemically, ipratropium bromide is a quanternary ammonium derivative of atropine. As such, it is poorly absorbed, is not rapidly removed from the site of deposition, and does not cross the blood-brain barrier, as does atropine. It is therefore the drug of choice in the parasympatholytic class. These traits give it a wider therapeutic margin, with fewer side effects.

Dosage. The dosage of ipratropium bromide per treatment is in the range of 40 to 80 µg for adults. Each puff of the MDI gives 18 µg of medication. It is also available as an inhalation solution of 0.02%. This gives 0.5 mg of medication in 2.5 ml. Dosages should be titrated by the physician when used on neonatal and pediatric patients.

Glycopyrrolate (Robinul®). Glycopyrrolate is another quaternary ammonium derivative of atropine. When aerosolized, it provides bronchodiliatory effects similar to atropine with fewer side effects. Experimentally, the drug has been nebulized in 1-mg dosages.[2] However, it was never released for aerosol therapy, and is not available for use.

Corticosteroids. The use of steroids in respiratory disorders is usually reserved for those cases in which other methods have not produced the desired results. This is because of the serious side effects of steroids, namely, suppression of immunologic and inflammatory responses. Patients on chronic steroid therapy may develop adrenal insufficiency and may be more prone to infection.

When aerosolized and delivered to the respiratory tract, steroids appear to reduce the inflammatory response of asthma. This effectively reduces the swelling, edema, bronchoconstriction, and increased outpouring of secretions seen during asthma attacks. It has been shown that steroids do produce short-term improvements in pulmonary function. The long-term effects of steroids on the neonate are unknown.

Aerosolized corticosteroids are delivered via MDI unless otherwise noted. All share the same indications, which are the treatment of bronchopulmonary dysplasis and asthma that does not respond to other conventional treatments. Steroids delivered via MDI share some common adverse reactions, which include hoarseness, dry throat, and mouth and oral *Candida* infections.

Common steroids and their dosages are listed below. Dosages are those prescribed for adults. Neonatal and pediatric dosages must be titrated to the individual patient as prescribed by a physician.

Beclomethasone (Vanceril®, Beclovent®)
Dosage. 1 to 2 inhalations of the MDI taken 3 or 4 times per day.

Flunisolide (Aerobid®)
Dosage. 1 to 2 inhalations of the MDI taken 2 times per day.

Dexamethasone (Respihaler®)
Dosage. 2 to 3 inhalations of the MDI taken 3 to 4 times per day.

Triamcinolone (Azmacort®)
Dosage. 1 to 2 inhalations of the MDI taken 3 to 4 times per day.

Other Drugs for Inhalation. This group of drugs includes those respiratory drugs that do not fit into the above groups.

Cromolyn Sodium (Intal®). The action of cromolyn sodium is to inhibit degranulation of the sensitized mast cell. Degranulation of the mast cell occurs following exposure to a specific antigen. It appears that cromolyn sodium stabilizes the membrane of the mast cell by blocking the entrance of calcium into the cell, preventing the release of asthma mediators. Cromolyn sodium is used to prevent bronchospasm and therefore has little effect as a bronchodilator.

Concentration and Dosage. Cromolyn sodium is provided as a dry powder, contained in a capsule with 20 mg of the drug. It is also available as a liquid for nebulization, 20 mg in 2 ml of liquid. The normal adult dosage is 20 mg of the drug, inhaled 4 times a day at regular intervals. If no relief is seen after a trial of 4 weeks of cromolyn sodium, the regime is stopped. Treatment should also be stopped if the patient develops an eosinophilic pneumonia.

Adverse Effects. Cromolyn sodium is used for prophylaxis and is of no value during an acute asthmatic attack. Possible adverse reactions to cromolyn sodium include bronchospasm, cough, laryngeal edema, pharyngeal irritation, and wheezing. The patient may also suffer headaches, dizziness, nausea, dysuria, rash, and joint swelling and pain.

Pentamidine Isethionate (Nebupent®, Pentam 300®)
Indications. Pentamidine is an antibiotic specifically used for the prophylactic treatment of protozoan infections. In particular, pentamidine has been designated for prophylactic treatment of *Pneumocystis carinii* pneumonia (PCP) in patients infected with HIV. Pentamidine must be delivered via a special nebulizer, described in Chapter 6.

Dosage. The inhalation dosage for primary or secondary prevention of PCP using the Respirgard II® jet nebulizer is 300 mg administered every 4 weeks. Another regimen uses the FISOneb® nebulizer with an initial loading dose of five 60 mg. doses given at 24- to 72-hour intervals over a 2-week period. This is followed by a maintenance dosage of 60 mg every 2 weeks.

Adverse Effects. The most commonly seen adverse effects with inhaled pentamidine are coughing and bronchospasm. Both can often be controlled by interrupting the treatment and administering a bronchodilator. Pretreatment with a bronchodilator may also reduce the incidence and severity of coughing and bronchospasm. Coughing has also been controlled by slowing the delivery of the aerosol stream. Other respiratory effects include laryngitis, shortness of breath, chest pain, congestion, and pneumothorax. Occasional adverse effects include rhinitis, hyperventilation, hemoptysis, gagging, cyanosis, and tachypnea.

Hepatic effects include elevated liver function tests, hepatitis, hepatomegaly, and hepatic dysfunction.

Adverse effects seen in the nervous system include neuralgia, confusion, hallucinations, and dizziness. Less often seen are tremors, anxiety, depression, memory loss, seizure, insomnia, loss of taste and smell, and fatigue.

Other adverse effects include hypocalcemia, fever, anaphylactic reactions, shock, conjunctivitis, eye discomfort, blurred vision, and blepharitis.

Exposure Risks and Precautions. The U.S. Centers for Disease Control and Prevention have issued an advisement for health care personnel to be aware of possible exposure to tuberculosis in HIV infected patients receiving pentamidine aerosol, due to the coughing that often accompanies it. Patients should be screened and anti-tuberculosis therapy initiated before beginning aerosolized pentamidine therapy.

Because the risk of potential effects of pentamidine on a fetus and pregnancy, as well as the risk of long-term exposure by health care workers is not totally understood, precautions should be taken by those who have contact with these patients. For pregnant, or potentially pregnant females, it is advised that any exposure to pentamidine be avoided. For all others, precautions such as the use of gloves, gowns, goggles, and masks should be followed. The patient receiving treatment should be isolated in a room or chamber and the air inside the room or chamber vented and filtered. Ideally the room or chamber will be negatively pressured to prevent the escape of the drug and exhaled droplets from the room.

Aerosolized Antibiotics. The aerosolization of antibiotics directly to the bronchial tree is advocated for treatment of organism colonization in the pulmonary tree. The advantage to this type of delivery is that it targets the specific site of infection and avoids systemic side effects. The aminoglycoside tobramycin, delivered at a dosage of 600 mg every 8 hours, has been successful in treating *pseudomonas*. Another antibiotic, colistin, has also been used in aerosol therapy, as well as gentamyacin.

INTRAVENOUS RESPIRATORY DRUGS

Methylxanthines. There still exists much controversy in the literature about whether theophylline or caffeine is the preferred respiratory drug of choice in premature infants. There are several general differences in the newborn system's ability to manage theophylline or caffeine, compared with adults. Theophylline has a greater tissue distribution and also has less protein-binding capacity in infants than in adults. Therefore, lower doses as well as a lower therapeutic range is necessary for infants.

Theophylline is not metabolized in premature and full-term infants via the same mechanism as it is in adults. In infants, theophylline is metabolized to caffeine, and serum concentrations of both theophylline and caffeine can and should be measured. In adults, caffeine is significantly metabolized, and, in contrast, most of the administered dose of caffeine (85%) is excreted unchanged in the urine in newborns.

Caffeine Citrate and Theophylline. Intravenous or oral solutions of caffeine citrate are not commercially available, and must be prepared by the pharmacist. Many oral solid and oral liquid dosage forms and strengths of theophylline are available. The intravenous formulation for theophylline is aminophylline (theophylline ethylenediamine), which is 80% theophylline.

Indications. Caffeine and theophylline are indicated for the treatment and management of neonatal apnea and for the treatment of acute and chronic bronchospasm.

Dosages for Caffeine Citrate. An initial loading dose of 10 mg/kg caffeine followed by a maintenance dose of 2.5 mg/kg administered once a day is recommended. Plasma caffeine levels ranging from 5 to 20 mcg/ml are associated with control of neonatal apnea.

Dosages for Theophylline and Aminophylline. For intravenous therapy an initial loading dose of 5 to 6 mg/kg theophylline (6.3 to 7.5 mg/kg aminophylline) followed by a maintenance dose of 3 to 6 mg/kg/day total dose of theophylline divided every 8 to 12 hours is used. Plasma theophylline levels ranging from 6 to 13 mcg/ml are associated with control of neonatal apnea.

Effects. Caffeine and theophylline exhibit their bronchodilatory effects by directly relaxing the smooth muscle of the bronchi and pulmonary blood vessels. The exact mechanism of relaxation that the xanthines produce is unknown; however, two mechanisms of action are currently accepted. The older of the two theories is based on the discovery that the xanthines inhibit the breakdown of cAMP by inhibiting phosphodiesterase. Phosphodiesterease is the enzyme that reduces cAMP to AMP. Therefore, if phosophodiesterase is inhibited, the cyclic AMP remains longer, exerting its effect of bronchodilation.

A newer finding suggests that the xanthines may block the action of adenosine. Adenosine is formed from intracellular AMP and has been shown to cause bronchoconstriction in asthmatics.

Other effects of the xanthines are stimulating the central nervous system, inducing diuresis, increasing gastric acid secretion, and as central respiratory stimulants.

Contraindications. Contraindications are hypersensitivity to xanthines and active gastritis or peptic ulcer disease.

Adverse Effects. Adverse effects are usually not seen with the xanthine-related products when appropriate serum levels are maintained. When normal serum levels are exceeded, adverse effects (in order of increasing toxicity) include nausea, vomiting, diarrhea, insomnia, irritability, tachycardia, cardiac arrhythmias, seizures, coma and death.

Precautions. Because of the effects of caffeine and theophylline on the heart, caution should be exercised in patients with severe cardiac disease, congestive heart failure, and severe hypertension. Routine monitoring of serum theophylline and/or caffeine levels should be performed.

ANTICONVULSANTS

Phenobarbital
Indications. Phenobarbital is indicated for the treatment of generalized tonic-clonic and cortical focal seizures and also for the acute control of convulsive episodes, including status epilepticus, eclampsia, meningitis, and tetanus. Phenobarbital is also indicated as a sedative for use in pediatric patients. Phenobarbital has been used for the management of narcotic withdrawal in the newborn.

Dosages. For the management of acute convulsive episodes, the recommended dose is 15 to 20 mg/kg administered intravenously immediately. The maintenance dose for the treatment of seizures or narcotic withdrawal is 1 to 5 mg/kg/day administered orally, intravenously, or intramuscularly every 8 to 12 hours. The recommended therapeutic serum levels are between 15 and 40 mcg/ml.

Effects. Phenobarbital is a drug in the barbiturate class. This class of drugs produces all levels of central nervous system alterations ranging from excitation to depression. Generally, barbiturates depress the sensory cortex causing a depression in motor activity, drowsiness, and sedation. Barbiturates can also cause respiratory depression in large enough doses.

Contraindications. Barbiturates are contraindicated in patients with impaired liver function or respiratory distress.

Adverse Effects. Barbiturates may cause a variety of adverse effects, including sleep disorders, nervousness, apnea, respiratory depression, vomiting, diarrhea or constipation, skin rashes, and liver damage with chronic use.

Precautions. Monitoring of liver and renal functions is recommended. The half-life of phenobarbital in the immediate newborn is very long, because of the immaturity of the newborn liver enzyme metabolizing system. As the age of the infant increases and the liver enzyme system matures, the half-life of phenobarbital decreases rapidly. For these reasons, monitoring of phenobarbital serum levels is highly recommended.

Phenytoin Sodium (Dilantin®)
Indications. Phenytoin is indicated for the control of grand mal seizures, for the prevention of seizures during or following surgery, and has been used investigationally (non-FDA approved use) as an antiarrhythmic agent.

Dosages. The recommended loading dose for neonates is 15 to 20 mg/kg administered via slow intravenous push in two divided doses separated by 20 minutes. The phenytoin maintenance dose for seizure control is 1 to 3 mg/kg/dose administered every 12 hours. The recommended serum levels for phenytoin are between 5 to 20 mg/ml. Even though oral suspension forms of phenytoin are commercially available, they should not be used in neonates owing to unpredictable absorption from the gastrointestinal tract.

Effects. The specific effects of phenytoin are not completely understood; however, it appears that phenytoin inhibits the spread of seizure activity in the motor cortex of the brain via multiple biochemical mechanisms.

Contraindications. Phenytoin should not be used in patients with sinus bradycardia, sinoatrial block, and second- or third-degree AV block.

Adverse Effects. There are many adverse effects associated with the use of phenytoin and many are related to long-term use of the drug. Major short-term adverse effects include motor twitching, irritability, insomnia, hypotension when rapidly administered intravenously, diarrhea or constipation, hepatitis, jaundice, liver damage, blood dyscrasias, and, occasionally, hyperglycemia.

Precautions. It is very important that intravenous doses of phenytoin be administered slowly to avoid some of the adverse effects of the drug. The pH of phenytoin injection is alkaline and irritating to the vein, and doses should be followed with normal saline for injection to flush the catheter. Due to the chemical composition of phenytoin, it is incompatible with the majority of IV solutions. For this reason, intravenous administration should be made as close to the catheter injection site as possible to avoid potential incompatibilities with IV solutions. Phenytoin should not be administered intramuscularly due to unpredictable absorption and pain and muscle damage at the injection site.

Felbamate (Felbatol®)
Indications. In the pediatric population, felbamate is used to control partial and generalized seizures associated with Lennox-Gastaut syndrome.

Dosage. In the child aged 2 to 14 years, felbamate is added at 15 mg/kg/day in 3 or 4 divided doses. If other antiseizure medicines are in use, they are reduced by 20% to control plasma levels. Felbamate is then increased 15 mg/kg/day at weekly intervals to a maximum dosage of 45 mg/kg/day.

Adverse Effects. The most commonly seen side effect is a rash. Acne is also occasionally seen.

Valproic Acid (Depakene®, Depakote®)
Indications. Valproic acid is indicated for the treatment of simple and complex absence seizures, including petit mal seizures.

Dosage. Valproic acid is dosed 15 mg/kg/day initially, and then increased as tolerated weekly 5 to 10 mg/kg/day until the optimal clinical response is achieved. The maximum dosage is 60 mg/kg/day.

Adverse Effects and Precautions. The use of this drug carries a risk of hepatotoxicity, especially within the first 6 months of therapy. The risk is highest in patients younger than 2 years of age. To avoid this problem, liver function tests should be performed before starting therapy and at regular intervals thereafter.

Carbamazapine (Tegretol®)
Indications. Carbamazapine is used for pediatric patients with epilepsy.

Dosage. For the child 6 to 12 years of age, 100 mg BID (twice daily) is given to start with weekly increases of 100 mg/day, up to a maximum of 1,000 mg/day in 3 to 4 divided doses. For the treatment of the child above age 12, the dose is started at 200 mg BID and increased 200 mg/day on a weekly basis up to a maximum of 1200 mg/day given 3 to 4 times per day.

Steroids. The steroid discussed in this section relates to its use outside the realm of respiratory disorders. Its use in the treatment of asthma and BPD is covered in the respiratory drug section of this chapter.

Dexamethasone (Decadron®).
Dexamethasone is the primary steroid that is used in neonates. It has less sodium retention activity than most of the other glucocorticoid steroids.

Indications. Dexamethasone is indicated for use in neonates for the treatment of tracheal edema, cerebral edema, and bronchopulmonary dysplasia (BPD). Dexamethasone is also indicated in the treatment of various dermatologic conditions, allergic conditions both systemically and topically, bronchial asthma, and inflammatory diseases.

Dosage. General neonatal recommendations for dexamethasone therapy are 0.2 to 0.5 mg/kg as an intravenous loading dose, followed by 0.1 to 0.4 mg/kg/day divided every 6 to 8 hours and administered either orally or intravenously. There are several guidelines for dexamethasone dosing in BPD. Each protocol is different in exact dosing, however, a gradual tapering of the dose over 7 to 21 days has been used and found effective.

Effects. Glucocorticoids exhibit their effects on virtually all body systems. Their mechanism of action is extremely complex and is involved with all levels of each cell's biochemical activity. This action includes the stabilization of cell membranes, inhibiting macrophage accumulation in inflamed areas, interference with the complement system, promoting gluconeogenesis, and suppressing the release of adrenocorticotropic hormone (ACTH).

Contraindications. Intravenously administered glucocorticoids are contraindicated in patients who are hypersensitive to them.

Adverse Effects. Some of the adverse effects associated with the short-term use of dexamethasone include hypertension, adrenal suppression, anaphylactic reactions, sodium and fluid retention, suppression of skin test reactions, and masking of the symptoms of infection.

Precautions. Dexamethasone therapy should be monitored by observing patients for weigh increase, edema, and hypertension.

SEDATION AND CONTROL OF VENTILATION

Chloral Hydrate (Noctec®)
Indications. Chloral hydrate is indicated when sedation of the patient is desired, to calm agitation, and to aid in sleep.

Dosage. Chloral hydrate is given orally or rectally at a dosage of 25 to 50 mg/kg. The oral preparation should be given after feedings or should be diluted to decrease the risk of gastric irritation.

Contraindications. Chloral hydrate should not be given in large doses in those patients with severe cardiac disease.

Adverse Effects. Chloral hydrate may cause CNS depression, gastric irritation, vasodilation, respiratory depression, cardiac arrhythmias, and myocardial depression. Because chloral hydrate does not provide any analgesic effect, a patient in pain may demonstrate a paradoxical excitement.

Precautions. Chloral hydrate should be used with caution on patients with renal and/or hepatic disease. In addition, caution must be employed when used with other CNS depressant drugs, furosemide, and anticoagulants.

Diazepam (Valium®)
Indications. Diazepam is used to relieve anxiety, for sedation, and as an anticonvulsant. Additionally, diazepam is used in the management of opiate withdrawal.

Dosage. Diazepam is given orally, intravenously, or intramuscularly at a dosage of 0.04 to 0.25 mg/kg, every 2 to 4 hours as needed. The maximal total dosage given should not exceed 5 mg/kg.

Contraindications. Diazepam should not be used on patients in shock or on patients with narrow-range glaucoma.

Adverse Effects. Adverse effects seen with the use of diazepam include hypotension, tachycardia, hypotonia, respiratory depression, elevated respiratory rate, increased risk of hyperbilirubinemia, urinary retention, constipation, and irritation at the site of administration.

Precautions. Caution must be used when delivering diazepam with other anticonvulsant drugs due to the additive effect of both drugs. Additionally, diazepam should be used cautiously on patients with renal and hepatic dysfunction.

Midazolam (Versed®)
Indications. Midazolam is a short-acting benzodiazepine that has a rapid onset of action. It is used as a sedative/hypnotic to reduce anxiety during invasive procedures, and to induce anesthesia.

Dosage. Midazolam is given intravenously (IV) or intramuscularly (IM) at a rate of 0.07 to 0.2 mg/kg over 2 to 5 minutes, repeated as required every 2 to 4 hours.

Adverse Effects and Precautions. Respiratory depression with apnea is commonly seen with administration of midazolam and personnel must be prepared to provide artificial ventilation if necessary. Other adverse effects include hypotension and seizures.

Morphine Sulfate
Indications. Morphine sulfate is indicated when analgesia from pain is desired, for sedation, and to induce respiratory depression, which enhances mechanical ventilation.

Dosage. Morphine sulfate is given subcutaneously, intramuscularly, or slow intravenous push at a dosage of 0.1 to 0.2 mg/kg, every 4 to 6 hours as needed.

Contraindications. Morphine sulfate should not be given when there is a known hypersensitivity to opiates and should not be administered to patients in shock, those with elevated intracranial pressures, or to those having convulsions.

Adverse Effects. Administration of morphine sulfate may cause hypotension, bradycardia, histamine release, increased intracranial pressure, respiratory depression, gastrointestinal irritation, muscle rigidity, and a dependence on the drug.

Precautions. Oxygen and ventilatory support should be kept at the bedside of patients receiving morphine sulfate. The drug should be used cautiously on those patients with renal and hepatic impairment and on those with cardiac arrhythmias.

Fentanyl Citrate
Indications. Fentanyl citrate is used to produce analgesia, sedation, and anesthesia in the patient. It is often used before performing an invasive procedure such as bronchoscopy.

Dosage. Fentanyl citrate is given intravenously by slow push at a dosage of 1 to 4 µg/kg, every 2 to 4 hours.

Adverse Effects. At dosages greater than 5µg/kg, respiratory depression may occur unexpectedly. Other adverse reactions include muscle rigidity, seizures, hypotension, and bradycardia.

Precautions. Fentanyl citrate should be used cautiously to avoid tolerance to the drug. The patient may additionally show signs of withdrawal when the drug wears off.

Pancuronium Bromide (Pavulon®)

Indications. Pancuronium is used as a adjunct to anesthesia to induce skeletal muscle relaxation, to facilitate ventilation by paralyzing the skeletal muscles, and to control muscle contractions during seizures.

Dosage. Neonates: pancuronium is given intravenously at an initial test dose of 0.02 mg/kg followed by a maintenance dose of 0.03 to 0.09 mg/kg. Children >1 year of age: an initial dose of 0.04 to 0.1 mg/kg is given IV followed by 0.01 mg/kg every 30 to 60 minutes as needed. Pancuronium may be reversed with neostigmine or edrophonium.

Contraindications. Pancuronium should not be used on any patient with a preexisting tachycardia.

Adverse Effects. Adverse effects of pancuronium include an increase in blood pressure, wheezing, and tachycardia.

Precautions. Whenever pancuronium is used, there must be full respiratory support immediately available. Extreme caution should be used when giving the drug to patients with poor renal perfusion or renal disease. Because pancuronium does not provide analgesia, the patient must be monitored for signs of pain and treated with appropriate analgesics.

Succinylcholine Chloride (Anectine®)

Indications. Due to its short duration of action, succinylcholine is indicated to induce skeletal muscle relaxation in order to facilitate intubation. It is also used as a muscle relaxant in concert with anesthetic agents.

Dosages. The dosage of succinylcholine in children is 1 to 2 mg/kg IV or 2.5 to 4 mg/kg IM.

Contraindications. Succinylcholine is contraindicated in those patients who have genetically determined disorders of plasma *pseudocholinesterase*. Additionally, succinylcholine should not be used on patients with myopathies which result in increased serum creatine kinase (CPK, for example) values or those patients with eye injuries.

Adverse Effects. Adverse effects include transient bradycardia, tachycardia, hypertension and hypotension, sinus arrest, respiratory depression, and wheezing.

Precautions. Whenever succinylcholine is used, full respiratory support must be immediately available. Succinylcholine should be used with extreme caution on patients recovering from severe trauma, electrolyte imbalances, those receiving quinidine or cardiac glycosides, and those with hyperkalemia.

EFFECTS OF MATERNAL DRUG ABUSE ON THE FETUS

The transfer of drugs across the placenta was previously discussed in this chapter. Abusable "street drugs" such as heroin, cocaine, and marijuana have the same potential teratogenic effects as do many prescription or over-the-counter drugs. Drug abuse not only includes the illicit use of street drugs but also the inappropriate and overuse of prescription drugs. Prescription drugs to lessen pain (narcotics) and those to aid in sleep disturbances (sedatives/hypnotics) are frequently prescribed during pregnancy and can lead to abuse, complications during delivery, fetal addiction, and birth defects.

Withdrawal from addictive drugs in the neonate may present itself with many signs and symptoms, many of which may be misinterpreted as meningitis, gastroenteritis, hypocalcemia, or intracranial hemorrhage. The most common withdrawal symptoms include restlessness, irritability, tremors, high-pitched cry, and vomiting. These symptoms will be noticeable within a few hours after birth. Phenobarbital is routinely used to treat the irritability, tremors, or twitching.

Neonatal addiction itself can be initially treated with tincture of opium (10% opium) administered as 1 to 2 drops per pound of body weight and can be increased until the symptoms dissipate. The tincture of opium is then gradually withdrawn over a 7- to 14-day period.

SUMMARY

The use of pharmacologic agents is a challenging science. It is more so in the pediatric and neonatal patient population because of the wide differences in metabolic rates, sizes, and weights in these patients. The response of a patient to any delivered drug is impossible to predict and two patients of equal age, and size, may respond totally opposite to the same drug given at the same dosage.

The effect of maternal drug use on the fetus has gained much attention in recent history. It is now well known that many drugs can reach 50 to 100% of maternal levels in the fetus. Depending on when the drug is taken, severe teratogenic effects may be seen in the fetus. Drugs taken late in pregnancy may make the baby flaccid and unresponsive when delivered. The best advice to follow is to avoid all medications during pregnancy, unless medically necessary.

Pharmacokinetics is the term used to describe the entire life of a drug, from when it enters the body, how it is distributed throughout the body, and how it exits.

One of the more common drugs to be used on the neonatal and pediatric populations, are antibiotics. Antibiotics fall into one of several categories, and each has a specific group of organisms for which it is effective. Proper use of antibiotics requires identification of the pathogen and use of the appropriate drug at the appropriate dosage, for the appropriate time period.

Cardiovascular drugs are used to control and treat cardiac arrhythmias, hypotension, congestive heart failure, pulmonary hypertension, and to close or keep open the ductus arteriosus.

Aerosolized respiratory medications are used in the neonatal and pediatric populations to treat reversible bronchospasm, improve mucus removal, reduce airway inflammation, and to treat or prevent infections. Other medications given intravenously are used to stimulate respirations, especially in neonates suffering from apnea.

Other common medicines used include those to control and prevent seizures, steroids to reduce edema, and sedatives to reduce agitation and anxiety.

References

1. Soranus. *Gynecology*. Baltimore: The Johns Hopkins University Press; 1956.
2. Rau, J. L., *Respiratory Care Pharmacology*. 5th ed. Chicago: Year-Book Medical Publishers Inc.: 1998.

Bibliography and Suggested Readings

Cottrell, GP, Surkin, HB *Pharmacology for Respiratory Care Practitioners*. Philadelphia: WB Saunders Co.; 1995.

Daglin, JH, Vallerand, AH *Davis's Drug Guide for Nurses*. 6th ed. Philadelphia: FA Davis; 1999.

Goetzman, BW, Wennberg RP. *Neonatal Intensive Care Handbook*. 3rd ed. St. Louis: Mosby; 1999.

Hazinski, MF *Manual of Pediatric Critical Care*. St. Louis: Mosby; 1999.

Hill, F *Delmar's Respiratory Care Drug Reference*. Albany, NY: Delmar Thomson Learning; 1999.

Marenstein, GB, Gardner SL. *Handbook of Neonatal Intensive Care*. 4th ed. St. Louis: Mosby; 1998.

PDR Nurses' Drug Handbook: 2001 Edition. Albany, NY: Delmar Thomson Learning; 2001.

The Physicians Compendium of Drug Therapy. Secausus, NJ: Compendium Publications Group Inc.; 1995.

2000 Physicians' Desk Reference. Oradell, NJ: Medical Economics Co. Inc.; 2000.

Young, TE, Mangum, OB *Neofax*. 8th ed. Columbus, Ohio: Ross Laboratories; 1995.

Posttest

1. Drug transfer across the placenta is affected by which of the following?
   I. concentration difference
   II. lipid solubility of the drug
   III. degree of ionization
   IV. diffusion coefficient
   V. molecular drug weight
      a. II, III
      b. I, III, V
      c. II, III, IV

    d. I, II, III, V
2. Teratogenic drugs generally have their greatest effect during:
    a. ovulation and fertilization
    b. the first trimester
    c. the second trimester
    d. the third trimester
3. A lipid-soluble drug has which of the following characteristics?
    I. readily cross cell membranes
    II. concentration is higher in tissues than in plasma
    III. high affinity for protein binding
    IV. 10% is bound to albumin
    V. distributed slowly to the heart and kidneys
        a. I, III
        b. I, III, V
        c. I, II, III, V
        d. I, II, III, IV, V
4. Of the following, which is *not* a type of biochemical reaction of drug metabolism in the liver?
    a. excretion
    b. conjugation
    c. reduction
    d. hydrolysis
5. Of the following antibiotics, which is considered to be bacteriostatic?
    a. tetracycline
    b. ciprofloxacin
    c. cefaclor
    d. penicillin
6. For each of the following antibiotic categories, list at least one drug that belongs to that category.
    a. penicillin
    b. cephalosporins
    c. aminoglycosides
    d. macrolides
    e. quinolones
    f. tetracyclines
    g. sulfonamides
    h. antifungals
    i. antivirals

Use the following list to answer questions 7 through 9.
    a. adenosine
    b. epinephrine
    c. digoxin
    d. indomethacin
    e. dopamine

7. Which drug would be most appropriate to treat congestive heart failure?
8. Which drug would be most appropriate to treat supraventricular tachycardia?
9. Which drug would be most appropriate to treat severe hypotension?
10. Acute bronchospasm would best be treated with which of the following drugs?
    a. atropine
    b. ipratropium bromide
    c. albuterol
    d. theophylline
11. Neonatal apnea is treated with which of the following?
    a. caffeine
    b. phenobarbital
    c. cromolyn sodium
    d. ribavirin
12. Which of the following best describe the effects of glucocorticoids?
    I. combat infections
    II. stabilize cell membranes
    III. inhibit macrophage accumulation
    IV. increase the release of adrenocorticotropic hormone
    V. promote gluconeogenesis
        a. I, III, IV
        b. II, III, IV
        c. III, IV, V
        d. II, III, V
13. The drug that inhibits mast cell degranulation is:
    a. theophylline
    b. dexamethasone
    c. atropine
    d. cromolyn sodium
14. Which of the following would be the drug of choice in sedating a neonate following surgery?
    a. pavulon
    b. chloral hydrate
    c. fentanyl
    d. morphine sulfate
15. Restlessness, irritability, tremors, high-pitched cry, and vomiting are all signs of:
    a. respiratory distress
    b. fetal drug withdrawal
    c. fetal drug addiction
    d. maternal heroin abuse

CHAPTER NINE

ASSESSMENT OF OXYGENATION AND VENTILATION

────── OBJECTIVES ──────

Upon completion of this chapter, the reader should be able to:

1. List the indications for obtaining an arterial blood gas sample in neonates and pediatric patients.
2. Identify the four methods of obtaining blood samples for analysis and describe why the UAC is the preferred blood sampling site.
3. Identify those arterial sampling sites that are preductal and postductal. Describe how a right-to-left shunt through the ductus arteriosus can be detected using blood gas PaO_2, transcutaneous monitors, or pulse oximeters.
4. Identify the hazards associated with each of the blood gas sampling methods.
5. Describe the importance of consistency in performance of the heel stick sampling.
6. Define "normal" and "safe" levels of PaO_2, $PaCO_2$, pH, base excess, and HCO_3. Describe why values in the midrange are desirable.
7. Compare total blood oxygen to PaO_2.
8. Describe the limitations of PaO_2.
9. Identify and discuss the detriments of $PaCO_2$.
10. Recognize the Henderson-Hasselbalch equation and the relationship between CO_2 and HCO_3 in maintaining proper pH.
11. Identify two possible causes each of respiratory and metabolic acidosis and alkalosis. Describe briefly the compensatory mechanisms for each of the disorders.
12. Describe the role of bicarbonate in buffering blood acids.
13. Define base deficit.
14. Briefly describe the mechanical aspects of a transcutaneous monitor (TCM).
15. Discuss how a TCM can be useful even if not reading arterial values.
16. List six factors that could cause a TCM to read lower than the actual PaO_2.
17. Describe how a TCM detects skin perfusion.
18. Explain the hazards of TCMs and how those hazards can be avoided.
19. Describe how a pulse oximeter determines arterial oxygen saturation.
20. Discuss the advantages and hazards of pulse oximetry.
21. Compare and contrast sidestream and mainstream CO_2 monitors.

22. Describe how increased deadspace ventilation and increased shunt perfusion can cause erroneous capnography readings.
23. List and explain the limitations of capnography.

KEY TERMS

calcaneus	logarithm	spectrophotometric infrared analysis
hyperalimentation	stratum corneum	

THE BASICS

The role of the respiratory care practitioner in obtaining and interpreting blood gases is critical in most NICUs. Not only is it important to understand how to obtain blood gas samples, it is vital that the respiratory practitioner understand when to obtain them and how to interpret the results. This chapter does not attempt to cover basic blood gas physiology, but assumes that the reader is fairly well versed in this area. The information provided here will serve to reinforce what is already understood and will apply that understanding to the neonatal and pediatric patient population.

There are many differences in interpretation between neonatal and adult blood gas values. With the arrival of new technologies and procedures, such as noninvasive transcutaneous monitoring, pulse oximetry, and capnography, the role of the arterial blood gas in the care of the neonate has changed. For this reason, this chapter will examine the use of these monitors and how that use has changed the care provided.

ARTERIAL BLOOD GAS ANALYSIS

INDICATIONS

Neonatal Patients. Before discussing the techniques of obtaining blood gases, it is important to understand when to obtain a blood gas. Premature neonates, in the first hours, days, and weeks of life, can make dramatic changes in their status very quickly, sometimes from one minute to the next.

It is very difficult to base therapeutic decisions simply on observation, especially when it comes to changes in oxygenation and ventilation. Some neonates may require blood gas analysis every 10 to 20 minutes, others may only need one every few weeks. The important fact to remember is that each neonate is different and will have different needs and requirements regarding the need for blood gases.

Keep in mind that a small preemie may only have 100 cc of blood in its entire body, and frequent blood gases can deplete that supply quickly. A fine line exists between getting too many blood gases and getting too few. If in doubt, it is better to get too many than not enough. Blood gas values are a very critical part of neonatal care, and many decisions affecting the outcome of the neonate are based on blood gas values.

There are certain rules that apply to most neonates that help determine when an arterial blood gas analysis is needed. They are presented here, not necessarily in order of their importance.

1. Any neonate showing signs of respiratory distress such as nasal flaring, retractions, grunting, and cyanosis should have arterial blood drawn for analysis.
2. Any neonate whose clinical course, appearance, vital signs, or condition have changed for no obvious reason should also have an arterial blood gas analysis. It is important not to wait for the blood gas results before reacting to and treating a problem. The patient should be treated first, then an arterial sample obtained. For example, if you notice that the patient is a dusky blue color or the HR has dropped, treat the patient first, then obtain the blood gas.
3. It is advisable to obtain an arterial blood gas analysis within 15 to 30 minutes after any change in ventilator or FiO_2 settings.
4. Once the neonate on a ventilator has stabilized, it is advisable to obtain an arterial blood gas analysis on a regular basis to ensure proper ventilator settings. Regular analysis also helps to document transcutaneous and pulse oximetry readings. The timing of blood gases should be made on an individual basis, as need dictates.

Specific units will have varying criteria for blood gases on long-term ventilator patients.

Pediatric Patients. The indications for arterial blood gas analysis on pediatric patients are basically the same as for adults. The primary indication for a blood gas analysis is to assess the oxygenation and ventilation status of the patient. Any patient who shows signs of distress, such as increased respiratory rate, retractions, and cyanosis, should have an arterial blood gas analysis.

In addition, blood gas analysis is indicated on pediatric patients being managed on a mechanical ventilator. Monitoring of PaO_2, $PaCO_2$ and pH allows for optimal settings to be achieved, as well as dictating proper changes in settings as needed.

Arterial blood gases are indicated as a follow-up to oxygen therapy or the administration of medications or therapy for the treatment of a pulmonary disorder. Follow-up blood gases show if inspired oxygen is adequate and if treatments and medications are effective.

CONSIDERATIONS IN OBTAINING SAMPLES

There are three sources of arterial blood in the neonate: umbilical, brachial, and radial. Capillary blood is another source; however, it is not arterial but rather a mixed sample. It is important to remember that at any time blood or blood products are to be handled, the possibility of contact exists and universal precautions must be observed.

UAC. The umbilical artery catheter (UAC) blood gas sample is the preferred method for obtaining arterial blood samples. This is because it causes no pain to the neonate, which may lead to erroneous values secondary to crying and agitation, and it is easily obtained. Arterial punctures can be very traumatic to neonates and can drastically change the blood gas values due to the crying and fussing of the patient. It should also be noted that punctures can damage the neonate's fragile skin.

If a right-to-left shunt is suspected through the PDA, a right radial arterial sample should be drawn simultaneously with the UAC blood gas to compare the pressure of oxygen in each sample. In normal cardiovascular anatomy (Figure 9–1), the right radial arterial blood will be preductal, and in the presence of a ductal shunt will reflect a higher oxygen tension than in the postductal location of the UAC.

An easier method of detecting a right-to-left ductal shunt is to place a transcutaneous PaO_2 monitor on the upper right quadrant of the chest and another on the abdomen (Figure 9–2). The higher PaO_2 on the upper right quadrant, compared to the lower abdominal PaO_2, would reflect the right-to-left ductal shunt. A relative uniformity between PaO_2 at these two sites helps to rule out right-to-left ductal shunting.

Several problems are associated with the use of the UAC. Most UACs rarely remain in place longer than 3 to 4 weeks in the neonate due to clot formation and problems with infection. A premature neonate may be on the ventilator or require supplemental oxygen for months. In these patients, the loss of the UAC makes the assessment of oxygenation and ventilation more difficult, as we must now rely on capillary samples and external monitors.

As discussed previously, the arterial blood obtained from the UAC may reflect a low PaO_2 from a ductal shunt. The arterial blood that supplies the head is normally preductal.

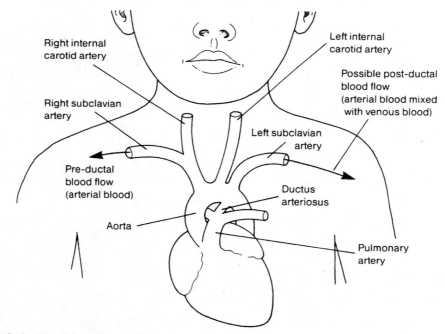

Figure 9–1 *Normal cardiovascular anatomy.*

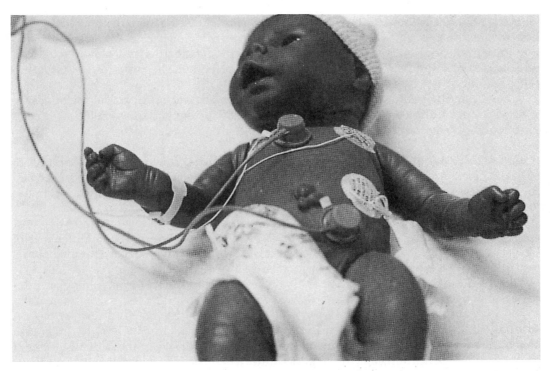

Figure 9–2 *Detecting a right-to-left shunt through the ductus arteriosus using two transcutanous monitors. The monitor on the abdomen measures postductal blood while the monitor on the right upper quadrant measures preductal blood.*

If the FiO_2 is increased in response to a low arterial PO_2 (caused by the ductal shunt), the arterial blood supplying the head and eyes increases to a dangerous level.

Complications associated with the use of a UAC include thromboembolism, hypertension, infection, hemorrhage, vessel perforation, and necrotizing entercolitis.

Procedure. To draw blood from the UAC line, two 3 cc syringes are obtained. One of the syringes is filled approximately two-thirds full with a special neonatal heparin flush solution. A clean gauze pad is placed under the stopcock and the empty 3 cc syringe is placed on the luer opening. The stopcock is then turned off to the incoming IV solution and 2 to 2.5 cc of blood is slowly withdrawn from the UAC. This clears the line of flush solution, which may contaminate the sample. The stopcock is then turned off one-quarter turn to stop flow from the artery and to prevent IV contamination of the sample. The blood gas syringe is next placed on the luer, and the stopcock is opened one-quarter turn to the artery and the sample withdrawn. The stopcock is now turned off to the luer and the blood gas syringe removed and capped.

Close attention must now be paid to the reinjection of the blood back to the patient. Place the syringe containing the withdrawn blood/flush mixture on the luer, turning the stopcock off to the IV line. Air bubbles that may be present in the luer are now removed by first flicking the stopcock with a finger and then slowly drawing back 0.25 to 0.5 ml of blood into the syringe, drawing any air out of the stopcock. The blood is now slowly reinjected into the UAC. The line is now flushed using the syringe with the heparin flush solution and following the same steps outlined above.

A newer, and possibly safer procedure has recently been introduced as a potential substitute for the traditional method of UAC line draws. This method uses a self-sealed compartment for the withdrawn flush mixture that is returned to the patient.

Radial Artery Catheter. An indwelling radial artery catheter can be a useful alternative to a UAC. The main advantage to the radial artery catheter is that the artery is accessible when the UAC has to be pulled out. It is also available in instances where the umbilical artery has lost its accessibility.

Another advantage is that right radial artery samples reflect preductal flow. In the presence of ductal shunting, knowledge of preductal PaO_2 is critical for proper maintenance of FiO_2 as it reflects the PaO_2 supplying the eyes. An additional advantage is that thrombosis formation, which is often seen when major vessels are used, is less common.

The hazards associated with radial artery catheters include infection, air embolism, arterial occlusion, infiltration of fluids, and nerve damage.

Arterial Puncture. When compared to the UAC, arterial punctures are fairly difficult to obtain in neonates. This is mainly due to the extremely small size of the neonate's arterial anatomy. When performing an arterial puncture on a neonate, one does not have the advantage of palpating the pulse to help locate the artery, as in adults. It is often done blindly, using only external landmarks to approximate the location of the artery. The distance from the skin to the artery is also deceiving, making it difficult to judge how deep to insert the needle.

One method that may enhance the capability of obtaining a radial sample is to use a transillumination light under the wrist to allow visualization of the artery. Care must be taken to not use a light, which may burn the patient.

Another problem with radial punctures is that it is not practical to do an arterial puncture as often as a UAC sample can be drawn. This is due to the trauma inflicted on the patient and the inaccuracies in the blood gas that are created from the crying and fussing. In these situations the use of transcutaneous monitors and pulse oximeters is invaluable.

Before performing a radial artery puncture on a neonate, an Allen's Test should be done to ensure collateral circulation. On the neonate, this is accomplished by first manually occluding both the radial and ulnar artery, then passively squeezing the hand closed, and then opening it while releasing the ulnar artery.

The primary complications found in arterial puncture include infection, bleeding, nerve damage, embolism, and hematoma.

Capillary Samples. Arterialized capillary samples are used primarily after the UAC has been removed and the patient requires ongoing blood gas monitoring.

Capillary samples are less hazardous to the patient and are more easily obtained than arterial punctures. Capillary samples are useful in assessing pH and $PaCO_2$, assuming adequate peripheral circulation. Capillary samples are not, however, reliable in the assessment of arterial PO_2.

Without arterial access, arterial PO_2 must be determined by pulse oximetry or transcutaneous monitoring. Another problem with capillary PaO_2 is that there are no defined normals. On some neonatal patients, a capillary PaO_2 of 35 mm Hg might be the equivalent of a 65 mm Hg PaO_2, and on another patient the capillary and arterial values might correlate closely.

Indications. According to the AARC Clinical Practice Guideline,[1] indications for capillary blood gas sampling are the following: an arterial blood gas analysis is indicated, but arterial access is not available; transcutaneous, pulse oximetry, or capnography readings are abnormal; assessing the patient following initiation, administration, or change in therapy; a change in the patient's status by history or physical exam; and monitoring the severity and progression of a documented disease process.

Contraindications. Contraindications as outlined in the AARC Clinical Practice Guideline[1] are that capillary punctures should not be performed on the following: the posterior curvature of the heel; the heel of any patient who has begun walking and has callus development; the fingers of neonates; previous puncture sites; inflamed, swollen, or edematous tissues; cyanotic or poorly perfused tissues; localized areas of infection; peripheral arteries; patients less than 24 hours old. Additionally, capillary samples should not be done when there is a need for direct analysis of oxygenation or of arterial blood. Relative contraindications include peripheral vasoconstriction, polycythemia, and hypotension.

The most reliable results from the arterialized capillary sample are obtained if the following steps are done consistently. The heel must be heated to the same temperature (ideally 45°C) for each puncture, and it must be heated for the same length of time (5 to 7 minutes). At the end of the appropriate time period, the equipment is readied and the heel is unwrapped and wiped with an appropriate antiseptic pad. The foot is grasped in the nondominant hand and the heel is punctured in the area outlined in Figure 9–3. Puncturing in the outlined area avoids lacerating the posterior tibial artery and additionally averts the accidental puncture of the *calcaneus*. The puncture should be made with a neonatal lance to avoid excess trauma to the heel. The blood should flow freely and quickly into the collection tube without needing to squeeze the heel.

Complications. Complications of capillary sampling are often related to improper procedure. Puncturing the calcaneus bone may lead to osteomyelitis or bone spurs. Other complications include infection, burns, hematoma, nerve damage, bruising, scarring, tibial artery laceration, pain, bleeding, and inappropriate patient management by relying on capillary PO_2 values.[1]

Pediatric Patients. The pediatric population offers the same arterial sampling sites as the adult, with one exception. It may be possible on the smaller pediatric patients to perform a capillary puncture on the heel or finger.

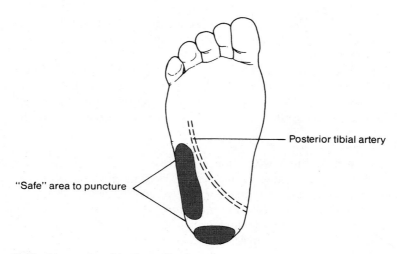

Figure 9–3 *The heel is punctured in the outlined area.*

The safest site for sampling pediatric arterial blood is the radial artery. Arterial blood can also be drawn from the brachial artery and the femoral artery. Other sites include the temporal artery and the dorsalis pedis artery. The femoral artery is always the last option, and should only be used in emergency situations.

Before performing a puncture on the radial artery, the practitioner should perform an Allen's Test to ensure good collateral circulation through the ulnar artery. The technique for performing arterial punctures on a pediatric patient is the same as on adult patients.

Indwelling arterial catheters are another method of obtaining arterial samples in the pediatric population. This method, however, is usually reserved for those patients on ventilators and others requiring numerous blood gases.

ARTERIAL BLOOD GAS ASSESSMENT

The assessment of blood gas status relies on an understanding of basic blood gas physiology and normal values. The physiologic concerns apply to both neonatal and pediatric patients. Differences in blood gas interpretation between these two groups are found in the normal (safe) values, which will be identified for each group.

An important point to remember when examining neonatal blood gas values is that there are no normal values. Values change over the first hours and days of life with changes in lung function and cardiac shunts. The neonatal normals listed here refer to what is considered to be the safe range.

PaO$_2$

Neonatal Safe Range
50 to 70 mm Hg

Pediatric Normal Range
85 to 100 mm Hg (sea level)
55 to 80 mm Hg (5000 ft.)

Basics of PaO_2. The arterial PO_2 tells something about oxygenation, but only that of arterial blood. The most important information would be tissue oxygenation, if it were available.

It should be remembered that PaO_2 is only one factor in oxygenation of arterial blood, representing the amount of oxygen dissolved in the plasma. According to the law of diffusion, movement through a membrane occurs following a concentration gradient. The larger the gradient, the more movement or diffusion takes place. The diffusion gradient for oxygen at the capillary level is represented by the PaO_2 in the blood being on the high end of the gradient and the PaO_2 of the tissues being on the low end. We can consider the PaO_2 as being the driving pressure for tissue oxygenation, not the total amount of oxygen present.

Total Blood Oxygen and PaO_2. The vast majority of oxygen is carried by binding to hemoglobin. How much oxygen is bound to hemoglobin is determined by how much enters the plasma from the alveoli. The more oxygen in the plasma (PaO_2), the higher the driving pressure causing more oxygen to attach to the hemoglobin. The amount of oxygen bound to hemoglobin is also affected by the position of the oxygen dissociation curve and the presence of pathologic species of hemoglobin such as carboxy- or methemoglobin.

Limitations of PaO_2 in Arterial Samples. The PaO_2 value of a pediatric or neonatal blood gas only reflects the level when the sample was drawn. At that moment, it may have been at a high, mid, or low point. It is for this reason that mid-range values are the safest when interpreting blood gas data. The patient's clinical status always needs to be considered before making any changes or accepting the validity of a value.

Use of Transcutaneous Monitors and Pulse Oximetry. During the acute and recovery phases of RDS, rapid changes in PaO_2 may be expected and particularly close monitoring of PaO_2 is required. With the advent of transcutaneous monitoring and pulse oximetry, the need for numerous blood gases has been diminished. The value of the blood gas in these patients is to verify the accuracy of the monitors.

If the PaO_2 on the transcutaneous monitor parallels that of the arterial blood, then PaO_2 can easily be monitored continuously, allowing the practitioner to make changes as needed to maintain adequate oxygenation.

Pulse oximeters can be reliably used to assess adequate arterial PO_2, as long as the practitioner understands the limitations, explained later in this chapter.

$PaCO_2$

Safe Range
(pediatric and neonatal) 35 to 45 mm Hg
Chronic Disease
<60 mm Hg

Basics of $PaCO_2$. Carbon dioxide is the byproduct of aerobic metabolism and is excreted by the lungs. As with oxygen, the $PaCO_2$ is the partial pressure of carbon dioxide in the plasma. It provides the "driving force" for the carbon dioxide to leave the plasma.

In the blood, 85% of the total carbon dioxide is carried as bicarbonate, 10% is bound to hemoglobin, and 5% is carried as a dissolved gas or carbonic acid.

$PaCO_2$ greater than 45 usually indicates alveolar hypoventilation with respiratory failure being indicated when $PaCO_2$ is greater than 60 mm Hg.

$PaCO_2$, then, defines the adequacy of alveolar ventilation, or that part of the tidal volume that is in direct contact with perfused alveolar surfaces.

Determinants of $PaCO_2$. The arterial $PaCO_2$ at any given time is the product of metabolism versus removal by the lungs. As metabolism increases, alveolar ventilation must also increase to remove the excess CO_2 in the blood. Any time there is an imbalance between alveolar ventilation and metabolism, $PaCO_2$ will increase or decrease.

Alveolar ventilation is determined by minute ventilation minus deadspace (V_D). Minute ventilation is the total of all gas moved into the patient's respiratory system in 1 minute. It is calculated by multiplying the respiratory rate and the tidal volume.

V_D is the volume of air moved in and out of the respiratory tract that does not come into direct contact with perfused pulmonary units. V_D is composed of gas occupying the nasal, oral, and pharyngeal passages, endotracheal tubes, and the trachea down to the respiratory bronchioles. V_D is also made up of ventilated alveoli that are not being perfused by blood.

With each inspiration, the first gas into the alveoli is from the deadspace, the gas that was left in the airways from the previous exhalation. Only after an inspiration large enough to move the deadspace volume into the alveoli does fresh gas begin to enter the alveoli. Gas exchange will not occur, then, if tidal volume does not exceed deadspace.

If shallow rapid respirations occur, the V_D may be all that is moved into the alveoli. Even though minute ventilation is high, alveolar ventilation is absent and $PaCO_2$ increases.

This shows that $PaCO_2$ is affected exclusively by alveolar ventilation, not minute ventilation. Alveolar ventilation may be increased by elevations in tidal volume or respiratory rate, as long as the tidal volume is greater than V_D. Tidal volumes that are inadequate or ventilator frequencies that are too low lead to a high $PaCO_2$.

In contrast, a low $PaCO_2$ indicates excessive tidal volumes and/or rates. In a spontaneously breathing patient, a low $PaCO_2$ is not a stimulus for ventilation and therefore indicates the neonate is hyperventilating in response to another drive. Stimulants that can cause hyperventilation include hypoxia, metabolic acidosis, hyperthermia, or a central nervous system disorder (asphyxia, intracranial hemorrhage).

pH

Safe Range
(neonatal and pediatric) 7.35 to 7.45
Acceptable Range
(neonatal and pediatric) 7.30 to 7.50

Basics of pH. The pH of the blood is a direct result of the number of hydrogen ions present. Hydrogen ions in the blood are the result of CO_2 reacting with water or are derived from lactic acid. The definition of pH is the negative *logarithm* of the hydrogen ion concentration. As pH becomes more acidic or alkalotic, the number of hydrogen ions increases or decreases logarithmically.

In the safe range of pH, enzyme systems function optimally and oxygen transport is in its physiologic range. The acceptable range is used for those patients with acute or chronic pulmonary disorders to serve as a guideline for initiation of support or to dictate changes in ventilator settings. A pH that falls below the acceptable range causes pulmonary vasoconstriction and a disruption of vital bodily functions.

Henderson-Hasselbalch Equation. To understand pH disorders, one must understand the Henderson-Hasselbalch equation. This equation compares the pH to the bicarbonate ion concentration and $PaCO_2$:

$$pH = 6.1 + \log \frac{HCO_{3^-} \text{ mEq/L} \quad \text{(base)}}{0.03 \times PaCO_2 \quad \text{(acid)}}$$

The $PaCO_2$ is multiplied by 0.03 to convert it to the same units as the bicarbonate.

With a normal blood pH of 7.40, the ratio of bicarbonate ions to dissolved carbon dioxide is 20:1. Alterations of blood pH can therefore occur whenever this ratio is changed. The pH increases whenever the bicarbonate concentration increases or the $PaCO_2$ decreases. Conversely, pH decreases whenever the bicarbonate decreases or the $PaCO_2$ increases.

Whenever these imbalances occur, the body attempts to correct the pH by returning the ratio of bicarbonate to $PaCO_2$ back to normal. This knowledge lays the groundwork for understanding pH disorders and how the body compensates for them.

Primary pH disorders may be the result of respiratory or metabolic disorders, or a combination of both, and may occur with or without compensatory mechanisms. Causes of various pH disorders are outlined in Table 9–1.

RESPIRATORY DISORDERS

Respiratory Acidosis. Respiratory acidosis is the result of increased levels of $PaCO_2$ and is caused by alveolar hypoventilation. Possible causes of respiratory acidosis include obstructive lung diseases such as BPD, meconium aspiration, and transient trachypnea of the newborn.

Alveolar hypoventilation could result from the effects of maternal anesthesia before delivery, depressed ventilatory drive from sepsis, intraventricular hemorrhage, and metabolic disturbances that affect the respiratory centers. Abnormalities or trauma to the thorax, including diaphragmatic hernia, pneumothorax, or paralysis, can lead to hypoventilation.

The response of the body to respiratory acidosis is to withhold the excretion of bicarbonate from the kidneys and to excrete H^+ ions. Each increase of 1 mm Hg in $PaCO_2$ results

---

TABLE 9–1 Causes of pH Disorders

Respiratory:
Acidosis—generated by the retention of CO_2 in the blood
    Causes—sedation, BPD, meconium aspiration, TTN, maternal sedation or anesthesia, sepsis,
    intraventricular hemorrhage, metabolic disturbances that affect the respiratory centers (hypo-
    glycemia), abnormalities or trauma to the thorax, diaphragmatic hernia, pneumothorax, and
    paralysis
Alkalosis—generated by a loss of CO_2 in the blood
    Causes—mismanagement of ventilator rates and volumes, RDS, stimulation of the central
    nervous system, and hypoxia-induced hyperventilation

Metabolic:
Acidosis—generated by an excess of hydrogen ions, a reduction in the loss of hydrogen ions, or a
loss of bicarbonate ions
    Causes—hypoxemia with resulting lactic acidosis, starvation, hyperalimentation, renal tubular
    acidosis, and diarrhea
Alkalosis—generated by an excessive loss of hydrogen ions or by the addition of bicarbonate to the
blood
    Causes—gastric suctioning, vomiting, diuretic use without adequate potassium replacement, IV
    administration of bicarbonate

---

in an increase of plasma bicarbonate of 0.1 mEq/L. This then restores the ratio of bicarbonate to $PaCO_2$.

Respiratory Alkalosis. Respiratory alkalosis occurs when the arterial CO_2 is blown off due to alveolar hyperventilation. Respiratory alkalosis is often caused by mismanagement of ventilator rates and volumes.

Respiratory alkalosis is also caused by restrictive lung diseases, such as early RDS, stimulation of the central nervous system, and hypoxia-induced hyperventilation. The body responds to respiratory alkalosis by eliminating excess bicarbonate through the kidneys, restoring the appropriate ratio of bicarbonate to $PaCO_2$. In acute cases of respiratory alkalosis, there is a 0.2 mEq reduction in bicarbonate for every 1 mm Hg decrease in $PaCO_2$.

METABOLIC DISORDERS

Metabolic Acidosis. Metabolic acidosis is the result of an increased production or reduced loss of hydrogen ions. It is also caused by an abnormal loss of bicarbonate. Metabolic acidosis is commonly due to hypoxia with resulting lactic acidosis. It may also be caused by starvation, *hyperalimentation,* or renal tubular acidosis, from the inability of the premature kidney to excrete acid and reabsorb bicarbonate. Diarrhea leads to a loss of bicarbonate and may lead to metabolic acidosis.

The response of the respiratory system to metabolic acidosis is to increase alveolar ventilation and reduce arterial $PaCO_2$. For every mEq reduction in bicarbonate, there is a 1.2 mm Hg reduction in $PaCO_2$.

Frequently, the neonate is unable to hyperventilate due to prematurity or the nature of the disease process.

Metabolic Alkalosis. Metabolic alkalosis is the result of an excessive loss of hydrogen ions from the gastrointestinal tract, or the kidneys, or by the addition of bicarbonate to the blood. Hydrogen ions are lost through gastric auctioning, vomiting, or with the overzealous use of diuretics without adequate potassium replacement.

The response of the respiratory system to metabolic alkalosis is a decrease in alveolar ventilation, causing $PaCO_2$ to increase. The response is about 0.6 mm Hg increase in $PaCO_2$ for every mEq increase in bicarbonate.

HCO_3-

Normal Range
22 to 26 mEq/L

Basics of Bicarbonate Levels. The level of bicarbonate in the blood is controlled by tissue metabolism and the function of the kidneys. There are two components to plasma bicarbonate: the respiratory portion, which is the smaller of the two, and the metabolic portion.[2]

In the bloodstream, hydrogen ions (H^+) combine with bicarbonate ions (HCO_3-) to form carbonic acid ($H^+ + HCO_3$- $= H_2CO_3$). Carbonic acid is then able to dissociate into carbon dioxide and water ($H_2CO_3 = CO_2 + H_2O$). The carbon dioxide is then removed from the blood by the lungs. The bicarbonate component of carbonic acid is said to be the respiratory portion.

The metabolic portion of bicarbonate is that component that is controlled by the kidneys. The kidneys have the ability to excrete bicarbonate ($KHCO_3$-) or to retain bicarbonate ($NaHCO_3$-) as needed to maintain the pH.

HCO_3- is calculated from the pH and $PaCO_2$. It is decreased in metabolic acidosis and respiratory alkalosis and increased in metabolic alkalosis and respiratory acidosis.

A level of 22 to 26 mEq/L shows adequate levels of buffering capacity. As the levels fall, the blood is less able to correct acid states. Conversely, as the levels rise, it signifies that the body has produced too much bicarbonate in relation to acid present, and an alkalotic state presents itself. An increase in CO_2 shifts the equation to the right by generating more H^+ and HCO_3- and lowering pH. A lowering of CO_2, shifts the equation to the left, thus lowering H^+ concentration and raising pH.

Application of the Henderson-Hasselbalch Equation. Understanding the application of the Henderson-Hasselbalch equation is facilitated by likening it to a balance with HCO_3- on one side and CO_2 on the other side (Figure 9–4A). As illustrated, a normal balance of 20:1 results in a normal pH. As bicarbonate increases or decreases (Figure 9–4B), the balance is offset and metabolic alkalosis or acidosis occurs. As the lungs now alter ventilation, CO_2 is either excreted or retained to counterbalance the effects of the bicarbonate (Figure 9–4C).

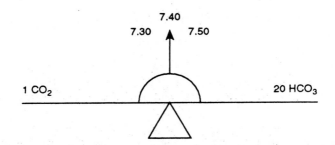

Figure 9–4A *The balance between HCO₃₋ and CO₂ results in a normal pH.*

When CO_2 increases or decreases, the balance is again offset and acidosis or alkalosis results (Figure 9–4D). The body then responds by either retaining or removing plasma bicarbonate, returning the balance to normal (Figure 9–4E).

BASE EXCESS/DEFICIT

Normal Range
±4 mEq/L

Basics of Base Excess. Base excess is a reflection of the nonrespiratory (metabolic) portion of the acid-base balance and reflects an excess or deficit of plasma bicarbonate. The buffering capacity of the red blood cells also has an effect on the base excess.[2]

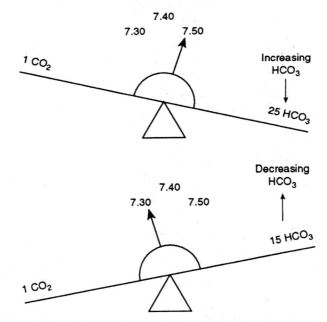

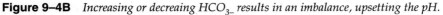

Figure 9–4B *Increasing or decreaing HCO₃₋ results in an imbalance, upsetting the pH.*

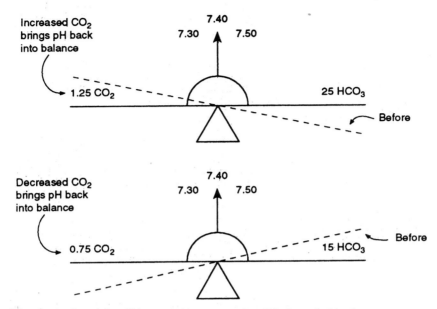

Figure 9–4C *Correction of the pH by retaining or removing CO_2 from the blood.*

Base excess must be viewed considering pH and $PaCO_2$, from which it is calculated, and the patient's clinical course. A base excess above 4 mEq/L indicates too much bicarbonate or too little acid in the blood. A negative value, called a base deficit, or a negative base excess, occurs whenever there is too little base or too much acid.

Base excess can be estimated by multiplying the calculated bicarbonate by 1.2 and then subtracting the normal value (24 mEq) from the product.[2]

Additionally, the bicarbonate binds with the hydrogen ions, forming carbonic acid, which then dissociates into carbon dioxide and water. If alveolar ventilation is not adequate, carbon dioxide levels increase and worsen the acidosis.

TRANSCUTANEOUS MONITORING

Frequent measurement of arterial blood gases is essential in the treatment and maintenance of oxygenation and ventilation in the sick neonate. However, traditional methods of assessing arterial blood gas status have inherent shortcomings that make them less than ideal. For example, the small neonate that requires frequent blood gas sampling may have a large portion of its blood volume depleted in a short period. Samples drawn from a catheter or by puncture show the status of the patient when the sample was obtained, but may be invalid within minutes due to the rapid changes that neonates can pass through.

The ideal situation would be the ability to monitor constantly arterial blood gas values as they exist in the artery without causing pain or diminishing the blood supply. Although

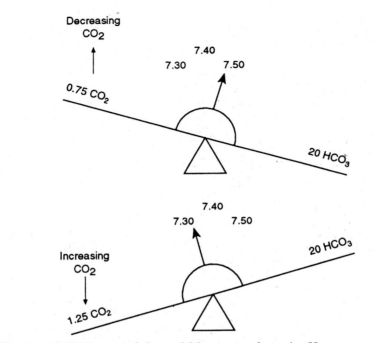

Figure 9–4D *As with HCO3_, an imbalance of CO2 causes a change in pH.*

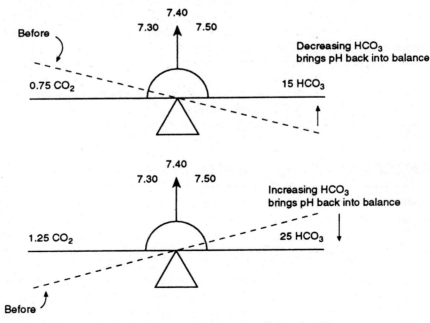

Figure 9–4E *Retaining or removing HCO3_ balances the CO2, normalizing the pH.*

this ideal situation is not available, transcutaneous monitoring offers a welcome alternative.

FUNCTIONAL DESIGN AND MECHANICS

Transcutaneous monitors (TCMs) evolved from the discovery in the early 1950s that oxygen diffuses through the skin from the capillaries. Modern TCMs use the same electrodes found in blood gas analyzers, except in miniature form.

Heating the area directly beneath the electrode results in three main effects. The heat changes the lipid structure of the *stratum corneum*, allowing a faster diffusion of oxygen through the skin. By heating the tissue and blood beneath the electrode, the oxygen dissociation curve is shifted to the right, enhancing the release of oxygen from the red blood cell. Finally, the heat causes a local vasodilation of the capillaries and causes an arterilization of the blood.[2]

Heat is provided by a small donut-shaped heater that surrounds the electrode. The temperature is regulated by a thermistor on the sensor that relays the temperature back to the monitor, which then supplies more or less power to the heater as needed. A cutaway view of a modern transcutaneous monitor is shown in Figure 9–5. Technology has now advanced to the point where both oxygen and carbon dioxide can be measured on one sensor, approximately the diameter of a quarter.

In general, transcutaneous PO_2 levels are lower than PaO_2 values. This could be due to the possibility that the TCM is measuring tissue oxygenation.

It is this author's experience that the $PtcCO_2$ tends to correlate more closely to arterial levels. This is possibly due in part to two factors. First, CO_2 diffuses easier than does oxy-

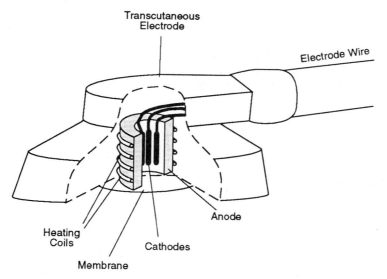

Figure 9–5 *Cutaway of a transcutaneous monitor probe.*

gen, and second, the surface area of the Severinghaus electrode that measures $PaCO_2$ is larger than the Clark electrode.

The result is a monitor or monitors that can be placed on the surface of the patient's skin, which give a continual readout of oxygen and carbon dioxide tensions that are reliable indicators of arterial values.

CLINICAL USES

Trending. An advantage in the use of a TCM is its ability to follow trends. The gradient between $PtCO_2$ and PaO_2 is most stable in noncritical patients. The unfortunate reality is that in critically ill patients, the gradient is highly variable.[3] In other words, the patient in whom we want the highest trending ability may be the one in whom we are least likely to get it. Before relying on the TCM in making critical therapeutic decisions, it must be determined that the monitor is trending adequately.

A patient on a ventilator whose $PaCO_2$ is trending downward can efficiently be weaned following the TCM values. Conversely, a patient with worsening status can be treated more quickly and effectively if the changes in oxygen and carbon dioxide can be continuously monitored. The TCM accomplishes this with minimal discomfort to the patient and, if used appropriately, with no harmful side effects.

The TCM should not be discontinued if it fails to correlate exactly with arterial values. A TCM has only lost its usefulness when its values are significantly different from arterial values and it does not tread in a reproducible way.

Factors that cause the $PtCO_2$ to measure lower than actual arterial PO_2 are those factors that reduce tissue perfusion. These factors, listed in Table 9–2, include shock, severe acidosis, hypothermia, severe cyanotic heart disease, severe anemia, skin edema, hyproxemia with PaO_2 greater than 100 mm Hg, and the use of Tolazoline given for pulmonary hypertension.

TABLE 9–2 Factors That Cause $PtCO_2$ to Read Lower Than Arterial Values

Shock
Severe acidosis
Hypothermia
Severe cyanotic heart disease
Severe anemia
Skin edema
PaO_2 greater than 100 mm Hg
Tolazoline delivery

Detection of Shunting Blood. Another clinical use of the TCM is in its ability to detect right-to-left shunting through the ductus arteriosus. This is done by placing one electrode on the right shoulder, which is fed by the preductal right subclavian artery, and placing another electrode on the lower abdomen or leg.

A shunt is indicated when the preductal PaO_2 of the right shoulder is significantly higher than the postductal PaO_2 of the abdomen.

Indicator of Skin Perfusion. The TCM can also be used as an indicator of skin perfusion.[4] If the monitor tracks the power required to heat the sensor to the preset level, changes in perfusion will show as changes in the amount of power required to maintain the probe temperature.

As perfusion increases, the blood carries the heat away more rapidly, requiring more power to maintain the temperature. Conversely, as perfusion decreases, less power is needed to maintain the temperature. Thus, the power output is a direct indication of perfusion at the electrode site.

LIMITATIONS

A task force on transcutaneous oxygen monitors identified seven limitations to their use.

1. $TcPaO_2$ may underestimate the PaO_2 in a hyperoxemic infant.
2. An inappropriate electrode temperature may adversely influence the performance of the monitor.
3. $TcPaO_2$ may underestimate the PaO_2 in infants with a compromised hemodynamic status or when there is excessive pressure on the electrode.
4. The performance of the $tcPaO_2$ may be suboptimal if placed over poorly perfused sites such as distal extremities, pressure points, and bony prominences.
5. $TcPaO_2$ may underestimate PaO_2 in infants with chronic lung disease.
6. The heated electrode may cause skin blistering, especially in very low birth weight infants and those with impaired perfusion.
7. $TcPaO_2$ cannot be used without periodic correlation with arterial blood gas analysis.

COMPLICATIONS AND HAZARDS

Thermal injury is the greatest hazard in the use of TCMs. Recommended temperatures may produce an erythema, or reddening of the skin that can last from several hours to days.

Temperature settings above 44°C may cause thermal injury to the skin. Blistering has been reported when the sensor has been left at one site too long or at too high a temperature. It can also occur if perfusion is diminished.[5] Thermal injury can be avoided by correct temperature selection and appropriate site change intervals every 2 to 3 hours.

The double-gummed disk adhesives used to hold the sensor in place may cause epidermal stripping when removed. When used on the very small preemie, it may be advisable to use a Velcro or Coban wrap to hold the sensor in place. In any case, removal of the sensor should be gentle, avoiding the tendency to pull the sensor off quickly.

Another potential hazard exists if the practitioner begins to rely on the TCM for total blood gas information. As advanced as technology has become, TCMs cannot be relied on alone in place of arterial blood gases. All TCMs are vulnerable to physiologic changes in skin perfusion that can cause erroneous readings. Whenever a TCM is being used to monitor and change oxygen or ventilator settings, blood gases must be done on a routine basis to verify the accuracy of the TCM.

PULSE OXIMETRY

Another exciting development in noninvasive blood gas monitoring is pulse oximetry. Pulse oximeters utilize light absorption to calculate the saturation of arterial hemoglobin. The pulse oximeter is placed on any location that allows the passage of light. The ideal location is on a toe, finger, or ear, as these areas are fairly thin on the neonate and allow easy passage of light.

Modern pulse oximeters contain both a light source and a photodetector on the probe. The light source uses light-emitting diodes, which transmit both infrared and red light. The pulse oximeter probe is placed on the patient with the light source and photodetector opposite each other, separated by the selected body part. Proper placement is depicted in Figure 9–6. As light passes through the skin it is partially absorbed by the tissues, muscle, bone, etc. These absorb a constant amount of the light, which passes through the body part. Blood pulsing through the arterioles absorbs more light every time a fresh supply of arterial blood passes the site. The result is a variable absorption of light reaching the photodetector.

Oxyhemoglobin (O_2Hb) and deoxyhemoglobin (Hb) are distinctly different in their capability to absorb red and infrared light. During systole, as the arterial blood pulsates between the light and photodetector, the pulse oximeter detects the variation in light absorption, and by comparing the ratio of infrared light to red light absorbed, calculates oxygen saturation.

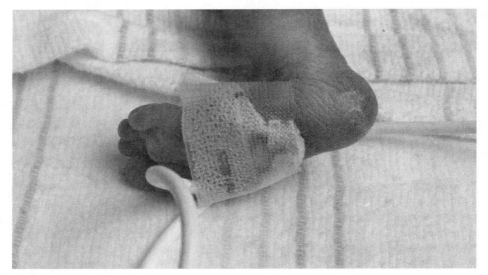

Figure 9–6 *Proper placement of a pulse oximeter probe.*

CLINICAL USES

Advantages. Pulse oximeters require no warm-up time and do not need to be calibrated. Probes used on pulse oximeters are available for use on different areas of the body and on different-sized patients. Pulse oximeters have been found to be accurate in critically ill patients whose arterial oxygen saturation exceeds 75%.[3]

For the larger pediatric patient, it may be desirable to use an ear probe or a finger probe specifically designed for that site. For the smaller patient, sensors come built into a small length of flexible plastic, shown in Figure 9–7, which can be wrapped around a finger, wrist, foot, or toe.

This type of sensor is held in place by small double-gummed adhesives, applied on each end of the sensor. These prevent the movement of the light source and photodetector on the skin surface and may or may not be used, depending on the maturity and health of the patient skin. The entire probe should then be secured to the body part using tape or a Velcro strap limb restraint.

External light sources, especially heat lamps and phototherapy lights, can interfere with the light detector. In these instances, if a limb restraint is not used, a cover should be placed over the sensor. It has also been noted that inaccuracies in measurement are seen in patients with heavy skin pigmentation.[3] Although the risk of skin trauma is small, the pulse oximeter probe site should be changed every 8 hours to prevent skin breakdowns and pressure sores.

Oxygen saturation is a better indicator of oxygen content than is PaO_2. A saturation of greater than 90% is usually indicative or normal oxygenation. It is important to remember, however, that the relationship between SaO_2 and PaO_2 is not linear and many factors affect

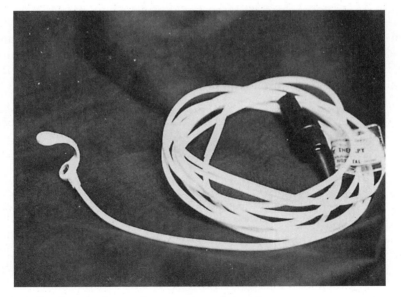

Figure 9–7   *A small pulse oximeter, used on preemies and neonates.*

that relationship.[3] The presence of different types of hemoglobin such as methemoglobin or carboxyhemoglobin in the blood will cause erroneously high readings on the pulse oximeter. This is because the pulse oximeter does not differentiate between different species of hemoglobin. Again, blood gas analysis should accompany the use of a pulse oximeter on a regular basis to ensure its accuracy.

The use of pulse oximetry has become routine in the emergency department and has been found to detect low saturations on patients who, by clinical evaluation, were not thought to be desaturated.[6] It is of interest to note also that pulse oximetry is being used to evaluate the presence of fetal hypoxia.[7]

CAPNOGRAPHY/CAPNOMETRY

The introduction of capnography, or capnometry, the measurement of exhaled CO_2, has added one more noninvasive tool to assess the blood gas status of a patient. It has been shown to provide an accurate estimation of $PaCO_2$, even in the presence of severe hypocarbia.[8] It has also proven helpful in confirming ETT position following intubation and during transport.[9] A typical $PetCO_2$ waveform is shown in Figure 9–8.

BASICS

Capnography uses *spectrophotometric infrared analysis* of the exhaled gas to determine end-tidal $PaCO_2$ ($PetCO_2$). There are two methods available to sample and analyze the end-tidal breath: sidestream and mainstream. The difference in the two methods is in how the sample is collected, not in the analysis itself.

Sidestream Analyzer. The sidestream analyzer removes a continuous sample of the exhaled gas through a small tube and carries it to the analysis chamber. Because it is small and lightweight, the sidestream analyzer may be less likely to cause inadvertent extubation. It can also be adapted for use in nonintubated patients.

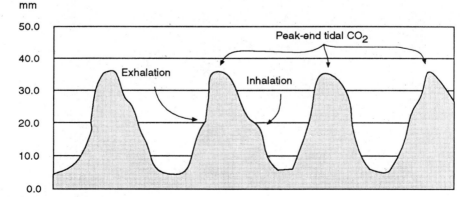

Figure 9–8 *A normal PetCO$_2$ waveform.*

There are several downsides to the sidestream analyzer. First, the sample must pass through the tubing and water trap before it reaches the sample chamber. This makes it less responsive to high respiratory rates. Additionally, the displayed $PetCO_2$ is behind in time from the actual breath. Water or mucus can accumulate in the sample tube and cause erroneous readings. Finally, the amount of gas sampled is important. If too much is drawn out, gas from the ventilator circuit may be entrained and dilute the sample. If used on a small neonate, excessive sampling may reduce the amount of delivered tidal volume.[10]

Mainstream Analyzers. Mainstream analyzers place the analyzing chamber at the airway. It is heated with a small wire to help prevent condensation in the chamber, reducing errors. An advantage to this type of system is that it gives current $PetCO_2$ readings, unlike the sidestream analyzer. This may make it more useful for patients with a high respiratory rate.

A disadvantage to this type of monitor is that the analyzing chambers are bulky and heavy, making the chance of accidental extubation a hazard. The chamber itself also has a large amount of deadspace, up to 15 ml, that could affect ventilation in the small neonate.

PHYSIOLOGIC FACTORS

$PetCO_2$ monitoring is valuable provided the practitioner understands the physiology of end-tidal CO_2 production and the factors that can alter it. $PetCO_2$ may be most valuable in the monitoring of trends over time. Changes in patient condition can be quickly observed and treated. Trend evaluation may also make weaning and extubation more exacting to patient conditions. The remainder of this section will describe those factors that are important to understand to properly use the $PetCO_2$ monitor in the clinical setting.

Physiology of CO_2 Production. Normal $PaCO_2$ in the healthy patient averages 40 mm Hg and reflects the amount of CO_2 dissolved in the plasma of arterial blood. As body cells metabolize, they consume oxygen and produce carbon dioxide as a byproduct. From the cell, the CO_2 diffuses into the venous blood to be carried back to the lungs for removal. This addition of CO_2 from the cells raises the $PaCO_2$ of venous blood to about 46 mm Hg. The pressure of CO_2 in the alveoli ($PaCO_2$) is lower owing to the inhalation of fresh atmospheric gas, which contains very little CO_2.

Upon reaching the alveoli, the CO_2 in the venous blood diffuses into the alveoli following a pressure gradient. The result is that the CO_2 in both the alveoli and in the blood equilibrate at a value of 40 mm Hg. Thus, in the healthy, well-perfused lung, end-tidal $PaCO_2$ ($PetCO_2$) levels are equal to arterial $PaCO_2$ levels, as depicted in Figure 9–9.

Unfortunately, most patients being monitored for $PetCO_2$ do not possess healthy, well-perfused lungs. The practitioner must understand the physiologic changes that occur in the diseased lung and what the effect will be on $PetCO_2$ to adequately manage the patient using the $PetCO_2$ monitor.

The Effect of Ventilation/Perfusion (V/Q) Imbalances. The basis of understanding $PetCO_2$ monitors is that ultimately they reflect changes in pulmonary perfusion. The $PetCO_2$ moni-

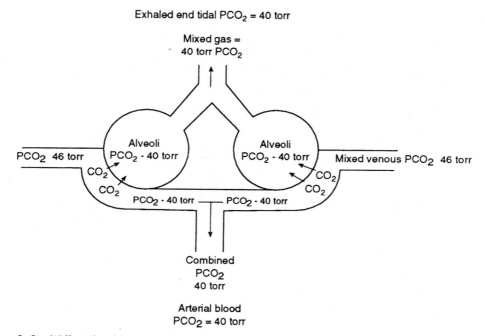

Exhaled end tidal PCO_2 = 40 torr

Mixed gas = 40 torr PCO_2

Alveoli PCO_2 - 40 torr

Alveoli PCO_2 - 40 torr

PCO_2 46 torr

CO_2

CO_2

Mixed venous PCO_2 46 torr

CO_2

CO_2

PCO_2 - 40 torr — PCO_2 - 40 torr

Combined PCO_2 40 torr

Arterial blood PCO_2 = 40 torr

Figure 9–9 *Well-perfused lungs resulting in a correlation between PetCO₂ and PaCO₂.*

tor looks at both lungs as though they were one respiratory unit. This is because exhaled gas at the level of the mouth is a mixture of all of the respiratory units in the lungs.

The healthy patient, with normal ventilation and perfusion, maintains 4 liters of ventilation for every 5 liters of blood flow. This produces a ratio of 4:5 or 0.8 when divided. Thus, for every liter of blood perfusion in the lungs, there is 0.8 liter of gas in the alveoli for exchange. We will now examine how changes in the V/Q ratio can alter PetCO₂ readings.

Deadspace Ventilation. Deadspace ventilation is at one extreme of the V/Q range. This type of abnormality has the greatest effect on the PetCO₂ monitor. Deadspace ventilation occurs when the lungs are adequately ventilated, but perfusion is interrupted to a portion of the lung, as depicted in Figure 9–10. In this situation, the gas that enters the nonperfused alveoli does not participate in gas exchange, while the perfused alveoli does. The result is that the gas in the nonperfused alveoli remains with atmospheric concentrations of CO_2, which is essentially 0. The perfused alveoli participate in gas exchange and produce an exhaled gas that has a typical $PaCO_2$ of 40 mm Hg.

As these two gases mix in the airways and are exhaled, the resultant mixed gas that exits the patient represents the average $PaCO_2$ of both gases, which is 20 mm Hg (40 mm Hg from the perfused alveoli, 0 mm Hg from the nonperfused alveoli). The arterial blood in this example has a normal $PaCO_2$ of 40 mm Hg. This is because the blood perfused good alveoli and participated in gas exchange, resulting in a normal $PaCO_2$. If this patient was monitored with a PetCO₂, the monitor would show a value of 20 mm Hg, when in reality the

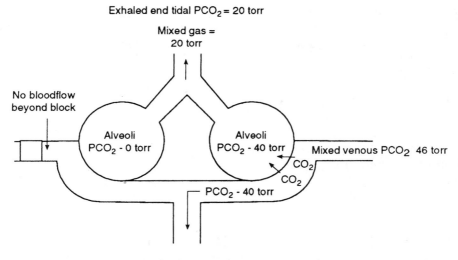

Figure 9–10 *Pulmonary embolism leading to deadspace ventilation.*

arterial $PaCO_2$ is 40 mm Hg. Thus, in the presence of increased deadspace ventilation, the $PetCO_2$ will read lower than arterial values.

Conditions Increasing Deadspace Ventilation. There are several clinical conditions that can lead to an increase in deadspace ventilation, listed in Table 9–3.

Pulmonary embolus, causing an occlusion to blood flow in the lung, is a cause of deadspace ventilation. Depending on the severity of the embolism, the effect of $PetCO_2$ may be minimal with a small emboli or drastic in the case of a large emboli.

Severe hypotension can lead to an underperfusion of the lungs and is another cause of deadspace ventilation. Mechanical ventilation with high airway pressures may overdistend alveoli and compress the nearby pulmonary capillaries, leading to deadspace ventilation. The higher the ventilator pressures, the more the compression and resultant hypoperfusion.

Shunt Perfusion. At the other extreme of the V/Q range is shunt perfusion. Shunts occur when blood perfuses areas of nonventilated alveoli. This type of mismatch does not have as drastic effects on the $PetCO_2$ monitor.

The maximal level that $PetCO_2$ can rise to is determined by the $PaCO_2$ of the mixed venous blood. Referring to Figure 9–11, if two arterial blood flows combine, one from an

TABLE 9–3 Conditions Leading to Increased Deadspace Ventilation

Pulmonary embolism
Hypotension
High pressures associated with mechanical ventilation

area of no ventilation, the other from an area of normal ventilation, the resultant $PaCO_2$ would be an average of the two, or 43 mm Hg. In this example, the $PetCO_2$ would reflect the ventilated alveoli and show a $PaCO_2$ of 40 mm Hg when the $PaCO_2$ is 43 mm Hg. Only in cases of severe, life-threatening shunting would the $PetCO_2$ be significantly lower than $PaCO_2$.

Conditions Causing Shunt Perfusion. Clinical situations that result in shunting are listed in Table 9–4 and include atelectasis and obstruction of the airways by foreign objects or mucus.

Limitations to Capnography. $PetCO_2$ monitors can only show a change in the patient's condition, not an improvement or deterioration. Consider the following scenarios, which further examine this limitation of capnography.

An increasing $PetCO_2$ may reflect a decrease in minute ventilation, a marked decrease in cardiac output, or a worsening of the V/Q ratio. All of these are considered a worsening of patient condition. Conversely, an increasing $PetCO_2$ may come from an improvement in alveolar deadspace disease, leading to an improvement in gas exchange. This condition would be a reflection of an improvement in patient status.

A decrease in $PetCO_2$ may be due to an improvement in ventilation or in the V/Q ratio, indicating an improvement of patient condition. However, a decreased $PetCO_2$ could also occur as alveolar deadspace increases, thus reflecting a worsening patient condition.

Another limitation of capnography is its inability to provide information on oxygenation. Arterial PO_2 may drop to dangerous levels, with little or no change in $PetCO_2$. Oxygenation must be monitored concurrently to get an overall view of respiratory status.

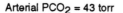

Figure 9–11 *The combination of flows from a ventilated and nonventilated area.*

TABLE 9–4 Causes of Pulmonary Shunts

---

1. Venoarterial (right-to-left) shunting
   a. Tetralogy of Fallot
   b. Atrial septal defect
   c. Tricuspid atresia
2. Atelectasis
3. Obstruction of the airway
4. Pulmonary consolidation

SUMMARY

In order to expertly care for the neonatal and pediatric patient, the practitioner must know how to properly obtain and then interpret data concerning the oxygenation, ventilation, and acid-base balance of the patient.

The most sure method of measuring these data is with arterial blood gas analysis. In order to get results that are of value, the blood must be obtained in a manner that does not contaminate the sample, and in which the patient is not traumatized. The most common method of obtaining arterial blood from a neonate is through an umbilical artery catheter (UAC). Because of the possibility of shunting through a patient ductus arteriosus (PDA), and the position of the catheter tip in the descending aorta, blood gas results may be lower than what the upper extremities and head are receiving. Understanding this possibility can help the practitioner make intelligent choices in the face of a low PaO_2 from the UAC. Another danger is in the possible dislocation of the catheter with resultant blood loss. In older patients, catheters may be inserted in the radial artery.

Other methods of obtaining blood for analysis are through arterial punctures and capillary samples. Because these inflict pain and usually result in an unhappy child, the results obtained may be skewed. Additionally, it must be remembered that capillary PO_2 does not adequately correspond to arterial PO_2 and should not be used to determine oxygenation status.

Once obtained, it is important for the practitioner to interpert the values correctly. The value for oxygen in the plasma, PaO_2 is often misused. It must be remembered that PaO_2 is only one determinant of oxygenation and that it is only a reflection of the amount of oxygen actually present. Ideally, PaO_2 is used with oxygen saturation measurements to give a more complete view of oxygenation status.

$PaCO_2$ reflects the adequacy of ventilation. If too high, ventilation is not adequate and respiratory acidosis may ensue. If too low, the patient is hyperventilating and respiratory alkalosis may occur.

The pH of the blood is a measurement of the number of hydrogen ions present. The relationship is inverse, with a low pH indicating a high amount of hydrogen ions and vice versa. A low pH is called acidosis, and a high pH is called alkalosis. The pH is affected by both metabolic acids and alkalis and by CO_2.

HCO_3-, or bicarbonate, is controlled by tissue metabolism and the kidneys and is responsible for maintaining proper pH balance. As more hydrogen ions become available, the bicarbonate quickly combines with them to form carbonic acid. Carbonic acid then dissociates into CO_2 and water, both of which are eliminated from the body. An excess or deficit of bicarbonate is reflected in the base excess/deficit measurement. A base excess above 4 mEq/L indicates too much bicarbonate, while a base deficit reflects too little bicarbonate to buffer the hydrogen ions.

Technology in the past decade has introduced several methods of noninvasive blood gas monitoring. One of the first to be introduced was the transcutaneous monitor (TCM). By measuring PaO_2 and $PaCO_2$ through the skin, constant monitoring can be accomplished and the amount of blood required for analysis reduced. If trending, the TCM can significantly aid in ventilator and oxygen management. Because of the risk of burning, the probe site must be changed every 2 to 3 hours.

Another technological advance is the pulse oximeter. In contrast to the TCM, which measure PO_2, the pulse oximeter measures the amount of oxygen bound to hemoglobin, a potentially more useful measurement. Because it is noninvasive, it can also be used continuously and is very helpful in monitoring for hypoxic spells.

Finally, capnography has been shown to accurately reflect arterial PCO_2. It does this by measuring a sample of the patient's exhaled breath through either a sidestream analyzer or a mainstream analyzer. In order to properly use the data, the factors affecting CO_2 production (such as ventilation/perfusion imbalances, deadspace ventilation, and shunt perfusion) must be understood.

References

1. AARC Clinical Practice Guideline: capillary blood gas sampling for neonatal and pediatric patients. *Resp Care*. 1994b; 39:1180–1183.

2. Merenstein, GB, Gardner, SL *Handbook of Neonatal Intensive Care*. 4th ed. St. Louis: CV Mosby Co.; 1997.

3. Durbin, CG Jr. Monitoring gas exchange: clinical effectiveness and cost considerations. *Resp Care*. 1994; 39:123–137.

4. Powerll, CC, et al. Subcutaneous oxygen tension: a useful adjunct in assessment of perfusion status. *Crit Care Med*. 1995; 23:867–873.

5. Avery, GB, et al. American Academy of Pediatrics Task Force on Transcutaneous Oxygen Monitors. Report of Consensus Meeting. *Pediatrics*. 1989; 83:122–125.

6. Maneker, AJ, et al. Contribution of routine pulse oximetry to evaluation and management of patients with respiratory illness in a pediatric emergency department. *Ann Emerg Med*. 1995; 25:36–40.

7. Luttkus, A, et al. Continuous monitoring of fetal oxygen saturation by pulse oximetry. *Obstet Gynecol*. 1995; 85:183–186.

8. Flanagan, JKF, et al. Noninvasive monitoring of end-tidal carbon dioxide tension via nasal cannulas in spontaneously breathing children with profound bypocarbia. *Crit Care Med*. 1995; 23:1140.

9. Bhende, MS, et al. Evaluation of a portable infrared end-tidal carbon dioxide monitor during pediatric interhopsital transport. *Pediatrics*. 1995; 95:875–878.

10. Monaco, F Patient monitoring. In: Barnhart, SL, Czervinske, MP, eds. *Prenatal and Pediatric Respiratory Care*. Philadelphia: WB Saunders Co.; 1995.

Bibliography and Suggested Readings

AARC Clinical Practice Guideline: transcutaneous blood gas monitoring for neonatal and pediatric patients. *Resp Care*. 1994a; 39:1176–1179.

Behrman, RE, Kliegman, RM, Jenson, HB *Nelson Textbook of Pediatrics*. 16h ed. Philadelphia: WB Saunders Co.; 2000.

Beske, VA Drawing blood from arterial lines in neonates. *Neonatal Network*. 1994; 13:79–80.

Burton, GG, Hodgkin, JE, Ward, JJ *Respiratory Care: A Guide to Clinical Practice*. 4th ed. Philadelphia: JB Lippincott Co.; 1997.

Cloherty, JP, Stark, AR, eds. *Manual of Neonatal Care*. 4th ed. Philadelphia: Lippincott; 1997.

Dantzker, DR, MacIntyre, NR, Bakow, ED *Comprehensive Respiratory Care*. Philadelphia: WB Saunders Co.; 1995.

Martin, RJ Transcutaneous monitoring: instrumentation and clinical application. *Resp Care*. 1990; 35:577–583.

Scanlan, CL, Wilkins, RL, Stoller, JK *Egan's Fundamentals of Respiratory Care*. 7th ed. St. Louis: Mosby, 1999.

Taussig, LM, Landau, LI *Pediatric Respiratory Medicine*. St. Louis: Mosby; 1999.

Watkins, JG Jr. *Arterial Blood Gases. A Self-Study Manual*. Philadelphia: JB Lippincott Co.; 1985.

Posttest

1. Of the following, which would *not* be an indication for obtaining a blood gas sample?
   a. signs of respiratory distress
   b. change in patient status
   c. departmental policy
   d. significant blood loss
2. Which of the following are common sites used to obtain arterial blood in neonates?
   I. umbilical artery
   II. radial artery
   III. femoral artery
   IV. capillary
   V. carotid artery
   a. I, II, IV
   b. I, III, V
   c. II, IV, V
   d. I, III, III, V

3. In the presence of right-to-left shunting of blood through the ductus arteriosus, arterial blood from the UAC would show:
   a. a low arterial PO_2
   b. a high arterial PO_2
   c. an alkalotic pH
   d. a low arterial $PaCO_2$
4. The complication of necrotizing enterocolitis is most prevalent in which of the following blood gas access sites?
   a. radial artery
   b. umbilical artery
   c. femoral artery
   d. carotid artery
5. Reliable values obtained from capillary samples require which of the following?
   a. heating the heel to at least 45°C
   b. consistency in the technique
   c. adequate squeezing or milking of the heel
   d. puncturing with a beveled needle
6. Which of the following best describes PaO_2?
   a. the total amount of oxygen present in the blood
   b. the amount of oxygen attached to hemoglobin
   c. the pressure of oxygen dissolved in plasma
   d. the best indicator of adequate tissue perfusion
7. Which of the following defines alveolar ventilations?
   a. tidal volume times respiratory rate
   b. minute ventilation minus deadspace ventilation
   c. minute ventilation minus tidal volume
   d. minute ventilation minus respiratory rate
8. As respiratory rate increases at a static tidal volume, which of the following occurs?
   I. $PaCO_2$ decreases
   II. $PaCO_2$ increases
   III. alveolar ventilation increases
   IV. alveolar ventilation decreases
       a. II, III
       b. I, III
       c. I, IV
       d. II, III, IV
9. At a pH of 7.40, which of the following represents the correct balance of bicarbonate to dissolved carbon dioxide?
   a. 1:10
   b. 10:1
   c. 15:1
   d. 20:1
10. In the presence of respiratory acidosis, which of the following is the amount of bicarbonate the body retains for each 1 mm Hg increase in $PaCO_2$?

   a. 1.0 mEq/L
   b. 0.1 mEq/L
   c. 0.01 mEq/L
   d. 10 mEq/L
11. Carbonic acid is formed by a combination of:
   a. HCO_3_ and CO_2
   b. HCO_3_ and H^+ ions
   c. HCO_3_ and H_2O
   d. CO_2 and H^+ ions
12. $NaHCO_3$_, if given too rapidly, could lead to:
   a. intraventricular hemorrhage
   b. cardiac arrest
   c. intestinal bleeding
   d. diminished PaO_2
13. The purpose of heating the skin at the attachment site of the TCM is to:
   a. decrease capillary shunting
   b. increase the tissue PaO_2
   c. increase the perfusion to the area
   d. cause the skin to sweat
14. Which of the following factors would cause $PtCO_2$ to measure lower than actual arterial PO_2?
   I. shock
   II. severe acidosis
   III. skin edema
   IV. hyperthermia
   V. severe anemia
       a. I, II, III, V
       b. I, III, IV
       c. III, IV, V
       d. I, II, III, IV, V
15. The greatest hazard associated with transcutaneous monitors is:
   a. erythema
   b. epidermal stripping
   c. hemorrhage
   d. thermal injury
16. Which of the following would cause erroneous pulse oximetry readings?
   a. presence of carboxyhemoglobin
   b. PaO_2 above 100 torr
   c. decreased hemoglobin levels
   d. increased hemoglobin levels
17. A major disadvantage of a mainstream end-tidal CO_2 monitor is:
   a. accidental extubation
   b. occlusion with condensed water
   c. increased risk of pneumothorax

  d. thermal injury
18. The greatest effect on the end-tidal CO_2 monitor is exerted by:
  a. a pneumothorax
  b. shunt perfusion
  c. deadspace ventilation
  d. hyperventilation
19. An increasing $PetCO_2$ may indicate which of the following?
  I. worsening oxygenation
  II. worsening V/Q ratio
  III. improving V/Q ratio
  IV. improvement in alveolar deadspace disease
  V. increasing alveolar deadspace
    a. I, II
    b. II, IV
    c. I, III, V
    d. I, III

CAUSES AND CARE OF ILLNESS IN PERINATAL AND PEDIATRIC PATIENTS

CHAPTER TEN

PERINATAL LUNG DISEASE AND OTHER PROBLEMS OF PREMATURITY

OBJECTIVES

Upon completion of this chapter, the reader should be able to:

1. Describe each of the following as it relates to RDS:
   a. Etiology
   b. Pathophysiology
   c. Clinical signs
   d. Treatment
   e. Complications
2. Describe the pathophysiology, diagnosis, and treatment of bronchopulmonary dysplasia.
3. Discuss the pathophysiology, clinical signs, and treatment of pulmonary dysmaturity (Wilson-Mikity syndrome).
4. Summarize the stages of eye development.
5. Identify and describe the factors that lead to retinopathy of prematurity (ROP), how diagnosis is made, and treatment.
6. Compare and contrast the pathophysiology and complications of intracranial and intraventricular hemorrhages.
7. Identify and describe the four stages of intraventricular hemorrhage.
8. Define asphyxia and identify its incidence in neonates.
9. Describe the pathophysiologic changes that occur with asphyxia, its consequences, and treatment.
10. Identify the cause of meconium release in utero and describe the diagnosis, pathophysiology, and treatment of meconium aspiration.
11. Relate the diagnosis and treatment of a pneumothorax to a pneumomediastinum and pneumopericardium.
12. Describe the pathophysiology and treatment of pulmonary interstitial emphysema.
13. Identify the factors that lead to pulmonary air embolism and subcutaneous air leaks.
14. Describe the etiology, diagnosis, and treatment of persistent pulmonary hypertension of the newborn (PPHN).
15. Identify and discuss those factors responsible for the onset of transient tachypnea of the newborn (TTN).

16. Compare and contrast central and obstructive apnea with regard to causes and treatments.

KEY TERMS

choroid plexus
cryotherapy
disseminated intravas-
  cular coagulation
germinal matrix

hypoxic-ischemic encephalopathy
micrognathia
ora serrata
periventricular leukomalacia
posthemorrhagic hydrocephalus
reflux
systolic ejection clicks

titration
tonic posturing
transillumination
vaso-obliteration
ventricular-peritoneal shunt
ventriculostomy
vernix

CONSEQUENCES OF PREMATURE BIRTH

The major factor of morbidity and mortality in the premature neonate is the degree to which the organ systems have not yet developed. The earlier in gestation that birth occurs, the higher the degree of morbidity and mortality. Although the fetus is capable of living outside the uterus as early as 23 to 24 weeks of gestation, it cannot survive without some degree of intervention to assist the underdeveloped organ systems. Of all the organ systems, the pulmonary system is most vulnerable to premature delivery and its complications.

RESPIRATORY DISTRESS SYNDROME (RDS)

Etiology. RDS, also called hyaline membrane disease (HMD), is the primary cause of respiratory disorders in the neonate. According to Avery, RDS is estimated to be the cause of 30% of neonatal deaths.[1] As much as 70% of all preterm deaths are also attributed to RDS. RDS was first reported in 1903 by the German physician Hochheim. Since its first report up to the present time, several names have been added to the RDS. Older terms include IRDS, for infant RDS, or idiopathic RDS. More current terminology is to simply use RDS, or NRDS for neonatal RDS.

The name hyaline membrane disease arises from the change in the alveolar membrane that occurs with the progression of the disease. The scar-like tissue that replaces the normal alveolar tissue is called hyaline membrane, thus the name.

The etiology of RDS is well understood. It is known that the underlying etiology of RDS in the neonate is a deficiency of surfactant production. Although many factors contribute to this deficiency, the main contributor is prematurity of the pulmonary system. Although surfactant is produced near gestational week 22, it is easily disrupted by hypoxemia, hypothermia, and acidosis, all of which plague the premature neonate. It is not until the mature surfactant is produced near week 35 that the above stressors do not disrupt the production and the fetal lungs are considered mature

Several risk factors have been recognized to help identify those neonates at risk for developing RDS (Table 10–1). At greatest risk are neonates born before 35 weeks. The shorter the gestation, the higher the risk involved. The presence of maternal diabetes is another risk factor, presumably because of the effect of diabetes on lung maturation and the high incidence of premature labor and delivery with diabetic mothers. A history of RDS in siblings also places the neonate at high risk. Males have a higher incidence of RDS, as does the second-born twin and infants born by cesarean delivery without labor. Neonates with poor Apgar scores are predisposed to RDS, possibly due to the associated asphyxia.

Pathophysiology. Continuing research on RDS has demonstrated that deficiency in surfactant production is not the only cause of the disease. Overall immaturity of other organ systems contributes to its development. The immaturity of the terminal air sacs and associated vasculature result in poor gas exchange. The immaturity of the chest wall allows very little stability. As a negative pressure is created for inspiration, the chest retracts inward, reducing the effectiveness of the inspiratory effort. Immaturity of the diaphragm and other muscles of respiration may cause further inspiratory difficulty.

Apnea is also common in the premature neonate due to the immaturity of the central nervous system. Add to these the effects of hypothermia, hypoxia, and acidosis on surfactant production, and RDS becomes a multifactorial process. The role of surfactant in the lung is covered in Chapter 1.

Focusing on the effects of a decreased surfactant activity, we will examine the pathogenesis of RDS (Figure 10–1).

TABLE 10-1 Factors That Increase the Incidence of RDS

---

1. Prematurity—incidence of RDS is inversely proportional to gestational age
2. Birth weight—incidence of RDS is greater in preemies weighing less than 1200 g
3. Gender—premature males outnumber females 2:1 in acquiring RDS
4. Persistence of fetal circulation
5. Atelectasis
6. Multiple gestations—higher incidence in the second and subsequent siblings
7. Prenatal maternal complications
   a. hypoxia
   b. hemorrhage
   c. shock
   d. hypotension
   e. hypertension
   f. anemia
8. Maternal diabetes
9. Abnormal placental conditions
   a. placental previa
   b. abruptio placentae
10. Umbilical cord disorders
    a. cord compression
    b. cord prolapse

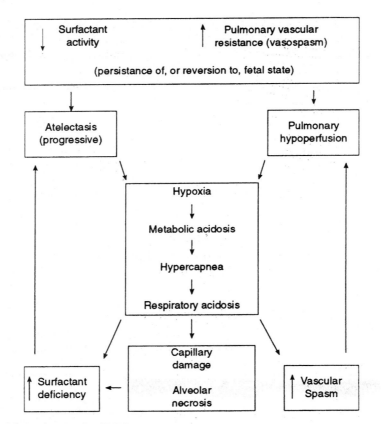

Figure 10–1 *The pathogenesis of RDS.*

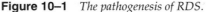

With decreased or absent surfactant in the alveoli, alveolar surface tension increases. As surface tension increases, the compliance of the lung decreases, and the lung becomes stiffer. The neonate now must generate tremendous negative intrathoracic pressures to inflate the lung. With each successive breath, the infant weakens and uses up vital energy stores.

The diminished surfactant supply leads to widespread atelectasis in the lungs, which in turn leads to a worsening of ventilation perfusion (V/Q) ratios and resultant hypoxia. Atelectasis also contributes to a decreasing functional residual capacity (FRC) in the lungs. FRC is the amount of gas left in the lungs following a normal expiration. It is made up of the residual volume (RV) and the expiratory reserve volume (ERV). A reduction in the FRC is mainly due to a decrease in the RV. As FRC decreases, the patient must work ever harder to create the negative pressures necessary to open the shrinking alveoli.

Along with hypoxia, hypercapnia develops and leads to respiratory acidosis. The lack of oxygen at the cellular level leads to anaerobic metabolism with resultant metabolic acidosis. The net effect of the hypoxia and combined acidosis results in damage to the capillaries and alveolar tissues. The condition is now worsened as the damaged alveoli and capillaries cause more surfactant deficiency.

The combined acidosis also leads to increasing pulmonary vasospasm. Pulmonary vasospasm is further enhanced by the hypoxemia, leading to pulmonary hypoperfusion. Hypoperfusion leads to a further worsening of the V/Q ratio and further hypoxemia.

The neonate is now caught in a vicious circle that begins again with worsening atelectasis, leading to more profound hypoxia and acidosis, increased pulmonary vascular spasm, and further hypoperfusion. If it continues unchecked, the cycle continues until the patient can no longer overcome the effects of the disease.

Clinical Signs and Diagnosis. The clinical manifestations of RDS usually begin at birth, or shortly thereafter. The patient has a respiratory rate above 60 breaths per minute (BPM), indicating some degree of respiratory difficulty. The patient then begins grunting, so named because of the sound created by the infant exhaling against a partially closed glottis. This obstruction of exhalation causes a back pressure in the alveoli, resulting in an increased FRC. This is an attempt by the neonate to combat the effects of volume loss in the stiffening lungs. It can be thought of as a natural PEEP in the airways.

The neonate with RDS will also begin to show chest retractions as the disease worsens. With ever-stiffening lungs, the patient must generate greater and greater negative pressures to open the alveoli. The increased negative intrathoracic pressure causes the spaces between the ribs and at the top and bottom of the thoracic cage to be pulled inward. This inward movement of the skin is called a retraction.

Another sign of worsening distress is the flaring of the external nares of the nose. This is an attempt by the neonate to get more gas into the lungs by widening the airway passage.

Cyanosis may also be present, especially if the patient is on room air. The blood gases are typical of respiratory distress with worsening PaO_2, increasing $PaCO_2$, and combined acidosis.

The chest x-ray helps establish a diagnosis with the lungs appearing underaerated bilaterally. Their appearance has been described as clouded, opaque, reticulogranular, and frosted or ground glass. As the atelectasis worsens, air-bronchograms appear in the lung periphery.

Other nonrespiratory signs may also be present in the patient with RDS. Hypothermia is a common problem in the RDS patient. Observation of the skin may reveal pallor or severe edema. The muscle tone may be flaccid, with a general hypoactivity. A relatively old method of determining the presence of pulmonary surfactant, the "shake" test, has been touted as a tool to rapidly diagnose RDS.[2]

In most cases, the symptoms of RDS gradually worsen for the first 48 to 72 hours followed by a stabilization and a slow recovery period. Stabilization of the disease is often associated with the onset of diuresis. The highest incidence of mortality from RDS occurs within the first 72 hours. If death occurs following 72 hours, it is usually secondary to complications such as barotraumatic air leaks, intracranial hemorrhages, or infections and not due to the lung disease.

Treatment. The ideal treatment for RDS would be to prevent it from occurring. The administration of glucocorticoids to the mother, if done at least two days before delivery, has been shown to promote fetal lung and surfactant development. It is of interest to note the use of antenatal steroids for reducing the need for blood pressure support in premature infants, in addition to promoting lung maturation.[3] No discussion of treating RDS would be complete without examining the use of artificial surfactant replacement. This subject is covered in detail in Chapter 16. As beneficial as surfactant replacement is, it apparently does not work on all patients equally. Many still require ventilatory support and others appear to get no effect from the surfactant. Therefore, we will examine conventional treatment of the RDS patient at this point.

The difficulty in treating RDS is in maintaining adequate alveolar ventilation without inflicting damage on the lungs. This then becomes the goal of treatment: to support the patient's respiratory system adequately while minimizing complications. This is easy to envision, but very hard to accomplish. The nature of the disease, and the means we have to treat it, often combine to create other problems that lengthen the recovery of the neonate. The overriding rule to follow when treating the patient with RDS is to treat the symptoms quickly, with pressures and FiO_2 as low as possible. However, never compromise the patient's status of using parameters that are too low. Use pressures and FiO_2 that restore blood gas values to acceptable ranges, whatever those pressures and percents may be. PaO_2 should be maintained between 50 and 80 mm Hg, with the $PaCO_2$ maintained below 60 mm Hg. The pH should be greater than 7.25 as a more acidotic pH leads to decreased surfactant production, organ dysfunction, and an increased risk of intraventricular hemorrhage.

Depending on the severity of the disease, the neonate may require positive pressure ventilation immediately or later in the course of the disease. Some institutions intubate and begin mechanical ventilation when the patient's condition begins to deteriorate, indicated by a $PaCO_2$ greater than 60 mm Hg and pH less than 7.25, or a worsening of clinical signs, such as grunting, flaring, and retracting. Others advocate the use of nasal CPAP before intubating the patient. Both of these modalities are covered in Chapter 14.

Regardless of the technique used, one must intervene before the onset of respiratory failure. By waiting too long to begin advanced support, the practitioner faces an uphill battle of trying to get ahead of the patient. Early intervention allows supportive steps to be taken that may reduce the amount of total support needed. Dexamethasone, administered early in the course of RDS has been shown in a study to improve pulmonary compliance and tidal volume, reducing the requirements for FiO_2 and mean airway pressure. Additionally, its use is associated with reduced time on the ventilator and a decreased incidence of chronic lung disease.[4] Short-term improvements in the respiratory mechanics of ventilated neonates are also seen with the use of salbutamol and ipratropium bromide given via MDI and spacer to ventilated neonates in a study by Lee and associates.[5]

Treatment of RDS also requires adequate hydration, including electrolyte balance. Diuretics are used widely in the management of fluid balance in the neonate. Furosemide (Lasix) is often used because of its excellence in unloading water off the patient. Ironically, researchers have demonstrated that furosemide appears to increase the incidence of patent ductus arteriosus (PDA) threefold.[6] However, it works so well as a diuretic that the benefit outweighs the risk of a greater incidence of PDA.

Of vital importance in the treatment of RDS is the maintenance of thermoregulation. A neonate who is not thermoregulated will not respond as well to treatment as a thermoregulated neonate.

The use of a pulse oximeter and transcutaneous monitor, along with supportive blood

PDA= patent ductus arteriosus

gases, allow for the *titration* of ventilatory support to meet the patient's needs and should be considered mandatory equipment for treating RDS.

Complications. Most complications of RDS are secondary to the use of ventilation. Successful management of the patient requires anticipation of potential complications. Anticipation can aid in prevention of some complications and rapid treatment in others.

Intracranial hemorrhage occurs in more than 40% of infants weighing less than 1500 g.[7] This risk increases significantly as positive pressure is initiated. The positive pressure inside the thorax is transmitted to the cranial cavity, where the immature vasculature of the developing brain may rupture, leading to intraventricular hemorrhage.

Barotraumatic injury that leads to pulmonary air leaks is a common complication in RDS. As the lung compliance drops, higher ventilator pressures are needed to maintain adequate ventilation and oxygenation. This can lead to rupture of the lung and the development of pneumothoraces and other barotraumatic diseases.

Disseminated intravascular coagulation (DIC) is an insidious disease caused by a disruption of coagulation factors, leading to profuse bleeding throughout the body. Neonates with RDS have an increased incidence of DIC.

Infection is a common complication, often due to the presence of an endotracheal tube in the trachea. Gram-negative organisms often infect the lung, causing low-grade, chronic pneumonias, which are very difficult to eradicate. The pneumonia further injures the lung tissue and makes additional ventilatory support necessary. Use of sterile technique when intubating and suctioning, along with sterile humidifiers and tubing, reduce the chances of a pulmonary infection.

PDA is another common complication of RDS. A PDA can lead to severe right-to-left shunting of blood, with accompanying hypoxemia. During the healing stages of RDS, a PDA can cause left-to-right shunting and subsequent right-sided heart failure. PDA is covered in detail in Chapter 11.

BRONCHOPULMONARY DYSPLASIA (BPD)

BPD was first described in 1967 by Northway and associates, who found secondary lung injuries following prolonged exposure to oxygen and high ventilatory pressures.[8] Most incidences of BPD occur following the treatment of RDS. Ironically, the treatment for RDS is considered to be the prime cause of BPD, that is, high pressures and high FiO_2 over a period of time. Symptoms of BPD present in a patient without the concurrent radiologic signs is termed neonatal chronic lung disease (NCLD).

Pathophysiology. The pathophysiology of BPD appears to be linked to four factors: 1) oxygen toxicity; 2) barotrauma; 3) presence of a PDA; and 4) fluid overload. Exposure to high concentrations of oxygen leads to edema and thickening of the alveolar membrane. As the exposure is prolonged, the alveolar tissues hemorrhage and become necrotic. The interstitial spaces become fibrotic as the disease progresses. As the lung attempts to heal itself, the new cells are damaged by the same factors, and the disease is perpetuated.

A study by Strayer and associates showed a strong link between the development of BPD and the presence of antisurfactant protein A antibodies in the neonate.[9] They found that levels of these immune complexes correlated well with the development of BPD, more strongly than even gestational age and birth weight. Another study showed that preemies who went on to develop BPD had a diminished ability to secrete cortisol. It is speculated that this inability leaves the preemie vulnerable to continued lung injury.[10] The effect of positive airway pressure on the development of BPD is well documented.[11] The incidence of BPD increases with higher peak airway pressures and declines as lower pressures and long inspiratory times are used.[12] The incidence of BPD has found to be higher also in those patients with PDA who subsequently develop congestive heart failure.[1,13] Patients with left-to-right shunting through the PDA develop pulmonary congestion with worsening compliance. The result is higher ventilatory pressures and oxygen percents needed to ventilate and oxygenate the patient. This may explain the higher incidence of BPD in these patients.

Neonates who have developed symptoms of fluid overload in the first few days of life have a higher incidence of BPD. This is especially common in very small preemies, in whom water balance is so difficult to manage. The predisposing factor may be an exacerbation of pulmonary edema in these patients. A study by Nickerson and Taussig linked a family history of asthma to an increased incidence of BPD.[14]

Despite rapid advances in scientific study regarding BPD, its exact etiology remains unknown. The key to understanding the development of BPD lies in the ability to understand the relationship between all of the mentioned factors and their role in its development.

Diagnosis. The diagnosis of BPD is made from the chronic need for oxygen therapy and ventilator support and is verified by chest radiographs and laboratory studies. The CXR characteristics in BPD were first described by Northway and coworkers as falling into four stages.[8]

In stage I, usually the first 3 days of life, the CXR is typical of RDS, with a bilateral frosted or ground glass appearance. In stage II (days 3 to 10 of the disease), the lungs become opaque with granular infiltrates that obscure the cardiac markings. Stage III occurs during the first 10 to 20 days of life and begins showing multiple small cyst formations within the lung fields with a visible cardiac silhouette. Stage IV occurs following day 28 of life and an increased lung density and the formation of larger, irregular cysts. A new scoring system to standardize the reading of chest x-rays in determining the severity of BPD has been proposed.[15]

Laboratory studies include arterial blood gas analysis, which shows evidence of chronic lung disease, that is, hypoxia, hypercarbia, and increased bicarbonate levels. As the patient progresses through the disease, the ECG will show a right axis deviation of the heart and possible hypertrophy of the right ventricle.

Pulmonary function studies will show an increased respiratory rate, decreased tidal volumes, and normal minute ventilation. Airway resistance, especially the lower airways, is increased and lung compliance is typically decreased as a result of airway and lung parenchymal damage.

Treatment
Prevention. The goal in treating BPD is to avoid or reduce those factors that lead to its development and perpetuation. Using the lowest possible airway pressures to achieve sufficient

gas exchange is the goal of mechanical ventilation. One recommendation is to use pressures, rates, and FiO$_2$ that maintain the PaO$_2$ at 50 to 70 mm Hg and the PaCO$_2$ at 45 to 55 mm Hg.[16] Transcutaneous monitors and pulse oximeters are used to maintain these parameters and avoid the need for numerous arterial blood gases.

Mechanical Ventilation. The endotracheal tube should be small enough to allow a small leak during the mechanical breath. This helps reduce the chance of subglottic stenosis in the long-term patient. If the patient requires mechanical ventilation for longer than 1 to 2 months, a tracheostomy may be more appropriate than endotracheal intubation.[17] Ideally, the patient should be extubated as quickly as tolerated: however, weaning should be done slowly and cautiously so as not to compromise the patient's status. The use of nasal CPAP may be of help in the transition off of mechanical ventilation.

High-frequency ventilation has shown some evidence of successful treatment of pulmonary interstitial emphysema associated with BPD.

Adequate humidification of inspired gases must be monitored closely. Patients with BPD requiring long periods of intubation must have the airway sufficiently humidified to avoid mucus plugging from thickened secretions.

Respiratory Therapy Procedures. Chest physical therapy is done as needed to prevent the accumulation of secretions and to maintain good bronchial hygiene. The frequency of treatment should be dictated by the amount and viscosity of the patient's secretions, not simply on a routine basis. Suctioning of the airway must be done aseptically to prevent the possibility of infection complicating the clinical course. Aerosolized bronchodilators may be used to improve bronchospasm. However, they have not been shown to reduce airway resistance in the small BPD patient.[18] This is possibly due to the immaturity of the bronchial smooth muscle in the preemie. Theophylline appears to be a better drug in reducing airway resistance, improving compliance, and shortening the duration of weaning in patients less than 30 days of age.

Fluid Therapy. Fluid therapy is aimed at maintaining adequate hydration and urination. Diuretics such as furosemide are often needed in addition to fluid restriction to reduce pulmonary edema and help in maintaining fluid balance. Patients receiving diuretic therapy may rapidly lose excess water in the body. In these instances, lung compliance may quickly improve, subjecting these patients to possible pneumothoraces if pressures and rates are not weaned. Close observation of urine output, breath sounds, and chest excursion will help the practitioner identify an improvement in compliance. Patients receiving long-term diuretics must have calcium and phosphorus levels maintained to avoid the weakening of bones.

Right Heart Failure. Symptomatic right-sided heart failure may be treated with digoxin in addition to diuretics. The effect of closure of the PDA, either chemically or surgically, on the development of BPD is not known, but it may reduce the degree of severity. Digoxin may be used to improve the effects of right-sided heart failure in the BPD patient. A patient with BPD must have frequent blood work, which depletes the blood volume to various degrees. In such instances, blood transfusions are given as needed to maintain a hematocrit above 40%.[7]

Nutrition. BPD patients must have adequate nutrition to meet increased metabolic needs. The patient with BPD may require 120 to 150 cal/kg/day to achieve growth and meet the needs of lung tissue repair.

Patients with inadequate nutrition may suffer a delay in the growth and development of new alveoli. Additionally, they may be very difficult to wean from the ventilator and are more prone to infection.[17]

Two precautions must be observed when administering a high number of calories to BPD patients. First, oxygen consumption increases in newborns as their caloric intake increases. The BPD patient has a limited ability to oxygenate and therefore may become more hypoxic as more oxygen is used to metabolize the added calories. Second, the metabolism of glucose results in increased CO_2 production. The BPD patient may be unable to remove the excess CO_2, resulting in hypercapnia and a worsening acidosis.

Vitamin E Administration. A deficiency of vitamin E has been shown to increase the incidence of oxygen toxicity. Additionally, the administration of vitamin E decreases lung injury caused by the administration of oxygen. Subsequent tests is BPD patients did not demonstrate conclusive evidence that vitamin E reduced the incidence of BPD.[1]

Future Outlook. Because of the relative newness of mechanical ventilation for neonates and subsequent BPD, few studies are available to examine the long-term effects of BPD in later life. Some have suggested that there is an increased risk of developing asthma and even chronic obstructive lung disease (COPD) later in life. These suggestions, however, have not been scientifically analyzed and documented. Early reports that BPD patients suffer from poor growth throughout childhood have recently been downplayed.[19]

PULMONARY DYSMATURITY (WILSON-MIKITY SYNDROME)

Wilson-Mikity syndrome is a disease of functional and structural pulmonary changes seen in premature neonates with no apparent underlying lung disease.

Pathophysiology. The underlying pathophysiology of Wilson-Mikity syndrome is unknown. The only common finding is prematurity, with a majority of afflicted neonates weighing less than 1500 g at birth.[1] One etiologic theory is that lung immaturity leads to emphysematous changes in the lungs. There may also be an association between maternal bleeding and asphyxia and the development of the syndrome.

The radiographic picture of the lungs is very similar to stage III and IV BPD, with the exception that the neonate with Wilson-Mikity has not been ventilated. Lung biopsies done on patients early in the course of the disease show little if any structural change in the pulmonary tissue. Later biopsies show immaturity of the alveolar septa, causing overexpansion and atelectasis of the lungs.[1]

Clinical Signs. The initial symptoms usually appear near the end of the first week or later and are usually mild. Early symptoms include hyperpnea, transient cyanosis, and retractions.

Arterial PO_2 begins failing, with a progressive hypercarbia and respiratory acidosis. The symptoms gradually worsen over the following 2 to 6 weeks, leading to the acute phase of the disease. The acute phase may last from days to weeks and presents as severe respiratory distress, poor feeding, and vomiting.

Two thirds of infants survive this acute phase and begin a gradual recovery with clearing of the disease by age 2.

Treatment. Treatment of Wilson-Mikity syndrome is supportive. The patient is mechanically ventilated to treat apnea and progressive hypercarbia. Oxygen is given to treat hypoxemia. Once ventilated, the disease becomes impossible to differentiate from BPD and is therefore treated as BPD would be treated.

RETINOPATHY OF PREMATURITY (ROP)

History. Retinopathy of prematurity, also called retrolental fibroplasia (RLF), was initially described by Terry in 1942.[20] The term literally means the formation of a scar behind the lens, which is the culmination of the disease. The term retinopathy of prematurity (ROP) was introduced by Heath in 1951.[21]

ROP is a more descriptive term of the actual events that the neonate passes through, leading to scar formation. The term ROP has now been expanded to include all stages of the disease, so that the term RLF is no longer used.

Following an epidemic of ROP that occurred in the 1940s and 1950s, a reduction in the use of supplemental oxygen led to a decline in the incidence of the disease. The reduction in oxygen use, however, led to an increase in mortality and cerebral palsy.[1]

More recent studies have identified a definite link between the development of ROP and oxygen use, but have also identified various other factors that contribute to its development. These include retinovascular immaturity, and circulatory and respiratory instability.[22]

ROP occurs in 25 to 35% of preemies up to 35 weeks, gestation, with 5 to 10% having stage 3 or more and 3 to 5% resulting in blindness.[22] Another study showed an ROP incidence of 26.5%, with 40% of those resulting in blindness or severely impaired vision.[23] In a study performed in 10 schools for the blind, 17.6% of all children with severe visual loss were found to have a history of ROP.[24] In recent years, while survival of the extremely low birth weight patient has increased, the rate of ROP has not been shown to increase proportionally.[25]

Physiology of the Developing Eye. An understanding of retinal development is basic to the understanding of ROP. The capillaries of the retina begin branching out at 16 weeks. Capillaries begin from the optic nerve and grow toward the *ora serrata*, the retina's anterior end. The capillaries do not completely reach the entire ora serrata until 40 weeks. As the capillary network expands, arteries and veins form in its path. The capillaries of a premature neonate have not had time to reach the ora serrata. Depending on several factors, the network can either develop normally or cease to grow and cause ROP.[26]

Pathophysiology of ROP. In the presence of high PaO_2, the retinal vessels constrict. If not relieved, the constriction leads to a necrosis of the vessels, called *vaso-obliteration*. In an attempt to reestablish a blood supply to the retina, those vessels that have not necrosed begin to proliferate. The proliferation may extend into the liquid portion of the eye, the vitreous, where the vessels hemorrhage, depicted in Figure 10–2. The result is the formation of a scar behind the retina with later traction, detachment, and blindness. It is important to note that at any time the process may stop, with no further damage occurring.

Although oxygen has long been implicated in the development of ROP, many downplay its role.[27,28] Studies of several risk factors led Lucey and Dangman to identify several factors that may contribute to the development of ROP.[29] Those factors include immaturity, hyperoxia, hypoxia, blood transfusions, intraventricular hemorrhage, apnea, infection, hypercarbia, PDA, prostaglandin synthetase inhibitors, vitamin E deficiency, lactic acidosis, prenatal complications, and genetic factors. Bright lighting in the nursery may also contribute to the development of ROP.[26] Additional factors related to the occurrence of ROP are early intubation, hypotension, and necrotizing enterocolitis.[23] A study by Wright and Wright showed that birth weight and duration of supplemental oxygen were significant predictors of stage 2 or higher ROP.[30] These data show the multifactorial processes involved in the development of ROP and help to illustrate why its development is difficult to prevent.

Diagnosis. ROP is classified into five stages, listed in Table 10–2. ROP is diagnosed by ophthalmologic examination of the internal eye anatomy. Capillary damage occurs in one of three zones shown in Figure 10–3. The extent of the disease is described by using the hours of a clock superimposed over the three zones. The disease is described by the stage number and the clock hours it is located in, for example, 3 clock hours of stage 2 ROP in zone 3. It appears that the most unfavorable outcomes are associated with injury involving zone 1 at a stage 3 or better.[31]

ROP appears between 35 and 45 weeks' gestational age and may progress from stage 1 to stage 5 in the next several weeks.

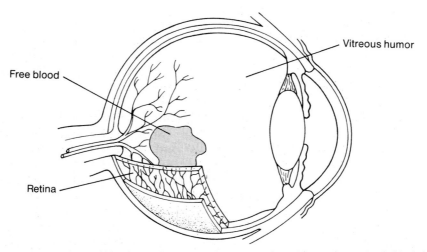

Figure 10–2 *Hemorrhage of blood into the vitreous humor resulting in scar formation behind the retina.*

TABLE 10–2 Stages of Retinopathy of Prematurity

Stage Number	Classification
1	A thin white demarcation line is seen separating the avascular retina anteriorly from the vascularized retina posteriorly.
2	A ridge is now formed and rises up from the plane of the retina. New vessels may be seen posterior to the ridge.
3	In this stage, there is a proliferation of extraretinal fibrovascular tissue. It is often seen posterior to the ridge or connected to the posterior aspect of the ridge.
4	In stage 4, there is a subtotal detachment of the retina.
5	Continued traction and buildup of fluids; the retina becomes completely detached.

Treatment and Prevention. The knowledge that vitamin E is a natural antioxidant led researchers to experiment with its use to prevent ROP. Studies concluded, however, that administration of vitamin E does not decrease the incidence or development of ROP.

The traditional treatment for stage 3 ROP is cryotherapy. *Cryotherapy* is performed by introducing a probe that has been cooled to –20°C with nitrous oxide behind the eye and freezing the avascular portion of the retina, preventing further abnormal vessel proliferation. Complications include retinal scarring, cell destruction, and possible retinal detachment.[32] Cryotherapy has also been linked to visual field changes later in life.[33]

Laser therapy is now being used as an alternative to cryotherapy. Either argon or diode lasers are used to photocoagulate the avascular portion of the retina. It is less invasive and

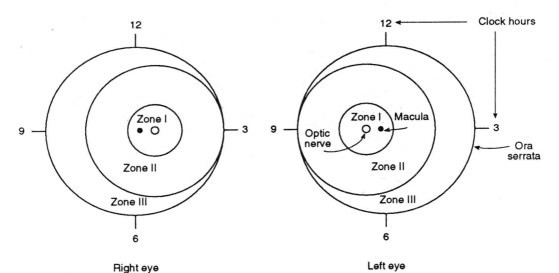

Figure 10–3 *The three zones of the internal eye.*

less traumatic to the eye than cryotherapy. Complications include scarring, choroidal hemorrhage and, rarely, pain.[32]

Surgical interventions, such as vitrectomy and lensectomy are also being investigated as possible treatments for severe ROP. There is some evidence that in stage 5 ROP, vitrectomized eyes function better than nonvitrectomized eyes.[34]

Until more is known about the development of ROP, prevention is based on cautious use of oxygen delivery to the patient. TCMs, pulse oximeters, and blood gases are all used to maintain levels of oxygen between hypoxia and toxicity.

INTRACRANIAL/INTRAVENTRICULAR HEMORRHAGE (ICH/IVH)

Bleeding in the cranium is a major source of morbidity in the premature population. It can occur in any one of several areas. Subdural or subarachnoid bleeds occur secondary to trauma or asphyxia, within the respective spaces of the cranial bone, shown in Figure 10–4. These bleeds are most commonly found in terms neonates following birth trauma.

Bleeding can also occur within the cerebellar tissue itself. This type of bleed is usually found in preterm neonates and is associated with the periventricular-intraventricular hemorrhages. The majority of cranial hemorrhages in neonates are the periventricular-intraventricular hemorrhages, or IVH. These bleeds occur in preterm neonates of between

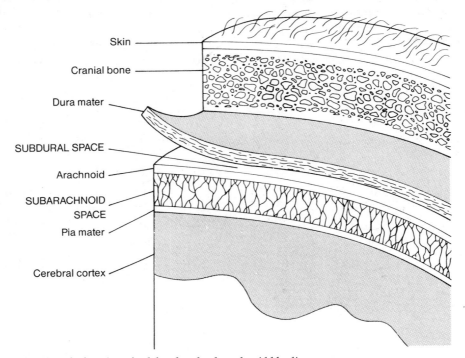

Figure 10–4 *The location of subdural and subarachnoid bleeding.*

24 and 32 weeks' gestation. Neonates with birth weights of less than 1500 g are also at a high risk.

Pathophysiology. In the developing fetus, the brain is perfused by highly vascular, extremely fragile areas. In the term neonate, the area of most frequent bleeding is called the *choroid plexus* of the lateral ventricles, shown in Figure 10–5. In the premature neonate, the *germinal matrix*, located in the subependymal region (Figure 10–6), is the most common source of bleeding.

The inability of the cerebral vascular system to regulate blood flow, probably due to immaturity, is the underlying cause of hemorrhage at these areas. Small bleeds may be confined to the immediate area, with no residual effect. With severe hemorrhages, the blood enters the ventricles, enlarging their size and compressing the parenchyma of the brain. Hemorrhaging may also extend into the brain tissue, resulting in further damage to the patient.

The triggering factors that lead to a fluctuation in blood flow include shock, acidosis, hypernatremia, transfusion of blood, seizures, and rapid expansion of blood volume.[11] Increasing intracranial pressure by placing the neonate in the Trendelenburg position or mechanical ventilation may also lead to IVH. It has also been reported that the premature infants of mothers who consume alcohol during pregnancy have a substantially increased

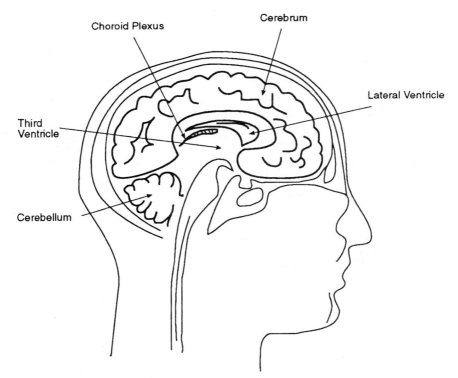

Figure 10–5 *The choroid plexus, common site of bleeding in term neonates.*

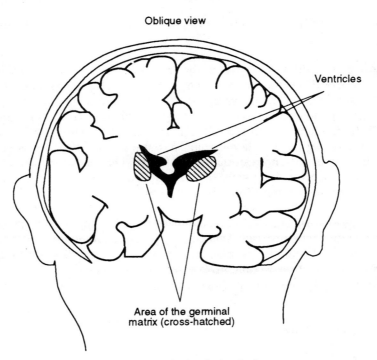

Oblique view

Ventricles

Area of the germinal
matrix (cross-hatched)

Figure 10–6 *The area of the germinal matrix in the developing brain.*

risk of developing IVH.[35] Table 10–3 lists a few specific factors that may lead to IVH. It lists some additional patient historical factors often seen with IVH.

While most IVHs occur one to several days postdelivery, it is possible that up to one third are congenital or are of immediate postnatal onset.[36]

The signs of the patient demonstrates depend on the severity of the bleeding. They range from severe, rapid deterioration in patient condition to having no apparent side effects. Some common signs of bleeding in the germinal matrix include apnea, hypotension, a drop in the hematocrit, flaccidity, bulging fontanelles, and *tonic posturing*.[11]

TABLE 10–3   Etiology and History of Intraventricular Hemorrhage

Etiologic Factors	*Historical Factors*
Hypernatremia	Less than 1500 g birth weight
Shock	Less than 34 weeks' gestation
Acidosis	Hyaline membrane disease
Blood transfusions	Coagulopathy
Seizures	Hyperviscocity
Rapid volume expansion	Hypoxia
Fluctuation in cerebral blood flow	Birth Asphyxia

IVH is classified into four grades diagnosed by CT scan or ultrasound. If no bleeding is present, it is categorized as grade 0. Hemorrhage that is limited to the germinal matrix is grade I. A grade II hemorrhage involves the germinal matrix with blood extending into the ventricles. With this degree of bleeding, there is no ventricular dilation. Grade III IVHs are comparable to grade II, with the exception that the ventricles are dilated. The most severe hemorrhages are grade IV. Grade IV hemorrhages dilate the ventricles and extend into the brain parenchyma. Grades I through IV are depicted in Figure 10–7.

Complications. Implications of IVH are related to the severity of the bleeding and the underlying causes. In general, the more severe the bleeding, the more severe the complications and sequelae.

The most serious complication of IVH is *posthemorrhagic hydrocephalus* (PHH). PHH is caused by the obstruction of cerebrospinal fluid (CSF) outflow and impairment of CSF resorption in the brain. Treatment of PHH is started to maintain a normal cerebral perfusion pressure at intracranial pressure rises. This is initially done by removing CSF by lumbar puncture. If PHH persists with the use of lumbar punctures, surgical placement of a *ventricular-peritoneal shunt* or a *ventriculostomy* with an external drainage is indicated.

Complications seen as the child grows include cerebral palsy, vision loss, hearing loss, epilepsy, and mental retardation.[37]

Treatment. The best treatment of IVH is to avoid those factors that lead to its occurrence. Careful avoidance of those factors that cause fluctuations in cerebral blood flow will help

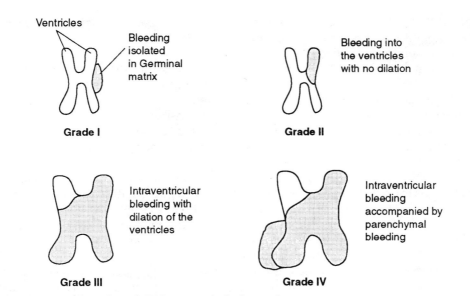

Figure 10–7 *Grades I through IV intraventricular hemorrhages.*

in preventing IVH. Caregivers must avoid wide fluctuations in blood pressure, oxygenation, and pH. Low-dose indomethacin, given prophylactically, has been shown to significantly lower the incidence and severity of IVH.

Treatment following an IVH is mainly supportive. Very little can be done to treat the IVH once it has occurred. Every precaution must be taken to prevent further hemorrhage and damage once a bleed has occurred.

Osmotic agents such as blood and plasma should be carefully and slowly administered. Caregivers should carefully monitor and treat the patient for hyperbilirubinemia, which is a common occurrence. Hypotension must be avoided in the presence of an elevated intracranial pressure to avoid a reduction in cerebral blood perfusion.

PROCESSES OF INTRAUTERINE ORIGIN

ASPHYXIA

Definition and Incidence. Asphyxia is a combination of hypoxia, hypercarbia, and acidosis in the fetus or neonate. It begins as either a lack of oxygen or a lack of perfusion to various tissues.

In utero, the placenta is the organ of respiration where the initial insult occurs, and in the neonate, it is the lung. Asphyxia is present in 1 to 1.5% of all births, increasing to 9% in neonates of less than 36 weeks' gestation.[7] Intrauterine growth retardation, breech delivery, and postmaturity also increase the risk of asphyxia.

Pathophysiology. Asphyxia in utero is a result of placental insufficiency with an inability to exchange oxygen and remove carbon dioxide from the fetus. Asphyxia after delivery is caused by pulmonary or cardiac problems.

During normal labor, the blood flow to the placenta is diminished during contractions with resultant diminished gas exchange. Compression of the umbilical cord may further interrupt blood flow, with resulting hypoxia to the fetus.

Both the mother and fetus have increased oxygen consumption secondary to the stress of the labor. Maternal hyperventilation may even further reduce placental blood flow. The net result of all these factors is reduced oxygen delivery to the fetus and ensuing decrease of oxygen reserve, even in the normal neonate.

Any maternal, placental, or cord problem that interferes with the exchange of gas in the placenta or fetus leads to asphyxia. These factors are listed in Table 10–4. In addition, impairment of maternal oxygenation will impair blood flow to the placenta and cause less oxygen to be available for the fetus, resulting in asphyxia. In the presence of asphyxia, blood is shunted away from the lungs, skeletal muscle, liver, kidneys, and gut. The blood flow is directed to the brain, heart, and adrenal glands.

Patient symptoms begin with a decreased heart rate and blood pressure. The fetus attempts to correct the asphyxia by starting a gasping reflex. If the asphyxia remains uncorrected, the fetus enters a period of apnea, known as primary apnea. With continuation of

---

TABLE 10–4 Factors leading to Fetal Asphyxia

---

1. Maternal hypoxia
   a. Maternal shock
   b. Acute asthma attack
   c. Carbon monoxide poisoning
   d. Anemia
   e. Oversedation
   f. Apnea from any cause
   g. Congestive heart failure
   h. Low ambient FiO_2
   i. Severe pneumonia
2. Disruption of uteroplacental blood flow
   a. Maternal shock
   b. Maternal vasoconstrictive states
   c. Inferior vena cava syndrome
3. Dysfunction of the placenta
   a. Placenta previa
   b. Abruptio placentae
4. Impairment of blood flow through the umbilical cord
   a. Compression of the cord
5. Intrinsic fetal disorder
   a. Fetal cardiac failure (hydrops fetalis)
   b. Fetal hypotension secondary to hemorrhage or drugs

---

the asphyxia, the heart rate and blood pressure continue to drop during primary apnea. The fetus then commences a series of deep, ineffective gasps, which gradually slow and, finally, cease. The fetus then enters a period of secondary apnea. If the asphyxia is untreated, the heart rate and blood pressure continue to fall, resulting in permanent damage or death.

Asphyxia in utero is detected by the fetal heart monitor and the presence of meconium in the amniotic fluid. The fetal heart monitor will show a loss of baseline variability, late decelerations, and prolonged periods of bradycardia.

Consequences and Treatment. The major complication of prolonged asphyxia is hypoxic-ischemic brain injury. In the term neonate, the resultant brain injury is called *hypoxic-ischemic encephalopathy*. It is the result of necrosis to the neurons of the cerebral cortex and basal ganglia. The injury in the preterm neonate is most often associated with hemorrhage into the ventricles of the brain. This entity is termed periventricular-intraventricular hemorrhage.

Another lesion that affects both term and preterm neonates is called *periventricular leukomalacia,* which is an area of infarct in the periventricular region. Victims of asphyxia may also suffer cardiac ischemia as a result of the insult. This is usually transient in nature with normal ECGs returning within 3 months.

The asphyxiated patient is also at risk of developing tubular necrosis of the kidneys and gastrointestinal effects such as bowel ischemia and necrotizing enterocolitis. Disseminated intravascular coagulation (DIC) may be present due to blood vessel damage. Severe asphyxia may also lead to liver damage, to the point that the liver may not provide its basic functions.

Asphyxic damage to the lung is manifest by increased pulmonary vascular resistance, hemorrhage, and possible damage to the production of surfactant with resultant RDS.

The treatment of asphyxia requires the immediate reversal of hypoxemia and acidosis. Asphyxia that occurs in utero requires the rapid delivery of the fetus, possibly by cesarean delivery if normal labor is not rapidly progressing. Once delivered, the neonate is dried, warmed, and stimulated. The airway is then opened and maintained while breathing is assisted using 1.0 FiO_2 and positive pressure. Circulation is assisted as needed with drugs and external massage. The neonate is then closely monitored and treated as needed for continuing hypoxia and hypercarbia. Prevention of asphyxia will prevent the need for treatment in the postdelivery patient. Clinical observation along with laboratory analysis of blood gases will help in avoiding asphyxia.

MECONIUM ASPIRATION SYNDROME (MAS)

Meconium aspiration syndrome is predominantly a disease of the term or postterm neonate who has experienced some degree of asphyxia either before or after the onset of labor. Meconium passage into the amniotic fluid occurs in 9 to 20% of all births.[38] Actual aspiration of meconium into the trachea occurs in about half of the neonates born with meconium staining the amniotic fluid and can occur before or during delivery, or with the first breath. Postterm patients are at a high risk, possibly due to diminished amniotic fluid levels, which dilute the meconium; and diminishing placental function, leading to increased asphyxia.

Meconium is the name given to the contents of the fetal bowel. It is a thick, tar-like dark green material that consists of swallowed amniotic fluid, bile salts and acids, squamous cells, *vernix*, and intestinal enzymes.

Pathophysiology. The sequence of events that results in the aspiration of meconium into the trachea involves a complex series of asphyxia-induced occurrences. During an asphyxial episode in utero, there is an apparent shift in blood distribution to the vital organs. The response to the fetal bowel is increased peristalsis and relaxation of the anal sphincter, resulting in the passage of meconium into the amniotic fluid.

In response to the asphyxia, the fetus begins gasping, attempting to relieve the asphyxia. With severe asphyxia, deep gasping movements may allow the passage of meconium into the oropharynx and tracheal tree.

Meconium that is aspirated into the tracheobronchial tree has two potentially devastating effects on the neonate. The physical presence of the meconium in the airways can lead to blockage of the airway and air trapping. This obstruction is enhanced by the ball-valve effect, illustrated in Figure 10–8, in which the airway dilates during inspiration owing to the negative pressures generated in the thorax. With the airway dilated, the meconium advances further into the airway. Upon exhalation, the airway constricts and traps the meconium in the lumen, trapping the gas behind the obstruction.

This leads to disruption of V/Q ratios and ensuing hypoxia and hypercarbia. Increasing obstruction leads to widespread atelectasis, which further impairs gas exchange, wors-

Inspiration

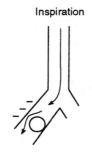

On inspiration, negative pressure external to the airway dilates the airway allowing gas to pass the obstruction.

Expiration

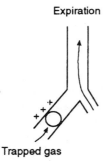

On expiration, positive pressure external to the airway closes the airway around the obstruction, trapping gas distal to the obstruction.

Trapped gas

Figure 10–8 *The ball-valve effect: inspiration dilates the airway, allowing gas to pass the obstruction; on exhalation, the airway collapses, trapping air distal to the obstruction.*

ening the hypoxia, and hypercarbia. Air leaks, such as pneumothoraces, occur as the trapped gas increases in volume and eventually ruptures the lung.

Another effect of meconium aspiration is an inflammatory response of the tracheobronchial epithelium to the presence of meconium. This is called a chemical pneumonitis and results from the irritating effect of the acidic meconium on the epithelium. The inflammation results in mucosal edema, decreasing lung compliance, and further impairment of gas exchange.

Vasospasm of the pulmonary vasculature occurs in many MAS patients in response to the effects of intrauterine asphyxia leading to persistent pulmonary hypertension (PPH). In these patients, blood flow follows fetal routes, bypassing the lungs and leading to an increased shunt and worsening arterial blood gases. It is important for the practitioner to ascertain the degree of PPH in these patients.

Persistent fetal circulation (PFC) in these patients is detected by several factors. Worsening cyanosis that does not respond to increased FiO_2 is a common sign. The patient may become tachypneic and develop retractions. Auscultation often reveals pulmonic *systolic ejection clicks* and a loud second heart sound. The chest x-ray (CXR) shows diffuse patchy infiltrates, which can be focal, general, symmetric, or asymmetric, hyperinflation, pleural effusions, and cardiomegaly.

A comparison of preductal and postductal PaO_2 shows the presence or absence of ductal shunting. One definitive test for the presence of pulmonary hypertension in the neonate is the hyperoxia-hyperventilation test. A positive test is when the patient has a PaO_2 of less than 50 mm Hg, which rises to above 100 mm Hg when the patient is hyperventilated to a $PaCO_2$ of 20 to 25 mm Hg.

Patients who have a severe hypoxemia despite being hyperventilated, as mentioned, are candidates for the powerful vasodilating drug tolazoline.

An additional problem is the potential for pulmonary infection that may occur following meconium aspirations. Broad-spectrum antibiotics started shortly after delivery may help prevent this occurrence.

Diagnosis and Treatment. The diagnosis of MAS is only made when meconium is aspirated from the trachea. It is suspected when the amniotic fluid is stained with the green meconium. The neonate is called meconium stained until meconium aspiration into the trachea is verified. It is possible that the aspirated meconium has advanced to the point where it cannot be suctioned out of the trachea. These patients may show classic signs of respiratory distress such as tachypnea and hypoxemia.

As the disease progresses, the severity of symptoms increases with ensuing hypercarbia and acidosis. The chest x-ray shows irregular densities throughout both lungs, similar in appearance to pneumonia. Hyperinflation may be present as the disease advances.

Treatment must begin with the obstetrician. If the amniotic fluid is merely stained and no particles of meconium are visible, it is classified as thin and watery and, as such, no special treatment is needed. In the presence of thick, particulate-laden amniotic fluid, the patient must be treated as though aspiration of meconium has occurred. This fluid often has the look of thick "pea soup."

Upon delivery of the head, before the delivery of the thorax, the obstetrician must thoroughly suction out the mouth and oropharynx and clear any meconium that is present using at least a 10 Fr. catheter. As soon as the fetus is delivered, the trachea must be intubated by a qualified practitioner. The largest endotracheal tube possible is used to aspirate the meconium. Upon completion of the intubation, suction is applied to the end of the endotracheal tube, either by mouth or by suction tubing attached to wall suction, as illustrated in Figure 10–9. The ET tube is withdrawn and examined for the presence of meconium. Attempts to suction meconium from the trachea by passing a suction catheter through the endotracheal tube should not be made. The small size of the catheter makes it ineffective to remove meconium.

If meconium is aspirated, the procedure must be repeated, using a new endotracheal tube, until no meconium is aspirated from the trachea. The general condition of the neonate must be taken into account while performing the intubations. The repeated intubation and suctioning of the patient must be performed rapidly, to reduce the effects of possible bradycardia and hypoxia. Exhaustive attempts to remove meconium that is beyond the carina are inadvisable.

Throughout the procedure, 100% oxygen should be blown by the patient's face, but under no circumstances should positive pressure be applied to the airways, until all meconium possible is removed. The instillation of sterile saline into the ET tube may dilute the meconium and cause it to enter further into the tracheobronchial tree.

Once the meconium has been removed from the trachea, as evidenced by a clear ET tube following intubation and suctioning, the neonate may be resuscitated using positive-

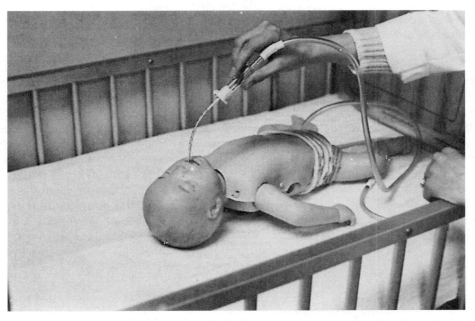

Figure 10–9 *Applying suction to the endotracheal adapter to remove meconium from the trachea.*

pressure ventilation to relieve any hypoxia and bradycardia. The patient is then treated according to the severity of symptoms.

Warmed, humidified oxygen is used to treat persistent hypoxia. Chest physiotherapy may be useful in removing remaining meconium. In patients with severe symptoms of hypoxia, hypercarbia, and acidosis, mechanical ventilation is indicated. In these cases, the presence of air trapping requires that longer expiratory times be utilized to allow adequate expiration of the gas. Utilization of PEEP may also aid in the exhalation of trapped gases. The presence of PEEP in the airways mechanically holds the airway lumen open and does not allow it to collapse. This may reduce the ball-valve effects to some degree and allow trapped gases distal to the plug to escape.

Low peak inspiratory pressures are desirable to prevent air leaks; however, the practitioner must use whatever pressure is needed to ventilate the patient. Treatment of the pulmonary vasoconstriction is often accomplished with tolazoline, a powerful vasodilator. Tolazoline must be used with extreme caution and only on selected patients. Because it dilates blood vessels throughout the body, a fall in blood pressure follows its administration.

Because meconium promotes the growth of bacteria, broad-spectrum antibiotics should be administered to those patients who present with infiltrates on CXR. Tracheal cultures should then be obtained to identify specific pathogens.

A relatively new procedure, amnioinfusion, involves the infusion of an artificial amniotic fluid into the uterus. Initially used to relieve variable fetal heart decelerations, it is now being proposed as an acceptable prophylactic treatment for meconium aspiration.[39,40] The theory is that the infusion of additional fluid dilutes the meconium and makes it less likely to block the airways if aspirated. Spong and associates feel that the benefit is a result of alleviating variable heart tones and not one of dilution of the amniotic fluid.[41]

BAROTRAUMATIC DISEASES: AIR LEAK SYNDROMES

Air leak syndromes appear with increased frequency in the newborn infant. The incidence is higher in patients with RDS, meconium aspiration, and transient tachypnea of the newborn. Most air leaks are caused by mechanical ventilation; however, some may occur spontaneously. Pulmonary air leak and its sequelae include pneumothorax, pneumomediastinum, pneumopericardium, pulmonary interstitial emphysema (PIE), subcutaneous emphysema, and air embolism.

All air leaks develop from a common event. The initial event is a rupture of the alveoli, usually secondary to uneven ventilation in the alveoli. Where the air goes after it leaks from the alveoli determines what kind of air leak will develop.

PNEUMOTHORAX

Pneumothorax is the most common of the air leaks, occurring in 1 to 2% of all newborns. A pneumothorax develops when the extraalveolar air ruptures to the external surface of the lung and into the pleural space.

Pneumothoraces are divided into two categories: spontaneous and tension. A spontaneous pneumothorax is an isolated pocket of free air in the pleural space that is not fed by a continuous inflow of gas from the point of the leak. Spontaneous pneumothoraces are the result of the rupture of a weak alveolar area and are often asymptomatic. It may resolve without complication and is frequently not detected.

A tension pneumothorax is so named because of the addition of new air through the rupture with each breath, creating a larger and larger air pocket that is under pressure. As the air accumulates in the pleural space, the lung collapses under the pressure. Additionally, the accumulated air causes the great vessels to shift toward the unaffected side and cardiac function becomes compromised.

Diagnosis. Physical symptoms are usually the first signs of a pneumothorax. The onset may be gradual or very rapid, depending on the severity of the air leak. Physical signs begin with an increase in respiratory distress, with retractions and tachypnea. The patient then becomes bradycardic, cyanotic, and may have periods of apnea and hypotension. Examination of the chest reveals asymmetry in chest excursion, a movement of the maximal impulse point of the heart, and a change in breath sounds.

Any patient showing a sudden demise in status should be transilluminated with a fiberoptic light source. *Transillumination* involves the placement of a high-intensity light source, usually fiber optic, on the thoracic surface. When the light is placed against the thorax of a neonate with normal lungs, the light is reflected to the surface of the thorax by the lung tissue, forming a uniform circle around the light. In the presence of free air in the thorax, the light is reflected at odd angles due to the collapse of the lung. The result is an irregular-shaped reflection on the chest wall, with fingers of light possibly appearing away from the light source, as seen in Figure 10–10.

Transillumination is a quick method of diagnosing a pneumothorax. However, a negative transillumination does not rule out a pneumothorax. Chest x-rays taken during expiration will show severe pneumothoraces. Taken in both AP and lateral views, the pneumothorax appears as a dark bleb with no lung markings present. The lung is often seen collapsed and unaerated. The mediastinum may be shifted away from the air pocket.

Treatment. Treatment of pneumothoraces depends on the severity of symptoms. Patients who are not on a ventilator and are in no respiratory distress can usually be managed by close observation. The patient in severe distress should have the trapped air removed through needle aspiration. Needle aspiration is an emergency procedure to be used only in a life-threatening situation until a chest tube can be inserted.

The patient with a continuous air leak who is receiving continuous positive pressure ventilation should have a chest tube placed as quickly as possible. This is only to be done by experienced nursery personnel trained under the direction of a physician. The chest tube is then attached to a one-way valve, water seal, or suction. The level of suction should range from –15 cm H_2O for small leaks to –25 cm H_2O for large air leaks.[7]

The chest tube is removed when the patient's respiratory disease is resolved, there has been no leakage from the tube for 24 to 48 hours, and the extrapulmonary air has been resolved for 24 to 48 hours. Often, the tube is clamped for 24 hours before removal to ensure complete resolution of the air leak.

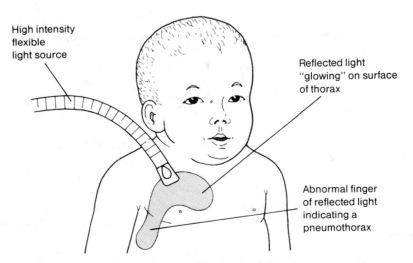

High intensity
flexible
light source

Reflected light
"glowing" on surface
of thorax

Abnormal finger
of reflected light
indicating a
pneumothorax

Figure 10–10 *The appearance of a positive transillumination indicating a pneumothorax.*

PNEUMOMEDIASTINUM

A pneumomediastinum occurs when extra-alveolar air dissects through the lung interstitium and ruptures into the mediastinum. Although rarely severe, it may compromise venous return and cause a tamponade on the heart in severe cases.

The symptoms depend on severity, with the most common sign being distant, crackly heart sounds. Diagnosis is made by chest x-ray, which shows free air in the mediastinal space. The air highlights the border of the heart, but does not surround the heart. Treatment involves close observation for other air leaks and, if possible, lower ventilatory pressures.

PNEUMOPERICARDIUM

Air that dissects through the perivascular sheaths to the great vessels may rupture into the pericardial sac, causing a pneumopericardium. Air may also rupture through mediastinal connective tissue, near the pleural-pericardial connection. As the air builds up in the pericardial sac, it compresses and tamponades the heart, impeding cardiac output and causing a severe, rapid demise in patient status. These patients may have severe bradycardia, with muffled or distant heart sounds. A chest x-ray shows the presence of air completely around the heart.

Treatment of symptomatic patients is by needle aspiration of the air in the pericardial sac. Because this is a dangerous procedure, it should only be performed by trained personnel.

PULMONARY INTERSTITIAL EMPHYSEMA (PIE)

PIE occurs when air dissects throughout the interstitial tissue of the lungs. It results from the chronic use of high PEEP, peak inspiratory pressures, and prolonged inspiratory times.

PIE develops into one of two classifications. If the air remains in the lung tissue, it is called intrapulmonary interstitial pneumatosis. Intrapleural pneumatosis is the name given when the extra-alveolar air is confined by the visceral pleura, forming blebs. Either or both forms may be present in the affected lung. PIE can lead to a pneumothorax, pneumomediastinum, and possibly pneumopericardium if the free air follows those routes.

Pathophysiology. As the air dissects and collects in the interstitium, the small airways and vessels are compressed. Widespread ventillation to perfusion mismatches follow and lead to a deterioration of blood gases. A vicious circle begins as higher ventilator pressures are required to correct the worsening blood gases. Higher pressures cause more air to leak into the interstitium and the mismatch of ventilation to perfusion worsens.

The chest x-ray of PIE resembles bubbly, cystic areas throughout the lung parenchyma. *(C XR)*

Treatment. PIE is best treated by prevention. Close attention to low ventilator pressures, while maintaining ventilation and oxygenation, may help avoid the onset of PIE. Mild cases may clear spontaneously with reabsorption beginning in 5 to 7 days.

The treatment of moderate and severe cases begins by lowering ventilator pressures while maintaining oxygenation and ventilation. Selective intubation of the unaffected or less affected lung may allow the injured lung time to heal. Several published studies report that high-frequency ventilation is successful in treating patients with pulmonary air leaks, including PIE.[42]

Survivors of PIE have a high incidence of BPD due to the necessity for vigorous mechanical ventilation.

PULMONARY AIR EMBOLISM

Air embolism is extremely rare but may occur when high pressures are being used to ventilate stiff lungs. It is thought that air enters the pulmonary vasculature through lacerations in the parenchyma. Infants suffering from air embolism have an extremely rapid deterioration of condition with eventual circulatory collapse. There is no effective treatment for air embolism.

SUBCUTANEOUS EMPHYSEMA

Subcutaneous air is usually secondary to other air leaks, with the air dissecting into the subcutaneous spaces. Clinically, it has little importance other than that it indicates the presence of a pulmonary air leak. Subcutaneous emphysema resolves when the causative air leak is treated.

OTHER RESPIRATORY DISEASES OF THE NEONATE

PERSISTENT PULMONARY HYPERTENSION OF THE NEONATE (PPHN)

PPHN is also known as *Aka* persistent fetal circulation (PFC) for reasons that will become apparent. PPHN is most frequently seen in term or postterm infants and often in patients suffering from asphyxia, meconium aspiration, sepsis, congenital diaphragmatic hernia, pulmonary hypoplasia, congenital heart disease, and premature closure of the ductus arteriosus.[43] Additional clinical disorders associated with PPHN include HMD, bacterial pneumonia, myocardial dysfunction, and pulmonary hypoplasia.[7]

Affected infants have severe, persistent pulmonary vasoconstriction, which causes increased pressures and decreased pulmonary blood flow. Right-sided heart pressures rise higher than arterial pressures. The result is a continuation of the factors that allow fetal circulation to occur, with blood shunting through the foramen ovale and ductus arteriosus and away from the lungs. This shunting is illustrated in Figure 10–11.

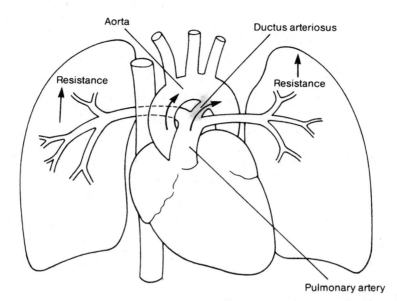

Figure 10–11 *Right-to-left shunting through the ductus arteriosus resulting from an increase in pulmonary vascular resistance.*

The profound mismatch in ventilation and perfusion that follows leads to metabolic and respiratory acidosis and hypoxia, which further worsen the pulmonary vasoconstriction.

Etiology. The underlying cause of the persistent vasoconstriction is unknown, but numerous factors that cause the initial constriction are involved to some degree. PPHN is primarily a disease of the term and postterm neonate. This is because the pulmonary arterial musculature does not develop until late gestation. The manifestations of PPHN suggest a dysfunction of pulmonary vasoregulation resulting in abnormally high pulmonary vascular resistance.[44] PPHN is also associated with chronic intrauterine events.[45]

Current theories surrounding the etiology of PPHN include chronic intrauterine hypoxemia, increased development of vascular smooth muscle, and perinatal factors that contribute to vasospasm.

Diagnosis and Treatment. In the presence of severe or worsening hypoxemia in a full-term neonate, one of three possible diagnoses should be considered: parenchymal lung disease, cyanotic congenital heart lesion, and PPHN. To help differentiate among the three disorders, a series of tests have been developed that can be done noninvasively at the patient's bedside.

The simplest test is the hyperoxia test. It is performed by administering an FiO_2 of 1.0 to the patient for 5 to 10 minutes. An arterial sample is then obtained and the PaO_2 is measured. In the PaO_2 is below 100 mm Hg, the diagnosis is a right-to-left shunt, found in both PPHN and cyanotic heart lesions. Because of the association between high PaO_2 and the development of ROP, the use of this test on premature neonates is questionable.

Right-to-left shunting is also detected by measuring preductal and postductal PaO_2 levels. In the presence of a significant right-to-left shunt, the preductal sample may be 15 to 20 mm Hg higher that the postductal sample. The difference between the two is increased when the FiO_2 is increased.

A third test, the hyperoxia-hyperventilation test, is the most accurate of the three to differentiate PPHN. The patient is hyperventilated to achieve a $PaCO_2$ of 20 to 25 mm Hg and raise the pH to 7.50 or greater. The alkalosis reduces the pulmonary vasoconstriction, improving lung perfusion and oxygen content. If the PaO_2 is less than 50 mm Hg before hyperventilation and rises to above 100 mm Hg follow hyperventilation, it is an almost certain diagnosis of PPHN.

With the increased presence of echocardiograms in the NICU, the diagnosis of PPHN has been advanced. The presence of PPHN is documented by an echocardiogram showing increased pulmonary artery pressures, right-to-left shunting at the ductal or atrial level, regurgitation through the tricuspid valve, and dilation of the right ventricle.[43]

The treatment for PPHN has traditionally been hyperventilation therapy. The risk of barotrauma is high when high ventilatory pressures and rates are used to hyperventilate the patient. Rates of up to 150 breaths per minute are recommended to allow lower inspiratory pressures. Care must be taken to allow sufficient time for exhalation to avoid lung ruptures, and thus, very short inspiratory times are required.

If hyperventilation is unsuccessful, drug-induced vasodilation may be attempted by the use of tolazoline. A positive response to tolazoline is indicated by a sudden flushing of the skin, followed by an increase in the PaO_2. Because a drop in systemic blood pressure may accompany the use of tolazoline, blood or plasma substitutes should be readily available to prevent shock.[7]

Dopamine has been used to support systemic blood pressure when tolazoline is being used. Other drugs that may be of some benefit in the treatment of PPHN include isoproterenol and prostaglandins E_1 and I_2.[7]

Neonatal patients with primary PPHN frequently meet the criteria for treatment with extracorporeal membrane oxygenation (ECMO). On these patients, ECMO supports the cardiopulmonary system and corrects the acidosis, allowing time for the hypertension to resolve. In one study, mortality was shown to be lower in those PPHN patients treated with ECMO over those treated medically.

High-frequency ventilation may prove to be beneficial in the treatment of PPHN. At this time, however, there is insufficient data supporting its use. Both ECMO and high-frequency ventilation are covered in detail in Chapter 16.

An exciting treatment for PPHN of recent discovery is nitric oxide (NO). NO is colorless and has the same density as air. Studies done on animals demonstrated inhaled nitric oxide (INO) to be a powerful, selective pulmonary vasodilator.[46] More recent studies have found this to be true.[47] Although this is still experimental in neonates, it has become a more mature therapy and will likely soon be approved by the FDA. It is being used in centers where ECMO is readily available. In addition to having PPHN as documented by echocardiogram, a patient must also be greater than 35 weeks' gestation, have a birth weight of at least 2000 g, and failed to respond to maximum conventional therapies.[43]

Typically, NO comes in an H-cylinder that contains 450 to 1000 parts per million (PPM) of NO mixed with nitrogen. When NO comes in contact with high concentrations of oxygen, it forms nitrogen dioxide (NO_2), which is very irritating to lung tissue. In order to minimize the production of NO_2, NO is usually delivered in very small quantities, 5 to 6 ppm. When delivered to a patient, NO is introduced to the inspiratory limb of the mechanical ventilator just proximal to the ETT. This further reduces the contact time between NO and O_2. In the bloodstream, excess NO is quickly absorbed by hemoglobin, forming methemoglobin.

When used inline with mechanical ventilation, the amount of NO introduced into the circuit is regulated by a flow controller. The concentrations of NO, NO_2, and FiO_2 are all measured inline near the ETT. Protocols for administration of INO vary among institutions. Ideally, the amount of inhaled NO and NO_2 are balanced to maximize the vasodilatory effects while minimizing methemoglobinemia and the toxic effects of NO_2. While it is generally thought that concentrations of 5 to 20 ppm of NO are considered usual, reports of concentrations up to 80 ppm with no side effects have been documented.[48,49]

TRANSIENT TACHYPNEA OF THE NEWBORN (TTN)

TTN is also called RDS Type II because of the similarities in patient symptoms. Although the exact etiology is unclear, the retention of fetal lung fluid following birth is felt to play a major role in the development of TTN. It most commonly occurs in near-term or term infants with a history of cesarean or precipitous deliveries. In either of these types of deliveries, the gradual compression of the thorax that develops during a vaginal delivery does not occur, possibly leading to the retention of lung water.

Diagnosis. Within the first few hours following delivery, the infant shows signs of respiratory distress including tachypnea, nasal flaring, retractions, and grunting. The patient may be cyanotic when in room air. Blood gases are usually normal but may show varying degrees of hypoxia. Hypercapnia is a rare occurrence.

The chest x-ray may mimic early RDS, with streaky infiltrates that radiate from the hilum of the lung. Fluid in the interlobar fissures is commonly seen. The chest x-ray gradually clears within 24 to 48 hours following the onset of symptoms.

The diagnosis of TTN is only made after other potential problems have been ruled out. It is important to rule out pneumonia as the source of the symptoms. The presence of an elevated white blood count, hyperglycemia, persistent metabolic acidosis, and poor perfusion all indicate a possible pneumonia.

Treatment. Treatment of TTN involves taking appropriate measures to treat the patient's clinical symptoms. Warmed, humidified oxygen is delivered via oxyhood to treat hypoxia. More severe symptoms may require the use of positive pressure to treat hypoxemia. Continuous positive airway pressure (CPAP) delivered via nasal prongs may be used to treat refractory hypoxemia. The use of mechanical ventilation may be necessary when nasal CPAP does not improve arterial oxygen.

Frequent turning of the infant with gentle chest physiotherapy may help in the absorption of lung fluids. Broad-spectrum antibiotics are given, as the symptoms of pneumonia are often mistaken for TTN.

APNEA

True apnea is defined as a cessation of breathing for a period sufficient to produce bradycardia and/or cyanosis. That period is usually 10 to 20 seconds or longer. Apnea is categorized into central or nonobstructive apnea, which is the absence of airflow and ventilatory effort, and obstructive apnea, which is the absence of airflow despite a ventilatory effort.

The mechanisms that provide for adequate ventilation and homeostasis are diverse. The respiratory centers in the medulla and pons receive information from numerous receptors and then send out impulses to the ventilatory muscles to maintain homeostasis. Apnea may be present when there is a dysfunction of any of the various mechanisms involved. We will briefly examine potential dysfunctions at each site. Causes of apnea are found in Table 10–5.

Central or Nonobstructive Apnea

Apnea of Prematurity. A common type of central apnea is identified as apnea of prematurity. As the gestational age of the preemie decreases, the incidence of apnea of prematurity increases. Apnea of prematurity is a result of one or more of the following factors.

Chemoreceptor Sensitivity. Evidence from apnea research has demonstrated that newborns, especially premature newborns, have a somewhat blunted response from peripheral chemoreceptors located in the aortic arch and the carotid artery. These receptors sense changes in PaO_2, pH, and $PaCO_2$ and send impulses to the respiratory centers to either increase or decrease ventilation.

Although both premature and term infants show an initial response to blood gas changes, the response is transient. It is not until around day 18 that the infant shows a sustained response to changes. This blunting in chemoreceptor sensitivity can potentially initiate an apneic spell or can prolong an apneic spell that is started by other factors.

Arousal Response. In the adult, periods of hypoxemia and/or hypercapnia during sleep cause arousal. There is some evidence that this response is not present in some infants who suffer apneic spells. The level of sleep also influences response to hypercapnia and hypoxemia. Nonrapid eye movement (NREM), or quiet sleep, has been shown to be controlled by metabolic and chemical factors, whereas REM, or active sleep, is controlled by behavioral and reflex mechanisms. Studies on infants suffering apneic spells have shown an apparent blunting of the sensitivity to CO_2 during NREM sleep.

Stimulation of Airway Reflexes. One of the protective mechanisms of the airways is to induce coughing, constriction, and apnea when a foreign substance is aspirated. This mechanism hopefully prevents the material from entering deeply into the tracheobronchial tree and occluding the airways. Apnea that is present in patients suffering from gastroesophageal reflux and infections such as RSV may be caused by an activation of this protective airway mechanism. Research indicates that as many as one third of patients diagnosed with apnea of prematurity in reality are suffering from apnea secondary to gastroesophageal reflux.[50] While the main response of the adult to airway stimulus is coughing, the response of the newborn is apnea.

TABLE 10–5   Causes of Apnea in Premature Infants

Respiratory

- RDS
- Congenital upper airway anomalies
- Airway obstruction
- Postextubation
- CPAP
- Pneumonia
- Hypoxia

Cardiovascular

- Congestive heart failure
- Patent ductus arteriosus
- Anemia
- Tachycardia and bradycardia
- Sepsis
- Polycythemia

Central Nervous System

- IVH
- Meningitis
- Seizures
- Pharmacologic sedation
- Kernicterus
- Immaturity of the respiratory centers
- Tumors

Gastrointestinal

- Necrotizing enterocolitis
- Gastroesophageal reflux

Metabolic

- Hypoglycemia
- Hypo- and hypernatremia
- Hypocalcemia
- Hypo- and hyperthermia

Environmental

- Increased environmental temperature
- Suctioning
- Feeding

Dysfunction of the Respiratory Centers. Dysfunction of the centers in the brain responsible for maintaining ventilation can be caused by several factors. In the preterm infant, inadequate development of the brain centers themselves may be the cause of dysfunction. The respiratory centers may also be damaged by trauma or bleeding in the brain, leading to hypoperfusion and increased pressures that damage the brain tissue.

The presence of certain drugs in the maternal or fetal circulation depresses the respiratory centers and leads to apnea.

Dysfunction of the Ventilatory Muscles. The muscles of ventilation, especially the diaphragm, may be dysfunctional and unable to increase ventilation in the face of hypercapnia and hypoxia, leading to apnea. At special risk are infants with chronic lung diseases that interfere with gas exchange. As $PaCO_2$ rises and PaO_2 falls, the muscles may not be able to respond by increasing ventilation due to chronic fatigue and underdevelopment. Studies have shown that fatigue of the ventilatory muscles leads to apnea in the newborn.

Dysfunction of the Peripheral Nervous System. Apnea may occur when a disease that affects neurotransmission to the ventilatory muscles is present. Diseases such as Guillain-Barré block transmission of the nervous system and may lead to apnea. The defect may be a maldevelopment of the motor neurons in the spinal cord as in Werdnig-Hoffmann disease. Toxins such as botulism and certain drugs disrupt and inhibit the neuromuscular junctions. Finally, trauma to the CNS leads to a loss of neurotransmission and subsequent apnea.

Other Factors That Cause Apnea. Other factors that have been linked to apnea in newborns are thermal instability, metabolid disorders, PDA, shock, anemia, sepsis, and NEC.

Treatment. Treatment of central apnea is accomplished by the administration of drugs that stimultae ventilatory mechanisms. The most commonly administered drugs are the methylxanthines, theophylline, and caffeine, which apparently stimulate the central respiratory chemoreceptors. Which drug is more effective is a matter of debate.

The drug primidone, chemically related to phenobarbital, is a drug that traditionally has been used to treat neonatal seizures. It is now being investigated as a possible treatment option for apnea in those cases that are resistant to theophylline.

Mechanical ventilation may be necessary to support the patient whose apnea leads to acute respiratory failure. In these patients, inspiratory pressures and ventilator rates are kept as low as possible to avoid barotraumatic injuries.

While apnea of prematurity can present a difficult challenge and may have long-term consequences in the presence of other events, it appears as though the apnea in and of itself is not associated with any significant developmental problems later in life.

Obstructive Apnea
Pathophysiology. In the adult, and in the healthy newborn, the upper airway is protected from obstruction by the presence of protective reflexes. During inspiration, negative intrapharyngeal pressures are countered by the presence of elastic fibers and smooth muscle in the pharyngeal wall to prevent collapse. Any time that negative intrapharyngeal pressures

exceed the force of the fibers and muscle, the pharynx will collapse. The most common cause of airway obstruction is the tongue.

Many infants who suffer from obstructive apnea have anatomic abnormalities that cause the obstruction. Prematurity or agenesis of the pharyngeal musculature may lead to pharyngeal collapse. Enlarged tonsils and adenoids, *micrognathia* (Pierre-Robin syndrome), and facial anomalies lead to airway obstruction. The presence of choanal atresia, laryngeal webs, and vocal cord paralysis have also been shown to cause apnea.

Obstructive apnea in suspect patients is documented by the use of the polysomnogram. The polysomnogram monitors chest wall and abdominal movement, oral and nasal airflow, heart rate and rhythm, arterial oxygen levels, and end-tidal CO_2 levels. The level of sleep is often determined by the use of electroencephalograms.

The pattern seen in obstructive apnea shows movement of the chest and abdomen, with no airflow at the nose or mouth. Significant apnea is present if the oxygen saturation drops 5% or more, the PaO_2 drops 8 mm Hg or more, or end-tidal CO_2 increases 2% or more. A polysomnographic tracing is shown in Figure 10–12.

Treatment. The treatment of obstructive apnea can range from pharmacologic agents to surgery. Antihistamines, decongestants, cromolyn sodium, and topical application of corticosteroids may help reduce the airway narrowing. Surgical correction normally involves the removal of the offending tissue or obstruction. Obstructive apnea may also be treated by the use of nasal CPAP during sleep periods to maintain a patent airway.

Nasal CPAP is used as an adjunct in the treatment of obstructive apnea, to stabilize and support the airway structures. The patients best suited for treatment with nasal CPAP are those suffering from obesity or those with enlarged or edematous tissues in the upper airways. CPAP mechanically holds the airway open during expiration, helping to prevent the airway collapse that leads to apnea.

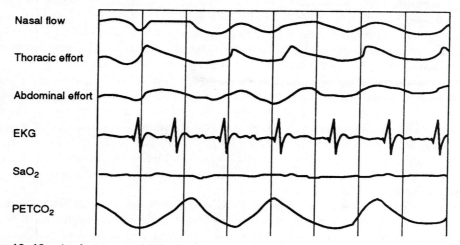

Figure 10–12 *A polysomnographic tracing.*

SUMMARY

As is apparent from the length of this chapter, the consequences of premature birth are many and complex. Prematurity affects all organ systems and the practitioner must be aware that interaction between the systems is also diminished.

Of all the problems associated with prematurity, none is as significant in its implications as RDS. The premature respiratory system is often unable to adequately provide oxygenation and ventilation for the neonate. The main reason for this is a lack of surfactant, which makes the lungs very noncompliant. As compliance worsens, atelectasis ensues with widespread V/Q mismatching the blood gas instability. Work of breathing also increases significantly, wasting the valuable energy reserves of the patient. The resultant hypoxia causes damage to the capillaries and alveolar tissue. Soon, the neonate enters a cycle of hypoxemia, damage, surfactant deficiency, and atelectasis that, if not corrected, leads to death.

A consequence of RDS is often BPD, also called neonatal chronic lung disease. The presence of BPD often requires the patient to remain on mechanical ventilation for long periods. Once off the ventilator, the patient often requires supplemental oxygen for long periods thereafter.

Pulmonary dysmaturity (Wilson-Mikity syndrome) is a disease similar to BPD; however, the patient often does not have RDS preceding its onset. Treatment of this, as well as the other pulmonary disorders, is mainly supportive with respiratory care procedures such as CPT and SVN used to aid recovery.

Retinopathy of prematurity is a disorder of the developing retina in which the retinal vasculature becomes constricted, leading to necrosis of the vessels. This is followed by a proliferation of new vessels in an attempt to reestablish the blood supply. This proliferation causes hemorrhage into the vitreous, scarring of the retina and possible detachment, and blindness. Treatment with laser is a promising technology.

Intraventricular bleeding is a major source of mortality and morbidity among the premature population. On the very tiniest of preemies, the very simple act of raising the hips to place a diaper under may increase intracranial pressure enough to cause a bleed. Prevention is the key, because little can be done once the bleed has occurred. The bleeding is graded from I to IV, with grades III and IV resulting in the most sequelae.

Problems occurring in utero also cause some significant problems for the neonate. Fetal asphyxia can be secondary to maternal hypoxia, disruption of uteroplacental blood flow, dysfunction of the placenta, umbilical cord compression, or an intrinsic fetal disorder. Asphyxia leads to meconium release into the amniotic fluid, gasping, fetal heart decelerations, and if long enough, encephalopathy. The release of meconium predisposes the fetus to aspiration of the meconium. This can lead to serious pulmonary problems such as air trapping and V/Q imbalances.

The presence of RDS with resultant positive-pressure ventilation, combined with the fragility of the premature lung, often leads to air leak syndromes such as pneumothorax, pneumomediastinum, and pneumopericardium. An air leak that remains in the lung tissue is called pulmonary interstitial emphysema (PIE). Because the air dissects into the lung tissue, this type of air leak can be very difficult to treat and has serious consequences.

Persistent pulmonary hypertension of the neonate (PPHN) is often seen in term or post-term infants. Increased vascular resistance in the pulmonary vasculature causes blood to shunt away from the lungs and leads to profound mismatch between ventilation and perfusion. Traditionally, PPHN is treated with hyperventilation, which raises pH. The increasing pH causes some vasodilation of the pulmonary vessels and allows more blood to enter the lungs. A relatively new treatment involves the use of nitric oxide, a powerful vasodilator. When inhaled in small quantities, nitric oxide has been shown to be successful in treating PPHN.

Transient tachypnea of the newborn, or RDS type II, is the result of retained lung water. It is often seen following cesarean delivery. Because it mimics RDS, the patient must be monitored closely and treated as needed. Most often, treatment involves only supplemental oxygen, but more aggressive treatments may be needed. CPT and postural drainage are often helpful in aiding the reabsorption of lung fluids.

Apnea in a newborn can either be the result of prematurity or obstruction. Either way, it can often avoid detection and is seen as frequent drops in the heart rate. Treatment involves the use of respiratory stimulants such as caffeine or theophylline, or correction of the obstruction. Polysomnography can be a useful adjunct in determining the cause and severity of apnea.

References

1. Avery GB, Fletcher MA, MacDonald MG. *Pathophysiology and Management of the Newborn*. 5th ed. Philadelphia: JB Lippincott Co; 1999.

2. Skelton R, Jeffery H. "Click test": rapid diagnosis of the respiratory distress syndrome. *Pediatr Pulmonol*. 1994;17:383.

3. Moise, AA, et al. Antenatal steroids are associated with less need for blood pressure supports in extremely premature infants. *Pediatrics*. 1995;95:845–850.

4. Durand M, et al. Effects of early dexamethasone therapy on pulmonary mechanics and chronic lung disease in very low birthweight infants: a randomized, controlled trial. *Pediatrics*. 1995;95:584.

5. Lee H, et al. Bronchodilator aerosol administered by metered dose inhaler and spacer in subacute neonatal respiratory distress syndrome. *Arch Dis Child 70*. 1994;F218–222.

6. Green TP, et al. Furosemide promotes patent ductus arteriosus in premature infants with respiratory distress syndrome. *N Engl J Med*. 1983;308:743–748.

7. Cloherty JP, Stark AR, eds. *Manual of Neonatal Care*. 4th ed. Philadelphia: Lippincott; 1997.

8. Northway WH, et al. Pulmonary disease following respiratory therapy for hyaline membrane disease. *N Engl J Med*. 1967;276:357.

9. Strayer DS, et al. Levels of SP-A-Anti-SP-A immune complexes in neonatal respiratory distress syndrome correlates with subsequent development of bronchopulmonary dysplasia. *Acta Paediatr*. 1995;84:128–131.

10. Watterberg IL, Scott SM. Evidence of early adrenal insufficiency in babies who develop bronchopulmonary dysplasia. *Pediatrics*. 1995;95:120–125.

11. Merenstein GB, Gardner SL. *Handbook of Neonatal Intensive Care*. 4th ed. St. Louis: CV Mosby Co; 1998.

12. Korones SB. *High-Risk Newborn Infants.* 4th ed. St. Louis: CV Mosby Co; 1986.

13. Jacob J, et al. The contribution of PDA in the neonate with severe RDS. *J. Pediatr.* 1979;96:79–87.

14. Nickerson B, Taussig L. Family history of asthma in infants with BPD. *Pediatrics.* 1980;65:1140–1144.

15. Weinstein MR. A new radiographic scoring system for bronchopulmonary dysplasia. *Pediatr Pulmonol.* 1994;18:284.

16. Hicks MA. A systemic approach to neonatal pathophysiology: understanding respiratory distress syndrome. *Neonatal Network.* 1995;14:29–35.

17. Carlo WA, Chatburn RL. *Neonatal Respiratory Care.* 2nd ed. Chicago: Year-Book Medical Publishers Inc; 1988.

18. Cabal L, et al. Effects of metaproterenol on pulmonary mechanics, oxygenation and ventilation in infants with chronic lung disease. *J. Pediatr.* 1987;110:116.

19. Vrlenich LA, et al. The effects of bronchopulmonary dysplasia on growth at school age. *Pediatrics.* 1995;95:855.

20. Terry TL. Extreme prematurity and fibroblastic overgrowth of persistent vascular sheath behind each crystalline lens [preliminary report]. *Am J Ophthalmol.* 1942;25:203.

21. Heath P. Pathology of the retinopathy of prematurity; retrolental fibroplasia. *Am J Ophthalmol.* 1951;34:1249.

22. Bossi E, Koerner F. Retinopathy of prematurity. *Intensive Care Med.* 1995;21:241–246.

23. Arroe M, Peitersen B. Retinopathy of prematurity: review of a seven-year period in a Danish neonatal intensive care unit. *Acta Paediatr.* 1994;83:501–505.

24. Gilbert CE, et al. Causes of blindness and severe visual impairment in children in Chile. *Dev Med Child Neurol.* 1994;36:326–333.

25. Keith CG, Doyle LW. Retinopathy of prematurity in extremely low birth weight infants. *Pediatrics.* 1995;95:42–45.

26. George DS, et al. The latest on retinopathy of prematurity. *MCN.* 1988;13:254–258.

27. Kushner BJ, Gloeckner E. Retrolental fibroplasia in full-term infants without exposure to supplemental oxygen. *Am J Ophthalmol.* 1984;97:148–153.

28. Schulman J, et al. Peripheral proliferative retinopathy without oxygen therapy in a full-term infant. *Am J Ophthalmol.* 1980;90:509–514.

29. Lucey JF, Dangman B. A reexamination of the role of oxygen in retrolental fibroplasia. *Pediatrics.* 1984;73:82–96.

30. Wright K, Wright SP. Lack of association of glucocorticoid therapy and retinopathy of prematurity. *Arch Pediatr Adolesc Med.* 1994;148:848–852.

31. Cryotherapy for Retinopathy of Prematurity Cooperative Group. The natural ocular outcome of premature birth and retinopathy. Status at one year. *Arch Ophthalmol.* 1994;112:903–912.

32. Hunsucker K, et al. Laser surgery for retinopathy of prematurity. *Neonatal Network.* 1995;14:21–26.

33. Kremer I, et al. Late visual field changes following cryotherapy for retinopathy of prematurity stage 3. *Br J Ophthalmol.* 1995;79:267–269.

34. Seaber JH, et al. Long-term visual results of children after initially successful vitrectomy of stage V retinopathy of prematurity. *Ophthalmology.* 1995;102:199–204.

35. Holzman C, et al. Perinatal brain injury in premature infants born to mothers using alcohol in pregnancy. Neonatal brain hemorrhage study team. *Pediatrics.* 1995;95:66–73.

36. Paneth N, et al. Incidence of timing of germinal matrix/intraventricular hemorrhage in low birth weight infants. *Am J Epidemiol.* 1993;137:1167–1176.

37. Aziz K, et al. Province-based study of neurologic disability of children weighing 500 through 1249 grams at birth in relation to neonatal cerebral ultrasound. *Pediatrics.* 1995; 95:837–844.

38. Houlihan CM, Knuppel RA. Meconium-stained amniotic fluid. Current controversies. *J Reprod Med.* 1994;39:888–898.

39. Dye T, et al. Amnioinfusion and the intrauterine prevention of meconium aspiration. *Am J Obstet Gynecol.* 1994;171:1601–1605.

40. Ericksen NL, et al. Prophylactic amnioinfusion in pregnancies complicated by thick meconium. *Am J Obstet Gynecol.* 1994;171:1026–1030.

41. Spong CY, et al. Prophylactic amnioinfusion for meconium-stained amniotic fluid. *Am J Obstet Gynecol.* 1994;171:931–935.

42. Goldsmith JP, Karotkin EH. *Assisted Ventilation of the Neonate.* 2nd ed. Philadelphia: WB Saunders Co; 1988.

43. Holowaty L. Nitric Oxide. *Neonatal Network.* 1995;14:83–86.

44. Kinsella JP, Abman SH. Recent developments in the pathophysiology and treatment of persistent pulmonary hypertension of the newborn. *J Pediatr.* 1995;126:853–864.

45. Fineman JR, et al. Chronic nitric oxide inhibition in utero produces persistent pulmonary hypertension in newborn lambs. *J Clin Invest.* 1994;93:2675–2683.

46. Frostell C, et al. Inhaled nitric oxide: a selective pulmonary vasodilator reversing hypoxic pulmonary vasoconstriction. *Circulation.* 1991;83:2038–2047.

47. Giacoia GP. Nitric oxide: a selective pulmonary vasodilator. *South Med J.* 1995; 88:33–41.

48. Finer NN, et al. Inhaled nitric oxide in infants referred for extracorporeal membrane oxygenation: dose response. *Pediatrics.* 1994;124:302.

49. Roberts JD, et al. Inhaled nitric oxide in persistent pulmonary hypertension of the newborn. *Lancet.* 1992;340:818–819.

50. Krishnamoorthy M, et al. Diagnosis and treatment of respiratory symptoms of initially unsuspected gastroesophageal reflux in infants. *Am Surg.* 1994;60:783–785.

Bibliography and Suggested Readings

Buhrer C, et al. Dose-response to inhaled nitric oxide in acute hypoxemic respiratory failure of newborn infants: a preliminary report. *Pediatr Pulmonol.* 1995;19:291.

Carey BE, Trotter C. The chest x-ray findings in retained lung fluid. *Neonatal Network.* 1994;13:65–69.

Chernick V, Boat TF. *Kendig's Disorders of the Respiratory Tract in Children.* 6th ed. Philadelphia: WB Saunders Co; 1998.

Goetzman BW, Wennberg RP. *Neonatal Intensive Care Handbook.* 3rd ed. St. Louis, Mo: Mosby; 1999.

Harwood R. *Exam Review and Study Guide for Perinatal/Pediatric Respiratory Care.* Philadelphia: FA Davis; 1999.

Kinsella JP, et al. Clinical responses to prolonged treatment of persistent pulmonary hypertension of the newborn with low doses of inhaled nitric oxide. *J Pediatr.* 1993; 123:103–108.

Kinsella JP, et al. Low-dose inhalation nitriic oxide in persistent pulmonary hypertension of the newborn. *Lancet.* 1992;340:819–820.

Koons AH, et al. Neurodevelopmental outcome of infants with apnea of infancy. *Am J Perinatol.* 1993;10:208–211.

Levin D, Morriss F, et al. *Essentials of Pediatric Intensive Care.* 2nd ed. St. Louis, Mo: Quality Medical Publishing, Inc.; 1997.

Ment LR, et al. Low-dose indomethacin and prevention of intraventricular hemorrhage: a multicenter randomized trial. *Pediatrics.* 1994;93:543–550.

Miller CA, et al. The use of primidone in neonates with theophylline-resistant apnea. *Am J Dis Child.* 1993;147:183–186.

Moore CS. Meconium aspiration syndrome. *Neonatal Network.* 1994;13:57–63.

Parker LA. Necrotizing enterocolitis. *Neonatal Network.* 1995;14:17–26.

Perez-Benavides F, et al. Persistent pulmonary hypertension of the newborn infant. Comparison of conventional versus extracorporeal membrane oxygenation in neonates fulfilling Bartlett's criteria. *J Perinatol.* 1993;13:181–185.

Taussig LM, Landau LI. *Pediatric Respiratory Medicine.* St. Louis, Mo: Mosby, 1999.

Walsh-Sukys MC, et al. Treatment of persistent pulmonary hypertension of the newborn without hyperventilation: an assessment of diffusion of innovation. *Pediatrics.* 1994; 94:3030–306.

Posttest

1. The underlying etiology of RDS is:
   a. surfactant deficiency
   b. pulmonary hypoperfusion
   c. hypothermia
   d. acidosis
2. Of the following, which are complications of RDS?
   I. DIC
   II. intraventricular hemorrhage
   III. infection
   IV. PDA
   V. Left ventricular failure
      a. I, II, IV
      b. I, II, III, IV
      c. I, III, V
      d. II, III, V

3. Oxygen toxicity, barotrauma, PDA, and fluid overload are all linked to the development of:
   a. RDS
   b. ROP
   c. BPD
   d. PIE

4. Which of the following is *least* likely to be used when treating BPD?
   a. high-frequency ventilation
   b. theophylline
   c. diuretic
   d. ECMO

5. The radiographic picture of Wilson-Mikity syndrome appears similar to:
   a. BPD
   b. RDS
   c. pneumothorax
   d. atelectasis

6. Which of the following best defines vaso-obliteration?
   a. necrosis of the optic nerve
   b. necrosis of retinal vessels
   c. proliferation of vasculature into the vitreous humor
   d. formation of scar tissue behind the retina

7. Prevention of ROP is based on:
   a. maintaining low $PaCO_2$ levels
   b. maintaining adequate blood pressure
   c. cautious use of oxygen
   d. maintaining PaO_2 above 100 torr

8. Intraventricular hemorrhage in premature neonates occurs most often in the:
   a. subdural space
   b. choroid plexus
   c. germinal matrix
   d. subarachnoid space

9. Bleeding in the brain ventricles, without evidence of ventricular dilation, describes:
   a. subdural hemorrhage
   b. subarachnoid hemorrhage
   c. grade I IVH
   d. grade II IVH

10. One of the initial signs of fetal asphyxia is:
    a. primary apnea
    b. bradycardia
    c. placental insufficiency
    d. increased blood pressure

11. Meconium passage into the amniotic fluid is precipitated by:
    a. bradycardia
    b. intraventricular hemorrhage

    c. asphyxia

    d. ventricular heart failure

12. Intubation of the trachea, followed by suction applied to the endotracheal tube while it is being removed, is indicated when:

    a. any meconium is present in the amniotic fluid

    b. thick meconium is present in the amniotic fluid

    c. thin meconium is present in the amniotic fluid

    d. the patient is apneic and flaccid

13. A ventilator patient's status suddenly worsens with bradycardia, cyanosis, retractions, and apnea. The immediate reaction of the respiratory care practitioner would be:

    a. order a stat chest x-ray

    b. check for signs of extubation followed by transillumination of the chest

    c. extubate and reintubate with a larger tube

    d. suction the patient

14. PIE can best be treated by:

    a. administration of antibiotics

    b. use of high pressures and rates

    c. high levels of oxygen

    d. low ventilatory pressures

15. A patient is suspected of having PPHN. Which of the following is the most accurate test to make the diagnosis?

    a. the hyperoxia-hyperventilation test

    b. measurement of preductal and postductal PaO_2

    c. the hyperoxia test

    d. hypoventilation to $PaCO_2$ ratio

16. Which of the following is a risk of treating PPHN with NO?

    a. hypoxemia

    b. methemoglobinemia

    c. patent ductus arteriosus

    d. retinal damage

17. Which of the following are indicative of TTN?

    I. deviated white blood cell count

    II. tachypnea

    III. cyanosis

    IV. metabolic acidosis

    V. normal PaO_2 and $PaCO_2$

        a. I, III, V

        b. II, IV, V

        c. II, III, IV

        d. II, III, V

18. Of the following, which is *not* a cause of central apnea?

    a. blunted chemoreceptor sensitivity

    b. stimulation of airway reflexes

  c. vocal cord paralysis
  d. dysfunction of the respiratory centers
19. Which of the following drugs would be used to treat central apnea?
  a. caffeine
  b. terbutaline
  c. antihistamines
  d. cromolyn sodium

CHAPTER ELEVEN

CAUSES OF PERSISTENT PERINATAL ILLNESS

OBJECTIVES

Upon completion of this chapter, the reader should be able to:

1. Explain how infections are acquired by the fetus and neonate.
2. Define chorioamnionitis and describe the various bacterial organisms seen in the neonatal population.
3. Review the etiology of acquired immune deficiency syndrome (AIDS), identify the number of pediatric cases, and discuss the five methods in which the fetus and neonate may become infected with the HIV virus.
4. Describe the clinical signs, diagnosis, treatment, and outcome associated with HIV infection.
5. Identify the effects of cytomegalovirus, rubella, herpes simplex, and toxoplasmosis on the developing fetus.
6. Describe the diagnosis, prevention, and treatment of infection in the neonate.
7. Describe the role of each of the following antibodies:
   a. IgA
   b. IgD
   c. IgE
   d. IgG
   e. IgM
8. Describe the pathophysiology, diagnosis, and treatment of the following:
   a. Tracheoesophageal anomalies
   b. Choanal atresia
   c. Diaphragmatic hernia
   d. Micrognathia (Pierre-Robin syndrome)
9. For each of the following cardiac anomalies, identify the defect from an artist's rendering and describe the diagnosis and treatment:
   a. Patent ductus arteriosus
   b. Atrial septal defect
   c. Ventricular septal defect
   d. Tetralogy of Fallot

e. Complete transposition of the great vessels
f. Subaortic stenosis
g. Coarctation of the aorta
h. Tricuspid atresia
i. Anomalous venous return
j. Truncus arteriosus
k. Hypoplastic left-heart syndrome
10. Describe the respiratory care of a neonatal patient with any of the above anomalies.

KEY TERMS

afterload
balloon septostomy
choanal atresia
chorioamnionitis
color flow mapping

disseminated
enzyme-linked immunosorbent
  assay (ELISA)
Fontan procedure
hypoplastic

immunoglobulins
petechiae
polyhydramnios
Western blot

INFECTIONS

A neonate is susceptible to infection from several routes. Prenatal infection of the fetus always follows some degree of maternal involvement, which may be asymptomatic. An infection may be acquired prenatally either through the placenta, or an infection may ascend upward through the birth canal. During delivery, the fetus may become infected from direct contact with infected maternal tissue in the birth canal. Following delivery, the neonate is at risk of acquiring infection from NICU personnel, other patients, or the equipment being used for treatment.

As in most circumstances, the earlier the gestational age, the more vulnerable the neonate is to picking up an infection.

ETIOLOGY: BACTERIA

Bacterial infections in the neonate are often caused by organisms found in the maternal intestinal and genital tracts. Prenatally, although some organisms may enter the uterus through an intact amniotic membrane, most bacterial infections ascend the birth canal and enter the uterus through a rupture in the amniotic sac. Amniotic membranes ruptured for more than 24 hours before delivery greatly predispose the fetus to infection.

Once in the uterus, the organisms may enter the fetal mouth and infect the lungs, intestinal tract, and may even enter the bloodstream from one of these sites. The presence of bacteria in amniotic fluid begins an inflammatory response known as *chorioamnionitis,* characterized by an outpouring of leukocytes into the fluid from inflamed amniotic tissues. Chorioamnionitis does not always lead to fetal infection, but greatly enhances the neonate's susceptibility. Chorioamnionitis is suspected when the neonate and birth fluids are malodorous and is diagnosed by culturing a tissue sample of the amniotic membrane.

Bacterial infections are also contracted from poor aseptic technique in the nursery or with equipment. One of the most common and challenging bacterial infections seen in neonatal care is pneumonia, covered in detail in Chapter 12. The various bacterial agents and their effects on the fetus are listed on Table 11–1.

TABLE 11–1   Common Disease-Producing Agents in the Fetus and Newborn

Organism	Abortion	Premature Birth	Intrauterine Growth Retardation	Congenital Disease	Neonatal Disease
BACTERIA/					
Anaerobic bacteria (*Bacteriodes, Clostridia, Peptostreptococcus, Veillonela*)	?	?	-	R	R
Escherichia coli	?	?	-	+	+
Group A streptococcus	+	+	-	+	+
Group B streptococcus	+	+	-	+	+
Group D streptococcus	-	-	-	R	+
Hemophilus influenzae	-	-	-	R	+
Klebsiella species	-	-	-	R	R
Listeria monocytogenes	+	+	-	+	+
Neisseria gonorrhoea	?	+	-	R	+
Neisseria meningitidis	-	-	-	-	+
Proteus species *Pseudomonas aeruginosa*	-	-	-	R	R
Salmonella species	-	-	-	R	+
Shigella species	-	-	-	R	+
Staphylococcus aureus	-	-	-	R	+
Staphylococcus epidermidis	-	-	-	R	R
VIRUS/					
Cytomegalovirus	?	+	+	+	+
Enterovirus (ECHO virus, poliomyelitis, coxsackie-virus A and B)	+	?,R	-	R	+
Hepatitis A	-	+	-	-	-
Hepatitis B	-	+	-	R	+

TABLE 11–1 *(continued)*

Herpes simplex (type I or II)	+	+	R	R	+
Human immunodeficiency virus	?	?	?	+	+
Measles	+	+	-	R	R
Respiratory syncytial virus	-	-	-	-	+
Rubella	+	+	+	+	R
Varicella	-	-	R	R	+

+, strong evidence for; -, no evidence for; R, rare association; ?, questionable association.
Source: Bruhn FW, et al. Infection in the neonate. In Merenstein GB, Gardner SL eds. Handbook of Neonatal Intensive Care. 4th ed. St. Louis: CV Mosby Co.; 1995:336. Reproduced with permission.

ETIOLOGY: VIRUS

Although viral infections are less common in the fetus and neonate, special attention is given them due to the serious effects that many of them have on the neonate. Refer to Table 11–1 for viral infections and their effect on the neonate.

Acquired Immune Deficiency Syndrome (AIDS). Since its first reported incidence in the early 1980s, AIDS has become an epidemic and continues to be a complex social, as well as biological, challenge to health care workers. There is also quite a bit of confusion remaining to be sorted out regarding the transmission of the disease and risk factors. As the disease continues to grow in its spectrum, it is essential that the health care provider remain abreast of the latest information regarding treatment protocols, risk factors, and preventive care. As with all of medicine, the understanding of HIV changes rapidly and by the time the information in this book gets into the hands of the reader, the information will be outdated. This discussion therefore will focus on the basic understanding needed to treat this disease.

The terminology surrounding AIDS is also a potential source of confusion. In discussing the disease as a whole, regardless of what symptoms are present, the patient is said to be HIV infected. Those who are infected and have symptoms, but do not meet the CDC definition of AIDS, are said to have AIDS-related complex (ARC). The term AIDS is used to describe the most advanced stage of HIV.

Risk Factors. A vast majority (89%) of neonatal HIV infection is acquired from an infected mother.[1] Therefore, risk factors for prenatal infection include: parents, and especially the mother, are IV drug users; maternal promiscuity or prostitution; and parental homosexuality. The remaining cases are acquired by exposure to infected blood products, exposure to infected breast milk, and a small percentage in which the cause is unknown.

Transmission. With regard to prenatal HIV infection, the virus passes transplacentally from the infected mother to the fetus. It apparently crosses early, as antibodies specific to HIV have been found as early as 9 weeks' gestation.[1] Not all HIV infected mothers pass the virus to the fetus. A study by Goedert and associates found that the presence of certain antibodies in the mother may prevent the transmission of the virus.[2] A reduction of nearly two thirds in the transmission rate was seen in a study where zidovudine was given before delivery to the mother, and then for 6 weeks to the neonate.[3]

During delivery, the fetus may acquire the virus by contact with maternal blood.[4] Postdelivery, feeding with infected breast milk, and transfusion with infected blood products serve as other transmission mechanisms. Unfortunately, sexual abuse by an infected adult is another possible cause of transmission that must be considered in older pediatric patients.

Factors that appear to affect transmission include the level of maternal immune suppression, whether or not there was continuous exposure during pregnancy, and whether the maternal disease is active or latent.

Pathophysiology. The causative organism of AIDS is the retrovirus HIV-1. Upon entering the body, it infects the T-helper lymphocytes (T4) by attaching to the CD4+ molecule. It also infects monocytes, macrophages, and cells of the central nervous system. Once the T4 cell is infected, it is destroyed by the virus. This results in abnormal humoral and cell-mediated immunity. This insidious destruction of the immune system makes the patient vulnerable to opportunistic infection that are usually kept in check by the immune system.

Manifestations. The time interval between initial infection and the development of AIDS, called the incubation period, is extremely variable, with a range reportedly from 6 weeks to 10 years.[1] The manifestations of AIDS in the infant and child are often different than those seen in the adult patient. Clinically, the patient may show a failure to thrive and be developmentally delayed. Other clinical signs include unexplained lymphadenopathy, chronic diarrhea, progressive neurologic dysfunction, hepatosplenomegaly, persistent oral/esophageal candidiasis, bacterial sepsis, and infection with hepatitis B. As in adults, the presence of opportunistic infections, such as Pneumocystis carinii pneumonia (PCP), Kaposi's sarcoma, tuberculosis, cytomegalovirus retinitis, and mycobacterium avium complex (MAC), indicate the presence of AIDS.

Diagnosis. Current methods to diagnose AIDS infection are based on the presence of serum antibodies against the HIV. The *enzyme-linked immunosorbent assay (ELISA)* and *Western Blot* tests, if positive, show the presence of antibodies against the HIV, not the actual presence of the HIV. Of the two, the Western Blot is more specific and has a higher sensitivity. It is always run following a positive ELISA test. Both tests are nondiagnostic in patients under 14 months, because both tests may be positive from antibodies passed transplacentally from the mother, when in reality, the infant has not been exposed to the virus.

Several new techniques are being used to diagnose HIV infection. These include polymerase chain reaction (PCR), which detects HIV DNA or RNA sequence, P24 antigen, HIV cultures, enzyme-linked immunospot (ELISPOT), in vitro antibody production assay (IVAP), and IgA and IgM assays.

Of the new techniques, PCR detects the presence of the virus and not the antibodies, making it more promising for diagnosis in newborns. Both the P24 antigen and HIV cultures take 2 to 5 weeks to get results, which is a disadvantage to their use. The ELISPOT technique detects antibody-secreting cells. HIV infection stimulates the infant's immune system to produce antibody-producing B lymphocytes, which can then be detected by IVAP. Finally, because both IgA and IgM molecules do not pass through the placenta, their increasing level in the infant signals HIV infection. When HIV is perinatally acquired, the infection can be diagnosed by the time the child is 4 to 6 months of age with the use of current tests available.

Treatment. HIV has the ability to escape detection by the body's immune system, which would normally attack and kill the virus. Therapy for AIDS utilizes a multifactorial approach with antiretroviral drugs, antibiotics, antifungals, antiparasitic drugs, and active and passive immunization.[5] Treatment is aimed at slowing progression of the disease and prophylactically treating against opportunistic infections.

The standard drug used to slow the progression of AIDS is the antiviral drug zidovudine (ZDV). It is usually started when the T cell count falls below 500 and then increased in dosage sequentially following the level of T cells. Other drugs used investigationally to slow AIDS progression include dideoxyinosine (ddl), and 2'3'-dide-oxycytidine (ddC).

Therapies used as prophylaxis against PCP include trimethoprim-sulfamethoxasole (TMP/SMX), dapsone, and aerosolized pentamidine. Therapy with corticosteroids in patients with PCP has been shown to reduce morbidity and mortality.[6] Didanosine has shown to be effective in pediatric patients over 12 weeks of age.

Serious bacterial infections are often seen in patients receiving ZDV therapy. A reduction of these bacterial infections has been identified in patients receiving TMP/SMX and in those not on TMP/SMX who received intravenous immunoglobulins.

Recommendations for prevention of HIV transmission in the health care setting have been outlined by the Centers for Disease Control and Prevention.[7] Hand washing, as always, is mandatory, as is the wearing of gloves, eye shields and masks, and clothing covers whenever contact with infected material is possible. Cleaning of equipment, countertops or other surfaces should be done with a 1:10 solution of 5.25% strength hypochlorite to kill the virus.

Outcome. Once diagnosed with AIDS, pediatric survival averages 62 months, as compared to 11 months for adults.[8] The level of disability varies greatly, depending on the severity of infection and the presence of opportunistic infections. It appears that more aggressive therapy may result in reduced morbidity and longer lifespan.

Psychosocial Implications. While education surrounding AIDS has improved, much work remains to be done. The implications of an AIDS diagnosis are extreme, not only to the patient, but to the family as well. Socially, it is not uncommon for the patient and family to be isolated and discriminated against. The stigma surrounding AIDS is difficult to eradicate and much work remains to be done. Financially, AIDS can be an overwhelming burden. Many patients come from an impoverished background, with no health care coverage. In these cases, the cost of treatment is often shouldered by public or government agencies. Even for those with coverage, the cost of treatment can be very high. AIDS causes a significant amount of stress to the family unit. Parents, siblings, extended family members, and even the patient all must learn to deal with the grief associated with the prognosis. As the disease progresses, the neurological dysfunction of the patient adds additional stress to the situation.

Above all, when treating children with AIDS, the respiratory care practitioner, and all other health care workers, must remember that these patients need and deserve much understanding and love.

Cytomegalovirus (CMV). CMV is a member of the herpes virus family and is passed transplacentally from the asymptomatic mother. CMV is most devastating to the fetus early in gestation, while having few, if any, effects on the term neonate. Patients with suspected CMV infections should not be treated by any pregnant personnel. The wearing of gloves when handling urine and secretions and good hand washing help prevent the spread of the virus.

Symptoms include intrauterine growth retardation, direct hyperbilirubinemia secondary to liver damage, hepatosplenomegaly, microcephaly, brain damage, and progressive sensorineural hearing loss.

Rubella. Rubella infections of the fetus in the first 5 months of gestation have a high incidence of congenital abnormalities. Rubella is preventable by appropriate vaccination of the mother before conception.

Symptoms of early gestation infection include cataracts, cardiac defects, hearing loss, intrauterine growth retardation, chronic encephalitis, direct hyperbilirubinemia, and microcephaly. The various organs of the growth-retarded fetus are hypoplastic as the rubella virus impairs the proliferation of cells, if acquired in early gestation. The combined presence of cataracts and congenital cardiac disease strongly suggests the diagnosis of congenital rubella infection.

Herpes Simplex Types I and II. Type I herpes is the common variety of the virus that causes recurrent lesions on the lips and on other parts of the skin above the waist. Type II is the variety most commonly acquired by the neonate.

The fetus is infected by the ascent of the virus up the birth canal, from infected genitalia, or from the direct contact with infected tissues during delivery. There may also be a rare transplacental passage of the virus. The fetus of a mother with known type II herpes, is best delivered via cesarean delivery, although the possibility of infection still exists.

In the infected neonate, symptoms are both *disseminated* or widespread, and nondisseminated, or localized. Neonates with disseminated symptoms have a 96% mortality rate, while those with nondisseminated symptoms have a 25% mortality rate. Disseminated symptoms include hepatosplenomegaly, hepatitis with jaundice, bleeding disorders, widespread skin lesions, and neurologic abnormalities. Convulsions, abnormal muscle tone, bulging fontanelle, lethargy, and coma are common neurologic abnormalities. The nondisseminated forms of the disease attack the eyes, central nervous system, and the skin.

Diagnosis is usually made from cultures of the virus from skin lesions. Some studies have shown a decreased mortality from herpes infections in the neonate with the use of adenine arabinoside (ara-A).

Several new antiviral drugs are available for the treatment of herpes simplex and zoster. Acyclovir (Zovirax®) is indicated for the treatment of neonatal herpes simplex, varicella zoster with CNS and pulmonary involvement, and herpes simplex encephalitis.[9] Two newer antiviral drugs, famcyclovir (Famvir®) and valacyclovir (Valtrex®) have shown significant effectiveness in the treatment of herpes and may gain use in the neonatal and pediatric populations in the future.

ETIOLOGY: PROTOZOA

Toxoplasmosis. *Toxoplasma gondii* is the protozoa organism responsible for toxoplasmosis infections. It is contracted by the mother via contact with cat feces or from eating raw meat. The organism is transmitted from the mother to the fetus through the placenta. The infected mother may be asymptomatic or may show influenza-like signs.

Transmission of the disease occurs mainly during the third trimester for unknown reasons. In the neonate, symptoms may be present immediately or may be delayed for several weeks. Those symptoms include neurological abnormalities such as microcephaly, coma, convulsions, and hydrocephalus. Other symptoms are hepatosplenomegaly, jaundice with both direct and indirect hyperbilirubinemia, *petechiae* of the skin, and pallor secondary to anemia.

Diagnosis is verified by the presence of specific toxoplasma IgM antibodies in the blood serum.

Pneumocystis carinii. As discussed previously in this chapter, *Pneumocystis carinii* is a protozoan infection that is seen primarily in immunocompromised patients, such as those with AIDS.

DIAGNOSIS AND TREATMENT OF INFECTION

In most instances, diagnosis of infection is made by isolating and identifying the antigen from specimens taken from the neonate or by serologic diagnosis, which shows an antibody response to the specific agent.

Viral diseases are treated by proper prevention of the disease in the mother. Proper immunization against rubella in the mother will prevent fetal infection. Toxoplasmosis is best prevented by avoidance of cat litter boxes and raw meat by pregnant mothers and by those attempting to get pregnant.

Bacterial infections are treated by administering broad-spectrum antibiotics such as ampicillin to the neonate until the pathogen is identified. Upon identification of the causative organism and its sensitivities, a specific antibiotic is selected. The ideal antibiotic will be the least toxic to the patient and lethal to the organism. Many institutions will administer broad-spectrum antibiotics for 48 to 72 hours any time the amniotic membranes have been ruptured for more than 24 hours, due to the high risk of infection imposed upon the fetus.

It is often very difficult to differentiate between bacterial pneumonia and RDS. For this reason, the practitioner must closely monitor the patient's ventilatory status and be prepared to ventilate the patient if the status worsens.

PREVENTION OF INFECTION

The most important factor in prevention of infection, both viral and bacterial, is proper aseptic technique. This includes proper hand washing, wearing of gloves when handling infected material, use of masks to prevent the spread of respiratory infections, and proper disposal of infected material. All equipment must be sterilized and aseptic technique followed when working with infected patients. Personnel may also further protect themselves by adhering to the standard precautions listed in Table 11–2.

FETAL IMMUNITIES

The fetus is endowed with certain immunities from its mother and also produces immunities of its own. These immunities are in the form of antibodies. An antibody is a type of protein produced by plasma cells in response to the presence of an antigen. An antigen is defined as anything that stimulates the production of antibodies.

The immunities that will be examined circulate in the plasma and are called *immunoglobulins* (Ig). Immunoglobulins are classified into five classes: IgA, IgD, IgE, IgG, and IgM. Of the five classes IgA, IgG, and IgM play major roles in the immunities of the neonate.

IgA ANTIBODY

IgA is not transported transplacentally and is not produced by the neonate until approximately 1 month of age. The importance of the IgA antibody lies in a subclass of antibody

---

Table 11–2   Standard Precautions

1. Gloves should be worn for direct contact with blood, body fluids and secretions, wounds, and for handling all items or surfaces that are contaminated with blood, body fluids, or secretions. Gloves should be worn for venipuncture and for handling vascular access lines or intravascular monitoring devices.
2. Gloves should be changed between patients, when they are torn, or whenever a perforation occurs, as with a needlestick injury. Hands should be washed whenever gloves are removed.
3. Hands should be washed immediately whenever contamination with blood or body fluids or secretion occurs.
4. Masks and protective eyewear or face shields should be worn during procedures in which splattering, splashing, or generation of droplets of blood, body fluids, or secretions is likely to occur.
5. Gowns or aprons should be worn under conditions described in item 4.
6. Precautions should be taken when handling needles and sharp instruments. Used disposable needless and syringes, scalpels, and other sharp items should be placed into puncture-resistant containers for disposal. Used needles should not be bent, broken, recapped, or cut.
7. Mouthpieces, resuscitation bags, and other ventilatory devices should be available to minimize the need for mouth-to-mouth resuscitation.
8. All blood and body fluid specimens should be placed into a sturdy, leakproof container for transport to the laboratory. The laboratory requisition form should be placed outside this container to minimize contamination.
9. Health care workers with exudative skin lesions should refrain from patient care activities.

called secretory IgA. Secretory IgA is found in tears, saliva, bronchial and intestinal secretions, and breast milk. Its presence enables the body to defend against antigens at the source of entry into the body. Breast-fed neonates gain immunity from the IgA in the milk while their own systems are maturing. Breast milk IgA protects the intestinal system from *Escherichia coli, Vibrio cholerae,* poliovirus, and rotovirus.[10] As the neonate grows, it begins producing and secreting its own IgA.

IgD ANTIBODY

The IgD antibody is a specialized protein found in serum tissue. The exact role of IgD is not known, but it increases in quantity in the presence of allergic reactions to milk, penicillin, insulin, and various toxins.

IgE ANTIBODY

IgE is concentrated in the lung, skin, and the cells of the mucous membranes. IgE is responsible for allergic reactions that cause the release of the allergic mediators from the mast cell. It provides the primary defense against environmental antigens.

IgG ANTIBODY

The IgG antibody is the only immunoglobulin that is transported through the placenta from mother to fetus. It accumulates in the fetus during the third trimester, reaching its highest level at birth. Because the majority of antibodies in the maternal circulation are of the IgG fractions the fetus receives a healthy portion of them.

The IgG antibody protects the neonate from infections to which the mother has acquired immunity. These infections include pneumococcus, streptococcus, meningococcus, *Hemophilus influenzae,* viruses, and the toxins of tetanus and diphtheria. The baby begins to synthesize its own IgG antibody as the maternal level falls to lower levels. This occurs around the third month following delivery.

IgM ANTIBODY

The IgM antibody is produced by the fetus around the 30th week of gestation and does not cross the placenta from the mother. Any IgM present at birth represents the baby's own synthesis of the antibody. The measurement of IgM levels in the neonate is used to detect the presence of infection. IgM levels do not rise for a week to 10 days following the appearance of disease. This makes it unreliable for early detection of infection. IgM levels rapidly increase during the first month of life and then gradually slow.

IgM synthesis is stimulated by most infectious organisms and is the main fetally produced antibody present in the baby.

CONGENITAL ANOMALIES

PULMONARY SYSTEM

Tracheoesophageal Anomalies. Atresia of the upper esophagus, with an accompanying fistula between the lower esophageal tube and the trachea, shown in Figure 11–1A, accounts for 75 to 80% of all tracheoesophageal anomalies. Other combinations of atresias and fistulas occur in much less frequency.

The next most common problem, accounting for about 8% of esophageal anomalies, is atresia of the esophagus, without any fistula attachment to the trachea, shown in Figure 11–1B. Other possible combinations, occurring very infrequently, are the so-called H-type fistula, illustrated in Figure 11–1C, esophageal atresia with attachment of the upper esophagus to the trachea, depicted in Figure 11–1D and attachment of the upper and lower portions of the esophagus to the trachea, represented in Figure 11–1E.

Diagnosis and Treatment. Diagnosis of esophageal-tracheal anomalies is usually based on the presence of three distinct clinical symptoms: 1) accumulation of secretions in the mouth;

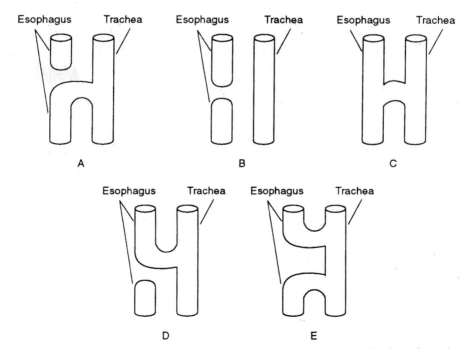

Figure 11–1 *A. The most common variety of tracheoesophageal anomaly. B. Esophageal atresia without a fistula to the trachea. C. The "H" type of tracheoesophageal anomaly. D. A lower esophageal atresia with upper attachment to the trachea. E. Upper and lower attchment of the esophagus to the trachea.*

2) sporadic or continuous respiratory distress, especially during feedings; and 3) repeated regurgitation of feelings.

In the presence of these signs, insertion of a nasogastric tube (NG) is attempted. Air is then injected into the catheter while listening with a stethoscope over the stomach. Absence of any sounds in the stomach requires the obtaining of a CXR. The air-filled pouch of the esophageal atresia can often be visualized on the x-ray.

Upon diagnosis of this disorder, the patient should be kept in a 30° upright position to help prevent aspiration. Treatment is always surgical repair of the defect. Although not an emergency procedure, the surgical repair of the defect should be done as quickly as possible. Surgical correction is done through an incision in the right retropleural area. The distal esophagus is divided from the trachea, and the ends of the esophagus are sutured together.

Caregivers should observe the patient for signs of worsening ventilatory status that may follow aspiration pneumonitis.

Choanal Atresia. The portion of the nasal cavity that opens into the nasopharynx is called the choana. *Choanal atresia,* illustrated in Figure 11–2, occurs when the membrane that separates the nasal cavity from the nasopharynx during embryologic development fails to disintegrate and blocks the passage of air.

This defect is apparent almost immediately in the neonate, as severe respiratory distress is usually present. The neonate's reliance on nasal breathing at its prime method of venti-

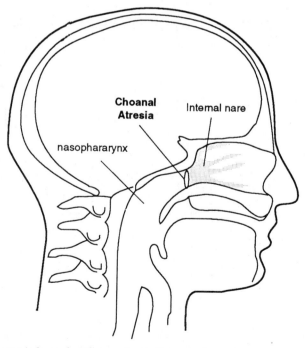

Figure 11–2 *Choanal atresia located at the opening to the nasopharynx.*

lation accounts for the severity of the distress. Choanal atresia is suspected as respiratory distress improves when the neonate cries. Diagnosis is verified by the inability to pass an NG tube past the obstruction.

Immediate treatment requires the use of an oral airway. Some neonates may require intubation to relieve the distress. Long-term treatment involves surgical removal of the membranes covering the choanae.

Diaphragmatic Hernia. Herniation of abdominal contents into the thorax is caused by an incomplete embryologic formation of the diaphragm. It most often occurs on the left side, slightly posterior and lateral, through the foramen of Bochdalek. It occurs less frequently in other locations on the left side and very rarely occurs on the right side. It occurs in approximately 1 in 2200 births.

When the herniation occurs on the left side, the stomach and intestines may enter the thorax and compress the lung, pushing the mediastinum to the right. Right-sided herniation may involve the liver and intestines, compressing the lung and pushing the mediastinum to the left.

The degree of distress noted in the neonate depends on the severity of herniation. As the neonate starts breathing, the presence of the abdominal contents compresses the lungs, making it extremely difficult for the neonate to inspire. Further distension of the intestines and stomach with air compresses the lungs even more, worsening the respiratory distress.

Symptoms. The presence of cyanosis, respiratory distress, bowel sounds in the chest, a flat abdomen, and the presence of *polyhydramnios* (excess amniotic fluid) are indications of a diaphragmatic hernia. The diagnosis is verified by a chest x-ray, showing the loops of bowel in the thorax. Right-sided hernias show a large density created by the liver in the right thorax. The mediastinal contents are pushed away from the affected side.

In left-sided hernia, heart sounds may be heard in the right chest. Mortality is high due to *hypoplastic* lungs and the inability to ventilate the patient.

Treatment. Immediately upon diagnosis, a nasogastric tube attached to suction should be placed in the neonate. If the patient must be ventilated, it must be done through an endotracheal tube and not by bag and mask.

The lungs of the neonate with this anomaly are in various stages of hypoplasia. The lungs are therefore very stiff and susceptible to barotrauma, especially pneumothoraces. When ventilating with a mask, the gas enters the esophagus and stomach due to the low compliance of the lungs. As the stomach fills with gas, it further compresses the lungs and makes ventilation extremely compromised.

Ventilation through an endotracheal tube should be done using rates near or above 100/min and low PIP and PEEP pressures to avoid barotrauma. An umbilical artery catheter should be placed to monitor blood gases and blood pressure. Surgical repair is done through the abdomen or chest to repair the defect.

Postoperatively, the patient is ventilated for at least 24 hours. As with the preoperative treatment, high rates and low pressures should be used to avoid barotrauma on the hypoplastic lungs. Monitoring of preductal and postductal arterial oxygen will help in the detection of right-to-left shunts. It is often desirable to paralyze the patient to facilitate ventilation.

Dopamine is started if cardiac output is diminished followed by the administration of colloids to maintain adequate cardiac output and perfusion.

The pulmonary status of the patient usually begins to improve by the third postoperative day. At this point, the medications and ventilator settings are slowly weaned.

Pierre-Robin Syndrome (Micrognathia). Pierre-Robin syndrome is hypoplasia of the mandible, which forces the tongue to be positioned posteriorly in the pharynx, creating an obstruction to breathing. It occurs in 1 out of 2000 births, with 50 to 70% having a cleft palate. The diagnosis is made by observation of a short jaw or receding chin during examination.

The treatment is to maintain the patient's airway patency until the mandible grows to its appropriate size, usually by 6 months to a year of age. This may require procedures such as facial slings, metal appliances passed through the lips to support the tongue, suturing the tongue to traction, and tracheostomy.

Care should be taken during feedings to prevent choking on the formula. Special feeders (Breck) are used to prevent aspiration. Often the patient's airway patency is maintained by having the neonate in a face-down position while sleeping.

CARDIAC SYSTEM

Congenital cardiac defects occur in approximately 1 out of 100 deliveries. Depending on the type and degree of defect, the patient may have mild signs that require no intervention or may have life-threatening symptoms that require immediate intervention. This section will look at the different types of cardiac defects, their signs, diagnosis, and treatment.

Patent Ductus Arteriosus (PDA). Anatomically, the ductus arteriosus connects the pulmonary artery to the aorta, shunting blood away from the lungs in the fetus. The smooth musculature that surrounds the ductus arteriosus develops toward the end of gestation. The vessel is maintained patent in the fetus by the presence of prostaglandins, which cause the smooth muscle to remain in a dilated state.

Closure of the ductus arteriosus following delivery is caused by several factors, including blood oxygen tension, levels of circulating prostaglandins, and the muscle mass present in the vessel. Studies have additionally connected the constrictive effects of acetylcholine, low pH, bradykinin, and catecholamines to ductal closure.[10] Closure of the ductus arteriosus usually occurs a few hours to a few days following delivery.

Pathophysiology. As the pressure in the pulmonary vasculature drops below arterial pressure, blood is shunted from the aorta through the ductus arteriosus into the pulmonary system, creating a left-to-right shunt, as shown in Figure 11–3A. The blood shunted into the pulmonary artery greatly increases intrapulmonary vascular and right-heart pressures. The result is a hyperperfusion and engorgement of the pulmonary vessels with resulting pulmonary edema. When large amounts of blood are shunted through the ductus, hypoperfusion occurs to all postductal organs and tissues, leading to necrotizing enterocolitis and other disorders. Right-sided heart failure may follow long bouts with a PDDA. If pulmonary vascular pressures exceed aortic pressures, blood is shunted from the pulmonary artery to the aorta, creating a right-to-left shunt, depicted in Figure 11–3B.

A PDA is not always undesirable. In the presence of certain heart defects, such as transposition of the great vessels, a PDA may be the only life-sustaining connection between pulmonary and systemic circulation. In this instance, it is desirable for the ductus arteriosus to remain open. This can be accomplished by the administration of prostaglandin E_1 (PGE_1), which can reopen a constricted ductus arteriosus and prevent the ductus from closing.

PGE_1 is indicated for any defect in which the left heart is obstructed or pulmonary perfusion is decreased. Following the administration of the drug, arterial oxygen levels improve and pulmonary congestion decreases, reducing the level of ventilatory support needed. Improvement in patient condition following administration of PGE_1 depends on the degree of ductal patency before the drug is given, with patients having total ductal closure showing the most dramatic improvements.

Diagnosis. Diagnosis of a PDA involves both clinical symptoms and laboratory data. The most common indication of a PDA is a loud grade I to grade III systolic murmur heard at the upper left sternal border. Some describe the murmur as sounding like a washing machine.

Positive identification of a PDA is made by ultrasound in which the ductus arteriosus is visible between the aorta and pulmonary artery. The use of *color flow mapping* can aid in detecting the direction of blood flow through the ductus. In the absence of color flow mapping, the direction of blood flow through the ductus can be determined using oxygen and noninvasive monitors.

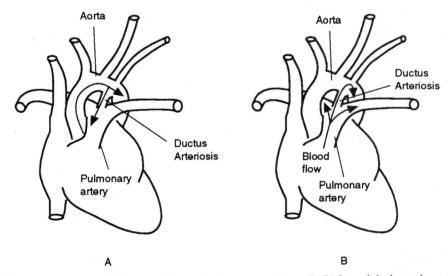

Figure 11–3 *A. Left-to-right shunt through the ductus arteriosus. B. Right-to-left shunt through the ductus arteriosus resulting from pulmonary vascular pressure exceeding aortic pressure.*

A right-to-left shunt through a PDA is indicated when low arterial oxygen levels do not change with increases in FiO_2. Placement of a pulse oximeter or $TcPO_2$ monitor preductally on the right arm and another postductally on the abdomen or lower extremities shows the higher preductal oxygen level, further indicating a right-to-left ductal shunt.

Left-to-right shunting is indicated by signs of congestive heart failure and pulmonary edema. The chest x-ray will show cardiomegaly with increased pulmonary vascularity.

Treatment. Treatment of a PDA is limited to those patients who show associated signs and symptoms. At the first sign of symptoms, usually the appearance of a significant murmur, a fluid restriction of <120 ml/kg/day is started. A continuation of the murmur along with bounding pulses, active precordium, and an unimproved or deteriorating respiratory status indicate additional treatment with the diuretic furosemide (Lasix). The benefit of digoxin for the treatment of PDA in the preemie is questionable.[11]

The Symptomatic infant of less than 1000 grams requires closure of the PDA either surgically or by the administration of *indomethacin* (Indocin).[12] Indomethacin is used to block prostagladin production in the ductus, allowing the smooth muscle to constrict. Two dangerous side effects of indomethacin administration are a constriction of renal vasculature with ensuing reduction in renal function and a reduction in platelet adhesion, leading to potential bleeding.

Symptomatic infants weighing over 1000 grams are placed on the previously mentioned fluid restriction for 48 hours. If ventilator parameters improve during that time, fluids are gradually increased. If the patient's condition worsens again, or if there was no improvement during the 48-hour trial, then methods to close the ductus should be considered.

Early closure of the PDA may decrease the incidence of BPD by reducing the amount of time spent on the ventilator.

Atrial Septal Defect (ASD). The most common type of ASD is an incompetent foramen ovale. This defect is called an osteum secundum defect and usually involves a failure of the tissue flap to cover the foramen, allowing the movement of blood between atria. Openings in the atria can also occur in the upper and lower atrial septum. Defects in the lower septum are often associated with clefts in the mitral or tricuspid valves.

Diagnosis. A majority of ASDs are symptomless and go undetected. Severe ASDs may result in left-to-right shunting with resultant right ventricular overload; however, this is uncommon. There may also be an increase in atrial arrhythmias as the patient matures.

Ventricular Septal Defect (VSD). Defects in the ventricular septum, seen in Figure 11–4, may be isolated, or may occur with other cardiac defects. VSDs are classified according to where they are located when looked at from the right ventricle. In the presence of normal pulmonary vascular resistance, a VSD leads to left-to-right shunting of blood from left ventricle to right ventricle.

As pulmonary resistance increases, as occurs with RDS, the left-to-right shunting may be minimal. Small VSDs may go unnoticed and be asymptomatic.

Diagnosis and Treatment. Diagnosis of a VSD is usually made by two-dimensional ultrasound. Treatment is usually withheld, unless the patient demonstrates a failure to thrive or congestive heart failure that does not respond to treatment. In these cases, the VSD is surgically closed by suture or patch.

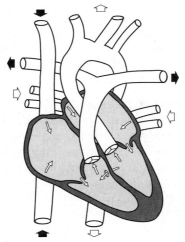

Figure 11–4 *Ventricular septal defect.*

Tetralogy of Fallot. This combination of defects is the most common cause of cyanotic cardiac disease. The four defects that make up tetralogy of Fallot, pictured in Figure 11–5, are: 1) VSD; 2) an overriding aorta; 3) hypertrophy of the right ventricle; and 4) obstruction to flow through the pulmonary artery.

Cyanosis is caused by decreased blood flow through the pulmonary artery and the resultant passage of venous blood into the aorta. Arterial pH and $PaCO_2$ values are typically normal with decreased PaO_2 in proportion to the amount of pulmonary artery obstruction. On the chest x-ray, the heart has been described as looking like a boot, with normal lung markings.

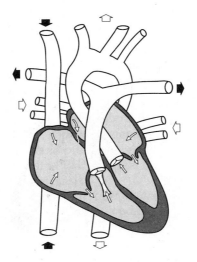

Figure 11–5 *Tetralogy of Fallot.*

Diagnosis and Treatment. Ultrasound is normally used to diagnose this disorder. The echocardiogram can detect the overriding aorta as well as the presence of the VSD. Cardiac catheterization is used to verify the diagnosis and to differentiate between pulmonary atresia, which has many of the same symptoms. Surgical repair includes closure of the VSD and relief of the pulmonary outflow obstruction.

Complete Transposition of the Great Vessels. In this defect the aorta arises from the right ventricle and the pulmonary artery arises from the left ventricle. Blood flow leaving the right ventricle is passed through the body and returns to the right atrium. Oxygenated blood from the pulmonary system enters the left atrium, the left ventricle, and is then passed through the pulmonary artery into the lungs again, as shown in Figure 11–6. Without an abnormal opening between the two systems, life is not possible.

Mixing of the two blood flows occurs through an ASD, a PDA, or through a VSD. The degree of cyanosis is usually profound with this defect, but may be minimal if a large shunt is present. The patient will often show signs of congestive heart failure. Blood gases show normal or slightly elevated arterial $PaCO_2$, normal or slightly acidotic pH, and an extremely low PaO_2 that is unaffected by oxygen administration.

Diagnosis and Treatment. Cardiac ultrasound is very useful in diagnosis, and cardiac catheterization verifies the diagnosis. *Balloon septostomy* is required during the cardiac catheterization to improve mixing of the two blood flows.

Surgical correction involves either the dissection of the aorta and pulmonary artery with reattachment to the correct ventricle or the redirection of atrial blood flows to the opposite ventricles. Administration of prostaglandin E_1 may be used to keep the ductus arteriosus open and improve oxygenation.

Subaortic Stenosis. This cardiac defect involves stenosis either at the aortic valve, above it, or below it, illustrated in Figure 11–7, causing an obstruction to the outflow from the left

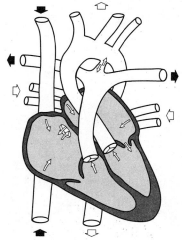

Figure 11–6 *Complete transposition of the great vessels.*

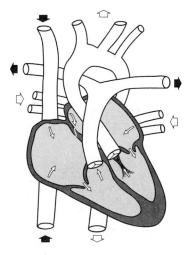

Figure 11–7   *Subaortic stenosis.*

ventricle. The cardinal findings in this defect are secondary to the reduction in cardiac output. The neonate has cool pale skin secondary to poor perfusion and diminished peripheral pulses. Severe stenosis may cause a dramatic decrease in blood pressure also.

Diagnosis and Treatment. Diagnosis is mainly accomplished by cardiac catheterization. A pressure difference of 50 mm Hg between the left ventricle and the aorta shows significant involvement. On ultrasound, the aortic valve appears thickened with an enlarged left ventricle and diminished stroke volumes. Blood gas values are typically normal. The chest x-ray will show a cardiomegaly, but is otherwise unremarkable. The only treatment for this defect is surgical intervention to repair the stenotic valve.

Coarctation of the Aorta. Coarctation of the aorta, seen in Figure 11–8, involves a constriction of the aorta that severely restricts blood flow. It can occur anywhere on the aorta from the aortic root to the abdominal aorta, but most commonly occurs near the entry of the ductus arteriosus into the aorta.

   The location of the stricture and the presence of other anomalies determine the clinical signs the patient demonstrates. The most common anomalies associated with coarctation of the aorta are PDA, VSD, and a defective aortic valve. Signs of this disease are associated with a decrease in cardiac output. The coarctation causes an increase in *afterload*, which leads to left-heart enlargement and increased pressures previous to the defect. With a coarctation distal to the aortic arch, it is possible to measure higher systolic pressures in the upper extremities than the systolic pressure in the lower extremities. CXR findings show cardiomegaly and increased vascular markings indicating pulmonary venous obstruction. Blood gases are typically normal and nondiagnostic.

Diagnosis and Treatment. Positive diagnosis is made by visualization of the stricture via ultrasound and followed up with cardiac catheterization. Treatment is surgical repair of the

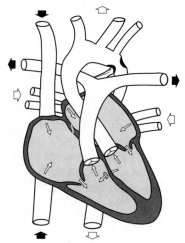

Figure 11–8 *Coarctation of the aorta.*

aorta by using the left subclavian artery to patch the aorta and increase its diameter. Prostaglandin E_1 is used to maintain ductal patency and increase blood flow to the descending aorta.

Tricuspid Atresia. Tricuspid atresia, shown in Figure 11–9, results from a complete agenesis of the tricuspid valve between the right atrium and ventricle. The result is that no blood flows between the two. The venous blood is therefore shunted through the foramen ovale or an ASD into the left atrium. Blood flow to the lungs must come from either a PDA or a VSD. The right ventricle and pulmonary artery may be hypoplastic if a large PDA exists. Cyanosis is present when there is a significant compromise in pulmonary blood flow. Blood

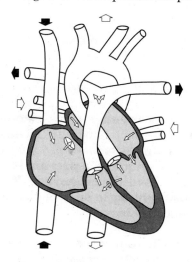

Figure 11–9 *Tricuspid atresia.*

gases show normal pH and $PaCO_2$. PaO_2 may be near normal in the presence of a large VSD or PDA, or may be tremendously low if there is little blood flow to the lungs.

Diagnosis and Treatment. On ultrasound the tricuspid valve is not seen, and color flows will show atrial shunting and the presence of a PDA or VSD. Immediate treatment involves cardiac catheterization with a balloon septostomy to improve mixing in the atria. Permanent treatment involves the surgical creation of a connection between the right atria and pulmonary artery or right ventricle (*Fontan procedure*), and the closure of any septal defects.

Anomalous Venous Return. This defect, presented in Figure 11–10, involves the return of pulmonary venous blood to the right atrium instead of the left atrium. An ASD must be present in order for the neonate to survive. These patients are typically cyanotic to some degree. The pH and $PaCO_2$ are near normal, with the level of PaO_2 depending on the degree of pulmonary blood flow. Ultrasound is usually nondiagnostic for this disease. Immediate cardiac catheterization with a balloon septostomy should be performed to increase intra-atrial mixing. Surgical correction is then needed to reimplant the pulmonary veins into the left atria.

Truncus Arteriosus. Truncus arteriosus (Figure 11–11) is a defect in which one large vessel arises from both right and left ventricles over a large VSD. The large vessel gives rise to the pulmonary arteries, the coronary arteries, and the systemic arteries and has one valve at its origin.

Cyanosis is usually present to some degree due to the pulmonary and systemic blood flows arising from a common vessel. Minimal cyanosis indicates adequate pulmonary perfusion. Blood gases may be normal or may show a decreased PaO_2 when pulmonary perfusion is decreased. On the chest x-ray, there are typically increased lung vasculature markings secondary to the increased pulmonary pressures.

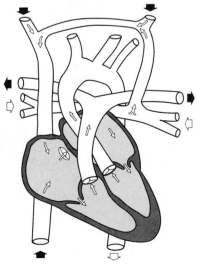

Figure 11–10 *Anomalous venous return.*

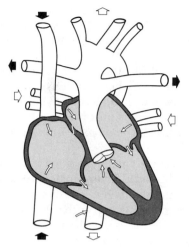

Figure 11–11 *Truncus arteriosus.*

Diagnosis and Treatment. Echocardiography is useful in diagnosis, and the presence of only one valve helps differentiate this condition from tetralogy of Fallot. Cardiac catheterization is used to verify the diagnosis. Surgical treatment involves separating the pulmonary artery from the large vessel, closing the VSD, and placing a valve between the right ventricle and pulmonary artery. Prognosis is poor with this defect, having a 40 to 50% mortality rate.

Hypoplastic Left-Heart Syndrome. This syndrome involves several anomalies including coarctation of the aorta, hypoplastic left ventricle, and aortic and mitral valve stenosis or atresia. These lesions lead to a diminished blood flow through the left ventricle and lead to an obligatory left-to-right atrial shunt and a right-to-left ductal shunt. Constriction of the ductus arteriosus leads to rapid hypotension and shock.

Diagnosis and Treatment. Diagnosis of hypoplastic left-heart syndrome is based on physical signs and laboratory data. Physically, the patient appears ashen and grayish as a result of hypoperfusion. A nonspecific systolic murmur may be heard. Signs of congestive heart failure, such as bounding pulses, an active precordium, and an enlarged liver, may be present.

Laboratory diagnosis is made by echocardiogram and cardiac catheterization showing a small left ventricle, abnormal aortic valve, and small ascending aorta.

There is no current medical treatment for hypoplastic left-heart syndrome. The only chance for survival is a risky surgical procedure.[12]

RESPIRATORY CARE OF THE PATIENT WITH CARDIAC DEFECTS

The various cardiac defects discussed differ in how they affect the pulmonary system. Cardiac defects either reduce blood flow to the lungs or increase pulmonary blood flow. Defects that reduce pulmonary flow include tricuspid atresia and tetralogy of Fallot. Defects that increase blood flow include VSD, coarctation of the aorta, subaortic stenosis, PDA, and anomalous venous return.

In neonates with decreased pulmonary blood flow, lung compliance is typically increased. The use of too high ventilatory pressures further compromises blood flow and worsens V/Q ratios. Changing the frequency of ventilation instead of inspiratory pressures will help keep mean airway pressure low and still meet ventilatory needs. Cautious use of oxygen is also required in these patients as high PaO_2 will increase the chance of the closure of the PDA, which may be the only source of pulmonary blood flow in these patients.

In contrast to patients with decreased blood flow, increased pulmonary blood flow decreases the lung compliance. In these patients, higher ventilatory pressures and PEEP are required to maintain adequate V/Q ratios. The higher pulmonary blood pressures are less affected by the increases in ventilatory pressures in these patients. Oxygen must also be used judiciously in these patients if the cardiac defect involves a necessary PDA.

A recent study evaluated the change in pulmonary function following the successful closure of a PDA. The authors concluded there is significant improvement in compliance and other ventilatory parameters in those patients with a successful closure.[13] It can probably be assumed that correction of the other heart defects that increase pulmonary blood flow would result in similar findings.

SUMMARY

While there are many disorders and diseases that cause persistent illness in the perinatal period, this chapter has summarized those that are most likely to be seen.

The fetus is susceptible to infection transplacentally, or by the organism ascending through the birth canal. During delivery, the fetus may come in contact with infected maternal blood, secretions, or lesions. Following delivery, the risk of nosocomial infection from personnel or equipment becomes a problem.

Bacterial infections are often acquired by the ascending route and lead to pneumonia, and less often, urinary tract infections and sepsis. Chorioamnionitis is a bacterial infection of the amniotic tissue and its presence indicates a high risk of fetal infection.

Viruses are unique in that they can lead to fetal malformation if acquired during certain developmental stages. In particular, rubella, CMV, and herpes can cause a great deal of problems in the developing fetus. Rubella affects the fetus in the first 5 months of gestation and causes cardiac defects, growth retardation, and hearing loss. CMV also affects the fetus during the early gestational period, causing brain and liver damage, growth retardation, and microcephaly. Herpes viruses are passed to the fetus during delivery, by contact with active genital lesions. Herpes may lead to severe neurologic problems, bleeding disorders, and liver problems. Prevention of infection in the mother is the only method of treatment often available, as little can be done once the damage has occurred.

A virus for which many volumes have been and will be written is HIV. This one virus has caused a significant portion of viral related morbidity and mortality and continues to defy methods of prevention and treatments. While the virus itself is not the cause of morbidity and mortality, by destroying the immune system, the patient becomes a victim of one of several opportunistic infections, such as *Pneumocystis carinii* pneumonia, Kaposi's sarcoma, and yeasts. As this virus continues to resist all attempts to control it, it will continue to play a major role in patient care efforts for the unforeseeable future. It is incumbent on the practitioner to be fully aware of the current preventive measures and treatments to competently take care of these patients. Above all, the practitioner must treat these patients with the same care and dignity as any other patient and, in addition, be aware of the special psychosocial needs of this special group.

Toxoplasmosis, a protozoan organism, affects the fetus during the last trimester of pregnancy and leads to severe neurological and hepatic disorders. *Pneumocystis carinii,* another protozoan organism, causes the opportunistic pneumonia seen in AIDS patients.

The fetus obtains some immunity transplacentally from the mother. The IgG antibody is the only one small enough to be passed transplacentally. It provides the fetus immunity to certain diseases that the mother has acquired immunity to. The IgM antibody is produced by the fetus around the 30th week of gestation. An increased level of IgM in the neonate is an indication that an infective process is present. The IgA antibody is produced by the neonate at about 1 month of life. Mainly a secreted antibody, it is found in the secretions of the gut, and respiratory tree. IgA is also found in breast milk and may aid in the protection of the gastrointestinal tract from bacterial invasion. The IgE antibody is the allergic response antibody and provides protection against environmental antigens. The last antibody, IgD, is present in serum tissue. Its exact role has yet to be determined.

Several anomalies can inflict the respiratory tract during fetal growth and development. Because the trachea and esophagus arise from the same germinal tissue, several defects can occur with either, or both. The most common type of anomaly is an atresia of the upper esophagus with an accompanying fistula between the lower esophagus and trachea. Other possible anomalies include esophageal atresia without any fistula, a normal esophagus and trachea with a fistula connecting the two ("H" type), lower esophageal atresia with the upper esophagus attaching to the trachea, and both upper and lower esophageal attachments to the trachea. Choanal atresia is a tissue blockage located at the posterior nasal chamber. Because neonates prefer to nose breath, this blockage can cause respiratory distress. Herniation of the diaphragm allows the abdominal contents, especially the stomach and small intestine, to enter the thoracic cavity. This compresses the lung on the affected side (almost always the left) and leads to significant respiratory distress. Intubation of these patients is mandatory to prevent air from passing into the stomach and further compromising lung status. Finally, Pierre-Robin syndrome (micrognathia) causes respiratory distress because of airway occlusion by the tongue. In this syndrome, the mandible fails to develop appropriately, causing the oral cavity to be too small for the normally developed tongue.

Cardiac defects are not uncommon, affecting 1 out of every 100 deliveries. Failure of the ductus arteriosus to close following delivery leads to the shunting of blood away from the lungs and difficulty in maintaining oxygenation. Another cardiac defect that leads to shunting is a defect in the atrial septum. Because of higher pressures in the left atrium, blood shunts from the left atrium to the right. Ventricular septal defects allow blood to shunt from the left ventricle to the right. One of the most well-known defects is tetralogy of Fallot. The tetrad of defects are ventricular septal defect, an overriding aorta, hypertrophy of the right ventricle, and pulmonary valve obstruction. Transposition of the great vessels occurs when the aorta arises from the right ventricle, and the pulmonary artery arises from the left ventricle. Coarctation of the aorta, involves a constriction of the aorta, which severely impedes blood flow. In tricuspid atresia, blood flow between the right atrium and right ventricle is interrupted and shunting through the foramen ovale occurs. Anomalous venous return involves the return of pulmonary blood flow to the right atrium instead of the left. In truncus arteriosus, one large vessel acts as both the aorta and pulmonary artery. Finally, hypoplastic left-heart syndrome is seen when outflow from the left ventricle is impeded by coarctation of the aorta and stenosis of the aortic valve. Respiratory care of these patients depends on an understanding as to whether the defect causes an increase or decrease of blood flow to the lungs. As changes occur, the practitioner must be ready to adjust ventilator settings to compensate for changes in compliance.

References

1. Shannon L. Clinical perspectives and current trends of HIV infection in the newborn and child. *Neonatal Network*. 1995;14:21–34.

2. Goedert JJ, et al. Mother-to-infant transmission of human immunodeficiency virus type I: association with prematurity or low anti-gp 120. *Lancet*. 1989;2:1351–1354.

3. Connor EM, et al. Reduction of maternal-infant transmission of human immunodeficiency virus type I with zidovudine treatment. Pediatric AIDS clinical trials. *N Engl J Med*. 1994;331:1173–1180.

4. Kuhn L, et al. Maternal-infant HIV transmission and circumstances of delivery. *Am J Public Health*. 1984;84:1110–1115.

5. Wu LR, et al. Therapy of pediatric AIDS. *Curr Opin Pediatr*. 1995;7:214–219.

6. Bye MR, et al. Markedly reduced mortality associated with corticosteroid therapy of pneumocystis carinii pneumonia in children with acquired immunodeficiency syndrome. *Arch Pediatr Adolesc Med*. 1994;148:638–641.

7. Notices to Readers: Publication of recommendations for prevention of HIV transmission in health-care settings. *MMWR Morb Mortal Wkly Rep*. 1987;36(suppl 2S).

8. Turner BJ, et al. A population-based comparison of the clinical course of children and adults with AIDS. *AIDS*. 1995;9:65–72.

9. Young TE, Mangum OB. *Neofax '93: A Manual of Drugs Used in Neonatal Care*. 6th ed. Columbus, Ohio: Ross Laboratories; 1993.

10. Avery GB, Fletcher MA, MacDonald MG. *Pathophysiology and Management of the Newborn*. 5th ed. Philadelphia: JB Lippincott Co; 1999.

11. Cloherty JP, Stark AR, eds. *Manual of Neonatal Care*. 4th ed. Philadelphia: Lippincott; 1997.

12. Merenstein GB, Gardner SL. *Handbook of Neonatal Intensive Care*. 4th ed. St. Louis, Mo: CV Mosby Co; 1998.

13. Stefano S, et al. Closure of the ductus arteriosus with indomethacin in ventiltaed neonates with respiratory distress syndrome: effects on pulmonary compliance and ventilation. *Rev Resp Dis*. 1991;143:236.

Bibliography and Suggested Readings

Blank A, et al. Maternal and pediatric AIDS in the United States: the current situation and future research directions. *Acta Paediatr Suppl.* 1994;400:106–110.

Levin D, Morriss F, et al. *Essentials of Pediatric Intensive Care.* 2nd ed. St. Louis, Mo: Quality Medical Publishing, Inc.: 1997.

Notterman DA, et al. Outcome after assisted ventilation in children with acquired immunodeficiency syndrome. *Crit Care Med.* 1990;18:18–20.

Spector SA, et al. A controlled trial of intravenous immune globulin for the prevention of serious bacterial infections in children receiving zidovudine for advanced human immunodeficiency virus infection. Pediatric AIDS clinical trials. *N Engl J Med.* 1994;331:1181–1187.

Posttest

1. Chorioamnionitis is caused by:
   a. viral infection of the placenta
   b. bacterial infection
   c. premature rupture of the membranes
   d. premature labor
2. Which of the following are routes of HIV infections in the fetus and neonate?
   I. transplacentally
   II. ascending route
   III. breast milk
   IV. contact with maternal secretions
   a. II, III
   b. I, II
   c. III, IV
   d. I, III, IV
3. Which of the following drugs is *not* used in the treatment of AIDS or its complications?
   a. pentamidine
   b. trimethoprim
   c. indocin
   d. azidothymidine
4. Hepatitis, jaundice, hepatosplenomegaly, and neurologic abnormalities are symptoms of which of the following fetal infections?
   a. disseminated herpes simplex
   b. CMV
   c. toxoplasmosis
   d. nondisseminated herpes simplex
5. Under what circumstances should prophylactic broad-spectrum antibiotics be administered to a neonate?
   a. upon positive identification of an antigen

b. all premature neonates

c. amniotic sac rupture over 24 hours before delivery

d. all cesarean deliveries

6. A fetus receives immunity from the mother by which of the following antibodies?

 a. IgA

 b. IgE

 c. IgG

 d. IgM

7. Which of the following are clinical signs of an esophageal-tracheal anomaly?

 I. accumulation of oral secretions

 II. sporadic respiratory distress

 III. regurgitation of feedings

 IV. absence of bowel sounds

 V. tracheal deviation

 a. II, III, IV

 b. I, II, IV

 c. I, II, III

 d. II, III, IV, V

8. The probable diagnosis of a neonate delivered with polyhydramnios, a flat abdomen, and respiratory distress is:

 a. choanal atresia

 b. diaphragmatic hernia

 c. esophageal-tracheal anomaly

 d. Pierre-Robin syndrome

9. A higher systolic blood pressure in the right arm over either leg would indicate which of the following?

 a. subaortic stenosis

 b. coarctation of the aorta

 c. tricuspid atresia

 d. ventricular septal defect

10. Which of the following heart defects is not compatible with life when an abnormal opening between the right and left heart does not exist?

 a. coarctation of the aorta

 b. tetralogy of Fallot

 c. transposition of the great vessels

 d. ventricular septal defect

11. With which of the following cardiac anomalies would one expect an increased lung compliance?

 a. subaortic stenosis

 b. ventricular septal defect

 c. tricuspid atresia

 d. anomalous venous return

CHAPTER TWELVE

PEDIATRIC DISEASES REQUIRING RESPIRATORY CARE

OBJECTIVES

Upon completion of this chapter, the reader should be able to:

1. Describe the pathophysiology, signs, symptoms, and treatment of the following disorders:
   a. Acute respiratory distress syndrome (ARDS)
   b. Asthma
   c. Cystic fibrosis
2. Compare and contrast progressive spinal muscular atrophy of infants (Werdnig-Hoffman paralysis), juvenile spinal muscle atrophy (Kugelberg-Welander disease), and muscular dystrophy.
3. Identify the causative organisms, signs, and treatment of the following:
   a. Guillain-Barré syndrome
   b. Tetanus
   c. Botulism
4. Describe the etiology and diagnosis of myasthenia gravis.
5. Discuss the etiology and treatment of spinal cord injuries.
6. Describe the pathophysiology and treatment of head injuries and near-drowning.
7. Identify and explain the manifestations of Reye's syndrome, its pathophysiology, and treatment. List and describe the five staging criteria for Reye's syndrome.
8. Describe, for each of the following infectious diseases, the causative organisms, symptoms, diagnosis, and treatment:
   a. Pneumonia
   b. Bronchiolitis
   c. Epiglottitis
   d. Croup
9. Discuss the pathophysiology, signs, diagnosis, and treatment of the following. Include the four phases of lung injury following chlorine gas inhalation.
   a. Aspiration
   b. Smoke inhalation
   c. Chlorine gas inhalation

10. Identify five factors that indicate a risk of developing SIDS.

--- **KEY TERMS** ---

azoospermia
bronchiolitis obliterans
decerebrate
decorticate
doll's eye reflex

electromyography
extrinsic
inotropic
intrinsic
intussuscection

leukotrienes
muscarinic
obtundation
oculcephalic
oculovestibular

VENTILATORY DISEASES

ACUTE RESPIRATORY DISTRESS SYNDROME (ARDS)

ARDS afflicts patients of all ages, including children. Despite advances in understanding and treatment of the disease, mortality remains near 60%.[1] Although research has broadened understanding of the pathophysiology of the disease, the key elements that initiate and potentiate ARDS have yet to be fully defined. Outcome is only improved by early recognition and intervention before the triggering factors are allowed to evolve. Table 12–1 lists the possible mediators of lung injury that can lead to ARDS.[2]

Pathophysiology. The classic conditions seen with ARDS are a severe mismatch between ventilation and perfusion, pulmonary hypertension, reduced compliance, and pulmonary infiltrates. These conditions lead to significant hypoxemia, hypercarbia, and acidosis. If not corrected, death ensues. ARDS is the result of either direct, or indirect injury to the pul-

---

Table 12–1 Possible Mediators of Lung Injury

Neutrophils
Platelets
Leukotriene-B$_4$
Platelet-activating factor
Bacterial peptides
Macrophage-derived chemotactic factor
Oxygen radicals
Proteolytic enzymes
Phospholipase products
Endotoxin
Kallikrein
Interleukin-1
Coagulation factors

---

monary system. Examples of direct injury are infection, aspiration, and embolism. Indirect injuries may be chest wall trauma, or bacteremia. Table 12–2 lists mechanisms that have been associated with the onset of ARDS.

ARDS has been divided into four distinct phases following the pathogenesis of the disease.[1] In the first phase, the patient becomes dyspneic and tachypneic. In this phase, the chest x-ray is normal and the patient's oxygenation status is normal. The second phase occurs within 12 to 24 hours. It is during this phase that alveolar damage begins and infiltrates begin appearing on the chest x-ray.

Research suggests that there are numerous pathways leading to the alveolar damage associated with ARDS. One study by Sivan and associates demonstrates that concept.[3] Several inflammatory pathways are activated in the lungs of the ARDS patient. The challenge is to determine which factors are primary causes of ARDS, and which are secondary responses to the initial insult.

Commonly seen changes include an increase of proteinases of neutrophil origin in the alveoli, components of the complement, kinin-forming, coagulation; and fibrinolytic cascades, and a change in pulmonary surfactant. These changes cause a fibrotic process in the lungs, similar to normal wound healing, that leads to impaired gas exchange and the need for extended care. Patients who survive ARDS appear to be those who have minimal fibrotic changes in the lungs.

As the ARDS worsens, phase 3 begins. During this phase, the alveolar/capillary membranes become leaky, resulting in fluid accumulation in the distal airways and alveoli. Damage to the alveoli also results in a decrease in surfactant production and a subsequent reduction in lung compliance. During phase 3, respiratory failure develops with worsening hypoxemia, hypercarbia, and acidosis. Diffuse infiltrates appear on the chest x-ray along with air bronchograms. Mechanical ventilation with high FiO_2 is often started at this point. It is possible that alveolar damage is increased by the high oxygen and mechanical

---

Table 12–2   Possible Triggering Mechanisms of ARDS

- Shock
- Thoracic trauma
- Pulmonary contusion
- Severe head injury
- Pulmonary embolism (fat, blood, or air)
- Aspiration syndrome
- Near-drowning
- Extensive burns
- Sepsis
- Diffuse pulmonary infection
- Transfusion of large amounts of stored blood
- Oxygen toxicity
- Disseminated intravascular coagulation
- Prolonged cardiopulmonary bypass
- Narcotic drug overdose

---

ventilation.[1] The fourth phase is described as progressive respiratory failure, fibrosis of the lungs, and recurrent, resistant pneumonias. Whether all of these changes occur in the pediatric patient has been questioned.

The role of vitamin E levels in the development of ARDS was studied by Richard and associates.[4] They concluded that the development of ARDS is associated with vitamin E deficiency and an enhancement of plasma lipoperoxidation. They also concluded that the vitamin E deficiency is a probable consequence of malnutrition.

Signs and Symptoms. Symptoms begin with signs of respiratory distress, crackles, increased respiratory rate, dyspnea, retractions, and possible expiratory grunting. The patient may also have signs of pulmonary edema, such as frothy pink secretions. Those patients who have conditions that predispose them to the development of ARDS should be carefully monitored for early recognition of the syndrome.

Initially, hyperventilation causes hypocapnia and respiratory alkalosis. As the disease progresses, arterial oxygenation begins to worsen to hypoxic levels, becoming resistant to oxygen therapy. As pulmonary insufficiency develops, the arterial PCO_2 rises and the patient becomes acidotic. Compliance begins to worsen as the lungs become stiffer. Crackles and rhonchi become more apparent during the acute stage of the disease.

As compliance drops, physiologic deadspace increases leading to decreased alveolar ventilation and a rise in minute ventilation. Intrapulmonary shunting increases and may exceed 20% of the cardiac output.[5] The chest x-ray becomes progressively worse, with diffuse, uneven infiltrations throughout both lungs fields.

Treatment. Treatment of ARDS is aimed at supporting the injured lungs, giving them time to heal. Early intervention may result in less severe lung injury with a shorter course and fewer complications. Hudson outlined three strategies for early treatment of ARDS: 1) correction of physiologic derangements; 2) suppression of alveolar inflammation; and 3) the prevention of complications.[6] It is crucial to resolve the source of infection, either medically or surgically, to reduce the inflammatory response.

The correction of physiologic derangement is achieved by several methods. As the patient begins to progress into respiratory failure, the patient is intubated and mechanical ventilation is initiated to reverse the hypoxemia and hypercapnia. High levels of PEEP may be needed to keep alveoli open and bring the functional residual capacity back up to normal, thus improving oxygenation and ventilation. However, Hudson indicated that early application of PEEP does not reduce the incidence of ARDS or alter the course of the disease.[6]

There is growing concern that mechanical ventilation causes further lung injury in the ARDS patient, worsening the course of the disease.[1] Nonconventional support therapies, such as high-frequency ventilation, ECMO, and liquid ventilation are possible answers to reducing lung injury. These modes are not without their own downsides. HFOV seems to be the most promising mode of therapy at this time.

The success in the use of artificial surfactant on neonates has sparked interest in this mode of therapy for victims of ARDS. To date, few studies have been performed, but those that have been done show promise.[1] Questions remain regarding the best surfactant to use, amount, and best delivery method. In virtually all studies done, there was short-term oxygenation improvement and decreased incidence of pneumothoraces.

Another technology, nitric oxide, may prove to be beneficial in the treatment of ARDS. Its main benefit is the ability to reduce pulmonary hypertension, while not causing systemic hypotension. Much research remains to be done, however, before nitric oxide is used as a treatment for ARDS.

The reduction of lung edema is another factor in the early treatment of ARDS. This has been accomplished by the use of diuretics, vasoactive and *inotropic* agents. Another approach is the use of terbutaline to enhance the clearance of alveolar edema by epithelial cells; however, this technique has not yet been applied to humans.[7] One hazard with the use of diuretics is the potential of lowering cardiac output and impairing tissue oxygenation.

The administration of prostaglandin E_1 (PGE_1) has been reported to increase survival in ARDS patients. A recent study, however, has shown that the use of PGE_1 does not alter the outcome.[8]

The use of antiinflammatory drugs, such as corticosteroids and nonsteroidal anti-inflammatory drugs (NSAIDs), has not been shown to decrease the onset or the severity of ARDS. The use of antiprotease, antioxidants, platelet-activating factor antagonists, and specific antibodies against toxic inflammatory agents is being investigated for potential use in the treatment of ARDS.

Aerosolized bronchodilators may reduce airflow resistance and improve oxygenation and ventilation in the ARDS patient. V/Q mismatch that is associated with ARDS has been shown to be improved by the use of Almatrine. Although not yet available in the United States, it appears to be helpful in the treatment of pulmonary vasoconstriction associated with ARDS.

The most common and severe complications of ARDS are infections. Two strategies being studied to reduce infections include the use of sucralfate to prevent gastric bleeding and selective decontamination of the digestive tract (SDD). Studies have demonstrated a lower incidence of pneumonia in ARDS patients treated with sucralfate. This reduction may be due in part to a prevention of bacterial proliferation by maintaining gastric acidity and the direct antimicrobial effect of sucralfate.

SDD involves the prevention of aerobic colonization of the upper airway and gut, allowing anaerobic organisms to remain. This is done by the selective use of gram-positive IV antibiotics and simultaneous topical and oral administration of tobramycin, polymyxin E, and amphotericin. Studies involving SDD are being conducted in Europe, and further research remains to be done.

ASTHMA

Asthma is an airway disorder in which a patient's hyperreactive airways spasm and constrict, swell, and pour secretions into the lumen, in response to various stimuli. The result is severe airway obstruction that may be life threatening.

Asthma is the most common pediatric disease, affecting 5 to 10% of children, and the most frequent cause of hospitalization in the United States.[9] The incidence of asthma in the adult population is 3 to 5%, with half of all patients acquiring the disease before age 10.[10] Asthma affects 1 in 12 school-age children in the United States.[11] Despite all that is known about asthma and its treatment, the mortality rate has continued to climb.

Although the exact etiology of the disease is unknown, several factors that precipitate acute attacks have been identified. They are listed in Table 12–3.

One study found that secondhand cigarette smoke aggravates asthma in children. Another study found a high incidence of reactive airway disease in infants who suffered bronchopulmonary dysplasia as neonates.[9]

Extrinsic or allergic asthma is a common variety of asthma that develops with exposure to allergenic substances. *Intrinsic* asthma is associated with respiratory tract infections.

Pathophysiology. The course of asthma includes two phases. In the acute allergic phase, the presence of a triggering stimuli on the airway causes the rupture or degranulation of the mast cell. The mast cell contains several chemical mediators that are released upon its rupture. These mediators include histamine, *leukotrienes* (formerly called slow-reacting substance of anaphylaxis or SRS-A), eosinophilic chemotactic factor of anaphylaxis (ECF-A), and prostaglandins. These mediators affect the smooth muscle of the tracheobronchial tree and result in bronchospasm, vasodilation, edema, increased secretions, and accumulation of eosinophils.

The second phase of the asthma attack is the inflammatory phase of the disease. Following the initial acute response, mediators are released by eosinophils, neutrophils, macrophages, and lymphocytes. These mediators initiate the inflammatory response of the airways.

As resistance to flow increases, work of breathing increases concurrently. Resulting ventilation and perfusion mismatches worsen blood gases and patient status. Because the airways are narrower during expiration, air trapping results with an incrase in the FRC. As a result, more negative intrapleural pressure is needed to maintain the same tidal volume and, thus, work of breathing increases.

Table 12–3   Factors That Precipitate Acute Asthma Symptoms

---

1. Allergens
   a. Molds
   b. Pollens
2. Outdoor irritants
   a. Smoke
   b. Air pollution
3. Indoor irritants
   a. Animal danders
   b. Dusts
4. Exercise
5. Viral infections
6. Foods
7. Emotions
8. Aspirin and related drugs

The narrowing of airways is unevenly distributed throughout the lungs and results in wide V/Q imbalances. V/Q mismatching leads to hypoxemia, which causes the patient to hyperventilate and become hypocarbic. The changes in respiratory function lead to derangement of both cardiovascular and metabolic function. The patient becomes dehydrated secondary to a decreased ability to take fluids and increased insensible loss from tachypnea and fever, if present. Lactic acidosis results from a combination of hypoxemia, dehydration, and increased metabolism caused by tachypnea. Hypocarbia limits the conservation of bicarbonate by the kidney and leads to metabolic acidosis.

After a time, the patient begins to exhaust from the energy spent attempting to maintain ventilation. The $PaCO_2$ begins to rise, and the patient enters acute respiratory failure, the terminal phase of illness.

There appears to be two distinct onset patterns to asthma, sudden-onset, and the more common, slow-onset. Immunohistologically, it has been observed that patients with sudden-onset fatal asthma had higher numbers of neutrophils and less eosinophils in the airway mucosa, raising the possibility that the mechanisms of inflammation and airway narrowing are completley different from those seen with slow-onset asthma.[12]

Signs and Symptoms. The patient suffering the effects of an asthmatic attack will often have a history of wheezing and shortness of breath mingled with periods of no symptoms. Many times the patient has a long history of hospital visits for treatment. A complete, thorough history is crucial to treat the asthmatic patient adequately. The success or failure of previous treatments is helpful in developing an appropriate plan. The presence of dehydration and concurrent infection can also be detected by the history.

Physical signs depend on the degree of the attack. A mild attack presents as a dry hacking cough, with little presence of wheezing. Patients suffering a moderate attack will have a productive cough, tachypnea, audible wheezes, tachycardia, and possible cyanosis. The patient with a severe attack has diminished breath sounds from lack of ventilation, retractions, rapid, shallow respiration, and may be stuporous and lethargic from hypoxia and hypercapnia.

Arterial blood gas results may be used to classify acute asthma attacks into four stages of severity. In stage 1, the blood gases are within normal limits. In stage 2, the $PaCO_2$ begins to decrease and the pH becomes alkalotic. There may or may not be signs of hypoxemia in stage 2. Stage 3 shows a normal $PaCO_2$ and pH in a fatigued, hypoxemic patient. These patients should be admitted to the ICU and observed closely. Stage 4 include those patients with a high $PaCO_2$, a low pH, and a low PaO_2. These patients require immediate intubation and mechanical ventilation.

Additional blood tests may reveal eosinophilia and increased polymorphonuclear cells. The IgE levels may also be elevated.

The measurement of peak expiratory flows helps to determine the extent of airway obstruction and the response to the therapy.

There are several causes of wheezing that have been misdiagnosed as asthma that should be ruled out whenever asthma is suspected. Those disorders most frequently misdiagnosed as asthma include left ventricular failure, endobronchial lesions, vocal cord dysfunction, and *bronchiolitis obliterans*.

Treatment. The primary treatment of an asthma attack is avoiding the precipitating factors that trigger the attack. In the presence of an actual attack, oxygen is nearly always indicated to treat hypoxemia. The PaO_2 should be kept above 55 mm Hg. Hypoxemia is often underestimated in the asthmatic patient, and under no circumstances should oxygen be withheld based on observation alone. The use of pulse oximetry may be helpful in assessing which patients require an arterial blood gas at presentation to the hospital. In a study by Carruthers and Harrison, they found that an oxygen saturation greater than 92% at presentation to the hospital suggested that respiratory failure is unlikely and an arterial blood gas not necessary.[13] They point out, however, that other parameters must be continually monitored and assessed in all asthmatic patients and arterial blood gases must be done whenever clinically indicated, regardless of the SpO_2.

The use of an 80:20 mixture of helium:oxygen (heliox) has been shown to be effective at reducing pulsus paradoxus and improving peak expiratory flow in acute asthmatics.[14] Pulsus paradoxus is an abnormal decrease in systolic pressure seen during inspiration. In asthma, its presence is indicative of severe disease. The use of heliox may diminish the tendency of inspiratory muscles to fatigue and thus improve the patient outcome.

Asthma is a multifactorial process that often requires the use of multiple drugs in its treatment. The treatment of asthma is best understood when the mechanics of airway regulation are understood. The tone of airway smooth muscle is maintained and regulated by three elements in the autonomic nervous system: the sympathetic (adrenergic), parasympathetic (cholinergic), and the nonadrenergic noncholinergic system (NANC) (see Figure 12–1). In addition, these nerves regulate mucus secretion, vascular permeability, blood flow, and the release of mediators from mast cells.[15]

The Nonadrenergic Noncholinergic System (NANC). While little is known about the NANC system, it is apparent that it plays a significant role in maintaining the airways. The NANC is believed to be the primary nervous system that inhibits bronchial smooth muscle contraction. The transmitters involved in the NANC system have not been positively identified but vasoactive intestinal peptide (VIP) and peptide histidine methanol appear to be the primary mediators. When the VIP receptors are stimulated, ATP is converted to cAMP by adenyl cyclase, resulting in bronchodilation. While VIP is a powerful bronchodilator, it has yet to be used successfully as an aerosol. It has been suggested that the hyperreactive airways seen in asthma are the result of a defect in the NANC system.

The Sympathetic System. The exact role of the sympathetic system in maintaining airway tone is not completely understood. While the smooth muscle of the airways has little, if any, sympathetic innervation, the airways themselves have an abundance of sympathetic β_2 receptors in the small peripheral airways. It is well known that stimulation of these β_2 receptors leads to bronchodilation, but the exact mechanism by which that occurs is poorly understood. The mchanism is similar to that of VIP receptors, in that stimulation of the β_2 sites causes the conversion of ATP to cAMP with the increase in cAMP leading to relaxation of the smooth muscle.

The Parasympathetic System. The parasympathetic system is the main system controlling airway smooth muscle and mucus secretion. The main receptor of the parasympathetic

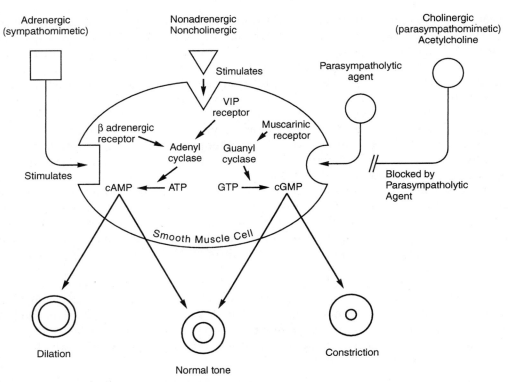

Figure 12–1 *Regulation of airway smooth muscle tone.*

system is the muscarinic receptor, which is stimulated by the transmitter acetylcholine. Muscarinic receptors are found almost exclusively in the large central airways. When the muscarinic receptor is stimulated, GTP is converted to cGMP by guanyl cyclase. The increased level of cGMP causes contraction of the bronchial smooth muscle, increased mucus secretion in the airways, and the release of mast cell mediators. These mediators lead to the inflammatory response with edema, increased muscle spasm, and mucus secretion into the airways.

Agents Used to Treat Asthma. Most drugs used to treat asthma are given by aerosol. This allows direct placement of the drug at the site of the problem, and allows for rapid onset of action. Based on the understanding of airway physiology (just reviewed) there are three main drug categories used to treat asthma.

Sympathomimetics (β_2-Adrenergic Agonists). The most commonly used medications are the sympathomimetic agents, those drugs that stimulate the β_2-adrenergic sites. In addition to causing bronchodilation, these drugs also have been shown to inhibit mast cell degranulation, reduce the permeability of the pulmonary vasculature, and improve the mucociliary transport of secretions.[15]

One of the oldest β_2 drugs used to treat asthma is epinephrine. Epinephrine, and two of its synthetic derivatives, isoproterenol, and isoetharine, were the standard medications used for many years. While providing rapid bronchodilation, these drugs have a limited duration, and often cause tremors, palpitations, and anxiety. For these reasons, newer medications that have a longer duration of action and fewer side effects have been developed. These medications include: bitolterol (Tornalate®); metaproterenol (Alupent®, Metaprel®); terbutaline (Brethine®, Bricanyl®); fenoterol (Berotec®); albuterol (salbutamol in Europe) (Proventil®, Ventolin®); pirbuterol (Maxair®); carbuterol (Bronsecur®); procaterol (Pro-Air®); salmeterol xinafoate (Serevent®); and formoterol.

Parasympatholytics (Anticholinergics). Drugs in this category are chemically similar to the neurotransmitter acetylcholine in that they actively bind to the muscarinic receptors. The difference, however, is that as an antagonist, these drugs do not stimulate any continuation of the nerve impulse, effectively blocking its transmission. The prototype parasympatholytic drug is atropine. Other drugs used in this category are derivatives of atropine and include atropine methonitrate, glycopyrrolate (Robinul®), ipratopium bromide (Atrovent®), and oxitropium bromide (Oxivent®).

Use of Sympathomimetics and Parasympatholytics. As understanding of lung physiology and asthma progresses, therapeutic drug treatment also progresses. In particular, the discovery that sympathetic innervation is mainly in the small peripheral bronchioles, and parasympathetic innervation mainly in the large airways, has led to the theory that it may be advantageous to delivery a parasympatholytic drug first, followed by a sympathomimetic.[16] By delivering the parasympatholytic drug first, the large airways are opened, allowing better penetration of the sympathomimetic drug to the peripheral airways.

Traditionally, aerosolized bronchodilators are given as a treatment that lasts 10 to 15 minutes, every 3 to 4 hours. A novel method of treating acute exacerbations of asthma, is the use of continuous aerosol therapy.[17] Fairly high doses of albuterol given by continuous aerosol have been shown to be safe and effective.[18]

Salmeterol xinafoate, one of the newer long lasting sympathomimetics, has been shown to be more effective when given twice daily, then albuterol administered 4 times daily.[19] The use of extended release oral theophylline in conjunction with an aerosolized sympathomimetic has also been shown to reduce asthma symptoms.[20] The result of longer dosing with the use of newer drugs, or by combination therapy, may improve patient compliance and reduce the need for more frequent treatment. Of interest to note, are studies indicating that MDI therapy using a spacer is at least as efficacious, if not superior to nebulizer therapy.[21,22]

Of major concern with the use of the sympathomimetic drugs is the possibility of overuse, resulting in asthma that is nonresponsive to treatment. This resistant asthma is thought to be the result of too frequent administration of inhaled β_2-adrenergic drugs causing rebound bronchoconstricton. Another theory is that too frequent use desensitizes the β_2 sites, making them increasingly less responsive to the medication. To offset this possibility, it has been suggested that asthmatic patients only use these medications on an "as needed" basis, treating only as their symptoms warrant.[23] However, a study by Chapman and associates showed that regular treatment with salbutamol resulted in less frequent asthma symptoms and did not appear to lead to worsening attacks.[24] There is still much to be understood regarding the treatment of asthma. The most prudent counsel may be to use the medication only as directed and seek medical help if asthma symptoms do not respond.

Corticosteroids. Corticosteroids have been shown to suppress the release of inflammatory mediators and are thus the drug of choice in the treatment of the inflammatory phase of asthma.[25]

Prophylactic reversal of airway hyperreactivity is best accomplished by the use of corticosteroids. Common steroids used include beclomethasone dipropionate, fluticosone (Flovent) triamcinolone acetonide, funisolide, and budenoside, which is not currently available in the United States. There are many who advocate that steroids should be the drug of choice when treating asthma and not used only when the beta agonists do not work.[25] A study by Salmeron and associates demonstrated that the use of inhaled beclomethasome dipropionate, 1500 μg/day, maintained optimal pulmonary function in asthmatic patients uncontrolled by albuterol and theophylline.[26] The rationale is that bronchial hyperreactivity is directly related to the degree of inflammation and that by treating the inflammation, the disease can be better controlled. Some have advocated changing the name to chronic eosinophilic bronchitis to indicate the inflammatory nature of the disease.

Other Medications to Treat Asthma. If mast cell degranulation is prevented, the inflammatory processes of asthma are averted. Two drugs, cromolyn sodium (Intal) and Nedacromil (Tiladc) stabilize the mast cell and prevent its degranulation. It is used as a prophylactic treatment for asthma.

Interestingly, aerosolized furosemide, a diuretic drug, has been shown to provide bronchodilation in children with mild asthma.[27] Anti-inflammatory drugs have shown some success in treating asthma; in particular, methotrexate and gold salts.[25]

Research is focusing on new medications aimed at treating the various aspects of asthma.[28] Cysteinyl leukotrienes released from the mast cell, and the immunoresponsive cells, cause bronchoconstriction, increased capillary permeability, and increase mucus secretion. Drugs aimed at blocking cysteinyl leukotriene receptors, and at inhibiting their production have been developed—Montelukast (Singular), Zafirlukast (Accolate), and Pranlukast (Ultair)—pending FDA approval. Drugs targeting platelet activating factor (PAF), and thromboxanes are being investigated. Drugs that inhibit lymphocyte-derived cytokines and augment cAMP are currently being investigated.

In the presence of purulent sputum, fever, or chest x-ray infiltrates, antibiotics are indicated.[29] Adequate hydration should be maintained, because asthmatics are frequently dehydrated, complicating the nature of the asthma. Conversely, excessive hydration may precipitate pulmonary edema in the asthmatic patient. Fluid administration should be based on clinical and laboratory indices of hydration. Epinephrine is often given subcutaneously during moderate and severe attacks. It has powerful bronchodilatory effects, but also has dangerous side effects.

Humidification of the airway may help loosen mucous plugs. This should not be done with ultrasonic nebulization, however, as there is a strong association between ultrasonic particles and the exacerbation of bronchospasm.

Decreased breath sounds with no wheezing may be an ominous sign, indicating respiratory failure. The definition of respiratory failure in an asthmatic is a refractory hypoxemia (PaO_2 < 60 mm Hg on FiO_2 of 0.5) or hypercarbia ($PaCO_2$ > 40 mm Hg). These patients are often the victims of status asthmaticus, also known as acute severe asthma. Status asthmaticus is a severe asthmatic attack that is refractory to sympathomimetic therapy. These patients require immediate attention and hospitalization.

In the patients in status asthmaticus were started on continuous intravenous isoproterenol and aminophylline. The rate of administration was gradually increased until the desired effect was achieved or the heart rate reached 200 beats per minute.[30] Constant cardiac monitoring was necessary to monitor for dysrhythmias. This method is no longer used due to the side effects. The accepted therapy consists of a continuous albuterol aerosol delivered at a rate of 10 to 50 mg/hr. Terbutaline has also been shown to be safe and effective delivered at a rate of 1 to 12 mg/hr as a continuous aerosol.

If the bronchodilators and aminophylline are not successful in relieving the symptoms, the patient should be intubated and ventilated mechanically. Sedation and paralysis are important to facilitate the intubation and ventilation and to reduce oxygen consumption. Pancuronium is the drug of choice for paralysis since both succinylcholine and tubocurarine are associated with histamine release.[29] A helium/oxygen mixture may be necessary to overcome the obstruction and facilitate ventilation of the patient.

Due to the increased resistance of the airways and the potential for airtrapping, short inspiratory times and long expiratory times may be needed to provide adequate ventilation and avoid complications of barotrauma.

Several studies have investigated various novel techniques in treating status asthmaticus. Johnston and associates showed a significant improvement in status asthmaticus when the inhalational anesthetic isoflurane was given.[31]

Another study concluded that patients who have suffered at least one episode of asthma induced respiratory failure are at a high risk of developing repeated episodes of respiratory failure.[32] Special attention should be paid to those patients in an attempt to avoid subsequent bouts with respiratory failure.

Magnesium sulfate ($MgSO_4$) has also been used via infusion as a bronchodilator in severe asthma that does not respond to conventional therapy. The bronchodilatory effects have been reported to last up to 2 hours; however, no controlled studies have been done to support these data.

Heliox (helium-oxygen mixture) has been shown to improve gas exchange in severe asthma by decreasing the turbulence of the gas flow due to the properties of the helium.

CYSTIC FIBROSIS (CF)

Cystic fibrosis is a hereditary disease (autosomal recessive) that affects all exocrine glands and leads to dysfunction in their secretions. Cystic fibrosis occurs in about 1 in 2000 live births, affecting mainly the Caucasian population. Cystic fibrosis is characterized by three clinically observable disorders: pulmonary disease, pancreatic insufficiency, and elevated sweat chloride concentrations.

The disease is passed to offspring as a Mendelian recessive trait, depicted in Figure 12–2 with both parents being carriers of the disease. Each offspring has a 25% chance of having CF, a 25% chance of being clear of the gene, and a 50% chance of being a carrier. A defective CF gene has been localized as a part of chromosome 7. It is only recently that the actual gene has been identified. The mutation that has been identified (delta F508) is only found in 68% of CF patients' chromosomes. It is estimated there are 10 to 12 additional mutations that cause CF. Another mutation (A455E) is associated with preserved pancreatic function and milder pulmonary disease.[33] Identification of these defective genes makes gene therapy an attractive treatment. With gene therapy, the defective gene is replaced by a normal gene, hopefully bringing with it a reversal of the disease process. Because the gene mutation is easily expressed, the target is accessible, and the results easily verifiable, replacement of the CF gene mutation by gene therapy is encouraging.[34]

With improved understanding of the disease, the median survival age has steadily increased.

Pathophysiology. Early in the development of the disease, the pancreas of the patient with CF dilates, fills with secretions that become hardened, and soon atrophies and becomes fibrotic. The resultant lack of bile secretion into the intestine from the pancreatic insufficiency leads to malabsorption and malnutrition, despite a voracious appetite. The stools become bulky and hardened. Newborns with CF may present with an obstruction of the bowel with thickened meconium, known as a meconium ileus.

As the disease progresses, the lungs become involved in 98% of patients.[35] The pulmonary glands begin secreting a thick, viscous mucus that plugs the airways and leads to airway obstruction and chronic infections. Inflammation of the airways has been detected in patients as young as 4 weeks, indicating that the mechanisms initiating lung disease in CF begins very early in the disease.[36] Once the lung injury occurs, the patient becomes susceptible to bacterial pneumonias. Younger CF patients are commonly infected with *Staphylococcus aureus*, whereas mucoid *Pseudomonas aeruginosa* is more prevalent as the patient gets older. Of interest to note is a study that sought to investigate why survival of females with CF is less than that of males. It was found that females contracted mucoid *P. aeruginosa* 1.7 years earlier than males. That earlier acquisition may contribute to the poorer sur-

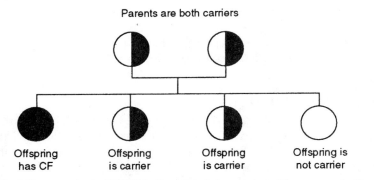

Parents are both carriers

| Offspring has CF | Offspring is carrier | Offspring is carrier | Offspring is not carrier |

Figure 12–2 *Mendelian recessive trait. With both parents being carriers of the gene, each offspring has a 25% chance of having the trait, a 25% chance of not having the trait, and a 50% chance of being a carrier of the trait.*

vival of female patients.[37] Another bacteria causing pneumonia in CF patients, *Burkholderia cepacia,* is associated with poor outcomes.

Other respiratory complications include chronic rhinosinusitis, nasal polyposis, pneumothorax, and hemoptysis. Cor pulmonale is often present as a result of chronic hypoxia and resultant increased pulmonary vascular resistance.

Death is often a result of hypoxia, which follows ever-worsening pulmonary congestion and infection, lung parenchyma and airway destruction, and cor pulmonale.

Diagnosis. A majority of patients with CF are diagnosed in childhood, but a few are not diagnosed until their mid to late teens. Late diagnosis is often due to either a lack of pulmonary manifestations or a previous misdiagnosis of the disease. A report by Dankert-Roelse and coworkers suggests that early diagnosis and appropriate treatment of CF may prevent serious deterioration and death at a young age and may reduce the extent of early irreversible lung damage.[38]

The most reliable diagnostic indicator of CF is the determination of sweat chloride levels. Ninety-eight percent of patients with CF have sweat chloride levels greater than 60 mEq/L. The basic defect in the sweat glands is an inability to reabsorb sodium and chloride ions. The defect is not structural, but is related to altered membrane transport mechanisms of both ions. The sample is usually obtained by stimulating the sweat glands of the forearm, collecting the sample, and analyzing the chloride content. There are a few rare conditions that can cause a false-positive sweat chloride. For this reason, a definitive diagnosis of CF is only made when a positive sweat test is accompanied by at least one of the following: a clinical history of respiratory tract infection, symptoms of pancreatic insufficiency, or a documented family history of CF.

Conversely, a normal sweat chloride test does not rule out CF altogether. It is possible for a patient to have classic intestinal and respiratory symptoms and still have normal sweat electrolytes. Some patients with the CF gene mutation who also had mild manifestations of the disease, have been found to have normal sweat chloride values.[39,40] Additionally, sweat chloride levels may be normal in very young CF patients. In light of these possibilities, any patient having chronic lung congestion, pancreatic insufficiency, failure to thrive, or respiratory colonization with *Pseudomonas,* should be suspected as having CF despite the presence of normal sweat chloride results.

Screening for CF is another possible tool to aid in the diagnosis, however widespread screening may be impractical due to the high number of false positives and false negatives. One such screening program, the measurement of immunoreactive trypsinogen, is described by Roberts and associates.[41]

The chest x-ray of the CF patient may appear normal at the onset of the disease, gradually showing bronchiectatic changes, hyperinflation, and air trapping as the disease progresses. The x-ray often shows bilateral upper lobe infiltrates and peribronchial thickening. The x-ray may also show a pneumothorax from a ruptured lung bleb.

The pulmonary function tests of a CF patient show a restrictive pattern early in the disease, progressing to an obstructive pattern with hyperinflation of static pulmonary volumes later in the course. It has been suggested that a restrictive pattern late in the disease correlates with a poor prognosis; however, a recent study by Ries and associates concluded that a restrictive pattern in CF does not necessarily indicate more severe disease and may actually be reversible in some.[42] Whenever PFT studies are done on CF patients, it is important to consider the within-subject variability that occurs within the day, from day to day, and from week to week. This is done by predetermining the variability of the individual, rather than using group data.[43]

On physical examination, the patient presents with a chronic cough, possible nasal polyposis, and chronic sinusitis. The patient may have nonrespiratory signs such as *intussusception*, the prolapse of one segment of bowel into the lumen of another segment, intestinal obstruction, idiopathic pancreatitis, or obstructive *azoospermia*, the lack of spermatozoa in the semen. The stools are often foul-smelling, oily, and high in fat and protein content. In the later stages of the disease, the chest may become barrel-shaped and the patient may have digital clubbing.

Treatment. Until a cure is found for CF, treatment is aimed at improving long-term survival and improving the quality of life. Because CF affects many body systems, treatment is a multidisciplinary effort. Treatment is focused not only on the respiratory system, but dietary and psychosocial areas as well.

Treatment of CF is often best handled at centralized facilities or CF clinics due to the need for various health care workers. The comprehensive plan of treatment by the team is to monitor the patient's condition, modify the therapy as needed, and hospitalize the patient as needed.

The treatment of pulmonary disease associated with CF makes up the bulk of therapy. Treatment is aimed at reducing infections and removing thick, viscous secretions.

As with all pulmonary diseases, oxygen is used on CF patients to relieve hypoxemia and improve the ability of the patient to exercise. The improvement of hypoxemia additionally slows the onset of cor pulmonale in the CF patient.

The treatment of pulmonary infections is handled on an acute or chronic basis. Acute antibiotic therapy consists of a combination therapy with an aminoglycoside and a broad-spectrum penicillin. Gentamicin, which is effective against *P. aeruginosa*, is the most common aminoglycoside used. The dosage of gentamicin used is often twice the normal dosage. This is due to an increase in the body clearance of aminoglycosides in patients with CF and a need for higher serum concentrations for adequate penetration into the thick pulmonary secretions. The penicillins with the best activity against *P. aeruginosa* are piperacillin, ticarcillin, azlocillin, and mezlocillin. Ceftazidime, a cephalosporin, has shown excellent results in CF infections.

The aerosolization of antibiotics has been suggested as a method of combating pulmonary infections. Short-term, high-dosage administration of aerosolized tobramycin was found to be safe and efficacious in treating stable CF patients infected with *P. aeruginosa*.[44]

Long-term antibiotic therapy is used on CF patients with severe pulmonary disease or who require frequent hospitalizations. Long-term therapy usually consists of oral antibiotics such as dicloxacillin, tetracycline, cotrimoxazole, cephradine, and chloramphenicol.

Bronchodilator therapy may be helpful in some CF patients, although many CF patients exhibit negative effects following bronchodilator therapy. It is therefore recommended that each CF patient receive a pulmonary function study before and after bronchodilator therapy to determine if the patient will respond favorably.

Several studies have been done to evaluate various bronchodilators and their effectiveness in treating patients with CF. Improvement in PFT results were seen in patients receiving large doses of inhaled salbutamol and ipratropium bromide in one study.[45] A delayed, but significant, improvement in PFTs was also seen in patients treated with inhaled theophylline.[46]

Other aerosolized drugs have been studied and shown to be helpful in treating the pulmonary symptoms of CF. Mucolytic type drugs that alter the adhesiveness of CF mucus, including human DNase I (rhDnase) and distearoyl phosphatidylglycerol, have been shown to improve pulmonary function.[47–50] An older mucolytic agent, acetylcysteine (Mucomyst®) is of limited clinical use and has been shown to cause bronchospasm. For this reason, it is not recommended for use with CF patients. Wetting agents such as saline and sodium bicarbonate may be helpful, but are not used as first line treatments. Agents that alter the ionic fluxes in the epithelium of the airways, such as amelioride and uridine 5'-triphosphate have been shown to increase mucus clearance and retard the decline in lung function.[48,51,52] Inhalation of the corticosteroid budesonide has shown to induce a small, but significant, improvement in the pulmonary status of patients with CF.[53]

Because the inflammatory response to the chronic infections associated with CF contributes to lung destruction, the use of antiinflammatory therapy has been proposed. In one study, high dose ibuprofen, taken consistently for four years, was shown to significantly slow the progression of lung disease in CF patients.[54]

A proven management tool in clearing the thickened bronchial secretions of CF is chest physical therapy (CPT). CPT modalities, discussed in Chapter 6, include traditional CPT (percussion, vibration, and postural drainage), positive expiratory pressure (PEP) therapy, autogenic drainage, forced expiratory technique (FET), high frequency chest percussion, and exercise. Much controversy persists over which method is best at clearing secretions. Using statistical methodology, a review of numerous studies regarding CPT showed that traditiona. CPT combined with exercise provided the best improvement in FEB_1.[55] Another similar review found traditional CPT and exercise effective, but included PEP therapy as an effective management tool.[56] When traditional percussion is used, there appears to be no difference between manual and mechanical percussion.[57]

Conventional mechanical ventilation in the CF patient presents special problems. With increased airway obstruction and frequent bacterial infections, the long-term prognosis is reduced once a CF patient is placed on mechanical ventilation. These problems are substantially reduced by the use of noninvasive ventilatory techniques. Noninvasive positive-pressure ventilation via nasal mask has been shown to be effective at providing ventilation.[58] Another useful noninvasive procedure to treat the CF patient is nasal CPAP, which has been shown to reduce shown to reduce respiratory disturbances and improve oxygen saturation during sleep.[59]

Dietary treatment of CF consists of supplying lipase, protease, and amylase to aid in the digestion of fats, proteins, and carbohydrates. Additionally, patients with CF are given twice the normal amount of protein and calories in their diet to maintain proper growth.

Finally, as a last modality of treatment for those patients with severe lung disease and cor pulmonale, heart-lung transplant is offered as a viable option. The cost involved in transplant is similar to that of medical treatment for the same patient, and mortality appears to be low following the procedure.[60]

Typically, patients are referred for transplant late in the course of their disease. The rate of successful transplants may increase if patients were referred earlier in the course.[61]

NEUROMUSCULAR DISORDERS

There are several neuromuscular disorders that either primarily or secondarily affect the pulmonary system. Most often, the disease affects the muscles of ventilation, making breathing difficult, if not impossible, for the patient. The various diseases affect the muscles in one of four ways: 1) defects in the muscle itself; 2) a defeat in the transmission of nervous impulses to the muscle; 3) a defect in the peripheral motor and sensory nerves; or 4) a defect in the central nervous system.

SPINAL MUSCULAR ATROPHIES

Diseases included in this category are identified by a progressive weakness in the skeletal muscles, gradually leading to their wasting away. These diseases are caused by a progressive degeneration of the anterior horn cells of the spinal cord and are inherited as autosomal-recessive traits.

Progressive Spinal Muscular Atrophy of Infants (Werdnig-Hoffmann Paralysis). This disorder is usually manifest at birth, with its most apparent feature being an inactive neonate. It is the most common and most severe form of the spinal muscular atrophy diseases.

The infant lies in a frog-like position with limited movement of the arms and legs. Breathing is diaphragmatic with sternal retractions present. The cry and cough are weak, and there may be a pooling of secretions in the pharynx. The neonate has an alert apperaance and sensation and intellect are normal.

The disease is diagnosed with *electromyography*, which shows a denervation pattern. Confirmation of the disease is made by muscle biopsy. Death is usually the result of respiratory failure or pulmonary infection from the aspiration of food.

Juvenile Spinal Muscular Atrophy (Kugelberg-Welander Disease). In contrast to Werdnig-Hoffmann paralysis, Kugelberg-Welander disease appears later in childhood or adolescence, and it has a slower progression. Some of the first muscles affected are in the pelvic girdle, with the arms and legs involved later. It is rare for victims of this disorder to have severe complications, and many have a normal life span.

MUSCULAR DYSTROPHIES

Muscular dystrophies are the largest group of muscle diseases that affect children. They all exhibit progressive, symmetrical weakness and wasting of skeletal muscles. The basic defect in these diseases is a degeneration of the muscle fibers. The most severe and most common type of muscular dystrophy seen in children is pseudohypertrophic (Duchenne) muscular dystrophy. Duchenne's muscular dystrophy usually appears during the child's third year. It first appears as a difficulty in running, riding a bicycle, or climbing stairs. A later manifestation of the disease is difficulty in walking, with an apparent abnormal gait. The name pseudohypertrophy is derived from an enlargement of the calves, thighs, and upper arms from fatty infiltration.

As the disease progresses, profound muscular atrophy occurs with ambulation becoming impossible. In its terminal stages, the muscles of ventilation, including the diaphragm, are affected.

ACQUIRED NEUROMUSCULAR DISORDERS

Infectious Polyneuritis (Guillain-Barré Syndrome). Guillain-Barré syndrome is characterized by a fairly rapid muscle weakness that usually begins in the legs and ascends upward in a symmetrical fashion. It may affect the respiratory muscles to the point that mechanical ventilation is required.

The cause of Guillain-Barré is unknown, but it has been linked to certain viral diseases, including infectious mononucleosis, hepatitis, influenza, and cytomegalovirus.

Affected muscles become flaccid and sensory changes may also be present. As the disease ascends, muscle weakness also ascends and affects the abdominal muscles, diaphragm, chest muscles, and possibly the muscles of the larynx and pharynx. The result of this degree of involvement is the inability to ventilate adequately to remove secretions and potential swallowing difficulty and aspiration.

Tetanus. Tetanus is a preventable neuromuscular disease caused by the endotoxin *Clostridium tetani*. It is acquired through a wound in the skin, particularly puncture wounds and burns. The disease is a result of a defect in the transmission of nerve impulses at the neuromuscular junction. In the neonate, infection may occur if delivery occurs in contaminated surroundings. Tetanus spores are found in soil and dust and are more prevalent in rural areas.

Incubation is generally less than 14 days, but may be longer, depending on the severity of the contamination. Initial symptoms are a progressive stiffness and tenderness of neck and jaw muscles. Progression of the disease causes rigidity of the abdominal and limb muscles. The patient has difficulty swallowing and is extremely sensitive to external stimuli. The slightest stimulus causes convulsive contractions that last from seconds to minutes.

As the disease progresses, the patient suffers from laryngospasm and tetany of the respiratory muscles. The patient is then predisposed to aspiration of retained secretions, pneumonia, and atelectasis.

The disease is best prevented by proper vaccination with the tetanus toxoid or antitoxin. These immunizations maintain protective antibodies for roughly 10 years and should be a part of a child's well-baby care.

Botulism. Botulism is the result of ingestion of food contaminated with the *Clostridium botulinum* organism. The most common source is improperly prepared home-canned foods.

Symptoms appear quickly, usually 12 to 36 hours following investion. The pediatric patient shows weakness, dizziness, headache, difficulty in speaking, and vomiting. As the disease progresses, the respiratory muscles become paralyzed with possible atelectasis, aspiration, and pneumonia. The patient must be monitored closely for signs of respiratory failure.

Infants can acquire botulism from the ingestion of the spores of *C. botulinum.* Although there is no common source of the organism, *C. botulinum* has been found in honey and therefore should not be given to infants. The infant patient becomes constipated and lethargic and feedings are poorly tolerated.

Treatment consists of administration of botulism antitoxin (which is controversial in infants) and general supportive measures.[62]

OTHER CAUSES OF NEUROLOGIC DISORDERS

Myasthenia Gravis. Although it is relatively uncommon in childhood, myasthenia gravis may appear in two forms: neonatal and juvenile. Transient neonatal myasthenia gravis occurs in infants of mothers who may not be aware they have the disease. There is general weakness, with depressed neurologic signs and a weak cry. Persistent neonatal myasthenia gravis is indisgtinguishable from the transient variety. It occurs in infants whose mothers do not have the disease.[62]

Juvenile myasthenia gravis is identical to that seen in adults. It usually appears after 10 years of age. Initial symptoms are paralysis of the optic muscles followed by difficulty in swallowing and speaking. There is also a generalized muscle weakness that is more pronounced following exercise and less pronounced following rest.

Diagnosis is made by observing the response following administration of anti-cholinesterase drugs. Two common drugs used are endrophonium (Tensilon) and neostigmine (Prostigmin). Following administration of the drug, muscle strength returns and lasts roughly 5 minutes.

Spinal Cord Injuries. Although not a common malady among children, spinal cord injuries do occur in infants and children, and an understanding of the pathophysiology involved is important for the respiratory care practitioner.

Etiology. Injury to the spinal cord is related to various accidents. Sudden hyperflexion or hyperextension of the neck during an automobile accident is a common cause of injury. Falls from trees, horses, and during sports are another cause of spinal injury. Injuries to the spine may occur in the neonate during breech deliveries. Gunshot wounds and stabbings are other possible causes of spinal cord injury.

Of most interest to the respiratory care practitioner are those injuries that affect the muscles of ventilation. The diaphragm is innervated by the *phrenic nerve,* which arises from the cervical plexus. The fourth cervical nerve is the main contributor to this plexus, with the third and fifth cervical nerves making secondary contributions. Injuries at or above this level result in loss of the use of the diaphragm and the need for long-term ventilatory assistance.

The intercostal muscles are innervated by the intercostal nerves, which arise from the 1st through the 11th thoracic vertebrae. Loss of these nerves by cord injury is not as devastating as a loss of the phrenic nerve; however, the patient will lose a portion of the pulmonary reserve when the intercostal nerves are damaged.

Treatment. The three goals of management of spinal cord injuries are: 1) preservation of neurologic function and prevention of further neurologic deteriorations; 2) maximization of neurologic recovery; and 3) prevention of intercurrent nonneurologic complications.

The role of the respiratory care practitioner in the early stages of the injury is to manage the ventilatory status of the patient and prevent pneumonias through vigorous pulmonary toilet and maintenance of the airway. In the later stages of the injury, the practitioner is vital in the rehabilitation of the pulmonary system. This is done by using breathing techniques and exercises that strengthen the diaphragm.

Head Injury. It is estimated that head injuries in children lead to over 500,000 hospitalizations a year. Of those injured, 3000 to 4000 deaths rsult and 15,000 require extended inpatient care. Several basic concepts in the care of head injuries may help to reduce morbidity and mortality in these patients.

Pathophysiology. When dealing with head injuries, it is important to understand there are two mechanisms that damage the brain. First is the primary insult, or the injury that occurs at the moment of the accident. How badly the brain is damaged is determined by the intenseness of the blow. Primary injuries are related to the physical impact of the brain against the cranial bone, resulting in fractures and contusions.

Secondary injuries are the result of the primary injury. They include hypoxia, hypotension, and hypercarbia, which worsen the brain ischemia, and associated swelling, and hematomas, which may cause herniation of the brain. The effect of the secondary injuries is to damage areas of the brain that may not have been affected by the primary insult. Eventually, the entire brain becomes involved, resulting in high morbidity and mortality. Treating and preventing secondary insults are a vital part of treating head-injured patients.

Often, a comatose pediatric patient with signs of brain stem injury has not suffered irreversible damage, but can still recover if proper treatment of intracranial pressure is initiated quickly.

Treatment. The treatment of a head injury must begin at the site of the accident, if recovery is to be expected. The most important aspect of treating a head-injured patient is to maintain and protect the airway from aspiration, and to provide adequate ventilation and oxygenation. Endotracheal intubation is the method of choice for maintaining the airway of the severely injured patient. Intubation should only be carried out by trained personnel who are able to intubate and/or ventilate without hyperextending the head and possibly exacerbating a neck injury.

The most reliable indicator of the severity of the injury is the consciousness level of the patient. Consciousness level can best be determined by the use of the *Glasgow Coma Scale.* The Glasgow Coma Scale, shown in Table 12–4, examines eye opening, verbal response, and

Table 12–4   The Glasgow Coma Scale

Test	Response	Rating
Eye Opening	Open spontaneously	4
	Open to verbal command	3
	Open to pain	2
	No response	1
Motor Response	Obeys verbal command	6
	Localizes to pain stimulus	5
	Withdraws from pain	4
	Decorticate posturing	3
	Decerebrate posturing	2
	No response	1
Verbal Response	Oriented	5
	Disoriented	4
	Inappropriate	3
	Incomprehensible sounds	2
	No response	1

motor response of the patient, with the motor response correlating best with the extent of the injury.

In each area, a point value is given depending on how the patient responds. The highest possible score is 15, with 3 points being the lowest. An adaptation to the Glasgow Coma Score in the verbal response area, depicted in Table 12–5, has been made for infants.

Diffuse swelling of the brain is the most common serious finding following a severe head injury, and its treatment is the keystone to neurologic recovery. The signs of cerebral edema,

Table 12–5   The Glasgow Coma Scale Modified for Infants

Test	Response	Rating
Eye Opening	Spontaneous opening	4
	Open to speech	3
	Open to pain	2
	No response	1
Motor Response	Normal spontaneous movements	6
	Withdraws to touch	5
	Withdraws to pain	4
	Decorticate posturing	3
	Decerebrate posturing	2
	No response	1
Verbal Response	Coos and babbles	5
	Cries irritably	4
	Cries to pain	3
	Moans only	2
	No response	1

obtundation, sweating, vomiting, and bradycardia, may occur rapidly or slowly, depending on the severity of the injury. The most severe injuries present in a deep coma immediately following the injury. There is often evidence of decorticate and decerebrate posturing, abnormal pupillary responses, and apnea. The diagnosis of brain swelling is confirmed by CT scan, which shows a decrease in the size, or even a total loss of the ventricles.

Immediate treatment of the brain swelling is essential. The immediate goal of the respiratory care practitioner is to hyperventilate the patient to a $PaCO_2$ of 25 to 30 mm Hg and a PaO_2 above 100 mm Hg. The purpose of the hyperventilation is to cause a constriction of the cerebral vessels and reduce cerebral blood flow. Hyperoxygenation reduces the chance of further hypoxic damage and may additionally cause vasoconstriction.

Hyperventilation is achieved with large tidal volumes and respiratory rates. Tidal volume should be set to allow adequate expansion of the lungs but avoid high inspiratory pressurs. The frequency of ventilation can then be used to maintain hyperventilation. Continuous monitoring of the $PaCO_2$ and PaO_2, by transcutaneous monitors, pulse oximetry, or end-tidal CO_2 will help the practitioner adjust the ventilator as needed to maintain the desired parameters. A recent study suggested the use of the ratio between conjunctival oxygen tension and arterial oxygen tension as a reflection of the reduction in cerebral blood flow. Suctioning should be done only as needed and should be done quickly to avoid increasing peak inspiratory pressures. Levels of positive end-expiratory pressures should be kept at a minimum, if used at all.

Increased intracranial pressure is further treated with furosemide mannitol, and pentobarbital to control combativeness and fighting of the ventilator, and elevation of the head 30 to 45°.

Near-Drowning. Drowning is an ever-increasing cause of mortality in the pediatric patient. Drowning is defined as death that occurs within 24 hours of suffocation due to submersion in water. The syndrome of near-drowning implies survival following submersion in water. It often leads to anoxic brain damage, a result of the pulmonary insult while underwater.

Factors associated with near-drowning and requiring special attention include hypothermia and the possibility of cervical spine injury if the victim had been diving. Another concern in the near-drowning patient is the potential of infection from aspirated water. Roughly 85 to 90% of near-drowning victims aspirate water or gastric contents. The other 10 to 15% are victims of *dry drowning,* in which laryngospasm prevents aspiration of water.

Substantial aspiration of fresh water may lead to a washout of surfactant, overhydration, and fluid overload as the hypotonic water is drawn into the tissues and blood. Salt water aspiration, conversely, may draw water out of the tissues and into the alveoli, leading to diffuse pulmonary edema. Salt water additionally causes a chemical injury to the alveolar tissue, enhancing inflammation.

Pathophysiology. Anoxia causes the brain to become edematous, greatly increasing intracranial pressure and reducing blood perfusion to brain tissues. Pathophysiologic changes seen in the lungs include decreased compliance, increased airway resistance, intrapulmonary shunting, increased deadspace, and severe ventilation to perfusion mismatches.

Treatment. The treatment of near-drowning begins at the scene of the accident. Artificial respiration is started as soon as the victim reaches the water's surface. If the patient has a history of trauma, a collar should be placed to stabilize the cervical vertebrae. CPR should be started immediately on the pulseless victim. A study by Nichter and Everett found that 68% of victims who received CPR went on to intact survival.[63] Interestingly, they found a high rate of mortality and neurologic damage in patients who received cardiotonic drugs during the initial resuscitation. They also found that age, sex, length of submersion, core temperature, arterial pH, absence of spontaneous ventilation, lack of pain response, and nonreactivity of the pupils are all unreliable indicators of outcome.

The hypothermia that often accompanies near-drowning may actually be of benefit in the survival of the patient. There have been many reports of survival in hypothermic patients who were submerged for 40 or more minutes. Total resuscitative efforts should continue until the core temperature has rewarmed to near normal levels.

The combination of increased intracranial pressure and diffuse lung involvement make a difficult situation for the respiratory care practitioner. The decreased lung compliance and increased resistance require high pressures to compensate. The high pressures then lead to an increase in intracranial pressure. In this difficult circumstances ventilator settings are maintained at levels adequate to provide desired oxygenation and ventilation, but low enough to avoid harmful increases in intracranial pressure. In the presence of increased brain pressures, the patient is treated pharmacologically and mechanically as previously discussed under head injury.

Reye's Syndrome. Reye's syndrome is a toxic encephalopathy first reported in 1963. It affects children from 2 months to adolescence, but the most common age group is 6 to 11 years. The etiology of Reye's syndrome is unknown, but most instances follow a viral illness. Many viruses have been implicated in the etiology of Reye's syndrome including parainfluenza, Epstein-Barr, coxsackie, mumps, rubella, adenovirus, herpes simplex, polio, influenza A and B, and varicella. Influenza A and B and varicella are most frequently associated with the onset of Reye's syndrome.

There may be an association between the ingestion of aspirin during the initial stages of illness and the occurrence of the syndrome. Because of this, the American Academy of Pediatrics has recommended that aspirin should not be used on children with varicella or suspected influenza.

Pathophysiology and Manifestations. The two most affected organ systems in Reye's syndrome are the brain and the liver. The disease apparently affects the mitochondria of the cells, as electron microscopy reveals large and swollen mitochondria in the brain and liver. The result in the liver is a net reduction in the enzymes that convert ammonia to urea, leading to hyperammonemia. Liver dysfunction is also manifest by the presence of elevated SGOT, SGPT, and LDH levels. The diagnosis of Reye's syndrome is often accomplished by performing a percutaneous liver biopsy. The biopsy reveals swelling of hepatocytes with minimal inflammatory response. Prothrombin levels are also diminished. A majority of patients also have a drop in blood sugar levels below 50 mg/dl, with reduced insulin levels. The child initially presents with symptoms of an upper respiratory viral infection or chicken pox. During the apparent recovery stage of the viral infection, the child develops recurrent vomiting and worsening CNS function.

Progression of the disease is variable, ranging from a few hours to a few days. Changes in sensorium deteriorate from lethargy in the early stages to coma. The patients may also become hyperexcited, with arms and legs thrown about. As brain damage worsens, the patient enters a state of *decorticate* posturing, with flexed upper extremities and extended lower extremities. The patient then begins more omnious signs, such as *decerebrate* posturing, where both upper and lower extremities are extended, muscle flaccidity, apnea, circulatory collapse, and death.

Treatment. Progression of the disease, as well as potential prognosis and evaluation of therapies, are all evaluated by the use of a staging system that follows the course of Reye's syndrome. The five stages are listed in Table 12–6.

Successful treatment of Reye's syndrome requires early detection and an aggressive approach to treatment. The progression of the disease and appropriate treatment are determined by the stage that the disease is in. Stage I disease requires supportive care, correction of hypoglycemia and acid-base disorders, and control of cerebral edema. The patient in stage II requires more aggressive monitoring. Special attention is focused on blood glucose level, coagulation studies, blood chemistries, and temperature. The patient should be made as comfortable as possible. Respiratory procedures such as CPT and suctioning may require sedation to prevent patient agitation.

Stages III through V are treated aggressively in the intensive care unit. The patient is electively intubated, preceded by the administration of thiopental and either succinylcholine or pancuronium. The patient is maintained in a pharmacologic paralysis to allow hyperventilation. The brain swelling is treated as described previously under head injuries.

Additional respiratory care includes appropriate pulmonary toilet to avoid pulmonary complications. The maintenance of analgesia is important because pain and anxiety may increase the intracranial pressure. A device to monitor intracranial pressure is placed, with

---

Table 12–6   Staging Criteria for Reye's Syndrome

Stage I—Vomiting, lethargy, and drowsiness; liver dysfunction; Type I EEG, follows commands, brisk pupillary reaction.

Stage II—Disorientation, combativeness, delirium, hyperventilation, hyperactive reflexes, appropriate responses to painful stimuli; evidence of liver dysfunction; Type I EEG, sluggish pupillary reaction.

Stage III—Obtunded, coma, hyperventilation, decorticate rigidity, preservation of pupillary light reaction and *oculovestibular* reflexes (although sluggish); Type II EEG.

Stage IV—Deepening coma, decerebrate rigidity, loss of *oculocephalic* reflexes, large and fixed pupils, loss of *doll's eye* reflex, loss of corneal reflexes; minimal liver dysfunction; Type III or IV EEG, evidence of brain stem dysfunction.

Stage V—Seizures, loss of deep tendon reflexes, respiratory arrest, flaccidity; Type IV EEG, usually no evidence of liver dysfunction.

the goal of maintaining the pressure less than 20 mm Hg. Dialysis or blood transfusions may be necessary to reduce blood ammonia levels.

Mortality rates have dropped from initial reports of 80% to more recent reports of 20%, probably due to early diagnosis and aggressive treatment. Recovery is rapid and without long-term effect in the presence of early diagnosis and treatment. The child may awaken disoriented and frightened, with no recollection of the hospitalization. Those who work with the recovering child must take steps to lessen the fear and confusion that may be present.

INFECTIOUS LUNG DISEASES

PNEUMONIA

Pneumonia is the most common serious infection that occurs in newborn infants. As a cause of death in neonates, it is second only to hyaline membrane disease in frequency.[64] Pneumonia may be acquired while the infant is still in utero. Infection of the amniotic fluid leading to congenital pneumonia is additionally a cause of premature labor.

Three factors that favor in utero infection are: 1) prolonged rupture of the amniotic membranes, usually more than 24 hours; 2) prolonged labor, even in the presence of intact membranes; and 3) excessive obstetrical manipulation. The most common causative organisms of perinatal infection are enteric organisms such as *E. coli* and also group B streptococcus.

Postnatal pneumonia is most often caused by contamination of the neonate's airway by infected humidifier reservoirs, poor hand washing, and contaminated incubators and other equipment. The most common organisms causing postnatal pneumonia are *S. aureus* and *S. epidermidis*. Other organisms causing pneumonia include *Klebsiella pneumoniae*, type b *H. influenzae*, *P. aeruginosa*, and *Candida albicans*.

Nonbacterial organisms that cause pneumonia are acquired by contact with an infected birth canal or by nosocomial infection. Those organisms acquired from the birth canal include herpes simplex virus, cytomegalovirus (CMV), *Chlamydia trachomatis*, and *Ureaplasma urealyticum*. Nosocomial infections often include respiratory syncytial virus (RSV), rhinovirus, and enteroviruses.

Diagnosis. The diagnosis of neonatal pneumonia is inexact, being based on the history, physical examination, chest x-ray results, and laboratory data. Symptoms of pneumonia often occur at birth, usually within 48 hours following delivery. The infant is tachycardic and shows signs of respiratory distress. Additionally, the infant may be flaccid, pale, and cyanotic. The amniotic fluid may be foul smelling, indicating the presence of infection. The white blood count is not consistent and may be depressed below 5000, or elevated above 15,000. Elevation of the patient's temperature is possible in term infants, whereas premature infants with pneumonia may be hypothermic.

The chest x-ray shows unilateral or bilateral streaky densities in the perihilar region.

Signs of a postdelivery pneumonia include an increasing tachycardia, poor feeding, and possible aspiration of feedings and lethargy.

Any infant who shows signs of a pneumonia, or who is at risk of developing a pneumonia, is started immediately on broad-spectrum antibiotics to combat any potential infection. Clinical symptoms are treated as they appear, and blood gas values are closely monitored and treated aggressively.

BRONCHIOLITIS

Bronchiolitis is a viral infection that leads to inflammation, swelling, and constriction in the bronchioles. The disease has its highest mortality and morbidity among infants less than 6 months old and those suffering from congenital cardiac defects, BPD, cystic fibrosis, and asthma. The most common causative organisms are RSV, causing approximately 75% of all cases, and the parainfluenza virus as well as *Mycoplasma pneumoniae*, rhinovirus, and adenovirus. RSV infection is highly contagious and requires extreme care in hand washing and other precautions to prevent nosocomial outbreaks in the hospital.

Diagnosis. Bronchiolitis begins as a typical upper airway infection with a runny nose, cough, and fever that lasts 2 to 3 days. With the onset of bronchiolar involvement, the cough worsens and the patient of less than 3 years begins showing signs of small airway obstruction and congestion. These signs include intercostal retractions, wheezing, rhonchi, crackles, and hyperinflation. Infants older than 3 years are seldom affected to the same degree.

Upon presentation of these symptoms, an RSV culture is obtained from the nasopharynx. It is important to rule out other processes such as cystic fibrosis and pertussis as part of the diagnostic workup. It has been suggested that infants with repeated bouts of bronchiolitis be considered to be asthmatic.

Treatment. Patients of less than 4 months may need hospitalization to control fluid intake and potential apnea. In those patients who require hospitalization, the level of distress and blood gas values determine the next step in treatment. Patients with severe distress, apnea, and worsening blood gas values are treated with ribavirin, which has a specific antiviral activity against RSV. While not recommended as a treatment for all bronchiolitis patients, ribavirin seems to benefit most the patient at high risk.[65] High-risk patients include those with a history of underlying disease, hypoxia, prematurity, young age, apnea, and pulmonary consolidation as seen on chest x-ray.[66] Ribavirin is given to the patient via a special small-particle aerosol generator called the Viratek SPAG-2 nebulizer, shown in Figure 12–3.

Treatment is done for 12 to 18 hours per day for at least 3 days and no more than 7 days. Ribavirin can be safely administered to mechanically ventilated patients; however, it does not appear to affect the immediate outcome in those patients.[67]

Extreme care should be taken by the health care worker when administering ribavirin to avoid inhalation of the drug. Precautions regarding the delivery of ribavirin are detailed in Chapter 8.

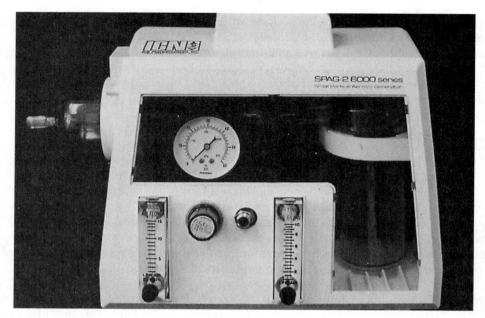

Figure 12–3 *The Viratek SPAG-2*

Sympathomimetic drugs and theophylline may be used to help reduce the associated bronchospasm and improve ventilation until the infection clears.

Mechanical ventilation is instituted when arterial blood gases show impending respiratory failure, or in the presence of frequent and severe apnea. Mechanically ventilated patients with bronchiolitis must receive adequate lavage and suctioning to remove excess secretions. Care must be taken to avoid barotrauma by using low rates and pressures, as tolerated. This sometimes requires accepting higher than normal $PaCO_2$ levels and lower than normal pHs.

Other treatments being proposed to treat bronchiolitis include alpha-interferon 2A, immunoglobulin A, both of which are still in the experimental stages.

Much work has been done to find a vaccine for RSV. At this time an immunoglobulin that is specific for RSV has been approved as prophylaxis for patients deemed at high risk. Some of the criteria used in determining patients at high risk include: prematurity, chronic lung disease, body mass less than 5 kg, congenital heart disease, T-cell immunodeficiency, and lower socioeconomic status. The medication is called Synagis® (palivizumab) and is infused once per month during RSV season with a dosage of 15 mg/kg body weight.

Outcomes. The long term effects of RSV infection is difficult to assess because the infection is universal in the first few years of life and as such, no uninfected control group exists.[68] One prospective study concluded that RSV bronchiolitis in the first year of life is an important risk factor for the development of asthma during the subsequent 2 years.[69]

DISEASES OF THE UPPER AIRWAYS

EPIGLOTTITIS

Epiglottitis is an acute inflammatory disease that affects not only the epiglottis, but also the surrounding aryepiglottic folds and arytenoid cartilages, illustrated in Figure 12–4. The most common causative organism of epigiottitis is type b *H. influenzae.*

Epiglottitis is a life-threatening disease that requires prompt diagnosis and appropriate treatment. Mortality from epiglottitis is due to the blockage of the trachea by swollen, inflamed tissues leading to asphyxiation. The rapid onset of tracheal blockage makes intubation extremely difficult and the probability of anoxic brain damage more pronounced.

Diagnosis. The patient with epiglottitis may present with symptoms similar to croup, making it important to differentiate between the two. Diagnostic differences for croup and epiglottitis are presented in Table 12–7.

Diagnosis is based on history, clinical signs, and x-ray. Because of its bacterial origin, epiglottitis has a rapid onset, usually less than 10 hours. The patient complains of a severe sore throat and demonstrates a high fever. Swallowing becomes difficult due to the swelling of the tissues and also the pain involved. The patient often leans forward and drools, rather than swallowing. The voice becomes muffled, with a soft inspiratory stridor.

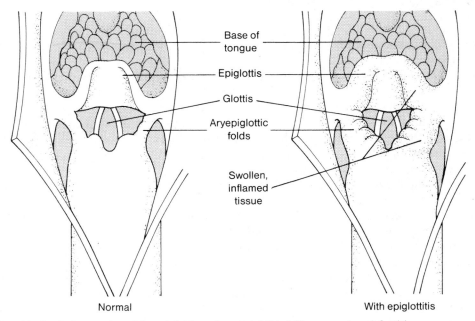

Figure 12–4 *Inflammation of the epiglottis and aryepiglottic folds as seen in epiglottitis.*

Table 12–7   Differentiating Between Croup and Epiglottitis

Presentation	Epiglottitis	Croup
Age	2–6 years	6 months–3 years
Rate of onset	Rapid (often only hours)	Slow (2–3 days)
Infectious origin	*Haemophilus influenzae* type b (bacterial)	Parainfluenza virus
Clinical presentation	High fever, anxious, leaning forward, drooling, low-pitched stridor, muffled voice, no cough	May be afebrile or febrile; hoarse, barky cough; tight upper airway stridor
X-ray examination	Swollen, edematous epiglottis (thumb sign), and supraglottic structures seen on lateral neck film	Narrowing of the subglottic airway (hourglass) seen on A-P neck film
Seasonal incidence	Any season	Usually winter

Diagnosis is verified by a lateral neck x-ray, which shows the epiglottis at the base of the tongue as extremely large and balloon shaped ("thumb sign"), with obliteration of the vallecula, depicted in Figure 12–5.

Direct visualization of the epiglottis should never be attempted, as this could irritate the inflamed tissues and cause complete airway obstruction.

From the moment of arrival at the hospital, all patients with suspected epiglottitis must be accompanied by personnel with the skill and equipment necessary to intubate the tracchea if needed.

Treatment. Epiglottitis is not a disease that can be given "wait-and-see" treatment. Because of its fulminant nature, epiglottitis is a true emergency.

The first priority, therefore, is the immediate establishment of an airway, either by intubation or tracheostomy, until the swelling subsides. Many centers routinely use nasotracheal intubation as the airway of choice in epiglottitis.

A physician well trained in the placement of tracheostomies must be present when the intubation is attempted. Insertion of the laryngoscope may cause the epiglottis to swell and occlude the airway, making intubation impossible. If that occurs, the physician has precious little time to insert the tracheostomy tube and avoid anoxic brain damage.

Once intubated, every precaution is taken to prevent accidental extubation. If necessary, the patient should be sedated with agents that produce sedation without respiratory depression. Drugs of choice include morphine sulfate, fentanyl, midazolam, and lorazepam. The patient's limbs should be restrained to avoid self-extubation.

Meticulous care is taken of the artificial airway to prevent further complications. Suctioning is done as needed, preceded by hyperoxygenation with 100% oxygen. Chest physiotherapy may be indicated in the presence of increased secretions to prevent atelectasis and infection. Adequate heating and humidification of the inspired gas are closely monitored. Arterial oxygen levels should be continuously monitored by transcutaneous monitors or pulse oximetry to maintain proper oxygenation and ventilation. Oxygen is given as

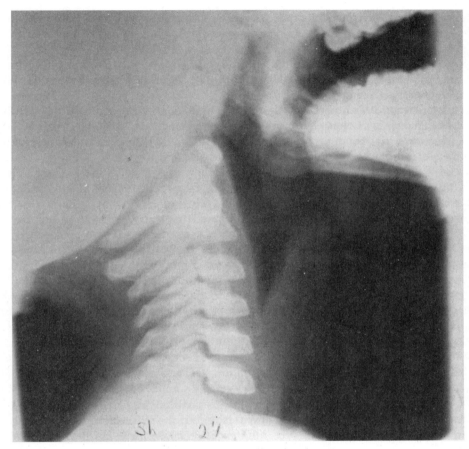

Figure 12–5 *The "thumb sign" of epiglottitis seen on a lateral neck x-ray.*

needed to maintain the patient in a normoxic state. Continuous cardiac monitoring should also be done while the patient is intubated.

Following establishment of the airway, the infection is treated with antibiotics, including ampicillin and third generation extended spectrum cephalosporines. Inflammation of the epiglottic region seldom lasts longer than 24 to 36 hours, at which point the patient may be extubated with no further danger of airway occlusion (Levin, 1997).[70]

Mechanical ventilation is required if paralyzation is necessary. Because the lung is basically healthy, very low pressures, rates, and FiO_2 are needed to maintain ventilation.

CROUP (LARYNGOTRACHEOBRONCHITIS—LTB)

Croup is the name given to a group of inflammatory diseases that affect the subglotitc area of the larynx. Three primary disorders fall in the category of croup. The most common manifestation of croup is laryngotracheitis. Spasmodic croup and laryngotracheobronchitis are less common manifestations seen in pediatric populations.

Diagnosis. Laryngotracheitis is the result of a viral organism, with parainfluenza virus accounting for 75% of all croup cases. RSV, influenzas, and *Mycoplasma pneumoniae* cause the remaining 25% of croup cases.

The onset is that of a common cold, with runny nose, cough, fever, and upper airway congestion. The onset of croup symptoms is much slower than is seen in epiglottitis, usually 3 to 4 days. The patient typically wakes in the night, with a tight, barky cough. The patient has upper airway stridor on inspiration and expiration and is in a degree of distress relative to the amount of airway obstruction. An anterior-posterior neck x-ray shows the narrowing of the airway at the level of the larynx. The trachea on these patients has been described as an hourglass, a pencil, and a steeple (Figure 12–6).

Spasmodic croup is an apparent allergic response that results in the sudden onset, usually at night, of a barky cough, shortness of breath, and stridor. The symptoms last for several hours and then subside. The distinguishing factor is in the history. The patient with spasmodic croup is typically healthy, with no signs of upper respiratory infection. There is also a frequent familial history of spasmodic croup and asthma.

Laryngotracheobronchitis is the name given to a bacterial superinfection of laryngotracheitis. As the name suggests, this category of croup involves not only the upper airway structures, but progresses to the bronchial airways and structures.

Treatment. Mild cases of croup may be successfully monitored and treated at home with room humidifiers, adequate hydration, and close observation. However, any sign of distress such as retractions, increased respiratory rate, and nasal flaring are indications for the need of medical invervention.

Because of its viral origin, common croup is treated by support and administration of drugs to reduce the subglottic swelling until the infection subsides. Primary medical treatment involves the nebulization of racemic epinephrine, 0.2 to 0.5 ml mixed with 2.5 ml of normal saline. Racemic epinephrine causes local vasoconstriction on the swollen tissues and reduces the edema.

If the stridor continues after the treatment, the patient is hospitalized and medication nebulizer treatments are continued as needed every 1 to 2 hours to relieve the airway occlusion. The treatments are then weaned to every 4 to 6 hours as the symptoms subside.

Steroids are often given, with Decadron being the popular choice due to its long half-life (36 to 72 hours) and because it is much more potent than hydrocortisone.[70]

Patients with severe obstruction of the airway may benefit from the use of an oxygen/helium gas mixture to provide oxygenation. Further treatment involves the use of cool mist tents to further reduce swelling and administer any necessary oxygen.

Severe manifestations of croup, such as labored breathing, decreased breath sounds, retractions, and worsening blood gases, may require intubation and the institution of mechanical ventilation. The use of glucocorticoid therapy for the treatment of croup has been strongly supported. In particular, nebulized budesonide has been shown to provide prompt clinical improvement in patients with mild to moderate croup.[71]

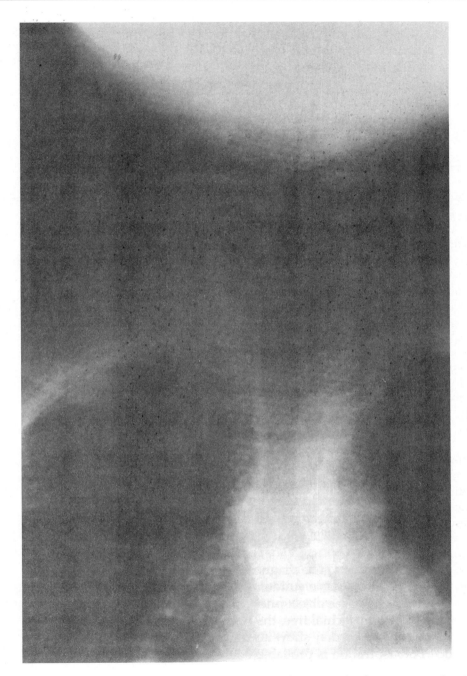

Figure 12–6 *An A-P neck x-ray showing the narrowing of the larynx. Notice the appearance of a steeple or an hourglass.*

Although it is not usually a life-threatening disease, any disease that causes swelling of the airway must be closely monitored for signs of worsening condition. The patient who appears to be at rest and comfortable may be semicomatose from exhaustion and the inability to ventilate. The nature of mist tents, with their high output of aerosol, further inhibits the ability to adequately visualize the patient. Because of these factors, the croup patient must be monitored for breath sounds, respiratory rate, and the presence of retractions at least every 4 hours until the airway swelling subsides.

ASPIRATION SYNDROMES

Infants are at a high risk of aspirating foreign objects owing to their insatiable desire to put objects in their mouth. This is further complicated by the narrowness of the airway, which makes even small objects potential airway obstructors. Aspiration of gastric contents is a common result of reflux in the newborn infant.

The pathologic result of aspiration is air trapping and tissue damage secondary to hydrocarbon aspiration. Air trapping is the result of the ball-valve effect, in which the aspirated object advances deeper into the airway during inspiration, as the airway dilates, and then becomes trapped during exhalation, when the airway collapses back to its original size. The result is the trapping of air behind the object, leading to hyperexpansion of the lung, reduced ventilation, and possible pneumothoraces.

The aspiration of hydrocarbons, such as gasoline, oils, turpentine, and kerosene, cause toxic damage to the epithelial lining of the lung called chemical bronchitis. Absorption of these toxic liquids into the blood leads to central nervous system disorders and toxic cardiomyopathies and hepatosplenomegaly. Chemical bronchitis leads to inflammation, edema, atelectasis, mucosal necrosis, and, if aspirated deeply, the formation of hyaline membranes.

Diagnosis and Treatment. The diagnosis of foreign body aspiration is made primarily on the history. The patient has a sudden onset of a dry, hacking cough. The patient may have been observed eating the object before the onset of symptoms. If the object is inhaled deeply into the tracheobronchial tree, the coughing may subside somewhat.

Chest x-ray examination may show air trapping distal to the obstruction during expiration. Hydrocarbon aspiration is probable when the symptomatic patient is found near an open container of hydrocarbon liquid and the patient has the strong odor of the liquid on the breath.

Treatment of an aspirated foreign body involves measures to remove the object. Chest physiotherapy may help dislodge the object from the airway. Severe cases may require the use of a bronchoscope to retrieve the object.

Treatment of hydrocarbon aspiration is nonspecific and consists mainly of support. However, if the substance has been swallowed, vomiting should not be induced. As symptoms dictate, the patient is given oxygen and bronchodilators, or intubation and mechanical ventilation are performed.

INHALATION OF NOXIOUS GASES

SMOKE INHALATION

Smoke inhalation is a broad category that covers a range of noxious gases produced in a fire. Most deaths in fires result from the inhalation of these noxious fumes, not from burns. Modern furniture and building materials give off many acids and aldehydes in their smoke when burned. These include carbon monoxide, sulfur dioxide, hydrochloric acid, phosgene, and hydrocyanic acid.

Carbon monoxide and hydrocyanic acid absorb into the bloodstream and cause serious toxicities in the blood and tissues. Carbon monoxide binds the carrying sites on the hemoglobin molecule, making it impossible for the red blood cell to carry oxygen at those sites. High levels of carbon monoxide lead to widespread tissue hypoxia and eventual death.

Hydrocyanic acid is chemically changed into cyanide, which prevents the uptake of oxygen from the blood by the tissues and leads to rapid death. The other gases and particles found in smoke damage the epithelial lining of the tracheobronchial tree, resulting in airway obstruction from edema, necrosis, sloughing of necrotic epithelium, and bronchospasm. Airway damage may also occur from thermal injury; however, thermal injuries are usually confined to the upper airways.

Diagnosis. Any patient who presents a history of being involved in a fire should be suspected of having suffered smoke inhalation. The patient with significant carbon monoxide poisoning may complain of headache, nausea, and vomiting with COHb levels of 20 to 30%. As the COHb climbs above 40%, the patient begins losing sensorium and becomes comatose.

Diagnosis is made by analyzing the carbon monoxide level of arterial blood with a CO-oximeter. Signs and symptoms of airway damage may be present immediately or may be delayed for hours. The patient shows signs of ever-increasing respiratory distress, with tachypnea, retractions, and cyanosis. As the airway obstruction increases, aeration decreases, widespread atelectasis forms, and the patient's status diminishes quickly.

Treatment. The treatment of any patient with smoke inhalation and carbon monoxide poisoning is immediate application of 100% oxygen, preferably under pressure.

In room air, the half-life of COHb is 5 hours, declining to 90 minutes in 100% oxygen. Hyperbaric oxygen administration reduces the half-life to less than 30 minutes.

Hyperbaric oxygen administration is the treatment of choice when the COHb is greater than 25%. If none is available, or at lower levels, oxygen is administered by a tight-fitting, nonrebreathing mask. The addition of a nasal cannula running at 5 to 6 lpm will help increase the FiO_2.

The hypoxia that results from carbon monoxide poisoning often affects the heart. Therefore, all smoke inhalation patients should have continuous ECG monitoring to observe for signs of myocardial damage.

Pulmonary edema is a frequent finding in patients suffering from carbon monoxide poisoning and smoke inhalation. This necessitates the frequent assessment of breath sounds and monitoring of the respiratory status.

The victim of smoke inhalation is at risk for development of RDS. This requires the practitioner to monitor the patient's status closely and be prepared for quick intervention if necessary.

Patients without obvious, immediate airway damage are monitored closely for signs of worsening respiratory status. When respiratory failure is apparent, the patient is intubated and mechanically ventilated to maintain oxygenation and ventilation.

Antibiotics are given to combat lung infections that take advantage of the damaged tissues. Meticulous attention to proper aseptic techniques will help in preventing nosocomial pneumonias. Attention is also given to adequate fluid and electrolyte balance, especially if the patient is suffering from skin burns, which tremendously increases water losses. Bronchoscopy may be needed to remove the epithelial debris that clogs the airways.

Nebulized bronchodilators, followed by chest physiotherapy, is helpful in maintaining the patency of the airways.

Mechanical ventilation is required on the comatose patient to establish an airway and administer oxygen. Ventilator parameters must be set at the lowest levels to achieve oxygenation and ventilation with correct I:E ratios to prevent possible air trapping and barotrauma. In addition, hypocarbia must be avoided because of the left shift of the oxyhemoglobin dissociation curve in the presence of alkalosis.

CHLORINE INHALATION

Chlorine is a greenish-yellow gas that is extremely irritating to the mucous membranes and skin. In the pediatric patient, inhalation is commonly the result of accidents at swimming pools, where the chlorine is used to disinfect the water. Chlorine is also found in a variety of household cleaning agents.

The injury to the respiratory tract following chlorine inhalation follows four phases. In phase 1, from zero to 6 hours following exposure, choking and coughing are present to some degree, but diminish following removal from the site. Minimal wheezing and slight oropharyngeal redness are present.

Phase 2 occurs between 6 hours and 8 days with the onset of pharyngeal and pulmonary edema, inflammation, and plugging of the bronchi with mucus. Atelectasis develops, as does significant respiratory distress from the combination of upper airway edema and lower airway blockage from sloughing epithelium and tissue debris.

Treatment at this point is mainly supportive, with intubation or tracheostomy often necessary. Large tubes are preferable to assist in the aspiration of airway debris. Mechanical ventilation is started when signs of impending respiratory failure are present. High levels of oxygen may be needed to treat hypoxemia. The use of bronchodilators helps reduce any bronchospasm that may be present.

Phase 3 occurs during weeks 1 to 4 with a gradual improvement in pulmonary function.

Phase 4 occurs after the fourth week, with further improvements in airway function and in blood gas status.

SUDDEN INFANT DEATH SYNDROME (SIDS)

Although much time and effort has been spent in the study of SIDS, it remains a relatively unknown entity and accounts for the highest number of deaths in infants of less than 1 year. The diagnosis of SIDS is not made until an autopsy is performed. A previously healthy infant who dies suddenly and unexpectedly during sleep, and on autopsy shows no apparent reason for the death, is diagnosed as a victim of SIDS.

In April 1992, the American Academy of Pediatrics recommended that infants not be placed in the prone position to sleep because of the association with SIDS; this initiative is known as the "back to sleep" program. While the exact relationship between the prone position and SIDS has not been determined, four factors have been identified which elevate the risk of SIDS in the prone position. They are: 1) the use of natural fiber mattresses; 2) swaddling; 3) recent illness; and 4) the use of heating in the bedroom.[72] The reduction in the number of infants sleeping prone was seen as a major contributing factor in a SIDS decline rate in Tasmania.[73]

Recently, risk factors associated with SIDS have been extensively studied. Traditional risk factors include black race, low birth weight, prematurity, 5 minute Apgar score less than 7, male gender, low maternal age and education level, multiple births, and maternal smoking. When examined statistically, the only risk factor independently associated with SIDS was maternal smoking.[74] This link between maternal smoking, passive smoke exposure, and SIDS has been corroborated in other studies.[75–77]

Several other factors that play a role in SIDS have been proposed. They include the following: increased levels of interleukin-6 in the cerebrospinal fluid[78]; surfactant abnormalities[79]; anaphylaxis[80]; variability in organ weights[81]; gastroesophageal reflux[82]; abnormal pulmonary inflammatory response[83]; maternal cocaine use[84]; and basement membrane thickening of the vocal cords.[85]

SIDS usually hits during winter and at night, and the most common ages are 1 to 3 months. Even with a knowledge of risk factors, it remains impossible to identify those infants who will die of SIDS. The incidence of SIDS remains at approximately 2 out of every 1000 births and continues to frustrate attempts to solve its cause.

The common event in all SIDS deaths is a quiet cessation of breathing during sleep. It is apparent that SIDS is a complex, multifactorial disorder that at the present time has no cure.

SUMMARY

The list of pediatric diseases requiring respiratory care is extensive. In general, they can be divided into groups comprised of ventilatory diseases, neuromuscular disorders, infectious lung diseases, problems associated with inhalation of noxious gases, and SIDS.

ARDS, as seen in the pediatric population, differs from RDS of the newborn. ARDS is predisposed by either direct or indirect trauma to the pulmonary system. ARDS is divided into four phases, starting with dyspnea and tachypnea, and worsening to pulmonary fibrosis, pneumonias, hypoxemia, hypercarbia, and acidosis. If intervention is not undertaken aggressively, death ensues.

Asthma continues to be a significant cause of respiratory distress in the pediatric population. The cause of asthma is complex and interrelated between many factors. Ideally, avoidance of triggering factors is of primary importance. Drug treatment is focused on preventing the release of inflammatory mediators, reversing of bronchospasm, and reduction of inflammation in the airways. Research focusing on new longer acting medications, which prevent or slow the onset of asthma, are promising.

Cystic fibrosis is an inherited disorder that causes the mucus secreting glands of the pulmonary tree to produce extremely thick, viscous mucus. This, in turn, leads to chronic infections, lung damage and eventual death. The diagnosis of CF is made by the presence of chronic lung congestion, pancreatic insufficiency, a failure to thrive, respiratory colonization with *Pseudomonas,* with or without elevated sweat chloride levels. Treatment is aimed at removing excessive secretions with CPT techniques, and aerosolized bronchodilators, mucolytics, and antibiotics. The goal is to reduce the number and severity of infections.

Neuromuscular disorders may be the result of atrophic disorders, muscular dystrophies, acquired disorders, and trauma. Respiratory care for these disorders varies from measures to prevent atelectasis and infection, in the case of paralytic disorders, to a reduction in cerebral blood flow, as with traumatic brain injuries.

Infectious lung diseases often require aggressive respiratory care to prevent unwanted complications. Pneumonias are treated with antibiotic therapy and also therapies aimed at removing excessive secretions and reinflating atelectatic lung.

Bronchiolitis is a viral infection that has its most dire consequences on young patients with underlying illness, hypoxia, prematurity, young age, apnea, and pulmonary consolidation as seen on chest x-ray. Treatment with ribavirin is indicated for these patients at high risk. Other treatments include aerosolized bronchodilators, alpha-interferon 2A, immunoglobulin A, and RSV immune globulin.

Epiglottis represents a true emergency. Epiglottitis, which is caused by *Haemophilus influenzae,* can cause complete closure of the patient's airway. Treatment includes intubation to secure the airway, and antibiotics to treat the infection.

Croup is an inflammation of the subglottic area caused by a virus. While usually not life threatening, croup can potentially occlude the airway and requires close monitoring. Because it is viral, croup does not respond to antibiotic therapy. Treatment is geared toward relief of the edema with aerosolized racemic epinephrine and cool mists.

Aspiration of a foreign body can be difficult to diagnose. It should be suspected in any patient with a recent onset of coughing with no other obvious cause. Chest x-rays may show air trapping beyond the foreign body, but often do not show the foreign body itself. Treatment may be conservative, with chest physiotherapy, or may require aggressive therapy such as bronchoscopy to remove the object.

The inhalation of noxious gases leads to damage of the epithelial lining of the pulmonary tree, and, in the case of smoke inhalation, carbon monoxide poisoning. Treatment is often prophylactic, with intubation being used to protect the airway from closure. Prevention of infection is another important aspect of care in these patients.

SIDS represents a major cause of mortality in patients up to age 1. While the exact cause of SIDS has yet to be identified, several risk factors have been identified. Of those, maternal smoking appears to the most closely associated with SIDS. Unfortunately, because the cause is not known, there is no treatment for SIDS, other than resuscitative efforts when it strikes.

References

1. Heulitt MJ, et al. Acute respiratory distress syndrome in pediatric patients: redirecting therapy to reduce iatrogenic lung injury. *Resp. Care.* 1995;40:74–85.

2. Burton GG, Hodgkin, JE, Wand JJ. *Respiratory Care: A Guide to Clinical Practice.* 4th ed. Philadelphia: JB Lippincott Co; 1997.

3. Sivan Y, et al. Adult respiratory distress syndrome in severely neutropenic children. *Pediatr Pulmonol.* 1990;8:104–108.

4. Richard C, et al. Vitamin E deficiency and lipoperoxidation during adult respiratory distress syndrome. *Crit Care Med.* 1990;18:4–9.

5. Idell S. The deadly danger of ARDS. *Emer Med.* 1989;21:67–68, 70, 72.

6. Hudson LD. The prediction and prevention of ARDS. *Resp Care.* 1990;35:161–173.

7. Maunder RJ, Hudson LD. Pharmacologic strategies for treating the adult respiratory distress syndrome. *Resp. Care.* 1990;35:241–246.

8. Russel JA, et al. Physiologic effects and side effects of prostaglandin E_1 in the adult respiratory distress syndrome. *Chest.* 19190;97:684–692.

9. Stachtiaris LE, Marino RV. The asthmatic child. *Emer Med.* 1989;21:119–120, 123–124.

10. Mitchell RS, et al. *Synopsis of Clinical Pulmonary Disease.* 4th ed. St. Louis: CV Mosby Co; 1989.

11. Zahr LK, et al. Assessment and management of the child with asthma. *Ped Nurs.* 1989;15:109–114.

12. Sur S, et al. Sudden-onset fatal asthma: a distinct entity with few eosinophils and relatively more neutrophils in the airway submucosa? *Am Rev Respir Dis.* 1993;148:713.

13. Carruthers DM, Harrison BD. Arterial blood gas analysis or oxygen saturation in the assessment of acute asthma. *Thorax.* 1995;50:186–188.

14. Manthous CA, et al. Heliox improves pulsus paradoxus and peak expiratory flow in nonintubated patients with severe asthma. *Am J Respir Crit Care Med.* 1995;151:310.

15. Howder CL. Antimuscarinic and β_2-adrenoceptor bronchodilators in obstructive airways disease. *Resp Care.* 1983;38:1364–1388.

16. Mathewson HS. Combined drug therapy in asthma [editorial]. *Resp. Care.* 1993;38:1340.

17. Colacone A, et al. Continuous nebulization of albuterol (salbutamol) in acute asthma. *Chest* 1990;97:693–697.

18. Fink JB, Jue PK. Humidity and aerosol therapy for pediatrics. In: Barnhart SL, Czervinske MP. *Perinatal and Pediatric Respiratory Care.* Philadelphia: WB Saunders Co; 1995.

19. D'Alonzo GE, et al. Salmeterol xinafoate as maintenance therapy compared with albuterol in patients with asthma. *JAMA*. 1994;271:1412.

20. Rivington RN, et al. Efficacy of Uniphyl®, salbutamol, and their combination in asthmatic patients on high-dose inhaled steroids. *Am J Respir Crit Care Med*. 1995;151:325.

21. Chou KJ, et al. Metered-dose inhalers with spacers vs Nebulizers for pediatric asthma. *Arch Pediatr Adolesc Med*. 1995;149:201–205.

22. Lin YZ, Hsieh KH. Metered dose inhaler and nebuliser in acute asthma. *Arch Dis Child*. 1995;72:214–218.

23. Spitzer WO, et al. The use of beta-agonists and the risk of death from asthma. *N Engl J Med*. 1992;326:501–506.

24. Chapman KR, et al. Regular vs as-needed inhaled salbutamol in asthma control. *Lancet*. 1994;343:1379.

25. Mathewson HS. Asthma and bronchitis: a shift of therapeutic emphasis. *Resp Care*. 1990;35:273, 275, 277.

26. Salmeron S, et al. High doses of inhaled corticosteroids in unstable chronic asthma: a multicenter, double-blind, placebo-controlled study. *Am Rev Respir Dis*. 1989;140:167–171.

27. Chin T, et al. Reversal of bronchial obstruction in children with mild stable asthma by aerosolized furosemide. *Pediatr Pulmonol*. 1994;18:93.

28. Mathewson HS. New avenues of asthma therapy. *Resp Care*. 1995;40:655–657.

29. Feinsilver SH. Respiratory failure in asthma and COPD. *Emer Med*. 1989;21:90, 93–94, 96.

30. Zimmerman SS, et al. *Critical Care Pediatrics*. Philadelphia: WB Saunders Co; 1985.

31. Johnston RG, et al. Isoflurane therapy for status asthmaticus in children and adults. *Chest*. 1990;97:698–701.

32. Newcomb RW. Respiratory failure from asthma: a marker for children with high morbidity and mortality. *Am J Dis Child*. 1988;142:1041–1044.

33. Gan KH, et al. A cystic fibrosis mutation associated with mild lung disease. *N Engl J Med*. 1995;333:95–99.

34. Colledge WH, Evans MJ. Cystic fibrosis gene therapy. *Br Med Bull*. 1995;51:82–90.

35. Burgess WR, Chernick V. *Respiratory Therapy in Newborn Infants and Children*. New York: Thieme-Stratton Inc; 1982.

36. Kahn TZ, et al. Early pulmonary inflammation in infants with cystic fibrosis. *Am J Respir Crit Care Med*. 1995;151:1075.

37. Demko CA, et al. Gender differences in cystic fibrosis: *Pseudomona aeruginosa* infection. *J Clin Epidemiol*. 1995;48:1041–1049.

38. Dankert-Roelse JE, et al. Survival and clinical outcome in patients with cystic fibrosis, with or without neonatal screening. *J Pediatrics*, 1989;114:362–367.

39. Stewart B, et al. Normal sweat chloride values do not exclude the diagnosis of cystic fibrosis. *Am J Respir Crit Care Med 151*. 1995;3(pt 1):899–903.

40. Highsmith WE, et al. A novel mutation in the cystic fibrosis gene in patients with pulmonary disease but normal sweat chloride concentrations. *N Engl J Med*. 1994;331:974.

41. Roberts G, et al. Screening for cystic fibrosis: a four year regional experience. *Arch Dis Child*. 1988;63:1438–1443.

42. Ries AL, et al. Restricted pulmonary function in cystic fibrosis. *Chest*. 1988;94:575–579.

43. Cooper PJ, et al. Variability of pulmonary function tests in cystic fibrosis. *Pediatr Pulmonol*. 1990;8:16–22.

44. Ramsey BW, et al. Efficacy of aerosolized tobramycin in patients with cystic fibrosis. *N Engl J Med*. 1993;328:1740–1746.

45. Sanchez I. The effect of high doses of inhaled salbutamol and ipratropium bromide in patients with stable cystic fibrosis. *Chest*. 1993;104:842.

46. Pan SH, et al. Bronchodilation from intravenous theophylline in patients with cystic fibrosis: results of a blinded placebo-controlled crossover clinical trial. *Pediatr Pulmonol*. 1989;6:172–179.

47. Fuchs HJ, et al. Effect of aerosolized recombinant human Dnase on exacerbations of respiratory symptoms and on pulmonary function in patients with cystic fibrosis. *N Engl J Med*. 1994;331:637.

48. Harris CE, Wilmott RW. Inhalation-based therapies in the treatment of cystic fibrosis. *Curr Opin Pediatr*. 1994;6:234–238.

49. Shah PL, et al. Medium term treatment of stable stage cystic fibrosis with recombinant human DNase I. *Thorax*. 1995;50:333–338.

50. Shak S. Aerosolized recombinant human DNase I for the treatment of cystic fibrosis. *Chest 107*. 1995;2(Suppl):65s–70s.

51. Tomkiewicz RP, et al. Amiloride inhalation therapy in cystic fibrosis. Influence on ion content, hydration, and rheology of sputum. *Am Rev Respir Dis 148*. 1993;4(pt 1):1002–1007.

52. Wilmott RW, Fiedler MA. Recent advances in the treatment of cystic fibrosis. *Pediatr Clin N Am*. 1994;41:431–451.

53. Van-Haren EH, et al. The effects of the inhaled corticosteroid budesonide on lung function and bronchial hyperresponsiveness in adult patients with cystic fibrosis. *Respir J Med*. 1995;332:848.

54. Konstan MW, et al. Effect of high-dose ibuprofen in patients with cystic fibrosis. *N Engl J Med*. 1995;332:848.

55. Thomas J, et al. Chest physical therapy management of patients with cystic fibrosis: a meta-analysis. *Am J Respir Crit Care Med*. 1995;151:846.

56. Boyd S, et al. Evaluation of the literature on the effectiveness of physical therapy modalities in the management of children with cystic fibrosis. *Pediatr Phys Ther*. 1994;6:70–74.

57. Bauer ML, et al. Comparison of manual and mechanical chest percussion in hospitalized patients with cystic fibrosis. *J Pediatr*. 1994;124:250.

58. Padman R, et al. Noninvasive positive pressure ventilation in end-stage cystic fibrosis: a report of seven cases. *Resp Care*. 1994;39:736–739.

59. Regnis JA, et al. Benefits of nocturnal nasal CPAP in patients with cystic fibrosis. *Chest*. 1994;106:1717–1724.

60. Scott J, et al. Heart-lung transplantation for cystic fibrosis. *Lancet*. 1988;2:192–194.

61. Ciriaco P, et al. Analysis of cystic fibrosis referrals for lung transplantation. *Chest*. 1995;107:1323–1327.

62. Wong D. *Whaley & Wong's Nursing Care of Infants and Children*. 6th ed. St. Louis: Mosby; 1990.

63. Nichter MA, Everett PB. Childhood near-drowning: is cardiopulmonary resuscitation always indicated? *Crit Care Med*. 1989;17:993–995.

64. Thibeault DW, Gregory GA. *Neonatal Pulmonary Care.* 2nd ed. Norwalk, Conn: Appleton-Century-Crofts; 1986.

65. Makela MJ, et al. Respiratory syncytial virus infection in children. *Curr Opin Pediatr.* 1994;6:17–22.

66. Wang EE, et al. Pediatric investigators collaborative network on infections in Canada (PICNIC) prospective study of risk factors and outcomes in patients hospitalized with respiratory syncytial viral lower respiratory tract infection. *J Pediatr.* 1995;126:212–219.

67. Meert KL, et al. Aerosolized ribavirin in mechanically ventilated children with respiratory syncytial virus lower respiratory tract disease: a prospective, double-blind, randomized trial. *Crit Care Med.* 1994;22:566.

68. Long CE, et al. Sequelae of respiratory syncytial virus infections. A role for intervention studies. *Am J Respir Crit Care Med.* 1995;151:1678–1680.

69. Sigurs N, et al. Asthma and immunoglobulin E antibodies after respiratory syncytial virus bronchiolitis: a prospective cohort study with matched controls. *Pediatrics.* 1995;95:500–505.

70. Levin D, Morriss F, et al. *Essentials of Pediatric Intensive Care.* 2nd ed. St. Louis, Mo: Quality Medical Publishing, Inc.; 1997.

71. Klassen ME. Nebulized budesonide for children with mild-to-moderate croup. *N Engl J Med.* 1994;331:285.

72. Ponsonby AL, et al. Factors potentiating the risk of sudden infant death syndrome associated with the prone position. *N Engl J Med.* 1993;329:377.

73. Dwyer T, et al. The contribution of changes in the prevalence of prone sleeping position to the decline in sudden infant death syndrome in Tasmania. *JAMA.* 1995;273:783–789.

74. Taylor JA, Sanderson M. A reexamination of the risk factors for the suddeen infant death syndrome. *J Pediatr.* 1995;126:887–891.

75. DiFranza JR, Lew RA. Effect of maternal cigarette smoking on pregnancy complications and sudden infant death syndrome. *J Fam Pract.* 1995;40:385–394.

76. Klonoff-Cohen HS, et al. The effect of passive smoking and tobacco exposure through breast milk on sudden infant death syndrome. *JAMA.* 1995;273:795–798.

77. Fleming PJ. Understanding and preventing sudden infant death syndrome. *Curr Opin Pediatr.* 1994;6:158–162.

78. Vege A, et al. SIDS cases have increased levels of interleukin-6 in cerebrospinal fluid. *Acta Pediatr.* 1995;84:193–196.

79. Masters IB, et al. Surfactant abnormalities in ALTE and SIDS. *Arch Dis Child.* 1994;71:501–505.

80. Holgate ST, et al. The anaphylaxis hypothesis of sudden infant death syndrome (SIDS): mast cell degranulation in cot death revealed by elevated concentrations of tryptase in serum. *Clin Exp Allergy.* 1994;24:1115–1122.

81. Siebert JR, Haas JE. Organ weights in sudden infant death syndrome. *Pediatr Pathol.* 1994;14:973–985.

82. Freed GE, et al. Sudden infant death syndrome prevention and an understanding of selected clinical issues. *Pediatr Clin N Am.* 1994;41:967–990.

83. Howat WJ, et al. Pulmonary immunopathology of sudden infant death syndrome. *Lancet.* 1994;343:1390–1392.

84. Fox CH. Cocaine use in pregnancy. *J Am Board Fam Pract.* 1994;7:225–228.
85. Shatz A. Age-related basement membrane thickening of the vocal cords in sudden infant death syndrome (SIDS). *Laryngoscope.* 1994;104:865–868.

Bibliography and Suggested Readings

Beachey W. *Respiratory Care Anatomy and Physiology.* St. Louis, Mo: Mosby; 1997.
Chipps BE, et al. Alpha-2A-interferon for treatment of bronchiolitis caused by respiratory syncytial virus. *Pediatr Infect Dis J.* 1993;12:653–658.
Cottrell GP. *Cardiopulmonary Anatomy and Physiology for Respiratory Care Practitioners.* Philadelphia: FA Davis; 2000.
DeBruin W, et al. Acute hypoxemic respiratory failure in infants and children: clinical and pathologic characteristics. *Crit Care Med.* 1992;20:1223–1234.
Des Jardins T. *Cardiopulmonary Anatomy and Physiology.* 3rd ed. Albany, NY: Delmar Thomson Learning; 1998.
Groothuis JR, et al. Respiratory syncytial virus (RSV) infection in preterm infants and the protective effects of RSV immune globulin RSVIG. Respiratory syncytial virus immune globulin study group. *Pediatrics.* 1995;95:463–467.
Harwood R. *Exam Review and Study Guide for Perinatal/Pediatric Respiratory Care.* Philadelphia: FA Davis; 1999.
Hess D. Neonatal and pediatric respiratory care: some implications for adult respiratory care practitioners. *Resp Care.* 1991;36:489–513.
Pilbeam SP. *Mechanical Ventilation: Physiological and Clinical Applications.* 3rd ed. St. Louis, Mo: Mosby; 1998.
Steinbach S, et al. Transmissibility of *Pseudomonas cepacia* infection in clinic patients and lung transplant recipients with cystic fibrosis. *N Engl J Med.* 1994;331:981.
Taussig LM, Landau LI. *Pediatric Respiratory Medicine.* St. Louis, Mo: Mosby; 1999.
Weltzin R, et al. Intranasal monoclonal immunoglobulin A against respiratory syncytial virus protects against upper and lower respiratory tract infections in mice. *Antimicrob Agents Chemother.* 1994;38:2785–2791.

Posttest

1. Which of the following is not considered one of the phases of ARDS?
   a. dyspnea and tachycardia
   b. progressive respiratory failure
   c. alveolar/capillary membranes become leaky
   d. significant barotrauma
2. Which of the following are possible strategies in the treatment of ARDS?
   I. maintain arterial PCO_2 below normal
   II. hyperventilation
   III. correct any physical derangements

    IV. suppress alveolar inflammation

    V. prevent complications

       a. I, III, V

       b. II, III, V

       c. III, IV, V

       d. I, II, IV, V

3. The release of mediators by eosinophils, neutrophils, macrophages, and lymphocytes is seen during:

    a. phase II of an asthma attack

    b. an exacerbation of ARDS

    c. Werdnig-Hoffman paralysis

    d. Guillain-Barré syndrome

4. The branch(es) of CNS that appear(s) to be primarily responsible for inhibiting bronchial smooth muscle contraction is (are) the:

    a. sympathetic

    b. parasympathetic

    c. nonadrenergic noncholinergic

    d. both a and c

5. Which of the following would be the drug of choice during the inflammatory stage of asthma?

    a. theophylline

    b. beclomethasone

    c. albuterol

    d. cromolyn

6. The most reliable diagnosis of cystic fibrosis involves:

    a. family history

    b. failure to thrive

    c. sweat/chloride levels

    d. evidence of pancreatic insufficiency

7. Which of the following are commonly used in the treatment of patients with cystic fibrosis?

    I. oxygen

    II. aerosolized antibiotics

    III. theophylline

    IV. mist tents

    V. CPT

       a. I, IV

       b. I, III, V

       c. II, III, V

       d. I, II, III, V

8. Which of the following is (are) inherited as autosomal-recessive traits?

    I. Kugelberg-Welander disease

    II. Duchenne-type muscular dystrophy

    III. Guillain-Barré syndrome

IV. Werdnig-Hoffman paralysis
    a. I only
    b. I, IV
    c. II, III
    d. II, III, IV

9. Edrophonium (Tensilon) is used to diagnose which of the following?
    a. myasthenia gravis
    b. Guillain-Barré syndrome
    c. botulism
    d. Duchenne-type muscular dystrophy

10. The diaphragm is primarily innervated by:
    a. the first cervical nerve
    b. the third thoracic nerve
    c. the fourth cervical nerve
    d. the first lumbar nerve

11. Secondary brain injuries include which of the following?
    I. hematoma
    II. brain fracture
    III. hypoxia
    IV. brain contusion
    V. hypotension
        a. I, III, IV
        b. I, III, V
        c. II, IV, V
        d. III, IV, V

12. Treating a patient with a head injury, the respiratory care practitioner receives the following arterial blood gas: pH = 7.48; $PaCO_2$ = 34 mm Hg; PaO_2 = 120 mm Hg. The appropriate response would be:
    a. continue with the present therapy
    b. increase the FiO_2
    c. increase ventilation and FiO_2
    d. increase ventilation only

13. Which of the following factors increase survival in near-drowning patients?
    I. rapid administration of CPR
    II. patients in a young age group
    III. short duration of immersion
    IV. male gender
    V. higher core temperatures
        a. I only
        b. I, II, IV
        c. III, V
        d. V only

14. Reye's syndrome is diagnosed by:
    a. patient history

  b. sputum culture and sensitivity
  c. CT scan
  d. liver biopsy
15. Which of the following would favor the development of an in utero fetal pneumonia?
  I. fetal asphyxia
  II. prolonged rupture of the amniotic membranes
  III. maternal exercise
  IV. excessive obstetrical manipulation
  V. prolonged labor
      a. I, II, III, V
      b. II, III, IV
      c. I, III, V
      d. II, IV, V
16. Which of the following organisms is the most likely to cause bronchiolitis?
  a. parainfluenza virus
  b. respiratory syncytial virus
  c. Haemophilus influenzae
17. A young patient presents in the ER with a history of a rapid onset of difficulty breathing. The patient complains of a severe sore throat and the voice is muffled. Which of the following would be appropriate at this time?
  a. lateral neck x-ray
  b. visualization of the tracheal opening with a laryngoscope
  c. MRI of the neck and thorax
  d. bronchoscopy
18. What treatment is preferred for the disease suspected in question 17?
  a. medication nebulizer with racemic epinephrine
  b. mist tent with oxygen as needed
  c. CPT and PD
  d. immediate intubation
19. When treating coup, which of the following would be the drug of choice?
  a. theophylline
  b. albuterol
  c. racemic epinephrine
  d. atropine
20. Which of the following gases is not released during a fire involving furniture and other building materials?
  a. carbon monoxide
  b. carbon dioxide
  c. sulfur dioxide
  d. phosgene
21. Coma is possible at carbon monoxide levels of greater than:
  a. 10%
  b. 20%

    c. 30%

    d. 40%

22. Development of atelectasis, edema, inflammation, and plugging of the bronchi occur during which phase of chlorine inhalation?

    a. phase 4

    b. phase 3

    c. phase 2

    d. phase 1

23. The incidence of SIDS is increased in which of the following?

    I. babies with low Apgar scores

    II. babies of mothers younger than 20 years old

    III. inadequate maternal prenatal care

    IV. maternal drug abuse

    V. babies who are small for gestational age

        a. I, II, III

        b. II, III, IV, V

        c. I, II, IV, V

        d. I, II, III, IV, V

CHAPTER THIRTEEN

INTERPRETATION OF CHEST X-RAYS

OBJECTIVES

Upon completion of this chapter, the reader should be able to:

1. Explain why x-rays alone cannot be used for diagnosis.
2. Describe the basic mechanics of how an x-ray is taken.
3. List and describe the three densities found on an x-ray.
4. Discuss the diagnostic usefulness and limitations of x-ray.
5. Describe how each of the following are determined when interpreting a chest x-ray:
   a. Patient identification
   b. Orientation of the x-ray
   c. Quality of the x-ray
   d. Patient position
   e. Determination of inspiration or expiration
   f. Proper heart size
   g. Proper position of the umbilical artery and vein catheter
   h. Congestive heart failure and right-to-left shunting
   i. Proper position of the endotracheal tube
6. Describe the cause and appearance of air bronchograms.
7. Describe the appearance of the following neonatal disorders on a chest x-ray:
   a. Respiratory distress syndrome
   b. Atelectasis
   c. Transient tachypnea of the newborn
   d. Pneumonia
   e. Meconium aspiration syndrome
   f. Diaphragmatic hernia
   g. Congenital lobar emphysema
   h. Pneumothorax
   i. Pneumomediastinum
   j. Pneumopericardium
   k. Pulmonary interstitial emphysema
   l. Bronchopulmonary dysplasia

8. Describe the radiographic appearance of the following pediatric disorders:
    a. Adult respiratory distress syndrome (ARDS)
    b. Foreign body aspiration
    c. Cystic fibrosis
    d. Asthma
    e. Epiglottitis
    f. Croup

KEY TERMS

air bronchograms
costophrenic angle
decubitus
densities
hilum

hyperlucency
MAS/KV
pseudocysts
radiopaque

reticulogranular
roentgenograph
scaphoid
thymus

BASIC CONCEPTS

X-rays have become a very important tool in managing newborns with lung disease because of their ability to give views of the effect of various disease processes on the internal body structures. When interpreting x-rays, it must be kept in mind that the disease itself is not seen. The radiograph represents a visual confirmation of the presence or absence of a disease process. The physical alterations resulting from a disease are seen on the x-ray film. For example, the air between the chest wall and the lung in a typical pneumothorax is not visible, but the lung tissue being pushed aside and compressed is visible. The space between both, filled with air, is distinct on the x-ray.

In most instances, a physician will be present to interpret the chest x-ray; however, there will be times when the physician is not available and other practitioners may be the first to view the film. In those instances, it is important that the practitioner be able to identify those abnormalities on the x-ray that could be vital in the care of the patient.

X-RAY PROJECTIONS

In order to fully visualize an abnormality in the chest of a patient, two x-ray views are required, frontal and lateral. If the patient is able to stand, the film is placed in front of the patient and the x-ray is projected from behind the patient. Because of the x-rays travel from the posterior to the anterior of the patient, this is called a posterior/anterior or PA view. On patients who cannot leave the bed, such as those being ventilated, the film is placed under the patient and the x-ray passes from anterior to posterior, creating an anterior/posterior or AP view.

It can usually be expected that a chest film of any newborn or intubated pediatric patient is an AP view, but the practitioner should always make sure which view was obtained. This is because PA and AP views cause the internal structures to appear differently and can cause a misdiagnosis if not understood. As an example, because the heart lies more anteriorly in the chest, it will appear larger on an AP film than on a PA film.

While the frontal view identifies whether an abnormality is on the right or left side of the chest, the lateral view identifies its position anteriorly or posteriorly. The lateral view is also used on the neck to identify an enlarged epiglottis.

MECHANICS OF THE X-RAY DEVICE

The basic mechanism of the x-ray is similar to photography. The x-ray is a frequency of light, outside the visible spectrum, that can penetrate most body substances. A film that is sensitive to x-rays is placed on the opposite side of the body from the x-ray "camera." The x-rays are then aimed through the desired part of the body (Figure 13–1). Some of the x-rays pass through and expose the film, while others are blocked from passing through. The film is developed and a transparent picture is obtained.

DENSITIES SEEN ON X-RAY

Three densities can be distinguished on x-ray, described below and listed in Table 13–1. First is an air or gas density. X-rays pass easily through gases, totally exposing the x-ray film and turning it black. Second are the fluid densities. Fluids partially absorb the x-rays and allow

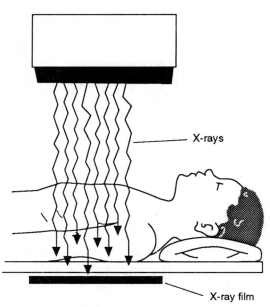

X-rays

X-ray film

Figure 13–1 *X-rays pass through the body, creating an image on film.*

Table 13–1   Densities Found on X-Rays

---

1. Air density—produces the darkest patterns
2. Fluid density—produces gray patterns
3. Bone density—produces the lighest patterns

---

only a portion of the x-rays to reach the film. The result is a grayish shade on the developed film. Various tissues of the body are largely liquid, and so create a hue similar to fluids on the x-ray. When such tissue is irregular in its density, the film will be patchy, stippled, or look like ground window glass. Third are the bone densities, which absorb a large position of the x-rays. If no x-rays reach the film, that area of the x-ray will be white. The amount of calcium in the bone will determine whether the bone is white or slightly transparent. Well-calcified bone is white on x-ray, compared to less calcified bone, which appears slightly more transparent.

DIAGNOSTIC USEFULNESS AND LIMITATIONS

It is important to remember that x-rays cannot be used to diagnose lung disease in newborns. The patient's diagnosis is made from physical examination, laboratory data, and clinical signs. Radiographs are then used to confirm the diagnosis. X-rays are also used to differentiate between diseases with similar signs and symptoms. They are limited by the fact that artifact, improper techniques in taking the x-ray, and patient movement may all lead to erroneous interpretation. The person examining the x-ray must be careful to avoid mistaking these factors for disease.

ANATOMIC CONSIDERATIONS

There are anatomic differences in the chest x-rays of neonates and children, which may cause confusion if not understood. First, the position of the carina—the point at which the trachea splits into the left and right mainstream bronchi—is higher than in adults. In a neonate, it is near the level of the third vertebrae and by age 10 it has descended to the level of the fifth vertebrae.[1]

The thymus is a gland located in the mediastinum extending from the lower edge of the thyroid gland in the neck to near the fourth rib. On x-ray, it appears less dense than the heart, but more dense than lung tissue. It is often confused with the heart border and can even appear as an upper lobe atelectasis or pneumonia. Often, it is triangular shaped and is called the "sail sign" when identified on x-ray. Its size in relation to the rest of the body is largest at about 2 years of age.

METHOD OF INTERPRETATION

Often, when reading an x-ray, our attention is drawn to a single overwhelming feature and we may overlook significant details. To avoid this, the caregiver should use a systematic approach when examining a chest x-ray, outlined in Table 13–2.

Table 13–2   Systematic Approach to Reading a Chest Radiograph

---

1. Confirm correct patient and date.
2. Correct orientation. Patient's left side should be on your right as you view the radiograph.
3. Check the quality of the radiograph. Check for over-or underexposure.
4. Confirm proper patient position.
5. Determine whether the radiograph is inspiratory or expiratory.
6. Examine the diaphragm.
7. Examine the abdomen.
8. Inspect the cardiac silhouette.
9. Examine the area of the lung hilum.
10. Inspect the respiratory tract:
    a. Trachea
    b. Position of the endotracheal tube
    c. Mainstream bronchus
    d. Lung fields
    e. Pleural surface

SYSTEMATIC APPROACH TO READING A CHEST X-RAY

Patient Identification and Date. Above all, check the patient identification stamp, date, and time. For accurate assessment of the patient's current problems, it is important to use the most recent x-ray. This may also save you some embarrassment when you present a dazzling interpretation of the x-ray, just to find out it is the wrong patient or the film is a week old.

Orientation. You should next orient the x-ray so that the patient's right side is on your left. This is often marked by the x-ray technician, but always check the anatomy yourself. Determining the infant's position at the time of the x-ray will help in orientation. Look for landmarks such as heart leads, a transcutaneous monitor, and chest tube sites. The heart should be centered but slightly to the left. If a stomach bubble is present, it should be on your right as you look at the film. Also, make certain that the film is not upside down. Many normal infants have mistakenly been diagnosed as having a diaphragmatic hernia, when the only problem was an upside-down film.

X-Ray Quality. Next check the quality of the x-ray. Determine if it is over-, under-, or normally exposed. Spaces between the vertebrae are visible and distinct when a proper exposure has been made. If the spaces between the vertebrae are not visible, too little energy was used and the film is underexposed. Too much energy overexposes the film, making the intervertebral spaces excessively dark. An x-ray that is over- or underexposed will be very difficult to interpret. The lung fields in an overexposed chest x-ray may look well aerated when in reality they are very underaerated. Conversely, the lung fields in an underexposed chest x-ray may appear vastly underaerated when in fact they are well aerated.

It is good practice to post the MAS/KV, the duration of exposure, and the energy used that resulted in a good exposure at the patient's bedside or on the incubator. This will help in consistently getting good exposures.

Patient Position. Next check the position of the infant on the film. The infant should be relatively straight on the film, and not rotated to either side. Rotation will alter the heart size and cover areas you may need to see. The clavicles should be examined for symmetry in relation to the spinal column. When the infant is straight, the clavicles and spine should form a "T," with both clavicles symmetrical and at right angles to the spine, as shown in Figure 13–2. The peripheral ribs should turn downward, and not be flat or turning upward. A rotated chest x-ray may give you the impression of an enlarged heart or shifted trachea.

Determination of Inspiration and Expiration. The next step is to determine if the film was exposed during inspiration or expiration. On an inspiratory x-ray the diaphragm should be at or below the ninth rib, as shown in Figure 13–3. Overdistention or hyperaeration will be near or below the 10th rib. A radiograph taken during expiration will show the diaphragm at the sixth or seventh rib. At this point take the time to examine the ribs for any deformities or fractures.

Examination of the Diaphragm. Now examine the shape of the diaphragm. It should be dome-shaped on both sides, with the right diaphragm usually being one rib higher than the left. This is caused by the liver pushing the diaphragm upward. If the diaphragm does not meet this description, there may be a water density in the lung adjacent to the diaphragm. Air trapping and hyperaeration will cause the diaphragms to become flat.

Examination of the Abdomen. Chest x-rays do not often include a great deal of the abdomen, but the practitioner should learn to examine the portion of the abdomen that is present. The presence of a stomach bubble helps to orient the film. A large air bubble in the stomach and excessive air in the bowel (Figure 13–4) are indicative of gastric distention. Excessive distention in the stomach can decrease the ventilation of the infant by pressing upward against the diaphragm.

Examining the upper right side of the abdomen, the posterior edge of the liver is seen as the lowest visible edge. The liver appears a gray-to-white shade on the film because it is a fairly thick tissue. The liver should not be more than 1 to 1.5 cm below the rib cage. A liver that is below that level may be an indication of blood engorgement resulting from right-sided heart failure.

If enough of the abdomen is showing, check the position of the umbilical artery or vein catheter. The tip of the umbilical artery catheter (UAC) should lie between the seventh and eighth thoracic vertebrae (T7-T8) or between the third and fourth lumbar vertebrae (L3-L4), as shown in Figure 13–5. One study found a higher incidence of leg blanching and

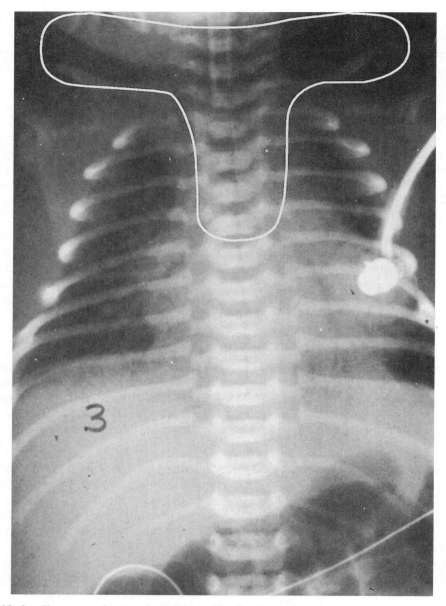

Figure 13–2 *Chest x-ray showing the "T" formed by clavicles and vertebrae.*

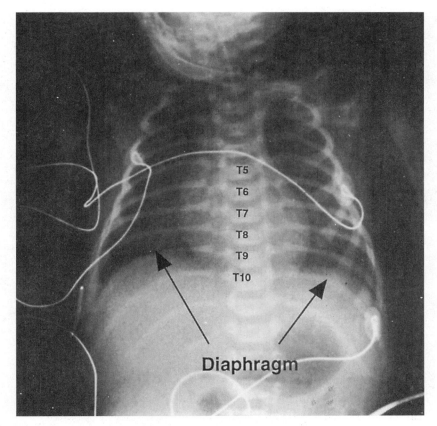

Figure 13–3 *Position of the diaphragm during inspiration.*

cyanosis in infants with the UAC tip at L3-L4. Finding the appropriate vertebrae can be done by locating the 12th thoracic vertebra (T12). T12 is the vertebra to which the last floating rib is attached. The next vertebra down is the first lumbar vertebra. Counting upward, T7 and T8 can be located. Placing the tip at T7-T8 positions the tip above the celiac arteries. Positioning the tip of the UAC between L3 and L4 places it above the division of the aorta into the legs and below the inferior mesenteric artery. These two positions prevent direct instillation of fluids and drugs into the celiac or mesenteric arteries. The L3-L4 position may also help prevent a possible hypoperfusion to the kidneys when blood is withdrawn from the catheter. The umbilical vein catheter is positioned in the interior vena cava, just above the diaphragm, as illustrated in Figure 13–6.

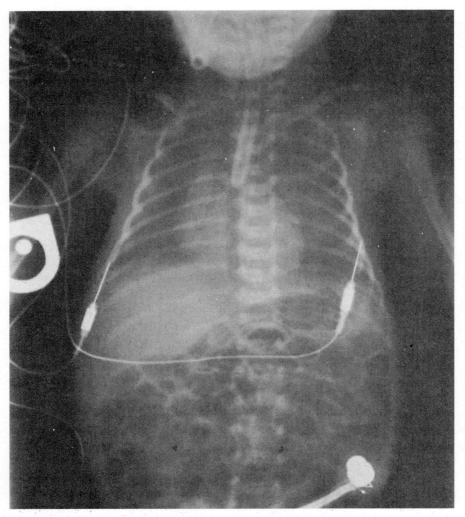

Figure 13–4 *Excessive gastric air resulting from an esophageal intubation.*

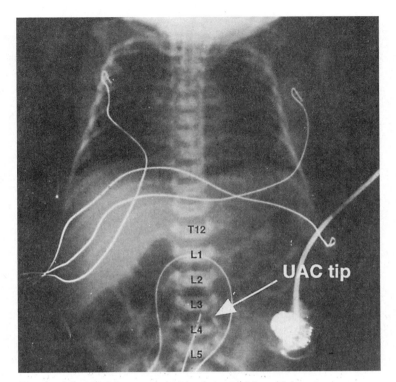

Figure 13–5 *The tip of the UAC in proper position between L3 and L4.*

umbil. art. cath.

Examination of the Cardiac Silhouette. The silhouette of the heart and thymus should now be examined. The cardiac silhouette (Figure 13–7) is extremely variable in size and should be less than 60% of the thoracic width. A cardiac silhouette larger than 60% implies an enlarged heart, but remember that the silhouette includes other structures in the mediastinum, including the thymus. Diagnosis of cardiomegaly is not done solely from the chest x-ray, but is verified by other clinical signs and symptoms the patient demonstrates.

Examination of the Hilum. Now examine the hilum area of the chest. The hilum, outlined in Figure 13–8, is the area where the trachea splits and enters both lungs. Of special concern in this area is the amount of vascularity that is visible. The blood vasculature appears as white streaks fanning out from the center of the cardiac silhouette. Excess vascularity is seen in congestive heart failure and certain congenital heart malformations. Undervascularity is seen in right-to-left shunting, resulting in a decreased pulmonary blood flow.

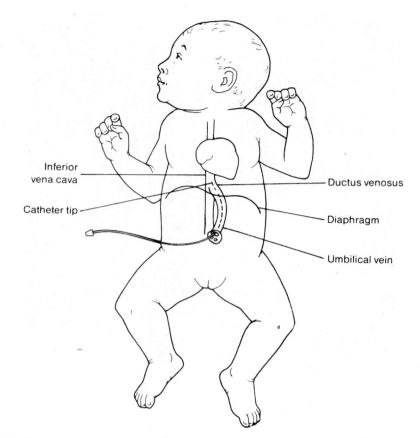

Inferior vena cava

Catheter tip

Ductus venosus

Diaphragm

Umbilical vein

Figure 13–6 *Proper position of the UVC catheter.*

Examination of the Respiratory Tract. We now focus attention on the respiratory tract.

Trachea. First, examine the trachea, beginning at the larynx and following it to the carina. The trachea often deviates slightly to the right, but should be located near the center of the spinal column. A trachea that is deviated significantly may indicate the presence of atelectasis or a pneumothorax. In the instance of atelectasis, the trachea will be deviated toward the affected side, whereas a pneumothorax will deviate the trachea away from the affected side.

Endotracheal Tube. If the patient is intubated, check the location of the tip of the endotracheal tube. It should have a radiopaque stripe on the tip, which makes it easily seen on the x-ray. The tip of the tube should be halfway between the carina and the clavicles, as shown

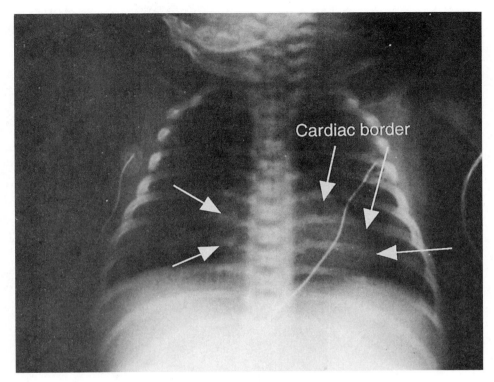

Cardiac border

Figure 13–7 *The cardiac silhouette as seen on the chest x-ray.*

in Figure 13–9. If the tube is in too far and near the carina, the chance of the tube entering the right mainstem bronchus is greatly increased. Conversely, if the tube tip is near the clavicles, the chance of extubation increases. The position of the tube tip may vary with the position of the patient's head. If the infant's chin is down at the time the x-ray is being taken, the tip of the ET tube may be higher in the trachea. When the chin is elevated, the tube may be pushed farther down the trachea.

Mainstem Bronchus. Now follow the trachea past the carina to the mainstem bronchi. The right bronchus may appear as an extension of the trachea, whereas the left angles off at almost a 90-degree angle. It is unusual to see the bronchi beyond the hilum of the lung because the air-filled lungs do not provide a contrast to the air-filled airways. However, if the lung tissue increases in density, such as in pneumonia, atelectasis, or aspiration, it may be possible to see the bronchi outlined into the lung periphery, as seen in Figure 13–10.

This is caused by two factors. First, as the lung consolidates, it begins appearing whiter on the x-ray film. The air-filled bronchus, passing through the lung, is contrasted against the lung and becomes visible on the x-ray.

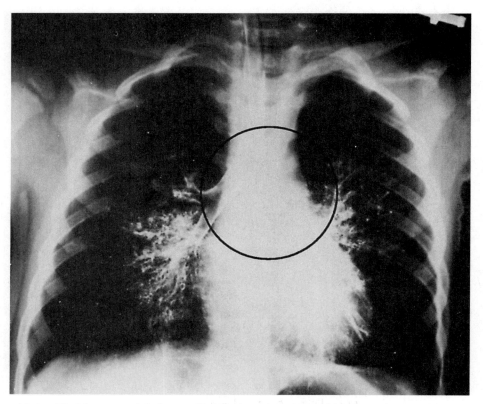

Figure 13–8 *The hilum area of the lungs. The bronchus are highlighted by the inhalation of radiopaque gas.*

Second, in the presence of atelectasis the bronchi may dilate, making them more visible against the lung fields. These visible bronchi are called air bronchograms.

Lung Fields. Next examine the lung fields. Generally speaking, the lung tissue should be expanded with air, if taken during inspiration, and thus appear dark on the x-ray (Figure 13–11). Lungs that appear more white are either underexpanded or are involved in some type of disease process that is making them atelectatic. The appearance of the lungs with different disease entities is examined in the following section. It is at this point that the practitioner should evaluate the lungs in light of the following descriptions.

Pleural Surface. The surface of the pleura should next be examined. This is best done at the interface of the peripheral lungs and the chest wall at a point between the ribs. Lung markings should extend to the outermost pleural border. Pneumothoraces are often detected only by the absence of lung markings in a section of the thorax. Chest tubes, if present, should be checked to make sure they are positioned to evacuate the free air in the thorax.

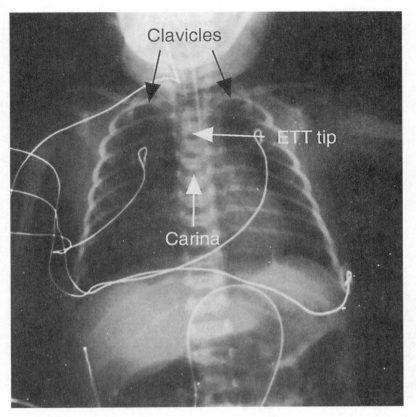

Figure 13–9 *Proper position of the endotracheal tube is determined by the tip being above the carina and below the clavicles as shown.*

RADIOGRAPHIC FINDINGS IN NEONATAL LUNG PATHOLOGY

RESPIRATORY DISTRESS SYNDROME (RDS)

RDS is the most common lung disease found in premature infants. Radiographic findings in RDS are quite characteristic. Fine reticulogranular patterns, alveoli with increased tissue and water densities surrounding small areas of aerated alveoli, are found in both lung fields. This is commonly called a ground glass or a frosted glass appearance (Figure 13–12).

Both lungs appear as opaque white density, reflecting the lack of lung aeration and expansion. Air bronchograms are prominently seen, particularly at the lung bases. Pleural fluid is absent, helping to differentiate the disease from an infectious process. Pleural fluid can be present in RDS, however, if the infant has been overloaded with fluid.

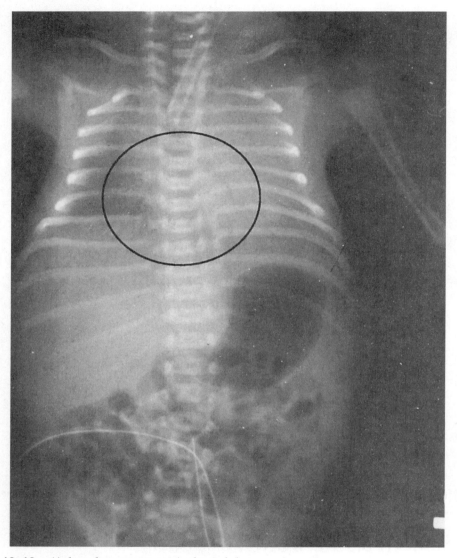

Figure 13–10 *Air-bronchograms as seen in the circled area.*

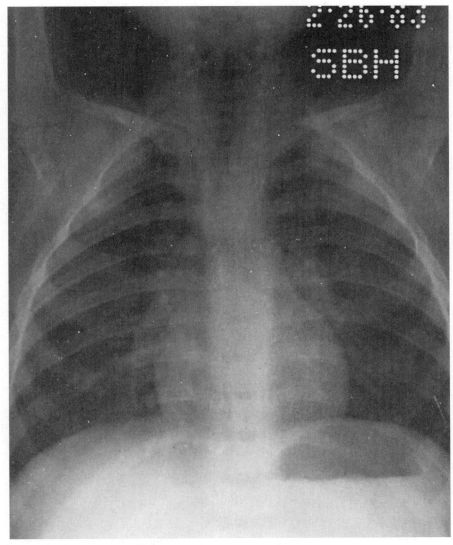

Figure 13–11 *Normally aerated lung fields.*

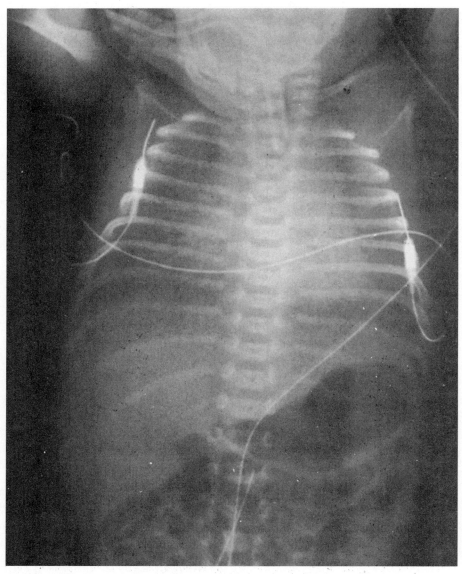

Figure 13–12 *The "ground glass" appearance of RDS.*

The bilateral opaque appearance continues until the lungs begin to recover. If the disease worsens, the lungs can become completely white on the x-ray film. This is called, fittingly, a white out, shown in Figure 13–13. White outs are due to an almost total absence of aeration, with massive atelectasis and collapsed lung segments. As the disease improves, lung clearing occurs over a period of a few days. Clearing usually starts with the apical and peripheral areas first, followed by the central and basal lung areas.

ATELECTASIS

Atelectasis is a consolidation of part or all of a lung due to a collapse of the alveoli. Radiographic atelectasis is shown in Figure 13–14. This loss of volume may be due to surfactant deficiency, as in RDS, bronchial obstruction, or scar formation. Bronchial obstruction may result from mucous plugging or from an aspirated object.

The signs of atelectasis include an elevated diaphragm on the affected side and a mediastinal shift toward the atelectatic area. There may also be a decrease in the spaces between the ribs, and possibly a hyperinflation of the adjacent lung lobes or of the opposite lung.

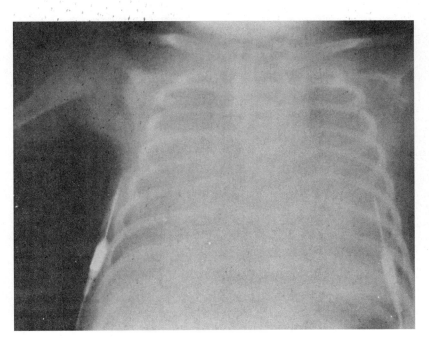

Figure 13–13 *Total "white out" of the lungs.*

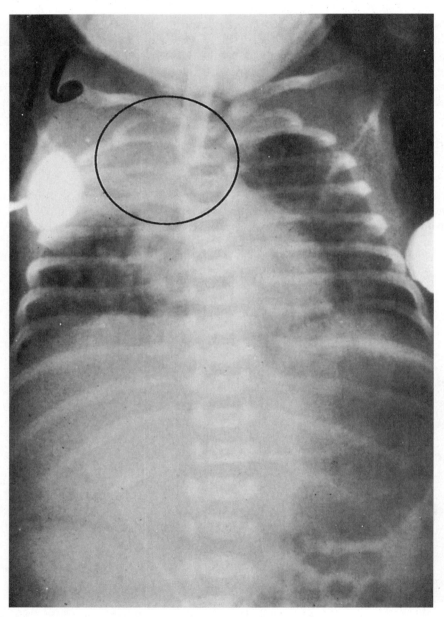

Figure 13–14 *Areas of atelectasis seen within the circled areas.*

TRANSIENT TACHYPNEA OF THE NEWBORN (TTN)

TTN is a common cause of respiratory distress in newborns, especially those born via cesarean delivery. Covered more in depth in Chapter 10, TTN is thought to be caused by a retention of fetal lung fluids. Radiographically, if seen within the first few hours of life, TTN may closely resemble hyaline membrane disease (Figure 13–15). A possible difference is that the lungs are hyperaerated rather than hypoaerated.

It is common to see small amounts of pleural fluid and symmetrical, stringy infiltrates in the hilar region, which may be due to engorged veins and lymphatic vessels. An important point in distinguishing TTN from other causes of respiratory distress is that the infiltrates clear rapidly, often within 24 hours.

NEONATAL PNEUMONIA

Contamination of the infant most commonly occurs just before, during, or after birth. Colonization of organisms on the infant's skin, gastrointestinal tract, or respiratory system may occur following premature rupture of membranes, dystocia, or the use of contaminated

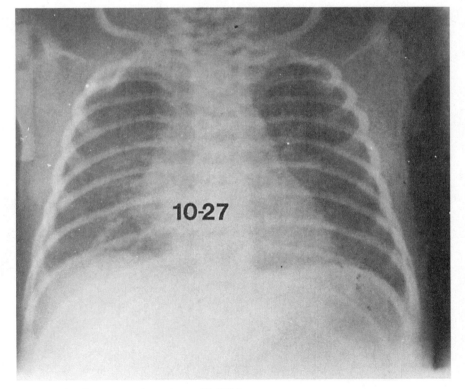

Figure 13–15 *The chest x-ray of a patient with TTN.*

equipment or hands on the infant. With pneumonias, the roentgenographic pattern may be variable. Neonatal pneumonia is very difficult to distinguish on the chest x-ray.

Lung markings are described as being diffuse, which may also describe many other lung diseases. A chest x-ray of pneumonia is depicted in Figure 13–16. The presence of pleural fluid helps establish the diagnosis of pneumonia. Consolidation of a lobe or segment, often seen in older patients, is very rare in neonates.

Often a pneumonia is diagnosed in a normal right lower lobe. This is because of a prominence of vessels and airways on the x-ray at that location, giving the appearance of consolidation. In contrast, a pneumonia in the lower left lobe may be difficult to see behind the cardiac shadow. A comparison of heart shadow densities from top to bottom and right to left may reveal increased density in the lower left region, indicating a pneumonia.

Group B hemolytic streptococci has recently become a common source of neonatal infection. The fetus may become infected while still in utero and present at birth with systemic symptoms of the disease. These symptoms may be indistinguishable from RDS in that the neonate may grunt, flare the nostrils, and have retractions. The chest x-ray may also appear as a complete white out and be mistaken for RDS, especially in the preterm neonate.

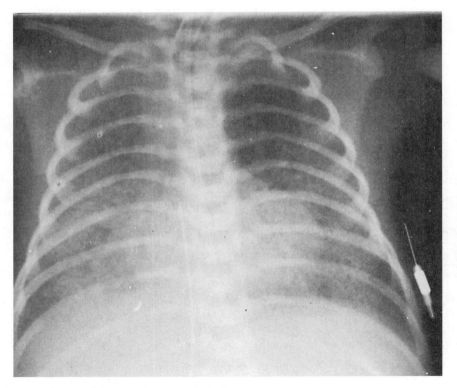

Figure 13–16 *Neonatal pneumonia as seen on x-ray.*

MECONIUM ASPIRATION SYNDROME (MAS)

The chest x-ray of an MAS patient may be normal, in mild cases, or very abnormal, in severe cases. Severe MAS shows bilateral infiltrates and air trapping. Air trapping predisposes the lungs to pulmonary interstitial emphysema, pneumomediastinum, and pneumothorax. With blockage of the airway by meconium, atelectasis results. Additionally, there may be signs of inflammation and edema caused by the chemical irritation of the meconium. Pleural effusions, indicated by a loss of the costophrenic angle (the angle between the diaphragm and the lateral chest wall) may also be present.

DIAPHRAGMATIC HERNIA

Diaphragmatic hernias may occur at birth or in utero. Diaphragmatic hernias that occur in utero cause severe damage to the lung by hampering its growth and development. Roughly 80 to 85% of diaphragmatic hernias occur on the left side. X-ray findings in congenital diaphragmatic hernia show the presence of the stomach and bowel loops in the left thoracic cavity (Figure 13–17).

Diagnosis is simplified when the stomach and intestines contain air. Air-filled intestines are easily identified when located in the thorax. The abdominal cavity will also be noticeably void of a stomach bubble or intestinal markings.

There is usually a severe deviation of the mediastinum and its contents away from the side of the hernia. If a gastric tube is present, the tip is commonly seen ending in the thorax instead of the abdomen. A diaphragmatic hernia is almost always accompanied by severe respiratory distress and a flat or sunken abdomen (scaphoid). X-ray findings are then used to verify the diagnosis.

CONGENITAL LOBAR EMPHYSEMA

X-ray findings in this disorder show a single lobe, commonly an upper lobe or the right middle lobe, becoming overdistended and emphysematous. The remaining lobes of the lung become atelectatic and collapsed. Depression of the diaphragm and displacement of the mediastinum to the opposite side is also seen. In later stages of the disease, atelectasis occurs in the opposite lung.

PNEUMOTHORAX

Radiographically, a pneumothorax is identified when the lung is displaced away from the chest wall by a dark band of air (Figure 13–18). The dark air space will have no lung markings, and, frequently, the border of the lung is seen as a sharp white line, medial to the air sack. In the presence of a tension pneumothorax, the diaphragm on the affected side will be depressed, and the intercostal spaces will be widened. The mediastinum is also displaced away from the pneumothorax.

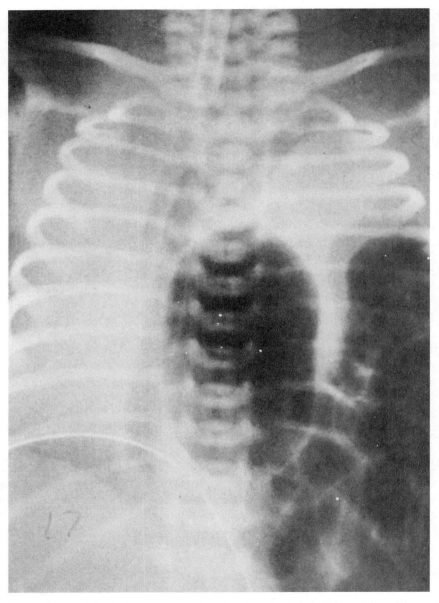

Figure 13–17 *Congenital diaphragmatic hernia. Note the stomach bubble and bowel loops in the left thorax.*

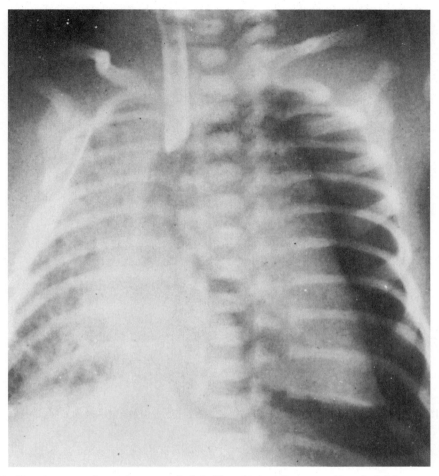

Figure 13–18   *A pneumothorax is seen on the left. Note the free air surrounding the left lung.*

It is sometimes possible to mistake a skinfold for a pneumothorax. Although skinfolds may appear as the border of the lung, the space surrounding the line will have lung markings, which is inconsistent with a pneumothorax. The skinfold may also be seen beyond the confines of the pleural cavity and into the soft tissues of the chest wall.

Patient symptoms are invaluable in diagnosing a pneumothorax. Lack of distress or other symptoms helps to rule out a pneumothorax when x-ray findings are inconclusive.

PNEUMOMEDIASTINUM

A pneumomediastinum is detected radiographically by the presence of air in the mediastinum, outlining the thymus and the lateral aspects of the heart (Figure 13–19). This

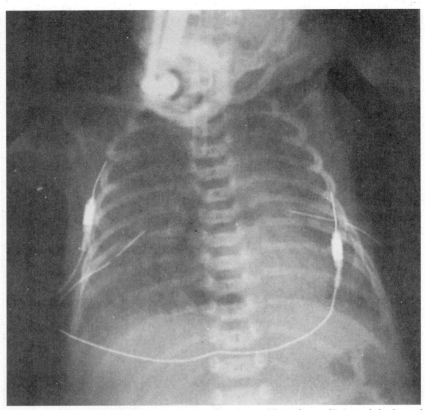

Figure 13–19 *A radiograph showing a pneumomediastinum. Note the outlining of the lateral edge of the heart. The free air does not surround the appex of the heart.*

outlining of the thymus has been called "bat wing" and "angel wing," because of its appearance as a wing. On a lateral view, the thymus is lifted, giving it the appearance of a sail. Collections of mediastinal air around the lung hilum are often confusing. They may be seen in areas of the lung not thought of as being the mediastinum. These collections, called pseudocysts, are often mistaken for other abnormalities, but are actually mediastinal air.

PNEUMOPERICARDIUM

The accumulation of air within the pericardial sac is called a pneumopericardium. On x-ray, the air completely surrounds the heart (Figure 13–20), in contrast to a pneumomediastinum, which only surrounds the lateral sides of the heart. The air pocket around the heart may appear as a halo. The amount of air present is of concern, because larger accumulations of air may tamponade the heart, reducing cardiac output and leading to shock.

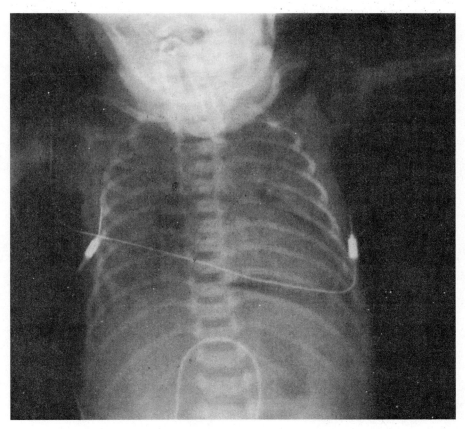

Figure 13–20 *A radiograph showing a pneumopericardum. Notice that the free air completely surrounds the heart.*

PULMONARY INTERSTITIAL EMPHYSEMA (PIE)

PIE is caused by air leaking from a lung rupture and migrating throughout the lung parenchyma. The radiographic appearance is unique to this disease. The interstitial air compresses the alveoli and bronchioles, leading to atelectasis and collapse. On x-ray, the lungs have small dark streaks and cysts, surrounded by the white of the lung tissue. Figure 13–21 shows a radiograph of PIE. Some have described its appearance as looking like black paint flicked onto a white background. It is also described as having a sponge-like appearance, or looking like ground hamburger with air in it.

PIE may affect one lung, but is most likely found in both lungs. PIE may show areas of air accumulations, as in a pneumothorax, or a cystic formation.

BRONCHOPULMONARY DYSPLASIA (BPD)

BPD is recognized when infant lungs show the presence of hyperaeration in association with alternating areas of dark cystic areas and strand-like densities. Radiologic characteristics of BPD have been classified into four stages.

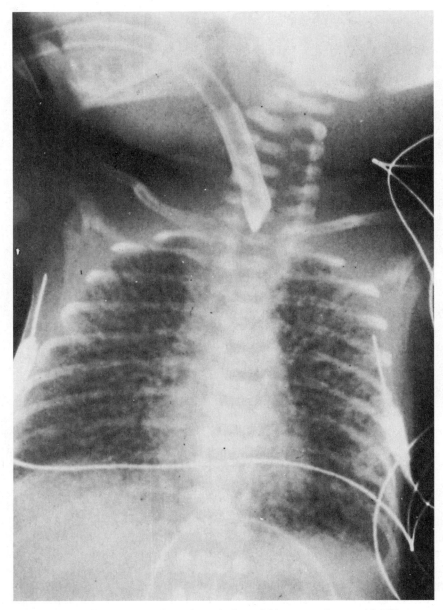

Figure 13–21 *The small cystic areas throughout the lung fields are consistent with PIE.*

Stage 1 (mild BPD): Stage 1 has an appearance similar to that of RDS and occurs within 2 to 4 days following delivery (Figure 13–22A).

Stage 2 (moderate BPD): The RDS appearance now changes to coarse, irregularly shaped densities that are often grouped together and contain very small cystic areas. The coarse infiltrates are often dense enough to obscure the cardiac markings. These areas are caused by interstitial edema, as well as alveolar septal edema, with subsequent atelectasis. The cystic areas represent early emphysematous changes. Stage 2 occurs 4 to 10 days following delivery.

Stage 3 (severe BPD): The small cysts now become arranged in generalized patterns. Dense cystic patches that appear are evidence of the progressive, emphysematous changes. In this stage, extensive repair is taking place in the alveolar walls. Fibrotic areas show up as irregular white streaks throughout the lungs. The size and number of irregular areas increases as the days pass. There may also be some areas of lung hyperexpansion. This stage occurs around 10 to 20 days following delivery (Figure 13–22B).

Stage 4 (chronic, advanced BPD): During this stage, lung hyperexpansion is less severe,

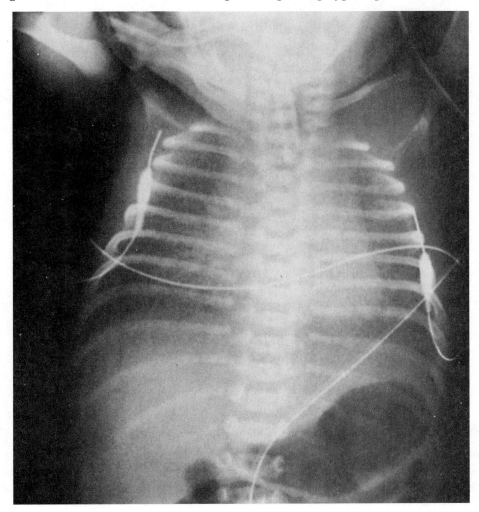

Figure 13–22a *Stage I BPD.*

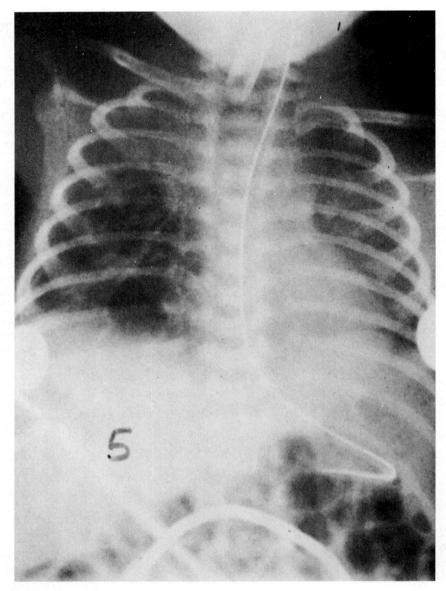

Figure 13–22b *Stage III BPD.*

as are the streaky opacities found between the large cystic areas. The lung field has a "bubbly" appearance caused by the continued enlargement of the cysts. Signs of chronic air trapping, with flattened diaphragms and hyperaeration, are usually present. The patient with stage 4 BPD has continued oxygen requirements that may persist for months. Occasionally, the infant requires mechanical ventilation for long periods, while the lungs slowly heal during stage 4.

RADIOGRAPHIC FINDINGS IN PEDIATRIC LUNG PATHOLOGY

ADULT RESPIRATORY DISTRESS SYNDROME (ARDS)

Depending on when the chest x-ray is obtained in the course of ARDS, the practitioner may see a variety of pathologic findings on the chest x-ray. The progression of ARDS involves an accumulation of lung pathologies, which result in acute widespread damage to the lung parenchyma.

Initially, the x-ray of the chest shows diffuse fluffy infiltrates due to the accumulation of fluid and debris in the alveoli. The infiltrates then give way to patchy, nodular densities as the disease progresses. As the lungs become fibrotic, the lungs take on a stringy interstitial pattern with diffuse areas of consolidation. The lung fields often become "whited out" secondary to diminished aeration as atelectasis progresses in the damaged lungs.

FOREIGN BODY ASPIRATION

The aspiration of a foreign body into the pulmonary tree is commonly seen in the pediatric population. Frequently, the aspirated object is not visible on the radiograph, making it necessary to look for signs of air trapping and atelectasis, which may be present distal to the object. If the object is causing a complete blockage of a major airway, air volumes in the areas distal to the blockage are often greatly diminished due to atelectasis.

A partial blockage of the airway leads to a ball-valve effect, in which gas passes the obstruction on inspiration but becomes trapped on exhalation as the airway collapses on the object. This results in areas of hyperlucency on the radiograph in those areas distal to the blockage. Of most value in this situation is an expiratory film, which more clearly shows areas of air trapping. An expiratory film may be obtained on younger patients by placing the patient in a decubitus position, where the lung on the downside is compressed into exhalation.

CYSTIC FIBROSIS

The chest x-ray of the patient with cystic fibrosis may be normal in the early stages of the disease. As the disease progresses with involvement of pulmonary glands, thickening of the peribronchial areas along with mucous plugging and hyperaeration begin to be seen. As the disease progresses, the chest radiograph shows areas of consolidation, cystic changes, and fibrosis of the lungs.

ASTHMA

The chest x-ray of an asthmatic patient appears normal with no signs of lung pathology in the absence of an acute attack. During an acute asthmatic attack, the classic lung radiograph is that of hyperinflation with a slight depression of the diaphragm and an overall hyperlucency of both lung fields. It must be noted, however, that even in the presence of an acute asthmatic attack, the lung fields may show little radiographic change.[2] In these cases, clinical and physical signs may be more diagnostic than the chest x-ray.

EPIGLOTTITIS

Epiglottitis is seen radiographically on a lateral neck x-ray (Figure 13–23). Epiglottic swelling of three to four times normal is seen at the base of the tongue and appears as if someone left a thumb print, thus the term "thumb sign," which is used to describe the swollen epiglottis. There is also involvement of the hypopharynx with swelling and thickening of the tissue.

CROUP

Croup is diagnosed radiographically with an anteroposterior view of the neck. The area of

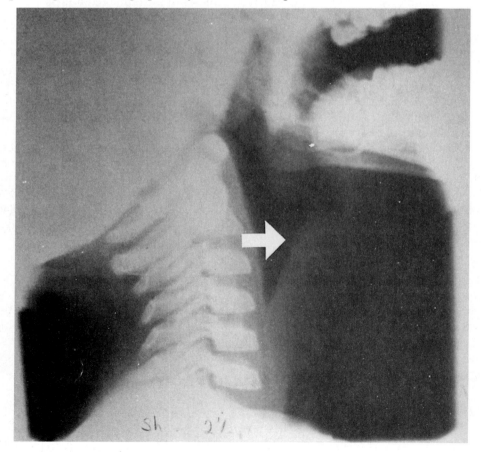

Figure 13–23 *Lateral neck x-ray showing epiglottitis. The arrow shows the swollen epiglottis, which appears as a thumb print.*

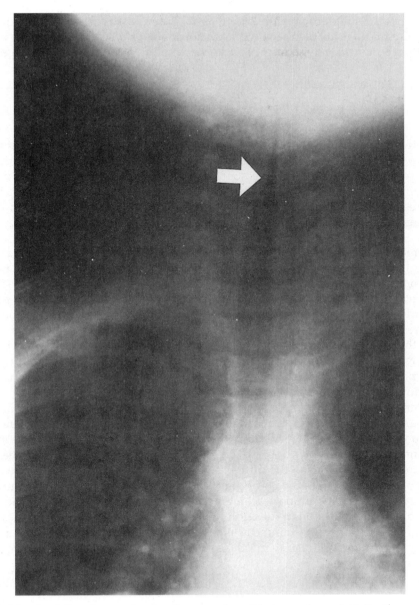

Figure 13–24 *An A-P neck x-ray showing the narrowing of the larynx (arrow). Notice the appearance of a steeple or an hourglass.*

the swelling in the subglottic region is seen as an "hourglass" or "steeple" (Figure 13–24). Because these findings are also seen with subglottic stenosis, severe symptoms in patients younger than 6 months may require bronchoscopy to provide a differential diagnosis.

SUMMARY

X-rays of the chest are one of the most commonly ordered tests in the neonatal and pediatric group of patients. An x-ray gives an internal view of the effect that a disease process is having on the organ systems. While not used alone for diagnosis, a chest x-ray is invaluable at verifying the presence of a process and monitoring its progression or improvement.

The three densities seen on an x-ray (air, fluid, and bone) form the details of the internal environment. Air spaces are seen as the darkest areas and bone is seen as the lightest areas. Fluid spaces are seen as the grays in between.

Anatomic differences in neonates and children can hinder proper interpretation if not understood in the proper context. For example, the carina is higher in the thorax in younger patients and may prove deceptive if the practitioner is used to looking for the carina lower in the chest. Additionally, the thymus gland adds an extra shadow to the chest x-ray of young patients, which may be mistaken for an enlarged heart or for lung pathology.

When reading a chest x-ray, it is important to follow a systematic approach. Begin by checking the name and date of the x-ray. Next orient the x-ray on the viewbox so the patient's right side is on your left. The quality of the x-ray is next evaluated for proper exposure. The position of the patient on the x-ray is then examined to ensure that no, or minimal, rotation has occurred.

Determination of expiration or inspiration, and examination of the diaphragm and abdomen are done next. Moving back to the thorax, the practitioner next examines the cardiac silhouette, the hilum, and respiratory tract. Placement of the endotracheal tube is evaluated on intubated patients, with the tip ideally placed between the carina and the clavicles.

Before the x-ray is obtained, the differential diagnosis has often been narrowed to two or three processes. The radiographic findings are then used to confirm or rule out the diagnoses. X-ray findings of commonly seen lung pathologies are characteristic and a knowledge of those findings is vital in identifying the disease process and its progression. The practitioner is encouraged to examine as many x-rays as possible, both normal and abnormal and to discuss the findings with others. By this mechanism, reading x-rays becomes almost second nature.

References

1. Karlson KH, Seibert JJ. Radiographic assessment techniques. In: Barnhart SL, Czervinske MP. Perinatal and Pediatric Respiratory Care. Philadelphia: WB Saunders Co; 1995.

2. Burton GG, Hodgkins J, Ward J. Respiratory Care: A Guide to Clinical Practice. 4th ed. Philadelphia: JB Lippincott Co; 1997.

Bibliography and Suggested Readings

Avery GB, Fletcher MA, MacDonald MG. Pathophysiology and Management of the Newborn. 5th ed. Philadelphia: JB Lippincott Co; 1999.

Barnhart SL, Czervinske MP. Perinatal and Pediatric Respiratory Care. Philadelphia: WB Saunders Co; 1995.

Bierman CW, Pearlman DS, Shapiro GG, Busse WW. Allergy, Asthma, and Immunology from Infancy to Adulthood. 3rd ed. Philadelphia: WB Saunders Co; 1996.

Chapman S. Essential Pediatric Radiology. Philadelphia: WB Saunders Co; 2000.

Chernik V, Boat TF. Kendig's Disorders of the Respiratory Tract in Children. 6th ed. Philadelphia: WB Saunders Co; 1998.

Cloherty JP, Stark AR, eds. Manual of Neonatal Care. 4th ed. Philadelphia: Lippincott; 1997.

Dantzker DR, MacIntyre NR, Bukow ED. Comprehensive Respiratory Care. Philadelphia: WB Saunders Co; 1995.

Flores MT. Understanding neonatal chest x-rays part I: what to look for. Neonatal Network. 1993;12:9–17.

Glanze WD, managing ed. Mosby's Medical, Nursing, and Allied Health Dictionary. 5th ed. St. Louis: CV Mosby Co; 1998.

Goodman LR. Felson's Principles of Chest Roentgenology. 2nd ed. Philadelphia: WB Saunders Co; 1999.

Hicks GH. Cardiopulmonary Anatomy and Physiology. Philadelphia: WB Saunders Co; 2000.

Merenstein GB, Gardner SL. Handbook of Neonatal Intensive Care. 4th ed. St. Louis: CV Mosby Co; 1997.

Posttest

1. Which of the following statements are true?
   a. Diagnosis of lung disease is made by x-ray alone.
   b. X-ray confirms the presence or absence of a disease process.
   c. Physical alterations of disease cannot be seen on x-ray.
   d. X-rays should only be done on neonates in an emergency.
2. Of the following, which are densities seen on x-ray?
   I. gas
   II. skin
   III. fluid
   IV. cartilage

V. bone
   a. II, III, IV
   b. I, III, IV
   c. I, III, IV, V
   d. I, III, V

3. Which of the following may limit the interpretation of a chest x-ray?
  I. artifact
  II. patient movement
  III. old film
  IV. improper technique
  V. the presence of bony material
   a. I, II, IV
   b. I, II, IV
   c. I, II, V
   d. II, IV

4. As you examine a chest x-ray, you note that the spaces between the vertebrae are visible and distinct. This film is:
   a. overexposed
   b. underexposed
   c. exposed correctly
   d. backwards

5. Flattened diaphragms seen on a chest x-ray indicate:
   a. meconium aspiration
   b. hypoaeration
   c. air trapping
   d. hyperventilation

6. The neonatal cardiac silhouette is considered normal size if it is less than what percentage of the thoracic width?
   a. 60%
   b. 50%
   c. 40%
   d. 30%

7. Undervascularization of the hilar region would indicate:
   a. heart failure
   b. right-to-left shunt
   c. RDS
   d. central vasospasm

8. As you examine a patient's chest x-ray, you note the tip of the endotracheal tube to be near the carina. You would:
   a. pull the tube back slightly
   b. push the tube in slightly
   c. leave the tube in its present position
   d. rotate the tube 90 degrees

9. Examination of a chest x-ray reveals a slightly elevated left diaphragm, with a slight

mediastinal shift toward the left. The left lower lobe appears whiter than the upper lobes with a slight hyperinflation of the right lower lobe. What is the probable diagnosis?

   a. atelectasis in the left lower lobe
   b. atelectasis in the right lower lobe
   c. left lung pneumothorax
   d. right lung pneumothorax

10. A newborn infant presents from delivery with severe respiratory distress. On examination, the abdomen is scaphoid. The radiograph shows a severe mediastinal shift to the right. The likely diagnosis is:
   a. diaphragmatic hernia
   b. pneumothorax
   c. pneumoperitoneum
   d. pneumonia

11. On examination of a chest radiograph, you note an air pocket on the right lateral heart border. This indicates (a) possible:
   a. pneumomediastinum
   b. pneumopericardium
   c. pneumothorax
   d. congenital lobar emphysema

12. Dense cystic patches arranged in generalized patterns that gradually increase in size and number describe which stage of BPD?
   a. stage 2
   b. stage 3
   c. stage 4
   d. stage 5

13. A decubitus film is best used to diagnose which of the following?
   a. croup
   b. epiglottitis
   c. foreign body aspiration
   d. cystic fibrosis

14. Which of the following is (are) true regarding the chest radiograph of an asthma patient?
   I. hyperinflation is common during an acute attack
   II. air trapping is chronically seen
   III. the chest x-ray may be normal
   IV. the lungs may appear hyperlucent during an attack
      a. I, III, IV
      b. I, II, III
      c. II, IV
      d. I, III

UNIT FOUR

MANAGEMENT OF VENTILATION AND OXYGENATION

CHAPTER FOURTEEN

CONCEPTS OF MECHANICAL VENTILATION

──────── **OBJECTIVES** ────────

Upon completion of this chapter, the reader should be able to:

1. Describe the goal of mechanical ventilation and the skills required to achieve the goal.
2. Define each of the following terms. Include a description of how each is determined and the ventilator parameters that determine each one.
   a. Peak inspiratory pressure (PIP)
   b. Positive end-expiratory pressure (PEEP)
   c. Frequency
   d. Inspiratory time
   e. Mean airway pressure
   f. Tidal volume
   g. Minute ventilation
   h. Deadspace
   i. Alveolar ventilation
   j. Opening pressure
   k. Driving pressure
   l. Functional residual capacity
   m. Diffusion Time
   n. Flow rate
3. Discuss the relationships that exist between ventilator parameters, using Figure 14–12 as a guide.
4. Define compliance and describe how lung compliance is measured.
5. Compare and contrast static and dynamic compliance.
6. State the range of lung compliance values in the neonate.
7. Describe the determinants of pulmonary compliance.
8. Discuss the compliance of the thorax and how it is developed.
9. Describe the relationship between the lungs and thorax that determines the overall compliance.

10. Compare and contrast the three positions on the lung compliance curve. Describe conditions that create each position.
11. Identify and discuss the various lung disorders that alter lung compliance.
12. List the four factors that create resistance and identify the factor that is responsible for airway resistance changes.
13. State range of airway resistance in the normal newborn and how it is measured.
14. List and describe three factors that increase resistance in the neonatal airway and how each can be countered.
15. Define a time constant. Discuss the significance of three time constants and expiratory time.
16. When given compliance and resistance values, calculate a minimal expiratory time needed.
17. Describe how changes in resistance and compliance change time constants.

KEY TERMS

compliance	elastic	static attraction
diffusion time	opening pressure	unstressed volume
driving pressure	resistance	viscosity

GOALS OF MECHANICAL VENTILATION

The goal of ventilation is to provide adequate alveolar gas exchange with minimal damage to lung tissue and minimal interference with the circulatory system. This can only be achieved with an understanding of the physiology and pathophysiology of the disease and the course the newborn infant is likely to take.

To gain this understanding, a knowledge of basic concepts of mechanical ventilation, the many options, modes, and settings that are available, is required. With such wide flexibility, the caregiver must be sensitive to the potential physiologic damage and changes that may occur with each setting change.

The caregiver must have the ability to interpret blood gas results and radiologic findings, which are assessed frequently throughout the course of the disease. The goals of mechanical ventilation are listed in Table 14–1.

DEFINITIONS

PEAK INSPIRATORY PRESSURE (PIP)

Most common neonatal ventilators use time cycling and pressure limiting. In other words, inspiration is stopped when a selected time period has been reached, and the maximum

Table 14–1   Goals of Mechanical Ventilation

Normalization and Maintenance of Blood Gases and Acid-Base Balance
PaO_2—Maintain arterial PO_2 above hypoxic levels and below hyperoxic levels.
P_aCO_2—Reverse hypercarbic states through adequate alveolar ventilation.
pH—Maintain blood pH within homeostatic range by managing the balance between $PaCO_2$ and HCO_3^-.

Prevention of Iatrogenic Complications
Barotrauma—Careful regulation of rate and pressures.
Infection—Following sterile technique whenever the airway is suctioned.
Sedation—Pharmacologic sedation and analgesia as needed to reduce anxiety and pain.

Support of the Patient's Respiratory Needs
Balance—Balance should be maintained to achieve acceptable blood gases without placing the patient at risk for barotrauma.

pressure exerted against the patient's airway during the breath is limited by the operator. This level of pressure limiting is the PIP level, illustrated in Figure 14–1.

The level of PIP is one determinant of the delivered tidal volume and is changed as needed to alter ventilation. Initially, PIP is set at a level that achieves good chest excursion, with patients having poor lung compliance requiring higher levels than those with good compliance. A suggested starting point for PIP is between 16 and 20 cm H_2O.[1]

POSITIVE END-EXPIRATORY PRESSURE (PEEP)

PEEP, depicted in Figure 14–2, is a positive pressure maintained in the patient's airway during the expiratory phase of ventilation. The maintenance of pressure during expiration pre-

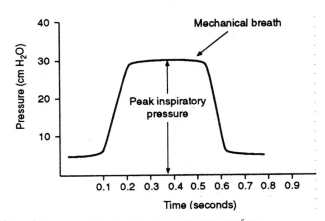

Figure 14–1   *Peak inspiratory pressure as seen on a pressure waveform.*

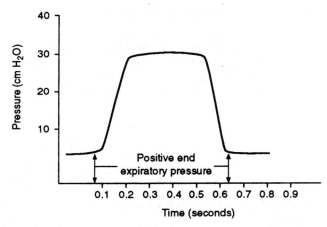

Figure 14–2 *Postive end-expiratory pressure (PEEP) seen on a pressure waveform.*

vents a collapse of the alveoli in the patient with RDS, thus increasing the functional residual capacity and improving compliance. PEEP improves oxygenation and allows lower levels of PIP and rate to be used. PEEP levels are usually kept between 4 and 6 cm H_2O.[1] Higher levels of PEEP often lead to increased deadspace and a reduction of cardiac output and are not recommended.

FREQUENCY

The frequency of ventilation, or rate, shown in Figure 14–3, is the number of inspirations that occur in 1 minute. With the determination of adequate PIP and PEEP levels, the rate is

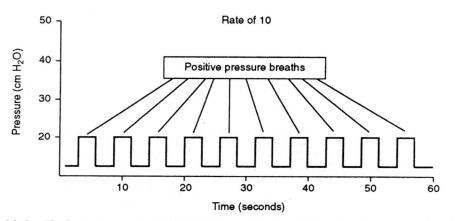

Figure 14–3 *The frequency or rate of ventilation is equal to the number of positive pressure breaths delivered per minute.*

set to achieve a minute ventilation that will maintain the desired $PaCO_2$. The initial breath rate varies but should be started at 20 to 40 BPM.[1,2]

Modern neonatal ventilators have the capacity of providing rates of up to 150 BPM. These high rates are reserved for those patients with extremely noncompliant lungs in an attempt to maintain adequate minute ventilation and also in the patient with persistent pulmonary hypertension who is treated with hyperventilation.

INSPIRATORY TIME (IT)

IT, depicted in Figure 14–4, is set by the operator to cycle off the inspiratory breath. The combination of IT and rate determines the I:E (inspiration and expiration) ratio. The IT further determines the amount of time the inspired gas is in contact with the alveoli. As ventilator rates increase, it becomes necessary to decrease the IT to prevent air trapping. The clinical use of IT and the determination of I:E ratios are discussed in Chapter 15.

MEAN AIRWAY PRESSURE (MAP)

MAP (Figure 14–5) is the average pressure exerted on the airway and lungs from the beginning of inspiration until the beginning of the next inspiration. It is usually calculated by electronic ventilator monitors that measure all pressure variables over a time period and then determine the average pressure. MAP can also be approximated by using the formula in Table 14–2.

MAP is the most powerful influence on oxygenation and must be carefully monitored because high levels of MAP lead to decreased cardiac output, pulmonary hypoperfusion, and increased risk of barotrauma. MAP is affected by PIP, PEEP, IT, and rate. Because MAP

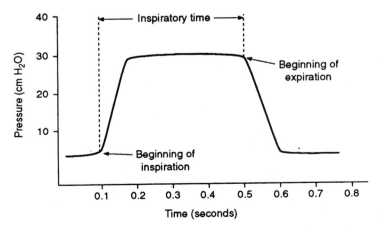

Figure 14–4 *Inspiratory time, measured from the onset of the inspiratory phase to the onset of the expiratory phase.*

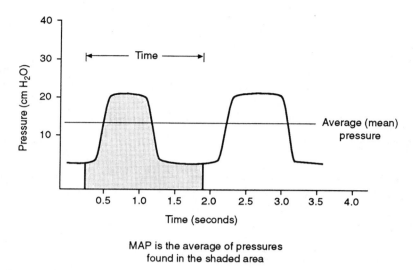

MAP is the average of pressures
found in the shaded area

Figure 14–5 *Mean airway pressure (MAP) is the average pressure in the airway over a time period. It is calculated by measuring all of the pressure variables during the time period and averaging the overall pressure.*

takes into account all of the factors that affect ventilation, it is the best indicator of balance between adequate ventilation and excessive pressures. MAP levels above 12 cm H_2O have been shown to contribute to barotrauma.[2]

TIDAL VOLUME

The amount of gas inhaled in a single breath is called the tidal volume. Adequate tidal volume can be assumed when there is appropriate chest expansion, good breath sounds, and acceptable blood gas values. During mechanical ventilation, the tidal volume is the volume of gas that enters the patient's lungs during the inspiratory cycle.

Table 14–2 Calculation of Mean Airway Pressure

MAP = (PIP) × (inspiratory time/total breath duration) + (PEEP) × (expiratory time/total breath duration)

For example, current ventilator settings:

PIP, 23 cm H_2O; PEEP, 5 cm H_2O; I:time, 0.51 second; E:time, 1.53 seconds; total breath duration, 2.04 seconds.

Inserting the above setting into the formula, we get:

23 × (0.51/2.04) + 5 × (1.53/2.04)
(23 × 0.25) + (5 × 0.75)
5.75 + 3.75
MAP = 9.5 cm H_2O

The two ventilator parameters that most directly affect tidal volume are PIP and PEEP. Referring to Figure 14–6, the delivered tidal volume is equal to the vertical distance from the baseline pressure to the PIP level. As PIP is increased, the distance between baseline and PIP increases, thus increasing tidal volume. If the baseline pressure, which is the PEEP level, is lowered or increased, the distance is again changed, and tidal volume changes.

MINUTE VENTILATION

Minute ventilation is equal to the tidal volume multiplied by the respiratory rate. Therefore, a change in either the PIP or PEEP, which alter tidal volume, or a change in frequency alter minute ventilation.

Minute ventilation is broken down into alveolar ventilation, the portion actually participating in gas exchange and deadspace ventilation, or that portion not taking part in gas exchange.

DEADSPACE AND ALVEOLAR VENTILATION

Deadspace is any gas that does not participate in gas exchange. Deadspace is divided into two categories: anatomical and alveolar.

Anatomic deadspace is the volume of tidal gas that fills the airways at the end of inspiration. It is comprised of the airways beginning at the nose and ending at the terminal bronchioles, as shown in Figure 14–7A. Anatomic deadspace in a neonate is roughly 2 to 2.2 ml/kg. Alveolar deadspace, depicted in Figure 14–7B, is that portion of the tidal gas that fills nonperfused alveoli. Alveolar deadspace, in contrast to anatomic deadspace, is impossible to determine and can vary tremendously from hour to hour in the same patient.

The total of anatomic and alveolar deadspace is called physiologic deadspace (V_D). When V_D is compared to tidal volume (V_T), the ratio ($V_D:V_T$) reflects the portion of the tidal

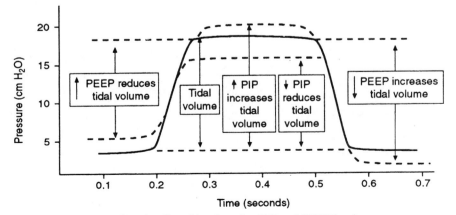

Figure 14–6 *Tidal volume directly affected by changing PIP and PEEP levels.*

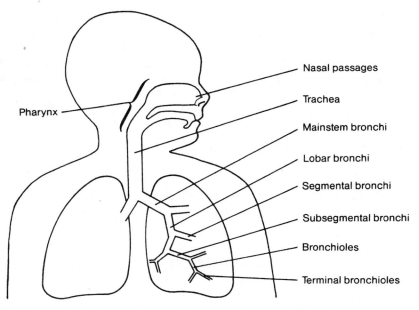

Figure 14–7a *Anatomic deadspace comprises the nose to the terminal bronchioles.*

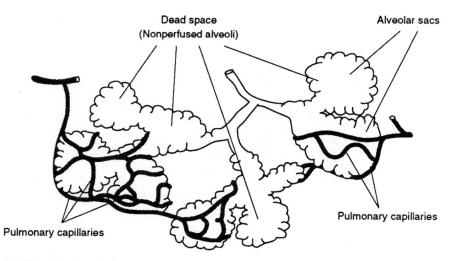

Figure 14–7b *Alveolar deadspace encompasses all nonperfused alveoli.*

breath that is not participating in gas exchange. This portion is called wasted ventilation. The amount of physiologic deadspace varies from patient to patient.

Alveolar ventilation, shown in Figure 14–7C, is the portion of tidal gas actually taking part in gas exchange. Anatomically, it comprises the respiratory bronchioles to the alveoli.

OPENING PRESSURE

To open and expand an alveolus, a certain amount of pressure must be applied to the alveoli. This pressure must overcome the surface tension that is causing the alveoli to pull inward. Surface tension is increased when there is a lack of surfactant, requiring a higher pressure to open the alveoli. To ventilate the lungs, the combined surface tensions of all the alveoli must be overcome. The pressure that must be applied to the airways to overcome the lumped tensions is the *opening pressure.*

It is not known exactly when opening pressure is reached, but it is clinically indicated when crackles are heard in the lungs during inspiration. As the wet alveoli are opened, the pulling apart of the alveolar walls creates the crackles.

DRIVING PRESSURE

The *driving pressure,* created by the ventilator, is the difference between the baseline pressure, or PEEP, and the PIP. If we are using a PIP of 20 cm H_2O with a PEEP of 3 cm H_2O, the compression pressure is 17 cm H_2O.

In theory, when mechanically ventilating a neonate, the driving pressure must be equal

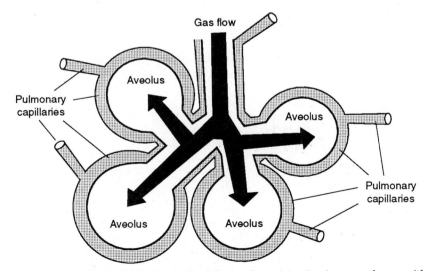

Figure 14–7c *Alveolar ventilation is the result of all alveoli participating in gas exchange with the blood.*

to the opening pressure to open and ventilate the alveoli. For example, if the opening pressure is determined to be 20 cm H_2O and we desire a PEEP of 3 cm H_2O, a PIP of 23 cm H_2O would have to be used to achieve a driving pressure that is equal to opening pressure. In this instance, if the PIP were set at 20 cm H_2O, the driving pressure would only be 17 cm H_2O, and in theory, the alveoli would not be ventilated.

In actual practice, the use of PEEP increases the diameter of the alveoli and reduces its surface tension. The opening pressure is thus reduced, and less driving pressure is needed to ventilate the lungs.

FUNCTIONAL RESIDUAL CAPACITY (FRC)

The FRC is the amount of gas remaining in the lungs at the end of a nonforced exhalation. In the presence of RDS, the lack of surfactant and subsequent collapse of the alveoli reduce the FRC (Figure 14–8A). As the alveoli get smaller, the surface tension increases and higher pressure is required to ventilate them.

The addition of PEEP prevents the collapse of the alveoli following exhalation and allows the FRC to increase (Figure 14–8B). The surface tension in the alveoli is reduced as FRC increases, resulting in less pressure being required to open the alveoli. The addition of PEEP, therefore, increases FRC and consequently increases lung compliance, decreasing opening pressures.

DIFFUSION TIME

Alveolar ventilation is also affected by the length of time that the gas is in contact with the alveoli, or the *diffusion time.* The longer the inflating gas is in contact with the alveoli, the more gas can diffuse to and from the blood. The diffusion time is controlled by the inspiratory time and peak flow.

Referring to Figure 14–9, the diffusion time is represented by the area under the volume curve. Increasing inspiratory time increases the duration of the volume curve and thus

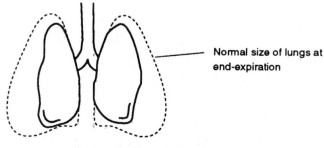

Normal size of lungs at end-expiration

Lower bronchus entering lungs

Figure 14–8a *Alelectatic lungs causing a decreased FRC at end-expiration.*

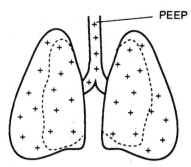

PEEP

PEEP prevents the lungs from collapsing down to their previous size (dotted line) at end-expiration

Figure 14–8b *FRC is increased as PEEP is added to the airways.*

increases the amount of time the gas is in contact with the alveoli. Increasing or decreasing peak flow changes the speed at which the gas enters the alveoli. At a constant inspiratory time, increasing the peak flow allows the gas to inflate the alveoli sooner. With a quicker opening of the alveoli, the gas is in contact for a longer time. Obviously, a change in peak flow has less of an effect on the diffusion time than does inspiratory time.

FLOW RATE

The flow rate used determines the wave pattern of the ventilator breath. Figure 14–10 shows the wave patterns that are achieved at high flow rates (wave A) and at low flow rates (wave B).

As can be seen, flow rate should be set high enough to achieve the desired pressure level, before inspiratory time is reached. If the flow rate is set too low, the inspiratory time may

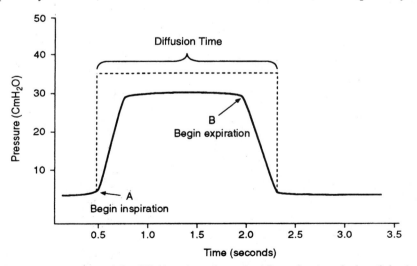

Figure 14–9 *A representation of the diffusion time, determined from the time the breath begins (point A) until pressure returns to baseline (point B).*

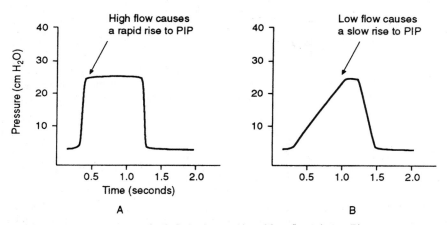

Figure 14–10   *Pressure patterns at high flows (wave A) and low flows (wave B).*

be reached before PIP is attained, thus limiting the plateau time. The result is a shortening of contact time between the gas and alveoli (Figure 14–11). A flow rate that is too high causes turbulent airflow, resulting in increased resistance and decreased tidal volume delivered to the patient.

Any adjustment made to the flow will alter the levels of PIP, PEEP, and CPAP. The practitioner must therefore make changes in those parameters to keep them at desired levels whenever flow is changed.

CLINICAL APPLICATIONS

An understanding of the clinical applications of the above-mentioned concepts will help the practitioner when actually caring for the ventilator patient. Changes in any ventilator parameter may be indicated by altered clinical signs, changes in the chest x-ray, or labora-

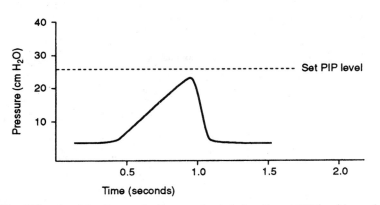

Figure 14–11   *If flow is set too low, expiration may begin before the set PIP level is reached.*

tory data. Any change made in a ventilator parameter will change another parameter to some degree. The exception to this is the FiO_2. Changes in FiO_2 do not change other parameters per se, but may necessitate other changes to be made. The interwoven relationship of all ventilator parameters is shown in Figure 14–12.

Referring to Figure 14–12, follow the changes when two common ventilator parameters are altered. A change in PIP will change both compression pressure and tidal volume, leading to a change in minute ventilation and an alteration of alveolar and deadspace ventilation. The alteration of alveolar ventilation leads to changes in $PaCO_2$, which changes pH and PaO_2.

A change in the PEEP level also changes compression pressure and tidal volume, leading to the same alterations mentioned with PIP changes. Additionally, changes in PEEP modify the FRC, which then changes compliance. A change in compliance then alters the time constant, expiratory time, and the I:E ratio.

If this discussion appears confusing, then it has served its purpose. The point is to show that all ventilator parameters influence one another to some degree. Ventilator management is no easy task and requires an understanding of these complicated interrelationships.

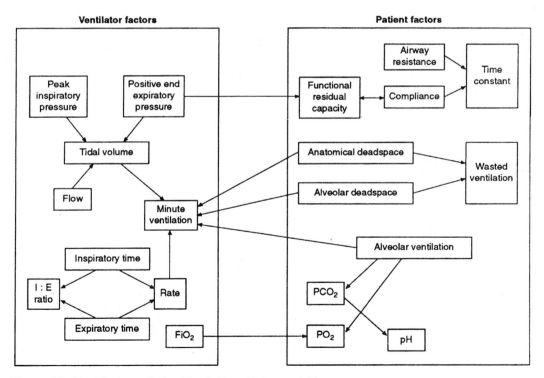

Figure 14–12 *The interrelationship of all ventilatory variables.*

PRESSURE-VOLUME RELATIONSHIPS (COMPLIANCE)

BASICS

The airways, lungs, and chest wall, like other body organs and structures, are elastic structures. An *elastic* structure, by definition, has the ability to resist deformation when a force is exerted against it, and thus produces a recoil force.

According to Hooke's law of elasticity, when an elastic substance is stretched, tension develops that is proportional to the degree of deformation that is produced. Thus, the more it is stretched, the more force it produces to recoil to its original size and shape.

To measure the elasticity of a hollow, spherical organ, such as the lung, it would be difficult to stretch the tissue and measure its recoil force. The recoil is instead measured by applying a known pressure to the lung and then measuring the change in volume that occurs. This relationship between a given change in volume and the pressure difference required to provide that volume change is called *compliance* and directly reflects the ability of the lungs to stretch.

STATIC AND DYNAMIC COMPLIANCE

Under static conditions, compliance reflects the elastic properties of the lungs alone. When measured understatically, or when there is no airflow, this compliance is called static lung compliance. Compliance measured during spontaneous breathing is called dynamic compliance. Dynamic compliance better reflects the elastic recoil of the lungs.

NORMAL COMPLIANCE

Lung compliance is measured in ml of volume change per cm H_2O of pressure applied to the trachea. Normal compliance in a newborn is approximately 2.5 to 5 ml/cm H_2O and can decrease to 0.5 ml/cm H_2O/kg with RDS.

COMPLIANCE CURVES

The amount of pressure required to increase the volume in the lungs is directly related to the number of elastic elements that are present in the lung tissue. The more elastic elements, the more pressure required to stretch them and the lower the compliance.

A graphic representation of the three possible compliance curves of the lung is shown in Figure 14–13. Figure 14–13 (curve A) shows the curve in a stiff, noncompliant lung, curve B is the normal lung compliance curve, and curve C shows a very compliant lung.

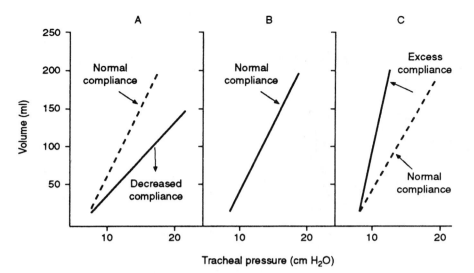

Figure 14–13 *Various compliance curves of the lungs. Curve A represents a stiff lung, Curve B represents a normal lung, and Curve C represents an excessively compliant lung.*

DETERMINANTS OF PULMONARY COMPLIANCE

The two main determinants of lung compliance are the alveolar surface forces and the elastic elements in the lung tissue. Alveolar surface forces are the direct result of surface tension in the alveoli created by the interface between the moist alveoli and the gas in them. (See Chapter 1 for a review of surface tension and surface forces.)

The degree to which surface tension affects lung compliance is illustrated in Figure 14–14. This graph shows a compliance curve of a normal lung when the air-liquid interface of the alveoli is removed by filling and then ventilating the lungs with normal saline, compared to the same lung when ventilated with air. Notice that the saline-filled lung is far more compliant than the air-filled lung. This difference is the result of alveolar surface tension.

In the healthy lung, these alveolar surface forces are counteracted by the presence of surfactant, which chemically reduces the surface tension of the alveoli. Elastic elements in the lung tissue remain fairly constant in the healthy lung, but in disease states may increase and contribute to a decrease in compliance.

COMPLIANCE OF THE THORACIC CAGE

The thorax, like the lungs, is an elastic structure. It differs from the lung in that it recoils inward or outward, whereas the lung only recoils inward. The direction of thoracic recoil depends on the volume in the thorax.

If all the organs were removed from the chest and the chest were reclosed, the ribs would be at a neutral point, neither recoiling or expanding. At this point, the pressure inside the

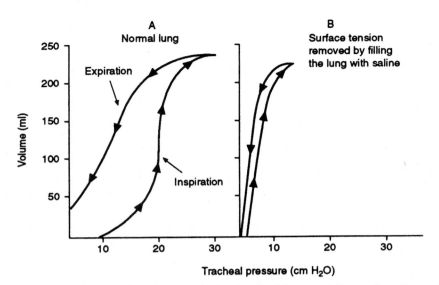

Figure 14–14 *The relationship between surface tension and lung compliance. Compliance dramatically increases when surface tension is removed (graph B).*

thorax is the same as outside the thorax. This is referred to as the *unstressed volume*. If we were to add volume to the thorax, the ribs would begin to pull inward as they are stretched beyond their unstressed level. This inward pull of the ribs increases the pressure inside the thorax. If volume is now removed from the thorax below the unstressed volume, the ribs attempt to recoil outward, which would decrease the pressure inside the thorax.

RELATIONSHIP BETWEEN THE LUNGS AND THE THORACIC CAGE

To ventilate the lungs adequately, both lung forces and chest wall forces must be overcome. The intimate relationship between the lungs and the chest wall is maintained by a thin layer of fluid found between the visceral pleura surrounding the lungs and the parietal pleura lining the chest wall. This thin layer of fluid creates a *static attraction* between the external surface of the lung and the internal lining of the lung. The net result is that the compliance of the chest wall and of the lungs, although two separate entities, become one compliance when ventilating the lungs.

FRC is determined when the inward pull of the lungs is balanced with the outward pull of the thorax and the unstressed volume in the chest is reached. At this point, the pressure in the thorax, and thus the lungs, is equal to atmospheric pressure. To inflate the lungs, the pressure inside the thorax must drop below atmospheric pressure, as occurs in spontaneous breathing, or atmospheric pressure must rise above thoracic pressure, as in mechanical ventilation.

As volume increases in the thorax, the elastic forces of both the lungs and the chest recoil inward, increasing the pressure in the thorax and allowing passive exhalation to occur. The gas then exits the thorax to the point that the unstressed volume is once again reached.

It is apparent, then, that if the compliance of the lung decreases, the inward pull of the lung exceeds the outward recoil of the ribs and a new unstressed volume is reached, which is less than the previous volume; thus the FRC has decreased.

COMPLIANCE CURVE OF THE LUNGS

The relationship between volume and pressure is graphically represented in Figure 14–15. The "S"-shaped curve represents the compliance of the lung, with pressure on the horizontal and volume on the vertical axis.

Point B in Figure 14–16 shows the location on the curve of the lung with a normal FRC. Notice that it is located on the steep portion of the compliance curve, indicating a high compliance. In other words, small changes in pressure produce large changes in volume.

With diseases such as RDS, as the alveoli lose surfactant, increased surface tension causes an increasing collapse of the alveoli and the FRC decreases. In this lung, the compliance is low. This is represented as point A in Figure 14–17. On the flat portion of the curve, increases in pressure produce only small changes in volume, indicating a very stiff noncompliant lung.

With the addition of PEEP, the alveoli are held open at the end of exhalation, causing an increase in FRC and moving the lungs back to point B on the compliance curve.

When the lungs are overexpanded, the FRC increases above normal and the elastic elements in the lung interstitium are stretched. The compliance becomes lower as the lung loses its ability to stretch further. The lungs are now at another flat portion of the compliance curve, represented by point C in Figure 14–18. Again, in this circumstance, changes in pressure produce only small changes in volume.

The hazard when ventilating at this portion of the curve is a tearing or rupture of the lung interstitium, because the lung cannot stretch any more in response to pressure increases. A high FRC (point C) can be caused by air trapping or from excessive levels of PEEP.

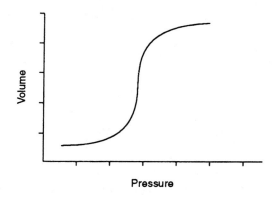

Figure 14–15 *The volume-pressure curve of the lung.*

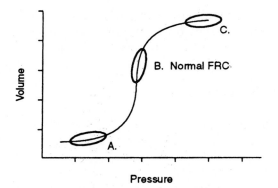

Figure 14–16 *The location of a lung with a normal FRC on the volume-pressure curve. Small changes in pressure cause large changes in volume.*

Successful ventilation techniques require the use of appropriate PEEP levels to keep the lung on the steep portion of the compliance curve.

CLINICAL APPLICATIONS

Any time mechanical ventilation is initiated on a patient, an understanding of lung compliance is vital. Diseases that increase surface forces in the alveoli (RDS) decrease compliance and increase the amount of pressure required to ventilate the lungs. As the alveoli shrink in size, the FRC is reduced. Higher pressure is now needed to inflate the alveoli. The addition of PEEP increases the FRC and allows the use of lower pressures.

Certain fibrotic diseases may cause an increase in the amount of elastic elements in the lung, thus altering compliance. Paralyzation of the chest wall reduces thoracic compliance and requires increased inspiratory pressures to overcome the increased stiffness.

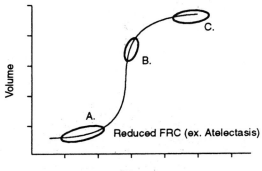

Figure 14–17 *The loss of FRC places the lung at the low end of the volume-pressure curve. Large pressure changes result in only small changes in volume.*

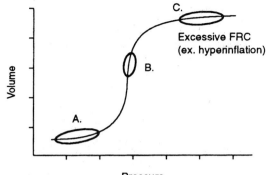

Figure 14–18 *An increase in FRC causes the lung to be at the high end of the volume-pressure curve. Large pressure changes result in only small changes in volume.*

With the need for increased pressure to open the alveoli, there is an increased risk of barotrauma. High pressure also further decreases cardiac output by reducing blood return to the right heart. Pulmonary vascular resistance increases as ventilatory pressures rise, resulting in diminished blood flow to the lungs and increasing V/Q mismatches.

An important goal when ventilating the lungs is to maintain the lung on the steep portion of the compliance curve, thus lowering inspiratory pressures and decreasing the chance of barotrauma and other mentioned effects on the cardiopulmonary systems.

PRESSURE-FLOW RELATIONSHIPS (RESISTANCE)

BASICS

There are several factors that determine the level of flow through a tube. They are: 1) the difference between the inlet and the outlet pressures, which is the driving pressure; 2) the radius of the tube; 3) the length of the tube; and 4) the *viscosity*, or thickness, of the gas or fluid, illustrated in Figure 14–19. This is the basic expression of Poiseuille's law. The pressure difference between the inlet and the outlet determines the rate of flow, with a greater pressure difference resulting in a greater flow and vice versa. The other three factors offer a *resistance* to that flow.

When dealing with the airways, the length of the airway and the viscosity of the gas remain relatively constant, so the only factor that changes resistance to airflow is a change in the radius of the airway.

MEASUREMENT OF RESISTANCE

Resistance is measured as the ratio between the driving pressure, measured in cm H_2O, and the amount of flow in liters per second. The basic definition of resistance is the driving pressure needed to move gases through the airways at a constant flow rate.

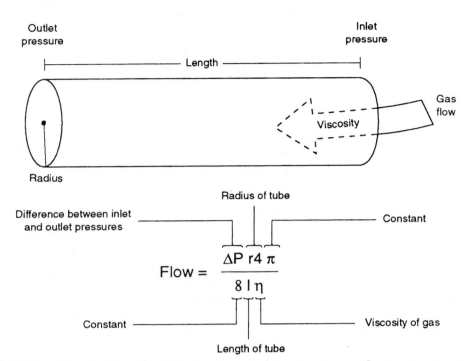

Figure 14–19 *Poiseuille's law determining flow through a tube. Flow is proportional to the viscosity of the gas and the length of the tube. Flow is inversely proportional to the fourth power of the radius of the tube.*

In the lung, the driving pressure is the difference between the pressure at the mouth (inlet pressure) and the alveoli (outlet pressure). We can then calculate resistance by measuring the driving pressure and dividing it by the flow of gas. The measurement of airway resistance is usually accomplished during pulmonary function studies. The normal airway resistance in a spontaneously breathing neonate is between 20 and 30 cm H_2O/L/sec.

OTHER CAUSES OF INCREASED RESISTANCE

Other factors lead to increases in airway resistance that are not associated with the normal anatomy of the airway. Neonates have an increased level of interstitial fluid in the lungs, which reduces the radius of the airway.

The presence of an endotracheal tube (ETT) and the associated ventilator tubing also increases resistance. The resistance offered by an ETT is directly related to its length and inversely related to its diameter. Turbulent flow is present in a 2.5 mm ID ETT at flow rates exceeding 3 lpm, and at flows exceeding 7.5 lpm in a 3.0 ETT. Subsequent changes in flow above these levels causes disproportionate increases in resistance, secondary to the increased turbulent flow.

CLINICAL APPLICATIONS

Of all the factors that affect resistance in the airway, by far the most powerful influence is a change in the radius of the airway. According to Poiseuille's law, for every decrease in the radius, resistance increases to the fourth power. Therefore, anything that reduces the radius of the airway, such as bronchospasm, mucus, edema, and swelling, increases the resistance to airflow. Table 14–3 lists possible causes of increased resistance.

Treatment is aimed at increasing the airway diameter and reducing the resistance to airflow. This is done with bronchodilators to relieve bronchospasm, vigorous chest physiotherapy and suctioning to mobilize and remove airway secretions, diuretics to reduce edema, and antibiotics and anti-inflammatories to reduce inflammation and swelling.

Resistance offered by the endotracheal tube is reduced by shortening the tube so only 4 cm of the tube extends beyond the lips. The shorter the tube, the less resistance it will offer. It is also desirable to use an endotracheal tube with the largest diameter possible, further reducing resistance.

To avoid extremes in turbulent airflow that increase resistance, attempts should be made to keep ventilator flow rates at or below those levels at which turbulence increases. The clinical implications of turbulent airflow are less pressure being delivered to the alveoli with a resultant reduction in tidal volume. This is especially prevalent when high rates and short inspiratory times are being used.

Additionally, the resistance offered by the ETT is greater than that of the upper airways, and spontaneous ventilation by the neonate through the ETT may require more work than the neonate is able to handle. The neonatal patient should be extubated when the IMV rate is weaned to a low rate with peak inspiratory pressure and should not be required to breathe spontaneously on CPAP.

TIME CONSTANTS (Kt)

Time constants reflect the amount of time required for alveolar and proximal airway pressures to equilibrate. In other words, time constants are the amount of time required for the lungs to inhale or exhale. Our focus in this section will be on expiratory time constants.

Table 14–3   Factors That Increase Airway Resistance

1. Bronchospasm
2. Airway secretions
3. Edema of the airway walls
4. Inflammation
5. Artificial airway
   a. Endotracheal tube
   b. Tracheostomy tube

CALCULATING TIME CONSTANTS

The two forces that determine the time required for exhalation are the elastic recoil of the lung and chest wall (compliance) and the opposition to airflow (resistance). The formula for calculating one time constant is to multiply compliance by resistance. Compliance must be changed to $L/cm\ H_2O$ before calculating the time constant.

The compliance and resistance of the respiratory system as a whole is used to calculate time constants. This is done realizing that we are using an average, when some alveoli having longer time constants and some shorter. A knowledge of time constants will help the caregiver choose the safest and most effective ventilator settings for each patient.

One time constant equals the time required for the alveoli to discharge 63% of the tidal volume. Three time constants are required before 95% of the tidal volume is emptied.

An example of calculating time constants, using a lung compliance of $0.006\ L/cm\ H_2O$ and a resistance of 25 cm $H_2O/L/sec$, is demonstrated in Table 14–4. In this instance, one time constant equals 0.15 second. This patient would therefore require a minimum of 0.45 second (3×0.15 sec) to exhale 95% of the tidal volume and avoid air trapping.

CLINICAL APPLICATIONS

All possible combinations of resistance and compliance changes, and the effect on time constants, are demonstrated in Table 14–5. We will briefly discuss three common clinical situations that demonstrate these relationships.

If airway resistance remains constant, a decrease in lung compliance results in a decreased time constant. This means that less time is needed to exhale, and shorter expiratory times can be tolerated by the patient. Shorter expiratory times allow for faster ventilatory rates without the risk of air trapping. This combination is often present in RDS, where the decreased amount of surfactant affects the alveolar compliance, but not the resistance of the airways.

If resistance increases along with a decrease in compliance, as would occur if bronchospasm accompanied RDS, the time constant would increase and expiratory times would need to be lengthened to prevent air trapping.

A possible clinical situation in which this could be dangerous is in a patient being mechanically ventilated at a high rate of RDS. If bronchospasm occurred, the time constant would increase and air trapping would result. To avoid air trapping, the expiratory time would need to be increased to allow the lungs time to empty. The administration of a bronchodilator may reduce the bronchospasm, reducing resistance and returning the time constants to previous levels.

Table 14–4 Calculation of Time Constants

Kt = compliance (L/cm H_2O) × resistance
Kt = 0.006 × 25
Kt = 0.15 sec
0.15 × 3 (amount of time to exhale 95% of the VT) = 0.45 sec needed for exhalation

---

TABLE 14–5   Effects of Compliance and Resistance Changes on Kt

Changes	Effect on KT
Compliance unchanged	
Increased resistance	Longer duration
Decreased resistance	Shorter duration
Resistance unchanged	
Improved compliance	Longer duration
Worsening compliance	Shorter duration
Improved compliance	
Increased resistance	Longer duration
Decreased resistance	No change
Worsened compliance	
Increased resistance	No change
Decreased resistance	Shorter duration
Increased resistance	
Improved compliance	Longer duration
Worsening compliance	No change
Decreased resistance	
Improved compliance	No change
Worsening compliance	Shorter duration

It should be apparent that the clinical disease state of the infant is continuously changing and must be closely monitored and anticipated so that appropriate ventilator changes can be made.

Another possible clinical situation surrounds the administration of surfactant. This example involves a preemie with RDS being ventilated at high pressures and frequency, receiving a dose of surfactant. The surfactant reduces the alveolar surface tension, increasing compliance. As the compliance improves, time constants also increase. The practitioner must be aware of these changes and slow the rate of ventilation to allow adequate expiratory time in the presence of longer time constants.

Procedures such as suctioning and reintubation with a larger endotracheal tube cause a decrease in resistance and decreased time constants. An understanding of these concepts will allow the practitioner to maintain the ideal patient/ventilator system.

SUMMARY

In order to appropriately manage a mechanically ventilated patient, the practitioner must understand the basic concepts involved in mechanical ventilation. Before committing a patient to a ventilator, the goals of the treatment must be understood. The overriding goal is to provide adequate alveolar gas exchange while causing minimal damage to the lungs and minimal interference with the circulation.

Understanding mechanical ventilation begins with an understanding of terminology. The peak inspiratory pressure (PIP) is the maximum pressure reached during the inspiratory phase. Positive end-expiratory pressure (PEEP) is the level of positive pressure applied to the airway during the expiratory phase. Frequency, or rate, is the number of inspiratory breaths delivered by the ventilator in one minute. The inspiratory time (IT) is the amount of time, usually measured in seconds or tenths of a second, that the inspiratory breath lasts. A slightly more difficult concept to grasp is that of mean airway pressure (MAP), which is the average pressure being applied to the airway throughout the inspiratory and expiratory cycle. The difficult part is that there are so many variables that make up MAP, such as rate, PIP, PEEP, and IT. In general, it is prudent to maintain MAP as low as possible in order to meet the ventilatory requirements of the patient.

Tidal volume is the amount of gas, measured in milliliters or liters, given to the patient during inspiration. When the tidal volume is multiplied by the rate of ventilation, the result is the minute volume, or the total amount of gas delivered to the patient in one minute. Deadspace is defined as those portions of the respiratory tract that do not participate in gas exchange. Deadspace is either anatomic or alveolar. Anatomic deadspace involves those airways not involved in gas exchange, basically from the terminal bronchioles upward. Alveolar deadspace includes those alveoli that fill with gas, but are not perfused with blood. The two together are called physiologic deadspace. Alveolar ventilation, therefore, is equal to the tidal volume, minus the physiologic deadspace.

The amount of pressure needed to open and expand the alveoli is called opening pressure. It is said to be achieved when crackles are heard during inspiration. The driving pressure of the ventilator is equal to the total amount of pressure rise during an inspiration, or PIP minus PEEP. Ideally, the driving pressure should be equal to or above the opening pressure in order to ventilate the alveoli. With the presence of PEEP, however, compliance is improved, opening pressure is reduced and less driving pressure is needed to provide ventilation.

The functional residual capacity (FRC), is the amount of gas remaining in the lungs at the end of inspiration. In the presence of surfactant deficiency, the FRC drops and compliance worsens. The addition of PEEP brings the FRC back to its appropriate level and improves lung compliance. The amount of time that the inspiratory gas is in contact with the alveoli is called diffusion time. The longer the contact time, the more gas is able to diffuse between the alveoli and the blood. Finally, the flow rate determines how quickly gas is delivered during inspiration. It can be likened to a water faucet in which the wider it is opened, the faster the flow escaping. Likewise, the more the flow valve is opened, the faster the gas will flow into the patient.

Terminology, as it relates to the structures of the pulmonary tree, is also important to understand. Compliance reflects the ability of the lungs to expand at any given pressure. At very high compliances, the lung expands at low pressures. Conversely, at low compliances, high pressures are required to make the lungs expand. Compliance is determined by alveolar surface forces and the elastic elements of the lungs. Low compliance is the result of increased alveolar surface forces, an increase in the elastic elements, or a combination of both. The compliance curve of the lung is useful to understand the role of FRC and its effect on lung compliance. As FRC increase above normal, the lung tissue is stretched beyond its normal length. As pressure is applied to the lungs, they can expand only a small amount and thus compliance is low. When FRC is below normal, the alveoli shrink due to their surface forces. Now as pressure is applied, a greater amount is required to overcome the surfaces forces. Again, compliance is low. At its normal volume, neither the lung tissues are stretched exceedingly, nor are the alveoli shrunk abnormally, and compliance is within its normal range. At that point, ventilation can be accomplished without having to resort to excessive pressures, which could damage the lungs and impede circulation.

As gas flows through the airways, its movement is resisted by several factors including the size and length of the airway. Of the factors affecting gas flow in the airways, all remain constant except for the size, or diameter. Therefore, the major factor in determining resistance to airflow is the changing diameter of the airways. As the diameter lessens, as in bronchospasm, resistance increases. The opposite is true when airway diameter increases.

The final term covered is time constants. The time constant is the amount of time required for alveolar and proximal pressures to equilibrate. Time constants are determined by the lung compliance and airway resistance. This is an important concept to understand when providing mechanical ventilation to a neonate. For example, if a patient has a long time constant secondary to increased airway resistance, a longer period of time will be required for exhalation to occur. If the expiratory time is too short, the next breath will be delivered while there is still gas remaining in the alveoli. The results could be air trapping and possibly air leaks.

References

1. Merenstein GB, Gardner SL. *Handbook of Neonatal Intensive Care.* 4th ed. St. Louis, Mo: CV Mosby Co; 1998.
2. Koff PB, et al. *Neonatal and Pediatric Respiratory Care.* 2nd ed. St. Louis, Mo: CV Mosby Co; 1993.

Bibliography and Suggested Readings

Chang DW. *Clinical Application of Mechanical Ventilation.* 2nd ed. Albany, NY: Delmar Thomson Learning; 2001.

Goldsmith JP, Karotkin EH. *Assisted Ventilation of the Neonate.* 3rd ed. Philadelphia: WB Saunders Co; 1996.

Levin D, Morriss F, et al. *Essentials of Pediatric Intensive Care.* 2nd ed. St. Louis, Mo; Quality Medical Publishing, Inc.; 1997.

MacIntyre NR, Branson RD. *Mechanical Ventilation.* Philadelphia: WB Saunders Co; 2000.

Pilbeam SP. *Mechanical Ventilation.* 3rd ed. St. Louis, Mo: Mosby; 1998.

Posttest

1. Which of the following is the goal of mechanical ventilation?
    a. the reversal of acute lung disorders
    b. maintain a patent airway in the presence of lung disease
    c. treatment and diagnosis of acute and chronic lung disorders
    d. provide adequate alveolar ventilation with minimal lung damage
2. Which of the following is the best definition of peak inspiratory pressure?
    a. the maximum pressure exerted against the patient's airway during inspiration
    b. a positive pressure maintained in the airway during expiration
    c. the pressure required to open the lungs to 75% of capacity
    d. the pressure generated by the ventilator before a tidal volume delivery
3. Of the following, which best describes wasted ventilation?
    a. alveolar deadspace
    b. physiologic deadspace
    c. the ratio of physiologic deadspace to tidal volume
    d. the amount of tidal gas that leaks around the endotracheal tube
4. Of the following, which alter the duration of ventilation?
    I. rate
    II. flow
    III. PIP
    IV. PEEP
    V. I:T
        a. II, V
        b. I, III, IV
        c. II, III, V
        d. I, II, III, IV, V
5. Assuming an alveolar opening pressure of 23 cm H_2O, which of the following combinations of PIP and PEEP would achieve the desired compression pressure?
    a. PIP-23, PEEP-3
    b. PIP-20, PEEP-5
    c. PIP-26, PEEP-3
    d. PIP-26, PEEP-5
6. Normal lung compliance in a newborn is:
    a. 2.5 to 5 ml/cm H_2O
    b. 7 to 10 ml/cm H_2O
    c. 10 to 15 ml/cm H_2O
    d. 25 to 30 ml/cm H_2O
7. Of the following, which are determinants of pulmonary compliance?
    I. elastic elements
    II. alveolar surface forces
    III. plateau pressure
    IV. airway resistance
    V. dynamic ventilatory pressures
        a. II, IV

b. I, III, IV

c. I, II

d. III, IV, V

8. As volume is extracted from the thorax at its unstressed volume, the ribs:

a. pull inward

b. spread apart

c. recoil outward

d. pull closer together

9. With overexpansion of the lungs caused by air trapping, lung compliance is:

a. normal

b. high

c. reduced

d. inverse to the level of airflow

10. RDS lowers lung compliance by:

a. increasing pulmonary blood flow

b. increasing airway resistance

c. increasing air trapping

d. increasing alveolar surface forces

11. Which of the following is the main factor that determines airway resistance?

a. airway radius

b. airway length

c. outlet pressure

d. viscosity of the gas

12. The normal airway resistance in a spontaneously breathing neonate is:

a. 10 to 20 cm H_2O/L/sec

b. 20 to 30 cm H_2O/L/sec

c. 20 to 30 mm Hg/cc/sec

d. 30 to 40 mm Hg/cc/sec

13. Endotracheal tube resistance can be reduced by:

a. lengthening the tube

b. increasing gas flow

c. shortening the tube

d. decreasing tidal volume

14. In the presence of which of the following scenarios could shorter inspiratory times and faster rates be used without the risk of air trapping?

a. RDS with bronchospasm

b. administration of surfactant to an RDS patient

c. improving RDS

d. RDS

15. With a compliance of 3.6 ml/cm H_2O and an airway resistance of 42 cm H_2O/L/sec, what would be an appropriate expiratory time?

a. 0.46 sec

b. 0.28 sec

c. 0.16 sec

d. 0.15 sec

CHAPTER FIFTEEN

MANAGEMENT OF THE PATIENT-VENTILATOR SYSTEM

OBJECTIVES

Upon completion of this chapter, the reader should be able to:

1. Identify and describe the indications for ventilatory support of the neonate and child.
2. Describe and contrast partial ventilatory support and full ventilatory support.
3. Describe how the following initial ventilator parameters are determined: mode, peak inspiratory pressure, set rate, sensitivity, PEEP, FiO_2, inspiratory flow, inspiratory time, I:E ratio, and tidal volume.
4. Describe volume versus pressure-controlled ventilation.
5. Describe how changes are made in ventilator settings based on blood gases and clinical evaluation.
6. Discuss the hazards of mechanical ventilation.
7. Discuss weaning and extubation of the neonatal and pediatric patient from mechanical ventilation.
8. Discuss extubation of the neonatal and pediatric patient.

KEY TERMS

Conditional variable

Control variable

Full ventilatory support

Mode of ventilation

Pallor

Partial ventilatory support

Pressure-controlled ventilation

Rebound effect

Volume-controlled ventilation

INDICATIONS FOR VENTILATORY SUPPORT OF THE NEONATE AND CHILD

The indication for mechanical ventilation is respiratory failure. This is commonly subdivided into three classifications: hypoxemic respiratory failure, hypercapnic respiratory failure, and mixed respiratory failure.

Hypoxemic respiratory failure is commonly manifested by a PaO_2 ≤50 mm Hg on an FiO_2

of ≥ 0.6 despite the use of continuous positive airway pressure (CPAP), or a decreasing PaO_2 (or SpO_2 <90–92%) despite an increase in FiO_2. Frequently, these patients will have an accompanying hypocapnia ($PaCO_2$ ≤ 30 mm Hg) and respiratory alkalemia (pH ≥ 7.5), as they attempt to compensate for hypoxemia by increasing minute ventilation. Clinical features include agitation, cyanosis, tachycardia or bradycardia, tachypnea (>70–80 breaths/ minute in neonates; >50 breaths/minute in children). Classic signs of distress in neonates also include nasal flaring, grunting, and retractions (substernal, sternal, intercostal, and suprasternal).

Hypercapnic respiratory failure is commonly manifested by a $PaCO_2$ ≥ 50 mm Hg, accompanied by acidemia (pH ≤ 7.25). The infant may appear apneic, listless, and cyanotic. Bradycardia or tachycardia may be present.

Mixed respiratory failure is manifested by both hypoxemia and hypercapnia. Acidemia will be present as well. Table 15–1 indicates the clinical conditions that may indicate mechanical ventilation of the neonate and child.

Once the decision is made to initiate mechanical ventilation, the airway is accessed with an appropriate endotracheal tube (see Chapter 16) and decisions are made concerning initial ventilator parameters.

It is generally accepted that mechanical ventilation is indicated when one or more reversible problems exist. However, not all problems in neonates or children are reversible and there is an ethical dilemma about whether to withhold or withdraw life support from these children. Diagnoses in which the decision is made to withhold life support include birth weight less than 800 g, severe intracranial hemorrhage, periventricular leukomalacia, severe necrotizing enterocolitis, hypoxic-ischemic encephalopathy, intractable respiratory failure, and major congenital anomalies or chromosomal abnormalities. In the presence of one or more of these problems, the pediatrician, neonatologist, and parents may choose to forego therapy because it may be futile, the abnormality may lead only to lifelong impairment, or the treatment may cause great suffering.[1, 2]

Table 15–1 Clinical Conditions That May Indicate Mechanical Ventilation

Category	Representative conditions
Neurologic alteration	Apnea of prematurity, intracranial hemorrhage, congenital neuromuscular disorders (i.e., Duchenne's muscular dystrophy), poisoning, phrenic nerve paralysis
Impaired respiratory function	Respiratory distress syndrome (RDS/ARDS), meconium aspiration syndrome (MAS), pneumonia, bronchopulmonary dysplasia (BPD), bronchiolitis, congenital diaphragmatic hernia, sepsis, radiographic evidence of decreased lung volume, asthma, trauma, inhalation injury
Impaired cardiovascular function	Persistent pulmonary hypertension of the newborn (PPHN), postresuscitation, congenital heart disease, shock
Postoperative	Central nervous system depression, atelectasis

From: AARC Clinical Practice Guideline. Neonatal time triggered, pressure-limited, time cycled mechanical ventilation. *Respiratory Care.* 1994;39:808–816.

MODES OF MECHANICAL VENTILATION

A *mode of ventilation* is described as the combination of control, phase, and conditional variables.[3] The *control variable* is that which does not change when compliance or resistance changes. In *volume-controlled ventilation*, if compliance or resistance changes, volume does not change; pressure changes. In *pressure-controlled ventilation*, when compliance or resistance changes, pressure does not change. This means that when compliance decreases or resistance increases, tidal volume decreases. The phase variables are trigger, limit, cycle, and baseline. Trigger variable refers to how a breath is initiated. Breaths that are begun only when dictated by an inspiratory timer are time triggered. The patient's inspiratory effort may be pressure, flow, or volume triggered. The limit variable is that which is reached before the end of inspiration and may include pressure, volume, time, or flow. The cycle variable is that which ends inspiration. Cycle variables include flow, time, pressure, or volume. The baseline variable defines expiration, which is usually pressure. *Conditional variables* describe the conditions that must exist for initiating a sigh breath, or a mandatory breath during synchronized intermittent mandatory ventilation (SIMV). A given mode may be classified in one of two categories, partial or full ventilatory support.

PARTIAL VENTILATORY SUPPORT (PVS)

Partial ventilatory support includes those modes indicated for patients who are capable of maintaining all or part of their minute ventilation. Included are CPAP, pressure support ventilation (PSV), intermittent mandatory ventilation (IMV) at low mandatory rates, and synchronized intermittent mandatory ventilation (SIMV) at low mandatory rates. CPAP and IMV are the primary modes used for neonates. CPAP, SIMV, and PSV, among others, are used in the mechanical ventilation of children.

CONTINUOUS POSITIVE AIRWAY PRESSURE (CPAP)

CPAP is the application of a continuous positive distending pressure to the airways. It is a technique that is used on spontaneously breathing infants and children suffering from respiratory distress syndrome in an attempt to prevent the need for continuous mechanical ventilation. It accomplishes this by increasing the functional residual capacity (FRC), increasing compliance, decreasing total airway resistance, and decreasing respiratory rate, which are the desired outcomes of nasal CPAP.[3]

In RDS, alveolar surfactant quantity and function are insufficient to maintain alveolar geometry, thus causing surface tension to increase. The increased surface tension in the alveoli cause an ever-decreasing FRC. With each breath, the patient must overcome the higher surface tension, and work of breathing increases. The administration of a continuous positive pressure to the airway physically holds the alveoli and airways open during exhalation and increases FRC, as shown in Figure 15–1. With an increase in FRC, lung com-

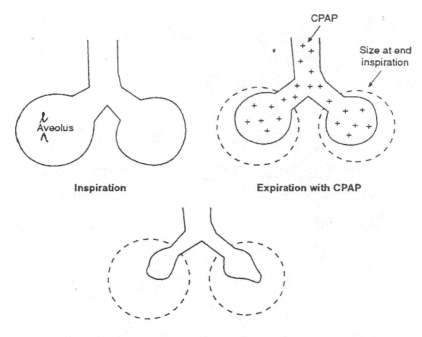

Figure 15–1 *The presence of positive pressure during the expiratory phase prevents alveolar collapse when surfactant is not present.*

pliance improves, easing the work of breathing, and PaO_2 increases while usually allowing a decrease in the FiO_2 and its accompanying toxic side-effects. CPAP may be administered to the neonate or infant through an endotracheal tube in the trachea. Alternative airways used on neonates include the use of a trimmed endotracheal tube in the posterior oral pharynx adjacent to the uvula, or through nasal prongs. To use the trimmed tube technique, an appropriately sized endotracheal tube is inserted into a nare and advanced until it is palpated adjacent to the uvula. Once there, it is trimmed outside the nare to decrease dead space, then taped in place above the upper lip. The endotracheal tube-ventilator circuit adapter is replaced and fitted to the ventilator circuit. The nasal prongs are attached to the ventilator circuit at the endotracheal tube adapter. The prongs are fitted into the nares and secured with tape to the infant's face.

CPAP is administered to a child through the endotracheal tube. A mask is not advised, because the child may aspirate air, leading to gastric distention, vomiting, and aspiration of gastric contents. The child may fear the mask and frequently dislodge it.

Indications. CPAP is useful for the treatment of conditions resulting in airway or alveolar instability. Five general indications for CPAP exist, as shown in Table 15–2. The first indication is any disease or condition that causes a decrease in the FRC. Causes of a decreased FRC include: infectious processes such as pneumonia; a loss of lung volume as seen with

---

Table 15–2   Indications for CPAP

A. *Decreased FRC*
Pneumonia
Atelectasis
Pulmonary edema
Thoracotomy
Meconium aspiration
Increased mucus
RDS
RDS type II (transient tachypnea of the newborn)
Left-to-right shunting

B. *Airway collapse*
Tracheobronchial malacia
Apnea

C. *Weaning from mechanical ventilation*

D. *Abnormal physical examination*
Increased respiratory rate (30–40%)
Retractions
Grunting
Nasal flaring
Cyanosis

E. *Abnormal arterial blood gases*
PaO_2 < 50 mm Hg at an FiO_2 of 60% (with adequate ventilation)

---

atelectasis, pulmonary edema, or thoracotomy; an inability for gas to reach the alveoli as occurs in meconium aspiration, or severe airway blockage with mucus; conditions that lower lung surfactant such as RDS; and other conditions, including RDS type II (transient tachypnea) and left-to-right shunting present with certain cardiac defects.

The second indication includes those processes that cause airway collapse. One of the primary causes of airway collapse is tracheobronchial malacia, in which the cartilage of the trachea is abnormal and does not offer the necessary rigidity to prevent collapse during inspiration and expiration. Airway collapse can also lead to apnea, making CPAP helpful in treating apnea.

A third indication is to assist in weaning the patient from mechanical ventilation. A study by Tapia and associates, however, failed to demonstrate any difference in extubation outcome whether CPAP was used or not.[4]

The fourth and fifth indications may be seen in the above conditions, but are not exclusive to them and are listed separately. An abnormal physical examination that shows a 30 to 40% increase in respiratory rate, retractions, grunting, flaring, or cyanosis is the fourth indication. The fifth involves blood gas abnormality. Assuming ventilation is adequate, the inability to maintain the PaO_2 greater than 50 mm Hg at an FiO_2 of 60% is an indication for CPAP.[5]

CPAP is most effective when it is instituted early in the progression of the disease. Initial pressures should start at between 4 and 5 cm H_2O. The pressure is increased in increments of 2 cm H_2O, as needed, to achieve the desired PaO_2 level, up to a CPAP of 10 cm H_2O.[3] CPAP is considered successful if the FiO_2 is stabilized at ≤0.6 with a PaO_2 ≥50 mm Hg or SpO_2 >90%, a decreased work of breathing, decreased retractions, nasal flaring and grunting, improved aeration on the chest radiograph, and subjectively improved patient comfort.

Nasal CPAP is considered to have failed when the PaO_2 remains below 50 mm Hg despite an FiO_2 of 0.80 to 1.0 on CPAP pressures of 10 to 12 cm H_2O. A $PaCO_2$ greater than 60 mm Hg with a pH less than 7.25, marked retractions on CPAP, metabolic acidosis that does not respond to treatment, and frequent apneic episodes while on CPAP are also indications that CPAP has failed. In this instance, intermittent mandatory ventilation is initiated.

Classification of Breaths and Waveforms. CPAP breaths are classified as pressure controlled, pressure triggered, pressure limited, and pressure cycled. The baseline variable is pressure. All breaths are spontaneous. That is, all breaths are initiated by patient effort and all breaths end owing to the patient's compliance and resistance characteristics. A representative pressure waveform is shown in Figure 15–2.

Hazards. The principal hazard of CPAP therapy is that associated with high pressures. In the presence of excessive pressures, pulmonary blood flow is diminished secondary to the compression of pulmonary vessels. Cardiac output may also be reduced owing to the decrease in venous return to the heart. For these reasons, CPAP is not useful in the patient with persistent pulmonary hypertension and other diseases where the problem is not one of alveolar instability.

Additional hazards include renal effects such as a decrease in glomerular filtration rate, sodium excretion, and urine output. CPAP also elevates intracranial pressure, increasing the incidence of hemorrhage. Further hazards include pneumothorax, nasal obstruction, gastric distention, and necrosis or erosion of the nasal septum. Nasal deformities from the use of nasal prongs has also been recognized.[6]

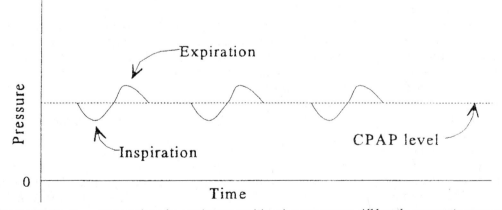

Figure 15–2 *Pressure waveform for continuous positive airway pressure. All breaths are spontaneous, pressure triggered, limited, and cycled.*

Contraindications. CPAP should not be used in the presence of upper airway abnormalities such as choanal atresia, cleft palate, or tracheoesophageal fistula, because it could be ineffective or dangerous. CPAP increases intrapulmonary pressure; therefore, it should not be used in cases of untreated air leaks such as pneumothorax, pneumomediastinum, pneumopericardium, and pulmonary interstitial emphysema. The increase in intrathoracic pressure may also further worsen cardiovascular instability and should not be used in those patients. Secondly, because the patient must maintain spontaneous ventilation, CPAP should not be used on the severely apneic patient who experiences episodes of desaturation or bradycardia. Any patient who cannot maintain an adequate spontaneous tidal volume and therefore have hypercapnic respiratory failure should not be treated with CPAP. Neonates with untreated congenital diaphragmatic hernia should not be treated with CPAP. One study raised the possibility of bronchiolitis being a contraindication for CPAP.[7]

Weaning from CPAP. As soon as the patient begins to show signs of clinical improvement, the FiO_2 is decreased in 0.05 decrements until the FiO_2 reaches 0.40 to 0.60. At that point, the CPAP is lowered in decrements of 2 cm H_2O, as tolerated and as indicated by the blood gas status. Continuous monitoring of blood gases with a transcutaneous monitor and/or a pulse oximeter is recommended during the weaning phase. CPAP is lowered until it reaches 2 to 3 cm H_2O, at which point the CPAP device is removed and the patient placed in an oxyhood at the preexisting FiO_2, which is then weaned as tolerated.

PRESSURE SUPPORT VENTILATION (PSV)

PSV is a mode of ventilation that supplements each patient effort with a clinician-selected pressure. PSV is indicated for any patient in whom a greater tidal volume (5–8 ml/kg) and decreased spontaneous ventilatory rate are desired during spontaneous breaths in the SIMV or CPAP modes. It is also used to overcome the resistance of the airways and ventilator circuit, or may be used to deliver a specified tidal volume (i.e., 10 ml/kg for FVS). Tidal volume is proportional to the PSV level and compliance, but inversely proportional to resistance.

BiPAP[TM] is the same as PSV with PEEP. It was popularized for patients with hypoventilation syndromes. Ventilators that incorporate this mode have settings for inspiratory positive airway pressure (IPAP) and expiratory positive airway pressure (EPAP). The pressure difference between EPAP and IPAP determines tidal volume. Breaths may be flow or pressure triggered, or the mode control may be set so time-triggered breaths can be delivered for patients with central apnea disorders.

A modification of PSV found on the Siemens Servo 300 ventilator, volume support (VS), is "compliance-sensitive." In VS, the user selects a tidal volume and the ventilator delivers successively higher pressures until the inspiratory tidal volume sensing mechanism senses the delivery of the desired tidal volume.[8] In the event of a decrease in compliance or increase in resistance, the ventilator automatically increases the PSV pressure until the desired tidal volume is restored. The ventilator automatically and continuously makes these adjustments. Waveforms are the same as in PSV. The correlate mode for patients who need time-triggered mandatory breaths is pressure-regulated volume control (PRVC).[9]

Hazards of PSV. It is important to realize that in PSV, there are no mandatory breaths, so the patient must have a reliable ventilatory pattern. If the patient becomes apneic, the ventilator must provide an alarm and/or may switch automatically to a mode of ventilation that provides mandatory breaths.

PSV Waveforms. Once a patient makes an inspiratory effort, the ventilator inflates the lungs until the pressure reaches the user-specified PSV level and holds it there until the gas flow tapers to approximately 25% of the peak flow, owing to the patient's airway resistance. PSV breaths are pressure controlled, flow, pressure, or volume triggered (not time triggered, except in the case of PRVC), flow limited, and flow or time cycled. The baseline variable is pressure, because PSV may be used with PEEP (Figures 15–3 A and B).

Weaning from PSV. To wean the patient from pressure support, the support pressure is gradually decreased, while ensuring that tidal volume is being maintained without an increase in ventilatory rate. Once the PSV level is 5 cm H_2O and the mandatory rate is discontinued, the patient should be assessed for extubation.

INTERMITTENT MANDATORY VENTILATION (IMV)

IMV is a mode of ventilation that provides mandatory breaths (a clinician-specified rate), which allows the patient to breathe spontaneously during the periods between mandatory breaths. The rate of mandatory breaths can be adjusted from 1 to 150 breaths/minute on several of the neonatal ventilators, so the time available for spontaneous breathing can vary widely, depending on the patient's ventilatory status. For IMV to be referred to as a mode of PVS, the mandatory rate must be low (<30 breaths/minute in the neonate) to allow for

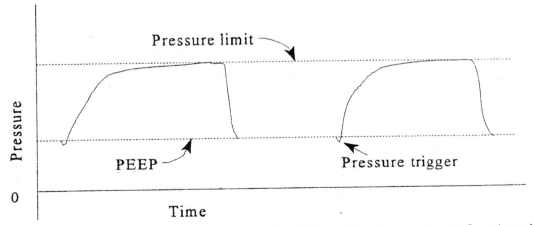

Figure 15–3a *Pressure waveform of pressure-support ventilation. All breaths are pressure or flow triggered from the baseline, which is often elevated, pressure limited, and flow cycled. Tidal volume depends on set pressure, resistance, and compliance.*

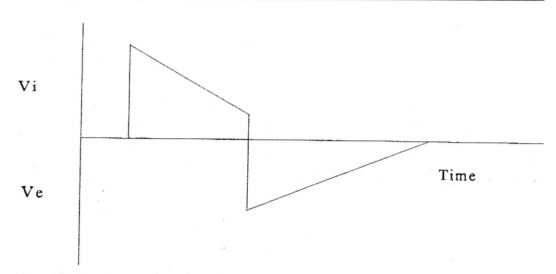

Figure 15–3b *Flow waveform of pressure-support ventilation. Inspiratory flow is above the baseline. Flow begins to taper in response to the patient's compliance and resistance. Inspiration ends at approximately 25% of peak flow. Vi = inspiratory flow; Ve = expiratory flow.*

effective spontaneous ventilation. The spontaneous breaths that occur during IMV are best described as CPAP breaths because the baseline pressure is nearly always above ambient. Neonatal ventilators provide a continuous flow of mixed gas from which the infant breathes spontaneously.

To initiate the IMV mode, the therapist need only turn the mode knob from CPAP to IMV/CPAP, which then powers the drive mechanism (see Chapter 16) to begin delivering mandatory breaths.

IMV is indicated when CPAP proves ineffective, or in any instance of hypercapnic ventilatory failure. Signs of the failure of CPAP include progressive hypoxemia, apnea, increased retractions, worsening tachypnea, tachycardia or bradycardia, and cyanosis. If the $PaCO_2$ rises above 60 mm Hg and pH decreases below 7.25, the patient's ventilatory demand has outpaced their ventilatory capacity and hypercapnic respiratory failure is evident. The set IMV rate depends on the patient's carbon dioxide production. The greater the carbon dioxide produced, the greater the $PaCO_2$, which means that to normalize the $PaCO_2$, the IMV rate will need to be increased. As the IMV rate is increased, this mode is more appropriately classified as a mode of full ventilatory support. There is no arbitrary mandatory rate at which FVS is commenced; however, it is usually begun at 30 to 40 breaths/minute. If the infant appears to have little or no ventilatory effort while being mechanically ventilated, FVS is assumed.

IMV Waveforms. Because IMV combines two breath types, each has its own classification characteristics. The mandatory breaths are pressure controlled, time triggered, pressure limited, and time cycled. The baseline variable is pressure. The spontaneous breaths are classified as described above in CPAP. The pressure waveform for IMV is shown in Figure 15–4.

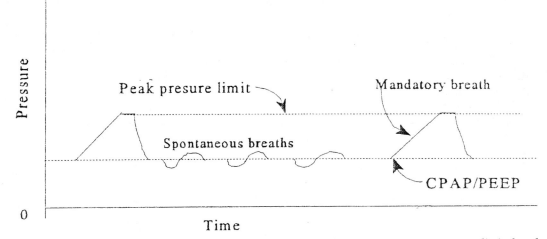

Figure 15–4 *Pressure waveform of IMV/CPAP. Mandatory breaths are time triggered, pressure limited, and time cycled. Spontaneous breaths are pressure triggered, limited, and cycled.*

Hazards of IMV. Because IMV increases the mean airway pressure more than CPAP, the hazards previously described may become more evident as peak, plateau, and mean airway pressures increase. A more complete discussion of the hazards of ventilation follows. Only that extent of peak pressure necessary to observe adequate chest expansion and auscult adequate breath sounds should be used. Otherwise, barotrauma and a decrease in cardiac output may occur.

Contraindications to IMV. IMV is only contraindicated when it is not necessary. If the infant is maintaining adequate blood gases and a ventilatory pattern within normal limits, IMV is unnecessary.

SYNCHRONIZED INTERMITTENT MANDATORY VENTILATION (SIMV)

SIMV differs from IMV in that in SIMV, the mandatory breaths are synchronized with the patient's inspiratory effort. In IMV, the ventilator delivers the mandatory breaths arbitrarily, according to the set total cycle time. In SIMV, the ventilator imposes a flexible "window" of time during which patient effort may trigger a mandatory breath. If the mandatory breath is not patient triggered, the window closes, and a time-triggered mandatory breath is given to maintain the mandatory rate. Ventilators that provide SIMV allow patient triggering by pressure, flow, or volume, which opens a demand valve to provide the volume for the patient's spontaneous breathing. SIMV has two advantages over IMV. First, breath stacking is avoided. Breath stacking occurs when the ventilator gives a mandatory breath arbitrarily during a patient's spontaneous breath, leading to discomfort, excessive tidal volume, and possibly, barotrauma. Second, because the patient breathes from the ventilator's demand flow system in SIMV, monitoring is considerably easier and more accurate because a continuous flow is unnecessary.

SIMV has been used as both a weaning mode and for continuous ventilation. The difference is in whether or not weaning is implemented and the magnitude of the mandatory rate. SIMV used for FVS will have a mandatory rate high enough so the patient has very little opportunity to take a spontaneous breath without causing iatrogenic hyperventilation, unless that is desired, as in closed head injury.

Because there are several breath types during SIMV, each breath type is individually classified. Mandatory breaths may be volume or pressure controlled. Volume-controlled breaths are usually time, pressure, or flow triggered. They are flow limited and time cycled, and the baseline is pressure. Pressure-controlled breaths are time, pressure, or flow triggered. Most of the newer neonatal ventilators provide a volume- or flow-triggering mechanism to provide SIMV as well as pressure-, volume-, or flow-triggered continuous mandatory ventilation (see below and Chapter 16). They are pressure limited and flow or time cycled, and the baseline is pressure. Spontaneous breaths are as described above in CPAP or PSV (Figure 15–5).

FULL VENTILATORY SUPPORT

Modes of *full ventilatory support* provide all of the required minute ventilation. They include synchronized intermittent mandatory ventilation (SIMV) at normal rates and continuous mandatory ventilation (CMV).

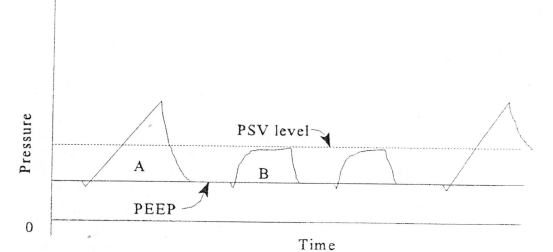

Figure 15–5 *Pressure waveform of SIMV-PSV. Breath A is a synchronized, pressure-triggered mandatory breath. Breath B is a pressure-triggered, pressure-supported breath.*

CONTINUOUS MANDATORY VENTILATION

Continuous mandatory ventilation (CMV) is indicated when all of the minute ventilation must be supplied by mandatory breaths. Each breath, regardless of trigger variable, has the same tidal volume or peak pressure. Time-triggered CMV is applied to patients who have been paralyzed traumatically or pharmacologically. Pressure- or flow-triggered CMV may be used to rest the muscles of ventilation in those patients who have muscle fatigue. The mode once known as assist/control is now classified as time- and pressure-triggered CMV. It is less commonly applied now than in past decades, with the advent of newer modes (i.e., SIMV-PSV) for patients who are able to partially support ventilation.

Breaths during CMV may be pressure or volume controlled. Volume-controlled breaths (VC-CMV) may be time, pressure, or flow triggered, flow limited, and time cycled. The clinician sets the mandatory rate and tidal volume (Figure 15–6).

Pressure-controlled breaths (pressure-controlled ventilation, PCV, PC-CMV) may be time, pressure, or flow triggered, pressure limited, and flow or time cycled. The clinician sets the mandatory rate and peak pressure.

Indications for PCV. PCV is indicated for patients (children and adults) with acute respiratory distress syndrome (ARDS) that results in a plateau pressure $\geq$35 cm H_2O or a peak pressure $\geq$40 cm H_2O while on volume ventilation. Sedation and paralysis may be indicated if the patient is unable to tolerate this ventilatory pattern.

PRESSURE-CONTROLLED INVERSE RATIO VENTILATION

CMV is usually administered with an inspiratory-to-expiratory time ratio less than 1:2 (1:3–1:4). A variation of CMV wherein I:E ratio is adjusted to $\geq$1:1 is inverse ratio ventilation (IRV). IRV may be pressure or volume controlled (PC-IRV or VC-IRV), and usually

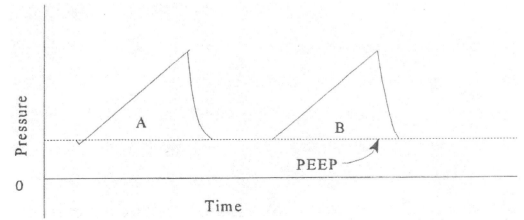

Figure 15–6 *Pressure waveform of continuous mandatory ventilation (CMV). Breath A is pressure triggered. Breath B is time triggered. Because these pressure waveforms are linear, it is implied that the flow waveform is square, so these breaths are flow limited.*

requires that the patient be sedated and pharmacologically paralyzed, because it is an uncomfortable ventilatory pattern. I:E ratio may be adjusted up to 4:1. IRV is indicated for those patients who fail to oxygenate despite high FiO_2 and PEEP. Patient management becomes more difficult in IRV because mean airway pressure rises precipitously. As mean airway pressure rises, there is a greater tendency for venous return, cardiac output, and blood pressure to decrease. IRV should not be used unless the patient care team is familiar with its use and the management of decreased cardiac output.

OTHER LESS COMMONLY USED MODES

Airway Pressure Release Ventilation (APRV). In this mode of ventilation, the patient is placed on a physiologic level of CPAP to restore his or her FRC. The patient is allowed to breathe spontaneously through the circuit. Ventilation occurs when the exhalation valve opens, allowing the pressure to fall to ambient, resulting in a patient exhalation. CPAP is restored the moment exhalation ceases. Mandatory breaths in APRV are pressure controlled, time triggered, pressure limited, and time cycled. Spontaneous breaths are pressure triggered, pressure limited, and pressure cycled. Breaths may be mandatory or spontaneous, depending on the patient's spontaneous effort.

Mandatory Minute Ventilation and Augmented Minute Ventilation. Both of these modes are similar in that they measure the patient's spontaneous breathing effort and provide assistance to the patient if he or she is unable to reach a predetermined minute volume. This is usually done by measuring the exhaled volume and comparing it to the desired minute volume. If the patient does not reach the desired volume, the machine provides assisted breaths, allowing the volume to be achieved. This mode is used mainly during weaning to prevent patient exhaustion during spontaneous breathing.

SETTING INITIAL VENTILATOR PARAMETERS

MODE

Once it is determined that the patient is in *respiratory failure*, the mode is often the first setting made on the ventilator. Remembering that the ventilator is a device that can supplement oxygenation and/or ventilation in parallel, modes can be selected that provide either or both, depending on the patient's needs. Modes that increase mean airway pressure (i.e., CPAP) are employed for hypoxemic respiratory failure. Modes that increase minute ventilation (i.e., SIMV, CMV) are employed for hypercapnic respiratory failure. On many newer ventilators, the mode setting guides the clinician to setting the other parameters. The clinician then determines the values for the parameters necessary to implement the chosen mode.

First, the choice is made between modes of partial versus full ventilatory support. If a patient is in hypoxemic respiratory failure, CPAP is usually the mode of choice. In this case, the patient relies on his own spontaneous ventilation to maintain the $PaCO_2$. When using CPAP, one sets the flow (on neonatal ventilators), FiO_2, and expiratory pressure (CPAP). If the patient is in hypercapnic respiratory failure, IMV, SIMV, or CMV is chosen to increase the patient's minute ventilation. This requires setting a sensitivity, flow, mandatory/set rate, and tidal volume/inspiratory time. An FiO_2 and end-expiratory pressure are chosen to maintain an adequate PaO_2. In combined respiratory failure, IMV or SIMV with CPAP/ PEEP or CMV with PEEP is chosen to support both ventilation and oxygenation.

Neonates who are in hypoxemic respiratory failure yet breathe spontaneously are first supported with continuous positive airway pressure (CPAP), described below. Should work of breathing increase and blood gases demonstrate hypercapnic respiratory failure as well, pressure-controlled ventilation in the form of intermittent mandatory ventilation is initiated to accompany the previously established CPAP. A decision tree representing guidelines for modes of ventilation for neonates is presented in Figure 15–7.

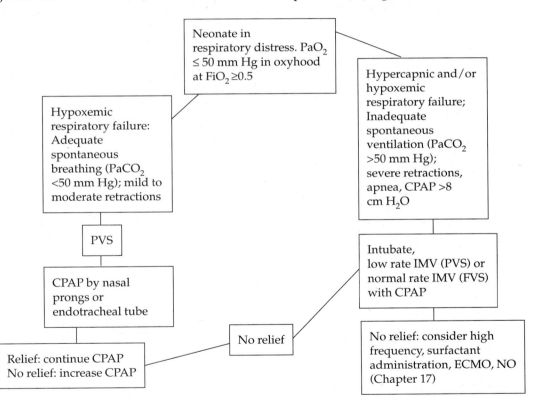

Figure 15–7 *Decision tree for modes of ventilation in neonates. After classifying the type of respiratory failure, partial versus full ventilatory support is chosen. In hypoxemic respiratory failure, CPAP is initiated and continued, provided that the PaO_2 normalizes.. If the PaO_2 remains inadequate, IMV at a low (PVS) or normal (FVS) rate may be necessary with additional CPAP to provide oxygenation and ventilation. If the PaO_2 remains low, more aggressive therapy may be required.*

Pediatric patients are usually ventilated similar to that of adults, with a lower tidal volume and higher ventilatory rate. A decision tree of guidelines for establishing ventilation for children is illustrated in Figure 15–8. These are only guidelines. The modes and techniques used will vary with severity of illness and the experience of the care team.

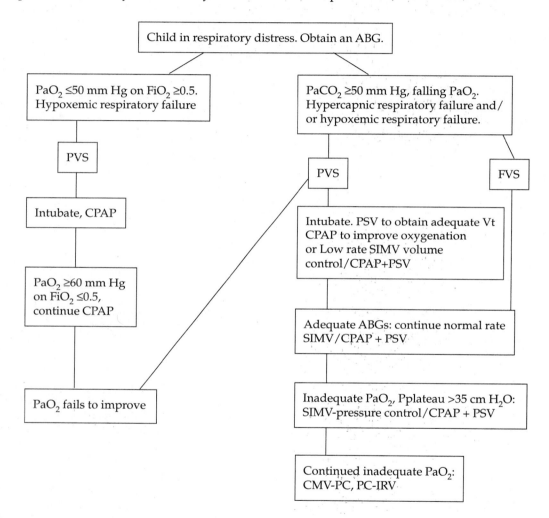

Figure 15–8 *Decision tree for initial mode of ventilation in children. After classifying the type of respiratory failure, partial versus full ventilatory support is chosen. In hypoxemic respiratory failure, the child is intubated and CPAP is initiated and continued, provided that the PaO$_2$ normalizes.. If the PaO$_2$ remains inadequate, SIMV may be necessary with additional CPAP to provide oxygenation. If hypercapnic respiratory failure is present, SIMV is necessary in either full or partial ventilatory support as dictated by the PaCO$_2$ and the child's response to the initial mechanical minute ventilation. If PaO$_2$ remains low and pressure is high, pressure-controlled ventilation is initiated. IRV is necessary only if PaO$_2$ remains low despite optimal PEEP and a high FiO$_2$.*

PEAK INSPIRATORY PRESSURE

In pressure-controlled ventilation (PC-IMV/SIMV, PC-CMV), the peak pressure is preset by the clinician. The inspiratory pressure is limited by a pop-off valve or by limiting the pressure applied to the expiratory valve and allowing excess pressure to vent through the expiratory side of the ventilator circuit. This pressure limit does not stop inspiration; it limits the inspiratory pressure. Once the inspiratory pressure limit is reached, flow is vented out of the pop-off valve or out the expiratory valve and flow to the patient ceases. The result is an inspiratory hold, where the volume in the lungs remains static until expiration occurs. This inspiratory hold promotes distribution of ventilation and increases mean airway pressure.

To set the PIP for a neonate, PIP is usually maintained at the pressure used during resuscitation, 15 to 20 cm H_2O.[10] The PIP is then changed slowly, if needed, until there is appropriate bilateral chest expansion, bilateral aeration on auscultation, and an adequate arterial $PaCO_2$.

For children, peak inspiratory pressure for PC-SIMV or PC-CMV is generally set to obtain a plateau pressure of ≥ 35 cm H_2O. This should result in a tidal volume of 8 to 10 ml/kg.

SET RATE

The initial ventilator rate for neonates is determined based on the ventilatory rate used during resuscitation to maintain the $PaCO_2$ within normal limits. It is usually set at 30 to 40 breaths per minute, but may need to be increased to as much as 150 breaths/minute in the presence of severe lung disease. In the event blood gases do not improve at this rate, high frequency jet ventilation or high frequency oscillation are considered. Rate may be decreased as the neonate's spontaneous effort increases. Neonates with RDS have been shown to tolerate high set rates without developing hyperinflation.[11]

The initial ventilatory rate for children is set in combination with an adequate tidal volume or pressure to achieve a $PaCO_2$ between 40 and 48 mm Hg in children with normal lungs.[12]

ALTERING RATE

Neonatal ventilators utilize either a rate or expiratory time control to set the IMV rate. When the determined time for exhalation has ended, the timing mechanism of the rate knob or the expiratory timer signals the closure of the expiratory valve. This occurs mechanically with a solenoid valve or a flow of gas, which pushes against a rubber diaphragm and seals off the expiratory side of the circuit. Other ventilators compress a diaphragm against an orifice at the end of the circuit, which occludes the end of the expiratory side of the circuit. With the occlusion of the expiratory side of the circuit, the continuous flow of gas increases pressure within the circuit and flow is diverted into the endotracheal tube and the patient's lungs. In most aspects the rate control and expiratory timer are similar, but one important difference bears discussion.

An expiratory timer determines a set expiratory time that remains fixed. Both inspiratory time and expiratory time must be set by the operator with appropriate I:E ratios in mind. When an expiratory timer is used, changes in inspiratory time changes the rate of ventilation because the total cycle time changes as well.

A rate control, on the other hand, automatically changes the expiratory time to maintain the desired rate, despite changes in inspiratory time. Figure 15–9 demonstrates this concept.

For example, if an expiratory time of 1.0 second was set using an expiratory timer, with an inspiratory time of 0.5 second, the resultant rate would be 40 breaths/min. This is determined by adding inspiratory and expiratory times and dividing into 60 (1.0 + 0.5 = 1.5 sec; 60/1.5 sec = 40 breaths/min). If inspiratory time is changed to 0.75 second, without changing the expiratory time, the rate would decrease to 34 breaths/min (1.0 + 0.5 = 1.75 sec; 60/1.75 sec = 34.3 breaths/min). A rate control, in the second scenario, would automatically decrease expiratory time to 0.75 second to maintain the set rate of 40 breaths/minute.

SENSITIVITY

The ventilator must be set to be sensitive to the patient's spontaneous inspiratory efforts. This is the trigger variable, which may be set to a pressure, flow, or volume. In pressure triggering, the sensitivity is set to –1 to –2 cm H_2O. In flow triggering the sensitivity is set to 0.15 to 1 L/minute. In volume triggering, the sensitivity is set to up to 3.0 ml. The sensitivity method is dependent on the ventilator being used (Chapter 16). Regardless, the sensitivity must not be set such that the ventilator triggers without patient effort. Nor should the sensitivity be set such that the patient who is making inspiratory efforts cannot trigger the ventilator. This artificially increases the work of breathing, and may lead to respiratory muscle fatigue and failure.

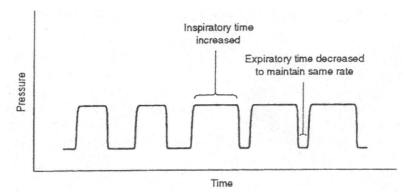

Figure 15–9 *The expiratory time is automatically adjusted by the rate timer whenever inspiratory time is changed. This results in the rate being maintained at the same level.*

POSITIVE END-EXPIRATORY PRESSURE (PEEP) OR CPAP

The PEEP is initiated at between 3 and 5 cm H_2O. PEEP is varied as needed to achieve optimal oxygenation and maintenance of FRC. Management of PEEP to obtain optimal oxygenation is described below.

FRACTION OF INSPIRED OXYGEN (FIO$_2$)

The required FiO_2 is determined during the resuscitation, as the amount needed to keep the baby pink. If a transcutaneous monitor or pulse oximeter is in place, FiO_2 is varied to keep the PaO_2 and SpO_2 within normal limits. In children, the FiO_2 is set depending on the pre-ventilation arterial blood gases. In the event the child is cyanotic, has cardiovascular instability, or is severely hypoxemic, an FiO_2 of 1.0 is set. Otherwise, an FiO_2 that maintains the PaO_2 greater than 60 mm Hg or SpO_2 greater than 90% is set.

INSPIRATORY FLOW

The initial flow on a neonatal ventilator is usually set at 6 to 8 L/min. The flow is then adjusted as needed for each patient. Excessive flow creates unnecessary turbulent flow that increases airway resistance. Inadequate flow will not provide adequate lung inflation in the short time allowed for inspiration.

The flow for a child is set to maintain an I:E ratio of 1:2 to 1:4. For the child who is triggering the ventilator, flow must be set to match the child's inspiratory effort. Otherwise, an increased work of breathing results. A flow of 25 to 30 L/min should deliver the set tidal volume within the recommended 1.0 to 1.5 second inspiratory time.

INSPIRATORY TIME

For neonatal ventilation, the inspiratory time is determined by an inspiratory time control and is set by the operator. The inspiratory time control begins timing the breath at the instant the expiratory time control signals the closure of the expiration valve. When the pre-determined inspiratory time has elapsed, the inspiratory time control opens the expiration valve and exhalation occurs passively from the patient's lungs.

The inspiratory time must be set to consider the desired set rate, the maintenance of a desired inspiration-to-expiration ratio (I:E), and lung condition. In RDS, the lungs are non-compliant. Therefore, a longer inspiration time may be needed to inflate the lungs. Expiratory time constants are decreased, and less time is needed for expiration. In diseases that are characterized by air trapping, expiratory time constants are longer, and therefore less time is needed for inspiration.

The inspiratory time for ventilation of children is often the result of the desired tidal volume and inspiratory flow, and should result in an I:E ratio that comfortably meets the patient's inspiratory needs. For example, if the child's tidal volume is 0.35 L and the inspiratory flow is set to 25 L/min, the inspiratory time is 0.83 second (Vt/flow = Ti; 0.35 L/0.42 L/sec =.83 sec). The extent to which the patient is comfortable with this flow is determined by noting a constant increase in pressure during inspiration, and by asking if the patient is comfortable.

I:E RATIO

The I:E ratio is not ordinarily set, but rather is derived once a pattern of ventilation is established. Once the I:E ratio is derived, it may be changed by manipulation of any of its components. Calculation of the I:E ratio is shown in Table 15–3.

Close attention to I:E ratio is required as the rate is increased. At the maximum rate of 150 breaths/minute, the inspiratory time would have to be decreased to 0.2 second to allow a 1:1 ratio (60 sec/150 breaths/min = 0.4 sec; 0.4 sec/2 = 0.2 sec inspiratory time). In diseases with a severe reduction in compliance, 0.2 second may be enough time for expiration, but in the presence of normal compliance or air trapping, 0.2 second would not allow adequate time for exhalation.

The proper setting of rate (or expiratory time) and inspiratory time requires not only an understanding of proper I:E ratios, but also an in-depth understanding of the disease process that is being treated.

TIDAL VOLUME

When ventilating neonates with pressure-controlled ventilation, the tidal volume is the result of the change in airway pressure between the peak and end-expiratory pressures, the lung-chest wall compliance, and the airway resistance. The desired tidal volume varies by birth weight from the very low birth weight infant at 4 to 6 ml/kg, to the term infant at 8 to 10 ml/kg.

Table 15–3   Calculation of the I:E Ratio

What is the I:E ratio, given the following data?
f = 50 breaths/minute, Ti = 0.4 seconds

1. Determine total cycle time.
   60/f = 60 sec/50 breaths/sec = 1.2 sec/breath
2. Determine the Te by subtracting the Ti from the TCT.
   Te = TCT − Ti
   Te = 1.2 − 0.4 = 0.8 sec
3. Determine the expiratory fraction of the I:E by dividing the expiratory time by the inspiratory time.
   Te/Ti = expiratory portion
   0.8/0.4 = 2
4. The I:E ratio is the ratio of 1 to the expiratory fraction.
   I:E ratio = 1:2

Children are usually volume ventilated. Tidal volume for children should be initially set to 8 to 10 ml/kg.

In recent years, ventilators have become more flexible in their tidal volume delivery (i.e., Siemens Servo 300), so that they can be used for neonates, children, and adults by alerting the ventilator's software to the range of patient size being ventilated. The term "seamless" is used to describe this flexibility. Once this is accomplished, the ventilator may be adjusted to meet the needs of the patient, rather than having to switch ventilators. The ventilatory needs of the pediatric patient—decreased lung compliance, small tidal volumes, high respiratory rates, high airway resistance requiring low flow rates, small dead space volumes, and the need for low compressible volumes in the ventilator circuit—are easily accommodated by the newer ventilators.

Suggested initial ventilator parameter settings are summarized in Table 15–4.

VOLUME VERSUS PRESSURE-CONTROLLED VENTILATION

Pressure-limited, time-cycled ventilation is the primary method of ventilating neonates. When using this method, the peak pressure is set so that it is achieved before the inspiratory time has elapsed. This traditional method has been effective for years, with excellent results, so there has not been a major concern about tidal volumes in neonates. Newer neonatal ventilators monitor the breath-to-breath tidal volume and minute ventilation so practitioners can affect tidal volume, if desired, to keep it within the recommended ranges for a given patient size. Mandatory breaths remain time cycled and pressure limited, but when changes are made to obtain a range of exhaled tidal volumes, those breaths become "volume targeted." While we continue to pressure ventilate, we are concurrently observing and making adjustments to target a range of tidal volume, as suggested in Table 15–4.

Table 15–4   Initial Ventilatory Parameters

Neonates		Children
PIP	15 to 20 cm H_2O	Keep Pplat <35 cm H2O
PEEP	3 to 5 cm H_2O	5 cm H_2O
FiO_2	Set to keep patient pink, or SpO_2 90–92%	1.0 or to maintain SpO_2 >93%
Rate	30–40 breaths/min	To maintain $PaCO_2$ 40–48 mm Hg
Flow	6–8 L/min	25–30 L/minute
Inspiratory time low birth weight infants 0.25–0.5 second term infants 0.5–0.6 second		1.0–1.5 seconds
I:E ratio 1:1.5–1:2		>1:2; maintain patient comfort
V_T Term 8–10 ml/kg Low birth weight 6–8 ml/kg Very low birth weight 4–6 ml/kg		8–10 ml/kg

Children who weigh less than 10 kg are usually ventilated as described above. Once a child's weight exceeds 10 kg, volume or pressure control is chosen, depending on lung condition. In children with normal lungs (i.e., postoperative ventilation, neuromuscular disease), volume-controlled ventilation with a tidal volume of 8 to 10 ml/kg and a rate to achieve a $PaCO_2$ within normal limits is instituted. However, in children with noncompliant lungs, pressure-controlled ventilation is instituted, as it is in adults with acute respiratory distress syndrome. The advantages and disadvantages of volume and pressure ventilation are outlined in Table 15–5.

ACHIEVING VOLUME TARGETED VENTILATION WITH A PRESSURE-CONTROLLED VENTILATOR

The easiest method to achieve volume-targeted ventilation with a pressure-controlled ventilator is to change the peak pressure limit until the desired range of tidal or minute volume is achieved. If the target ventilation cannot be achieved by increasing the peak pressure, the inspiratory time or inspiratory flow may also need to be increased.

Another method of volume targeting involves increasing the peak pressure limit above that which can be reached during the set inspiratory time. Then, tidal volume can be increased by increasing the inspiratory time or flow. Tidal volume may be decreased by decreasing the inspiratory time or flow. Care must be taken to ensure that the I:E ratio does not exceed normal limits. Tidal volume then becomes the product of inspiratory time and inspiratory flow, as shown in Table 15–6.

RECOGNIZING A DECREASED COMPLIANCE OR INCREASED RESISTANCE

Signs of a decrease in compliance include an increase in auscultated crackles, a decrease in chest wall excursion, a decreased slope of the pressure-volume loop and a decrease in mon-

Table 15–5   Advantages and Disadvantages of Volume and Pressure Controlled Ventilation in the Neonatal and Pediatric Population

| Volume-controlled ventilation | | Pressure-controlled ventilation | |
Advantages	Disadvantages	Advantages	Disadvantages
Delivers a set tidal volume despite changes in compliance or resistance. Consistent minute ventilation. Better control of $PaCO_2$.	Potential for volutrauma. Leaking around cuffless endotracheal tubes. High mean airway pressure.	Lower mean airway pressure Avoids volutrauma.	Inconsistent minute ventilation. Changes in tidal volume with changes in compliance and resistance.

Table 15–6 Calculating Tidal Volume Using a Pressure-Controlled Ventilator

---

Infant weighs 2.3 kg and is being ventilated at 20 cm H_2O above PEEP of 5 cm H_2O (PIP = 25 cm H_2O). Are the inspiratory flow and time appropriate for delivery of a 6 to 8 ml/kg V_T?

Tidal volume is calculated by multiplying the inspiratory time by the flow rate as follows:
  Inspiratory time = 0.4 second
  Flow rate = 6 L/min (flow must be converted to ml)
  6 L/min = 6000 ml/min or 100 ml/sec
  Tidal volume = 0.4 sec × 100 ml/sec = 40 ml

Volume lost due to tubing compliance:
  Pressure = 20 cm H_2O × tubing compliance of 1.5 ml/cm H_2O = 30 ml lost volume
  Measured V_T is 40 ml –30 ml lost volume = 10 ml
  Desired V_T is 16 ml; if flow is increased to 7 L/min (117 ml/min), delivered V_T should be 46.8 ml; subtracting 30 ml lost volume = 16.8 ml (7.3 ml/kg), which is within the desired range.

---

itored tidal volume. An increase in airway resistance is indicated by an increase in secretions and the presence of wheezing. The practitioner may need to make appropriate changes to the ventilator (i.e., increase the peak pressure) while investigating and correcting the causes of decreased compliance or increased resistance.

INITIATION OF PRESSURE-CONTROLLED VENTILATION

Initial parameters are usually set according to the disease process and clinical evaluation of the patient who weighs less than 10 kg and who is ventilated with pressure-limited, time-cycled ventilator. Peak inspiratory pressure is set to that which obtains good chest excursion and good lung aeration as heard on auscultation.

The mandatory rate is set considering the time constants present in the lung. Noncompliant lungs and those in which resistance is low have a shorter *time constant* than do lungs with normal compliance and can therefore sustain shorter expiratory times and faster rates. In contrast, compliant lungs and those with increased resistance have longer time constants and require longer expiratory times and slower rates. The inspiratory time is set to maintain an I:E ratio of 1:2 with the selected frequency. Flow should be set to allow the peak inspiratory pressure to be reached before the end of inspiratory time.

INITIATION OF VOLUME-CONTROLLED VENTILATION

Under most circumstances, pediatric patients should be ventilated at a tidal volume of 8 to 10 ml/kg. It is also necessary to use a noncompliant circuit when using volume-controlled breaths on pediatric patients to minimize volume loss due to tubing compliance.

The compliance of the ventilator circuit can be calculated and used to determine the actual delivered tidal volume. Tubing compliance is calculated by delivering a known volume (usually less than 300 ml) into the circuit with the patient connection occluded. The pressure generated is measured from the manometer and is divided into the volume, resulting in the compliance of the circuit. The set tidal volume can be set to deliver the desired tidal volume and the additional tubing loss volume in order to ventilate the patient with the proper volume. The method of calculating corrected tidal volume is shown in Table 15–7.

CHANGING VENTILATOR PARAMETERS IN VOLUME AND PRESSURE VENTILATION

When making changes on the ventilator, one must remember how each parameter affects the blood gas values. Ventilation, reflected by the $PaCO_2$, is affected by changes in the minute ventilation; that is, the ventilatory rate × tidal volume. The tidal volume in pressure-controlled ventilation is determined by the difference in pressure between the PIP and PEEP (the ΔP), resistance, and compliance. $PaCO_2$ is also affected by inspiratory time, because the longer the alveoli are inflated, the more diffusion takes place between the blood and alveoli.

PaO_2 is a function of the FiO_2 and the end expiratory pressure. It is also affected by the mean airway pressure. Calculation of the mean airway pressure was discussed in Chapter 14. The end-expiratory pressure is the most important parameter determining mean airway pressure, because the relationship between mean airway pressure and end-expiratory pressure is 1:1.

CHANGING $PaCO_2$

The $PaCO_2$ is changed by manipulating the ΔP or set rate. Once the PIP is set, as described above, it is usually held constant, unless the patient's compliance or resistance changes. In the event of a decrease in compliance or increase in resistance, PIP may need to be increased

---

Table 15–7   Determination of Corrected Tidal Volume

A patient weighing 35 pounds is to be mechanically ventilated.

Step 1:   Determine the weight in kg:
 35 lb/2.23 lb/kg = 15.69 kg. This will be rounded to 17 kg.
Step 2:   Determine the desired tidal volume by multiplying the patient's weight in kg by 9.0 ml/kg:
 17 kg × 9.0 = 153 ml desired tidal volume
Step 3:   Determine volume loss due to tubing compliance:
 (PIP − PEEP) × circuit compliance = volume lost due to tubing compliance
   (23 cm H_2O − 5 cm H_2O) × 2 ml/cm H_2O = 36 ml
Step 4:   Determine actual tidal volume:
 set V_T − lost volume = actual V_T
 150 ml − 36 ml = 116 ml (6.8 ml/Kg)
Step 5:   Increase the set V_T by the valve of the lost volume to arrive at the corrected tidal volume.
 150 ml + 40 ml = 190 ml (11.1 ml/kg)

The addition of tidal volume may increase the PIP and therefore compressible volume, which may necessitate a further increase in tidal volume.

---

in 2 cm H_2O increments to maintain tidal volume and good breath sounds. In the event that compliance increases or resistance decreases, PIP may need to be decreased to avoid overdistension and baro/volutrauma. If the clinician is satisfied with the PIP but the $PaCO_2$ is high, the set rate is increased, usually in increments of 2 to 5 breaths/minute until a satisfactory $PaCO_2$ is obtained. Likewise, if the $PaCO_2$ is low, the rate may be decreased until a satisfactory $PaCO_2$ is obtained. Flow also affects $PaCO_2$. Because pressure-controlled ventilation in neonates is time cycled, the tidal volume is determined by the product of the inspiratory time and the inspiratory flow. Should the pressure limit be reached before the end of the inspiratory time, flow will continue to be delivered until the end of the inspiratory time, thus affecting tidal volume. Pressure or flow waveform graphics may assist the clinician in determining the presence of this phenomenon.[13] Should the inspiratory time be too long, it may be decreased so as to limit the duration of a plateau pressure (which also increases the mean airway pressure). In RDS accompanied by high peak or plateau pressures, it may be desirable to allow the $PaCO_2$ to rise above 50 mm Hg, as long as the pH does not decrease below 7.25. This technique, permissive hypercapnia, allows a reduction in tidal volume, and assists in avoiding baro/volutrauma.

In summary, the set rate is the primary parameter used to alter the minute ventilation, and therefore, $PaCO_2$. Other parameters to consider are PIP, flow, and inspiratory time.

In volume-controlled ventilation, $PaCO_2$ is also affected by minute ventilation. The tidal volume (or inspiratory time) is set directly and peak pressure is a function of resistance and compliance. As previously mentioned, the tidal volume is set in the 8 to 10 ml/kg range for children. Once that is established, it is not usually changed. A factor that may influence the need to increase tidal volume would be persistent atelectasis or air hunger, despite an optimally adjusted sensitivity and flow. The major factor that would contribute to the need to decrease tidal volume would be the desire to institute permissive hypercapnia in ARDS.

Once the clinician is satisfied with the tidal volume, the remaining factor determining minute ventilation and therefore $PaCO_2$ is the mandatory rate, which is increased if the $PaCO_2$ rises and decreased if $PaCO_2$ is low. Rate is usually changed in 1 to 3 breaths/minute increments. The higher the rate is, the greater the increment. For example, if the rate is set at 20 breaths/minute, effecting a 20% change in minute ventilation would require a change of 4 breaths/minute. If the rate is set at 8 breaths/minute, effecting a 20% change in minute ventilation would require a change of 1 to 2 breaths/minute.

An additional factor affecting minute ventilation is the extent of spontaneous minute ventilation during CPAP or PSV breaths. If the tidal volume during CPAP (without PSV) are ≥5 ml/kg, then this fraction of the minute ventilation is contributing to a normal $PaCO_2$. If these tidal volumes are less than 5 ml/kg, this fraction of the minute ventilation is contributing to dead space, and the $PaCO_2$ may increase. It is for this reason that PSV is useful. Initiation of 5 to 8 cm H_2O PSV will usually increase the spontaneous tidal volume to ≥5 ml/kg and decrease the spontaneous ventilatory rate, both contributing to normalizing the $PaCO_2$.

CHANGING PaO_2

The PaO_2 is changed by manipulating the FiO_2, end-expiratory pressure (PEEP/CPAP), and subsequently, the mean airway pressure. The decision to use the FiO_2 or the end-expiratory pressure depends on the cause of hypoxemia. In case of V/Q inequality (pneumonia, bronchiolitis), hypoxemia generally responds to an increase in FiO_2.

In the case of capillary shunting (RDS, ARDS), the PaO_2 responds to an increase in end-expiratory pressure, not an increase in PaO_2. This is referred to as refractory hypoxemia. In refractory hypoxemia, alveoli are collapsed, fluid-filled, or smaller than normal, resulting in a decrease in alveolar surface area and functional residual capacity. Therefore, an increase in FiO_2 alone will have little effect on the PaO_2.

An increase in PEEP is usually indicated if the PaO_2 is inadequate despite a PEEP of 3 to 5 cm H_2O and FiO_2 of ≥ 0.5. PEEP may be increased in 2 to 3 cm H_2O increments until the PaO_2 increases. This indicates alveolar surface area recruitment and restoration of the functional residual capacity.

In neonates, a PEEP of 12 to 15 cm H_2O is rarely exceeded. There are two reasons for this. One is that, owing to the cuffless endotracheal tube, additional PEEP would be lost. Second is the decrease in cardiac output and pulmonary barotrauma that may occur as a result of high PEEP. If a PEEP of 12 to 15 cm H_2O fails to provide adequate oxygenation, high-frequency ventilation, nitric oxide, or extracorporeal membrane oxygenation are considered, as appropriate for the etiology of hypoxemia.

Excessive PEEP is also avoided in children for the same reasons. Higher PEEP may be used in children who have a cuffed artificial airway. The highest PEEP that should be used is referred to as optimum PEEP. This is defined as the PEEP that results in a PaO_2 greater than 60 mm Hg that does not result in cardiac output depression. Some method of cardiac output measurement, such as thermal dilution or a continuous cardiac output pulmonary artery catheter, is necessary when using this method. Another method of obtaining the best PEEP level is to measure the static lung-thorax compliance (static compliance, lung-thorax compliance = exhaled tidal volume/Pplateau-PEEP) at the initial PEEP level. The Pplateau is the end-inspiratory pause pressure. The PEEP is increased in 3 to 5 cm H_2O increments. After each increase in PEEP, the lung-thorax compliance is calculated. The best PEEP is that pressure where lung-thorax compliance is greatest. If PEEP is adjusted above this level, intrathoracic pressure increases, lung-thorax compliance will decrease, cardiac output may decrease, and the child will be susceptible to other forms of barotrauma.

Under most circumstances, hypoxemia will respond to less than 10 cm H_2O of PEEP, at which time the FiO_2 may be decreased slowly in decrements of 0.05 to 0.3–0.4. Weaning of PEEP may occur when the FiO_2 has been decreased to a safe value and the patient is hemodynamically stable. PEEP is decreased 2 to 3 cm H_2O, no more than every 6 hours. After a decrease in PEEP, the PaO_2, SaO_2, or SpO_2 are observed for acute deterioration. If the saturation decreases below 90% or PaO_2 decreases below 60 mm Hg, the previous PEEP level should be restored and the patient monitored for acceptable oxygenation.

Mean airway pressure is increased by increasing PEEP, PIP, set rate, or inspiratory time, or by decreasing expiratory time (increasing the I:E ratio). Changing the mean airway pressure other than by increasing PEEP is considered a secondary method of changing the PaO_2. It is the mechanism whereby PaO_2 is improved when using inverse ratio ventilation.

In extreme cases, where an FiO_2 of 1.0 is insufficient to maintain oxygenation, several alternatives may improve the oxygenation status. The hypoxemia may be due to blood shunting away from the lungs through the PDA. In this case, a decrease in the MAP by lowering the PIP, PEEP, rate, or inspiratory time may allow more blood to perfuse the lungs by lowering the pulmonary vascular hypertension and thus increase oxygenation.

VENTILATOR CHANGES USING CLINICAL INFORMATION

The practitioner may rely on the patient's clinical signs to make appropriate ventilator changes. The adequacy of minute ventilation is best determined by auscultation of breath sounds and the observance of chest excursion. With each mandatory breath, there should be air movement heard in both lung fields, indicating sufficient aeration. In addition, the chest should rise and expand with each mandatory breath. The determination of suitable chest excursion is subjective and changes from patient to patient. The size of the patient and the nature of the lung disease alter the amount of chest excursion. In most circumstances, however, a rise in the chest during inspiration is a sign of adequate lung expansion.

Changes in lung mechanics may be estimated by auscultating changes in the breath sounds and observing chest excursion. In the presence of worsening compliance, breath sounds diminish, fine crackles may be auscultated, and chest excursion may decrease. The slope of the pressure-volume loop may decrease. An increased resistance may be noted by the observation or auscultation of secretions in the airway and/or the auscultation of wheezing. An increase in airway resistance will also increase the PIP. Once the cause is determined, therapeutic measures are implemented. In the meantime, minute ventilation or FiO_2 may need to be increased until the problems are reversed.

In contrast, an improvement in breath sounds and chest excursion from baseline indicates an improvement in compliance or resistance. In this example, tidal volume or rate can be weaned to avoid hyperventilation and barotrauma.

HAZARDS OF MECHANICAL VENTILATION AND HOW TO AVOID THEM

The hazards of mechanical ventilation (Table 15–8) can be categorized into the various parameters that constitute total ventilation. The hazards are basically the same for neonates and children, with exceptions noted as needed.

HAZARDS OF OXYGEN, CPAP, AND PEEP

Hazards of high oxygen concentrations include oxygen toxicity (one factor in the development of bronchopulmonary dysplasia, BPD) and possible absorption atelectasis. Oxygen toxicity may enhance the appearance of hyaline membranes and cause or worsen ARDS in the pediatric patient, making the lung less compliant. Retinopathy of prematurity (ROP) is caused by an excessive PaO_2. Only that FiO_2 necessary to maintain a PaO_2 within normal limits for a given patient is appropriate. An $FiO_2 \geq 0.5$ is hazardous, and every effort must be made to decrease it, including the application of PEEP/CPAP and increased mean airway pressure (i.e,. inverse ratio ventilation). Misapplied levels of CPAP and PEEP can lead to hypoventilation with resulting respiratory acidosis, decreased cardiac output from a decreased venous return, and air leak syndromes (pneumothorax, pneumomediastinum, pneumopericardium). PEEP/CPAP is increased until the FiO_2 can be decreased to less than 0.5, contingent on a stable cardiovascular status (normal cardiac output, SvO_2).

Table 15–8 Hazards of Mechanical Ventilation

Oxygen

Oxygen toxicity
Hyaline membrane formation
BPD
ROP

PEEP and CPAP

Excessive pressures
    a. Hypoventilation from excessive FRC
    b. Decreased cardiac output
    c. Barotrauma

Peak Inspiratory Pressure

Barotrauma
    a. Pneumothorax
    b. Pneumomediastinum
    c. Pneumopericardium
    d. Pulmonary interstitial emphysema
BPD
Hyperinflation
    a. Hyperventilation
    b. Respiratory alkalosis
    c. Hemodynamic depression

Respiratory Rate

Respiratory alkalosis
Air leaks
Decreased ventilation-to-perfusion ratios
Increased intrapleural pressure
Decreased pulmonary perfusion
Diminished cardiac output

General Hazards

Infection

Hypoxic-Ischemic Injuries

Intracranial hemorrhage in the neonate
Gastric distention
Complications of endotracheal intubation

HAZARDS OF PEAK INSPIRATORY PRESSURE (PIP)

Complications of excessive PIP include barotrauma leading to air leak syndromes and BPD, and respiratory alkalosis from alveolar hyperventilation. In the pediatric patient, PIP is the direct result of the tidal volume and lung compliance, with higher volumes and stiffer lungs causing higher pressures to be generated. The transmission of PIP to the surrounding vasculature varies depending on the disease state. In the normally compliant lung there is a maximal transmission of pressures to the environment; therefore, the degree of hemodynamic depression is directly related to the level of PIP and PEEP. Lungs with decreased compliance, as in ARDS, allow for a lesser transmission of pressures, and so the effect on the hemodynamics is not as great until higher pressures are reached.

In pressure-controlled ventilation, PIP should be set such that plateau pressure does not exceed 35 cm H_2O. For neonates, PIP is increased only to the point where there are adequate breath sounds and chest excursion. In volume ventilation, tidal volume should not exceed 10 ml/kg. In ARDS, tidal volume should not exceed 6 to 8 ml/kg. Should PIP exceed 40 cm H_2O, pressure ventilation should be instituted.

HAZARDS OF FREQUENCY/I:E

Respiratory alkalosis is a possible hazard of an unnecessarily high rate or short expiratory time. Inappropriately high I:E ratios lead to air leaks from air trapping, decreased ventilation-to-perfusion ratios, increased intrapleural pressure leading to decreased pulmonary perfusion, and diminished cardiac output.

The mandatory rate should be maintained to keep the $PaCO_2$ within normal limits. I:E should be maintained at less than 1:2 to allow for sufficient expiratory time.

GENERAL HAZARDS

General hazards of mechanical ventilation include infection, hypoxic-ischemic injuries, intracranial hemorrhage in the neonate, gastric distention, and complications of endotracheal intubation.

Infection is avoided by careful attention to standard precautions and changing of ventilator circuits no more than every 48 hours. Hypoxic injuries may be avoided by ensuring oxygenation during suctioning. Gastric distention is avoided by placing a gastric tube. The hazards of endotracheal intubation are avoided by paying careful attention to technique during intubation, insertion of the proper size endotracheal tube, and properly securing it once in place.

WEANING AND EXTUBATION

Appropriate management of the patient-ventilator system usually results in a patient who is ready to be removed from ventilation and ready to be extubated. The goal of removing the patient from ventilatory support should have been in place since the time of intubation and commitment to the ventilator. Weaning or gradual withdrawal of ventilatory support should, therefore, have been in progress since the initiation of support. This section defines weaning as the final process of discontinuing the ventilator and removal of the artificial airway.

When making the decision whether to wean and extubate, two factors must be considered: 1) the ability of the patient to spontaneously maintain adequate gas exchange; and 2) the ability of the patient to maintain the airway and clear secretions. Each of these factors must be approached separately and decisions involving weaning and extubation must be made with these factors in mind.

The success of weaning and extubation depends on many elements. Foremost is that there has been significant progress toward the resolution of the original disease or condition that required mechanical ventilation in the first place. Perhaps the most difficult element is customizing the weaning process on each individual patient. This means that the patient must be closely monitored, and adjustments made as the patient's condition dictates. Too often, we follow a rigid set of guidelines that may not suit a particular patient.

In the older child, it may be necessary to psychologically prepare the patient for weaning and extubation. Following a prolonged time on mechanical ventilation (usually months), the patient may have become both physiologically and psychologically dependent on the ventilator. Failure to realize these important aspects will result in failure and the necessity of prolonged ventilation.

NEONATAL PATIENT

Upon stabilization and improvement of the infant's condition, the ventilator parameters are slowly weaned to allow the neonate to assume responsibility for ventilation.

CLINICAL INDICATIONS FOR WEANING

Signs that the neonate is ready to be weaned include blood gas values within normal limits, the presence of adequate spontaneous respirations, and increased muscle tone and activity that allow weaning of the FiO_2.

WEANING VENTILATOR PARAMETERS

The decision as to which parameter to wean is based on the patient's condition and the level of support provided by each parameter. The FiO_2 should be weaned to ≤0.4 in 0.2 to 0.5 increments before starting to wean other parameters. The purpose of weaning is lost if high FiO_2 is needed to provide adequate oxygenation ($PtcO_2$ 60–80 mm Hg or SpO_2 90–92% on FiO_2 ≤0.4) as PIP and rate are lowered. Once the FiO_2 is ≤0.4, PEEP is decreased in 1 to 2 cm H_2O increments to 3 to 4 cm H_2O before considering extubation.

When adequate arterial oxygenation is ensured, PIP can then be slowly weaned, usually in increments of 1 to 2 cm H_2O to 15 to 18 cm H_2O.

Following reduction of PIP, rate can be lowered in increments of 1 to 5 to allow the patient to assume ventilation. On those patients who have required high set rates, rate may be decreased faster, as previously discussed.

Gas exchange, often by arterial blood gas analysis, must be monitored after each ventilator change to assess the response of the patient. Provided there is good correlation between ABGs and noninvasive monitors of gas exchange, the transcutaneous monitor and/or pulse oximeter make weaning a much easier process and greatly decrease the number of blood gas samples needed.

DURATION OF WEANING

The speed at which weaning takes place is dictated by patient response. Generally, the longer the patient has been on the ventilator, the slower will be the weaning. Careful attention to the speed of weaning will help prevent a *rebound effect*, which is a negative reaction to a weaned parameter that requires not only a reinstitution of the parameter but often reinstitution to a level higher than was set before the weaning.

The disease state also dictates the speed at which weaning takes place. In RDS, the lungs often begin stabilizing 48 to 72 hours after birth, resulting in improvement in lung compliance. In these patients, PIP, rate, and FiO_2 are weaned as tolerated to prevent barotrauma and effects of hyperoxia.

As lung compliance improves, the transmission of excessive pressure, and the depression of hemodynamics that follows, is averted by appropriate weaning of pressures.

Not all neonates respond to the weaning of parameters. Patients with BPD, PDA, and neurologic damage may require long periods of ventilatory support and do not respond well to weaning attempts. This is indicated by the dependence on any of the ventilatory parameters, with a rapid decline in blood gas levels when those parameters are weaned.

CLINICAL INDICATIONS OF A FAILURE TO WEAN

Tachycardia, bradycardia, *pallor*, retractions, hypercapnia, and cyanosis during weaning indicate a failure to wean. The ventilator parameters used before the weaning attempt should be restored and the cause of weaning failure investigated and treated.

EXTUBATION

When the PIP is weaned to 15 to 18 cm H_2O, the PEEP to 3 to 5 cm H_2O, the rate to less than 10, and an FiO_2 of 0.3 to 0.4, the patient can be extubated. Feedings should be withheld for several hours before extubation to reduce the risk of aspiration. Before extubation, tracheobronchial hygiene should be ensured to remove as much mucus as possible. A leak should be audible at the end of a mandatory breath to help assess the absence of airway edema. In the presence of edema (no leak), a racemic epinephrine aerosol is administered.

The patient is prepared to extubation by hyperoxygenating and then carefully removing the tape and holder that are securing the endotracheal tube. Following successful completion of the above preparations, the manual resuscitator is used to deliver several breaths. During one of these breaths, the endotracheal tube is withdrawn. Following removal of the endotracheal tube, oral secretions are removed using a suction device.

RESPIRATORY CARE FOLLOWING EXTUBATION

Following extubation, blood gas values and patient status are closely monitored to ensure safe adaptation off the ventilator. Oxygenation is maintained by the use of an oxyhood, nasal CPAP, or nasal cannula, as dictated by the PaO_2 or SpO_2. One recent study supported the use of nasopharyngeal SIMV postextubation in a sample of 22 very low birth weight infants.[14] The incidence of postextubation respiratory failure was significantly lower in the SIMV group than in the nasal CPAP group, thus preventing reintubation. Stridor caused by inflammation and edema from the endotracheal tube can be treated with nebulized racemic epinephrine. Chest physiotherapy is performed as indicated to assist with removal of secretions.

PEDIATRIC PATIENT

WEANING

As with the neonate, plans should be made for weaning and extubation as soon as the patient is placed on the ventilator. Weaning then begins when the patient has met the following criteria: 1) the disease process is stabilized and past the acute phase; 2) the cardiovascular system is stable; 3) gas exchange is stable without the need for high pressures or FiO_2; and 4) the patient is alert with minimal sedation.

Successful weaning requires good communication with and psychological preparation of the patient. The patient must understand what is happening and that he or she has the choice to rest when necessary. When it is determined that the patient is ready to be weaned, the FiO_2 is lowered to ≤ 0.4 and PEEP to ≤ 5 cm H_2O. The set rate is then weaned slowly to allow the patient to assume the work of breathing. Depending on the duration of mechanical ventilation, this may take a short or long period of time.

It is important to closely monitor the patient during weaning to ensure that the patient does not become anxious or exhausted. A patient who shows signs of tiring or anxiety should be rested on the ventilation by increasing the set rate for a period of time before resuming weaning.

FAILURE TO WEAN

Several cardiorespiratory problems contribute to a failure to wean. These factors and possible solutions are shown in Table 15–9.

Table 15–9   Factors Associated with Failure to Wean and Potential Solutions

Factor	Solutions
Increased work of breathing	Ensure appropriate PSV
	Increase artificial airway diameter
	Ensure optimal bronchodilation
	Tracheobronchial hygiene
	Ensure ventilator synchrony
Atelectasis/secretions	Ensure adequate hydration
	Tracheobronchial hygiene
	Chest physiotherapy
	Frequent position changes
Agitation/dyspnea	Reassure the patient
	Check ABGs for acute deterioration
	Antianxiety agents
	Relieve excessive work of breathing
Respiratory muscle weakness	Slow wean using PSV
	Check electrolytes
	Ensure optimal position
	Ensure proper nutrition
	Respiratory muscle rest on ventilator

The mandatory rate is decreased to 3 to 5 breaths/min. The PEEP is decreased to 3 to 5 cm H_2O during this time. PSV is decreased to 5 cm H_2O, or may be discontinued if the patient is able to completely support the tidal volume. At this point, the patient is placed on CPAP and observed to determine satisfactory aeration. An ABG is frequently obtained to determine tolerance of CPAP/PSV.

In a study of 213 children, ages 32 to 64 months, several respiratory variables were found to predict weaning success or failure. Table 15–10 lists these variables and the threshold values for low (<10%) and high (>25%) failure to remain extubated following a course of mechanical ventilation. Subjects in this study were ventilated from less than 3 days to in excess of 7 days.[15]

This study represents the scarce evidence in this area. Extubation failure was defined as the need to be reintubated within 48 hours of extubation. Several of the parameters that are useful in predicting successful extubation in adults such as ventilatory rate, maximum inspiratory pressure, the rapid-shallow breathing index, and the compliance-rate-oxygenation-pressure (CROP) index, were also examined and found to be not predictive in the pediatric population.

Several parameters were predictive of successful extubation. There was a low risk of extubation failure if the spontaneous tidal volume indexed for body weight (ml/kg) was ≥6.5 ml/kg., FiO_2 <0.30, mean airway pressure <5.0 cm H_2O, oxygen index (OI = mean airway pressure × (FiO_2/PaO_2) × 100) ≤1.4, fraction of minute ventilation by the ventilator (FrVe%) ≤20%, peak inspiratory pressure on the ventilator of ≤25 cm H_2O, dynamic compliance (Vt/PIP – PEEP) ≥0.9 ml/kg/cm H_2O, and mean inspiratory flow of ≥14 ml/kg/sec.

Table 15–10 Threshold Values for a Low (<10%) and a High (>25%) Failure of Extubation*

Variable	Low-risk value	Failure (%)	High-risk value	Failure (%)
V_{Tspont} (ml/kg)	≥6.5	9.9	≤3.5	25.9
FiO_2	≤0.30	8.1	>0.40	24.1
Mean Paw (cm H_2O)	< 5	6.7	>8.5	26.1
Oxygen Index	≤1.4	6.7	> 4.5	30.4
FrVe%	≤20	8.5	≥30	27.5
PIP (cm H_2O)	≤25	7.3	≥30	26.4
C_{dyn} (ml/kg/cm H_2O)	≥0.9	9.1	<0.4	25
V_T/Ti (ml/kg/sec)	≥14	9	≤8	27.2

V_{Tspont}, spontaneous tidal volume indexed to body weight; FrVe%, fraction of total minute ventilation provided by the ventilator; PIP, peak inspiratory pressure; C_{dyn}, dynamic compliance; V_T/Ti, mean spontaneous inspiratory flow. (From: Kahn N, Brown A, Venkataraman ST. Predictors of extubation success and failure in mechanically ventilated infants and children. *Crit Care Med.* 1996;24:1576.) *All values were measured just before extubation and were on or off the ventilator as appropriate.

Because these parameters are easily measured at the bedside, practitioners using these data may be more confident of a successful extubation in children.

EXTUBATION

Once it is concluded that the patient may be ready for extubation, a leak test is performed. The oral pharynx is suctioned and the endotracheal tube cuff is deflated. The presence and quantity of a leak past the cuff is assessed during a mandatory breath. If there is no leak, laryngeal edema is assumed. This must be treated with racemic epinephrine and/or intravenous steroids before extubation is attempted. Otherwise, the airway may close following extubation, precipitating respiratory failure and reintubation, which may be traumatic. Extubation is only performed if a leak is present.

The patient is prepared for extubation by first hyperoxygenating and then thoroughly suctioning the endotracheal tube, followed by reoxygenation. The tape or other securing device is loosened from the face and tube. If present, the endotracheal cuff is deflated in preparation for removing the tube. The patient is given a positive pressure breath with a manual resuscitator, and at peak pressure the tube is removed from the trachea.

Following extubation, oxygen is administered to maintain SpO_2 greater than 92%. The patient is observed closely for signs of edema or subglottic stenosis. Aerosolized racemic epinephrine or dexamethasone may be given as needed to reduce postextubation edema. Incentive spirometry is often done following extubation to prevent atelectasis.

SUMMARY

This chapter discusses the use of conventional modes of ventilation of the neonate and child. It begins with a discussion of the forms of ventilatory failure (hypoxemic, hypercapnic, and mixed) and examples of each. Modes of ventilation are discussed as they are classified into either partial or full ventilatory support. Partial ventilatory support occurs when the patient is responsible for all or part of his or her minute ventilation. Full ventilatory support occurs when the ventilator is responsible for all of the minute ventilation. The use of full versus partial ventilatory support is based on the patient's physiologic status and ability to support his or her own minute ventilation. The rationale for these modes is discussed and each mode is graphically depicted. The concepts of control, phase, and conditional variables are discussed.

Once the decision is made to utilize full or partial ventilatory support, and a particular mode is chosen, initial values for the parameters of ventilation are selected. These parameters include peak inspiratory pressure, tidal volume, set rate, sensitivity, PEEP, FiO_2, inspiratory flow, inspiratory time, and I:E ratio. The need to set any of these parameters rests with which mode of ventilation has been selected. Once the patient has been established on mechanical ventilation, decisions are made about how to vary the parameter values to accomplish the goals of ventilation—adequate ventilation and oxygenation. Usually, this is done by obtaining and analyzing arterial blood gases and by clinical observation of the patient's synchrony with and toleration of ventilation. Changes in oxygenation and ventilation are accomplished by manipulating the controls of the ventilator until adequate arterial blood gases are achieved and there is patient-ventilator synchrony. Once the original indication for mechanical ventilation has been treated, consideration of how to liberate or wean the patient is made. The fraction of minute ventilation supplied by the ventilator and the FiO_2 and PEEP are decreased. The spontaneous parameters of ventilation and oxygenation as they pertain to neonates and children are discussed, as are the considerations involved in the extubation and postextubation therapy of these patients.

Bibliography and Suggested Readings

1. Partridge JC, Wall SN. Analgesia for dying infants whose life support is withdrawn or withheld. *Pediatrics* 1997;99(1):76–79.

2. Partridge JC, Wall SN. Death in the intensive care nursery: physician practice of withdrawing and withholding life support. *Pediatrics* 1997, 99(1):64–70.

3. Chatburn RL. Classification of mechanical ventilators. *Respiratory Care* 1992;37:1026–1044.

4. Tapia JL. et al. Does continuous positive airway pressure (CPAP) during weaning from intermittent mandatory ventilation in very low birthweight infants have risks or benefits? *Ped Pulmon* 1995;19:269.

5. American Association for Respiratory Care. Application of continuous positive airway pressure (CPAP) to neonates via nasal prongs or nasopharyngeal tube. *Respir Care* 1994; 39(8):817–23.

6. Loftus BC, et. al. Neonatal nasal deformities secondary to nasal continuous positive airway pressure. *Laryngoscope* 1994;104(8pt1):1019–22.

7. Smith PG, El-Khatib MF, Carlo WA. PEEP does not improve pulmonary mechanics in infants with bronchiolitis. *Am Rev Respir Dis* 1993;147:1295–98.

8. Siemens-Elema Life Support Division. *Servo ventilator 300 operating manual*, v 7.1. Art. No. 6027416E313E. 1994:84–85.

9. Siemens-Elema Life Support Division. *Servo ventilator 300 operating manual*, v 7.1. Art. No. 6027416E313E. 1994:82–83.

10. Bloom RS, Cropley C. *Textbook of neonatal resuscitation*. Dallas. American Heart Association/American Academy of Pediatrics, 1994.

11. Kano S. et. al. Fast versus slow ventilation for neonates. *Am Rev Respir Dis* 1993;148:578.

12. Wilson BG. Mechanical ventilation of the infant and child. In: Aloan CA, and Hill TV, eds.. *Respiratory care of the newborn and child*, 2nd ed. Philadelphia, Lippincott, 1997:327.

13. Waugh JB, Deshpande VM, Harwood RJ. *Rapid interpretation of ventilator waveforms*. Upper Saddle River New Jersey, Prentiss Hall, 1999:97.

14. Freidlich P, Lecart C, Posen R, Ramicone E, Chan L, Ramanathan R. A randomized trial of nasopharyngeal-synchronized intermittent mandatory ventilation versus nasopharyngeal continuous positive airway pressure in very low birth weight infants after extubation. *J Perinatol* 1999;19(6 pt 1):413–418.

15. Kahn N, Brown A, Venkataraman ST. Predictors of extubation success and failure in mechanically ventilated infants and children. *Crit Care Med* 1996;24(9):1568–1579.

Posttest

1. CPAP increases FRC by:
   a. physically holding the alveoli open during exhalation
   b. increasing inspiratory time and decreasing expiratory time
   c. reducing time constants
   d. increasing PaO_2 and decreasing $PacO_2$
2. Of the following, which is the most common device used to apply CPAP to the neonate?
   a. headbox
   b. face chamber
   c. nasal mask
   d. nasal prongs
3. Which of the following would indicate a failure of CPAP?
   I. PaO_2 less than 50 mm Hg with an FiO_2 of 0.80 to 1.0 and CPAP of 10 to 12 cm H_2O
   II. $PaCO_2$ greater than 55 mm Hg
   III. marked retractions
   IV. frequent apnea spells
   V. reduced FiO_2 needs
       a. I, II, V
       b. II, III, IV
       c. I, III, IV
       d. I, II, III

4. Determination of adequate levels of PIP is initially determined by:
   a. chest excursion, breath sounds, and PaO_2
   b. patient weight and gestational age
   c. FiO_2 requirements
   d. flow and inspiratory time to be used

5. Changing which of the following ventilator parameters would *not* alter minute ventilation?
   a. PIP
   b. expiratory time
   c. rate
   d. PEEP

6. Which of the following parameters has the greatest influence on mean airway pressure?
   a. PIP
   b. PEEP
   c. flow rate
   d. inspiratory time

7. The respiratory care practitioner receives blood gas results on a ventilated infant. The $PaCO_2$ is 48 mm Hg and previously it was 43 mm Hg. A proper ventilator change would be:
   a. decrease the rate by 5 BPM and the PIP by 3 cm H_2O
   b. increase the rate by 5 BPM or the PIP by 2 cm H_2O
   c. increase the inspiratory time and flow
   d. decrease the flow rate and the FiO_2

8. The main advantage in using volume-cycled ventilation with neonates is:
   a. reduced barotrauma
   b. improvement in lung compliance
   c. reduction in airway resistance
   d. delivery of a consistent tidal volume

9. A 6-year-old female patient weighing 40 pounds is being ventilated at a tidal volume of 280 ml and a rate of 20 breaths/min. The PIP is 38 cm H_2O with a PEEP of 4 cm H_2O. The compliance of the circuit tubing is measured at 2.5 ml/cm H_2O. Which of the following accurately describes this patient's corrected tidal volume?
   a. 9.5 ml/kg
   b. 10.8 ml/kg
   c. 12 ml/kg
   d. 13.4 ml/kg

10. Which of the following modes of ventilation should not be used on a spontaneously breathing patient?
    a. IMV
    b. APRV
    c. Inverse ratio ventilation
    d. SIMV

11. Which of the following is not considered a hazard of mechanical ventilation?
    a. barotrauma
    b. infection
    c. intracranial hemorrhage
    d. diaphragmatic paralysis

12. The first parameter weaned from a mechanically ventilated infant should be:
    a. FiO_2
    b. rate
    c. PIP
    d. flow

13. Which of the following are clinical signs of a failure to wean?
    I. increased chest excursion
    II. bradycardia
    III. retractions
    IV. tachycardia
    V. pallor
       a. I, III, IV
       b. II, III, IV, V
       c. III, IV, V
       d. I, III, V

14. Which of the following are predictive of a low risk of the need for reintubation in the pediatric patient?
    I. spontaneous tidal volume of 3.2 ml/kg
    II. FiO_2 of 0.45
    III. mean airway pressure of 4.0 cm H_2O
    IV. PIP of 20 cm H_2O
    V. V_T/Ti of 16 ml/kg/sec
       a. I, II, III only
       b. II, III, IV only
       c. III, IV, V only
       d. I, III, V only

15. What arterial blood gas change is most likely to be observed when the mean airway pressure is increased?
    a. increased PaO_2
    b. increased $PaCO_2$
    c. decreased $PaCO_2$
    d. decreased PaO_2

16. What mode of ventilation should be instituted if the physician requests an increase in the spontaneous tidal volume during SIMV?
    a. APRV
    b. MMV
    c. PSV
    d. IRV

17. The respiratory therapist observes a PaO_2 of 52 mm Hg on an infant despite nasal CPAP of 8 cm H_2O and 60% oxygen. What is the therapist's most appropriate action?
    a. increase the CPAP pressure to 12 cm H_2O
    b. increase the FiO_2 to 0.8
    c. intubation and ventilation in the IMV/CPAP mode
    d. replace the CPAP with an oxyhood at an FiO_2 of 0.8
18. What is the most accurate classification of neonatal mechanical ventilation?
    a. volume controlled, flow limited, time cycled
    b. pressure controlled, pressure limited, flow cycled
    c. volume controlled, flow limited, volume cycled
    d. pressure controlled, pressure limited, time cycled
19. How is hypercapnic respiratory failure identified?
    a. a decreased pH
    b. an increased $PaCO_2$
    c. a decreased PaO_2
    d. a decreased bicarbonate
20. How is tidal volume increased during pressure-controlled ventilation?
    a. increase the PEEP
    b. increase the ΔP
    c. increase the PEEP and ΔP by the same value
    d. increase the expiratory time

CHAPTER SIXTEEN

COMMON VENTILATORS AND MONITORS

OBJECTIVES

Upon completion of this chapter, the reader should be able to:

1. Identify and discuss, for each of the following ventilators, the classification, control switches and timers, internal mechanisms, and features:
   a. Babybird
   b. Babybird 2
   c. V.I.P. BIRD/V.I.P. GOLD
   d. Bio-Med MVP-10
   e. BEAR Cub
   f. Hamilton Veolar
   g. Infant Star 500/950
   h. Newport Breeze
   i. Sechrist IV-100
   j. Sechrist IV-200 SAVI
   k. Siemens Servo 900C
   l. Siemens Servo 300/300A
2. Calculate FiO_2 and flow rate when given the necessary information and data.
3. Describe the features and uses of the following ventilator monitors:
   a. BEAR NVM-1
   b. Partner volume monitor
   c. Sechrist airway pressure monitors, Models 400 and 600

KEY TERMS

analog
anemometer
assist/control
automode
bias flow

CPAP
cycle
demand flow
duration of positive
   pressure

flow transducer
fluidic
LED
limited parameter
linear drive

microprocessor	pressure regulated	sine wave
minute ventilation	volume control	termination sensitivity
MMV	pressure support	transducer
peak flow	PSIG	volume assured pressure
pneumatic	rise time	support
pressure control	sensitivity	volume support
	SIMV	

COMMON NEONATAL VENTILATORS

INTRODUCTION

All ventilators, whether designed for use on adults or neonates, are classified following designated criteria. The classification criteria that we will use for each ventilator are: 1) what powers and controls the ventilator, that is, electrical, pneumatic, or a combination; 2) what initiates a mechanical breath; 3) what ends the inspiration, also known as the cycling mechanism, that is, pressure cycled, volume cycled, time cycled; and 4) what pressures and flows are available during the expiratory phase, that is, PEEP. Our goal, then, is to classify common neonatal ventilators and examine their characteristics, options, and unique features.

Because most neonatal ventilators are classified as time cycled and pressure limited, we will only mention classification as it deals with initiation of the breath and expiration characteristics.

BABYBIRD VENTILATOR

Basic Mechanisms. The Babybird ventilator, shown in Figure 16–1, is pneumatically powered and controlled by a 50 psi gas source. Because it does not have a built-in oxygen blender, the powering gas source must come through a blender, which is then attached to the inlet on the top of the ventilator.

The Babybird ventilator has the option of controlled IMV breaths or spontaneous breathing, which is selected by turning a rotary switch on the face of the ventilator. When spontaneous breathing is selected, the blended gas is diverted in a continuous flow into the ventilator circuit, allowing the patient to draw a spontaneous breath from the circuit.

When IMV ventilation is selected, the flow of gas is diverted into a device known as the Bird Mark 2, illustrated in Figure 16–2. The Bird Mark 2 is a combination of two spring-loaded valves that oppose each other in a small cylindrical housing. As gas flow is diverted into the expiratory chamber of the Mark 2, the increasing pressure opens the spring valve and allows flow to be diverted into the second chamber, the inspiratory chamber, and also to the expiratory valve. As pressure builds in the second chamber, the inspiratory chamber valve opens. Opening this valve allows the expiratory side to vent, closing the expiratory valve and starting the cycle again.

Thus, by altering the flow into the two chambers by the inspiratory and expiratory time

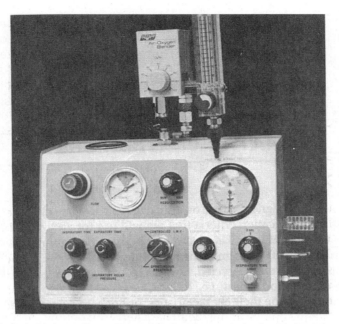

Figure 16–1 *The Babybird ventilator. (Reproduced with permission by Bird Products Corporation, Palm Springs, CA)*

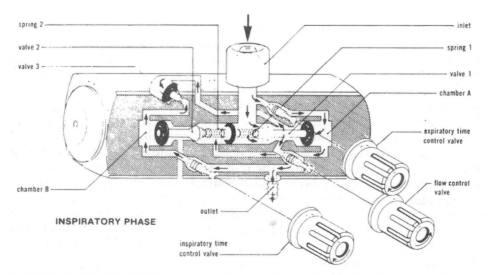

Figure 16–2 *The Bird Mark 2. (Reproduced with permission by Bird Products Corporation, Palm Springs, CA)*

controls, duration of inspiration and expiration are determined. Inspiration is initiated when the pressure in the Mark 2 valve triggers the inspiratory phase and is controlled by the expiratory time control.

Both inspiratory time and respiratory rate are set by independent inspiratory and expiratory timers on the face of the ventilator. The I:E ratio is a result of the settings on the two timers.

PIP is regulated by the inspiratory relief pressure control on the face of the ventilator. It controls the amount of gas that is allowed to push against the expiratory diaphragm. The more the gas flow, the higher the PIP that will develop. Pressure builds in the circuit until the pressure exerted on the expiratory diaphragm is exceeded, at which point excess pressure is vented to the atmosphere.

PEEP and CPAP are generated by turning a small red lever located on the expiratory valve assembly. Turning the lever left to right physically moves the exhalation port against the diaphragm. Exhalation gases must then build pressure in the circuit to open the expiratory valve, thus creating PEEP and CPAP.

Unique Features. The Babybird has several unique features. It utilizes a Bourdon gauge to measure flow rates, controlled by a flow regulator. Total flow to the patient is determined by setting the flow regulator to the desired flow indicated on the gauge.

The flow then passes the nebulization control. This valve determines whether a majority of the flow is directed to the nebulizer jet, if one is used, or if the majority of flow is diverted directly into the nebulizer. If a 500 cc nebulizer is used in place of a humidifier, then turning the control clockwise diverts a majority of the flow to the nebulizer jet, creating a high quantity of aerosol. Turned all of the way counterclockwise, most of the flow is diverted into the nebulizer and the amount of aerosol produced is low.

When a humidifier is used in place of the 500 cc nebulizer, both outputs are connected together and directed to the inlet of the humidifier. Regardless of where the flow is directed, total flow to the patient is determined by the flow regulator, not the nebulization control.

Another unique feature found on the Babybird is the expiratory flow gradient control. This control allows a flow of gas to be diverted to a venturi in the expiratory valve. As flow to this venturi is allowed, the negative pressure created draws the exhalation gases through the circuit, resulting in the removal of inadvertent PEEP. Care must be taken, however, to ensure that a negative pressure does not occur in the circuit, which may lead to massive atelectasis.

The inspiratory time limit control is another feature unique to the Babybird. This control sets a maximal inspiratory time limit that prevents a dangerously long inspiratory time from occurring. The operator sets the control by turning the control knob to the desired limit. The control has a 3-second setting, but otherwise is uncalibrated and can limit inspiration from 0 to infinity. If the inspiratory time exceeds the limit set by this control, the inspiration stops and a flow of gas is directed to a reed valve on the bottom of the ventilator, which whistles, indicating that the alarm has been violated. Inspiration will not commence again until the silver reset button is pushed.

The original Babybird circuits included a resuscitation bag, called the AIRbird, attached to the expiratory valve assembly. The concept is to enable the operator to ventilate the patient manually through the expiratory tubing.

BABYBIRD 2 AND 2A

Basic Mechanisms. The Babybird 2 (Figure 16–3) and 2A, are pneumatically powered and electronically controlled. Mechanical breaths are initiated by the electronic closure of a solenoid valve, which, when closed, diverts gas flow through the right output of a fluidic flip-flop valve to the inspiratory pressure control and then to the expiratory diaphragm, closing the exhalation valve.

The rate of ventilation is determined by a frequency control on the front of the ventilator. The frequency control is simply an electric timer that signals the solenoid valve to close. It allows a frequency of 0 to 150, with rates above 75 requiring the frequency multiplier to be in the x2 position.

Expiration begins when another electric timer, the inspiratory time control, opens the solenoid valve. The inspiratory time is set between 0.1 and 3 seconds by the operator. During expiration, when the solenoid valve is open, gas flow is directed through the left output of the flip-flop valve to the PEEP/CPAP control, then to the expiratory diaphragm, exerting a pressure against the exhalation valve and generating the PEEP or CPAP.

Unique Feature. The Babybird 2 and 2A ventilators have a relief pressure control that limits, as an alarm condition, how high the inspiratory pressures can reach. If the relief pressure is exceeded, inspiration is stopped and the patient overpressure alarm on the front of the ventilator is triggered. This alarm condition remains until the cause of the overpressure is relieved, and the relief pressure control is reset by pushing in the relief pressure control knob.

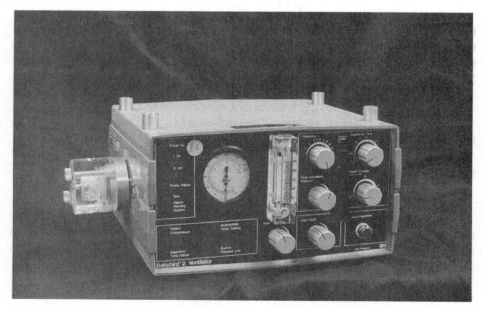

Figure 16–3 *The Babybird 2 ventilator. (Reproduced with permission by Bird Products Corporation, Palm Springs, CA)*

The ventilator incorporates other alarms that are somewhat unique to the ventilator. A loss of electrical power triggers the power failure alarm, which is both audio and visual. If the power fails, the alarm is corrected by depressing the failure warning system switch. Ventilation can then proceed using the manual inspiration button, which remains functional. In this circumstance, the relief pressure control is nonfunctional, and the potential for extreme inspiratory pressure requires close monitoring.

The audiovisual incompatible timer setting alarm is triggered any time the expiratory time is less than 0.2 second. When this alarm is violated, the ventilator immediately cycles into a 5-second expiration, and then begins mechanical breaths at 10 to 12 per minute.

If inspiratory times reaches 4.25 seconds, the inspiratory time failure alarm sounds and cycles the ventilator into expiration. The source pressure low alarm is activated when the gas entering the ventilator reaches 38 psi.

V.I.P. BIRD VENTILATOR

Basic Mechanisms. The V.I.P. BIRD ventilator is a new-generation ventilator marketed as a neonatal and pediatric ventilator with the capacity to treat newborn to 30-kg patients.

The V.I.P. ventilator (Figure 16–4) is microprocessor controlled and pneumatically powered. It can be set to deliver time-, pressure-, or volume-cycled, and pressure or flow limited breaths. With the addition of the Bird Partner monitor, flow triggering is also possible. The V.I.P. also offers pressure support ventilation.

Time Cycled. In the time-cycled mode, the operator has the option of (S)IMV, assist/control (optional), and CPAP. When in the time-cycled mode, the tidal volume, assist *sensitivity,* and pressure support controls are disabled. Inspiratory time is set with the inspiratory time control from 0.10 to 3.00 seconds. Breath rates from 0 to 150 BPM are available using the breath rate control.

When in the (S)IMV/CPAP mode, a continuous flow of 3 to 40 L/min is determined by the operator using the flow rate control. This continuous flow supports spontaneous breaths as well as delivered breaths. In the time-cycled mode, the assist sensitivity control is deactivated and is maintained at a factory preset level of –1 cm H_2O. If the patient draws in an inspiratory flow that causes pressure to drop 1 cm H_2O below the baseline pressure, a demand flow system augments the baseline flow up to 120 L/min depending on patient need. These augmented breaths are pressure triggered, limited, and cycled. When in the (S)IMV/CPAP mode, mechanical breaths are pressure controlled, flow triggered, pressure limited, and time cycled. In the assist/control mode, mechanical breaths are flow triggered (assuming the patient is breathing spontaneously), time triggered (in the absence of spontaneous breaths), pressure limited, and flow cycled.

The high-pressure limit control serves as the peak inspiratory pressure control in the time-cycled mode. When the selected PIP is reached, the exhalation valve opens and "servos" at this pressure until the inspiratory time is reached. It offers a range of 3 to 80 cm H_2O of PIP when time cycled.

PEEP and CPAP are established with the PEEP/CPAP control at levels ranging from 0 to 24 cm H_2O.

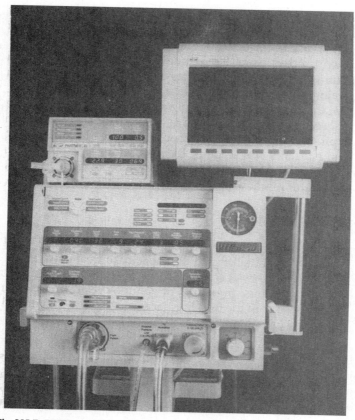

Figure 16–4 *The V.I.P. BIRD ventilator (Courtesy Bird Products Corportation, Palm Springs, CA)*

The ventilator provides a manual breath button, which is used to deliver a single, operator-initiated breath. In the time-cycled mode, the delivered breath is given at the preset inspiratory time, peak flow, and PIP levels. Manual breaths are available in both the IMV and CPAP modes but are ignored if the operator attempts to give a breath during the inspiratory phase of ventilator breath. If given during the expiratory phase, the ventilator delivers the breath at the end of a minimum time frame.

Volume Cycled. In the volume-cycled mode, the V.I.P. offers the choice of assist/control, SIMV, or CPAP. In the assist/control mode, the patient is delivered a breath with each spontaneous inspiratory effort, assuming the assist sensitivity control is properly set (see following). If the patient does not trigger an assisted breath, the ventilator delivers controlled breaths at the rate set by the operator on the breath rate control. SIMV allows spontaneous breathing by the patient with additional synchronized mandatory breaths delivered at the rate set on the rate control. Again, proper setting of the assist sensitivity control is vital to achieve synchronized breaths. The CPAP mode requires the breath rate control to be set to zero while the mode selection is in the SMIV/CPAP position.

The tidal volume control sets the volume of delivered ventilator breaths in the assist/control and SIMV modes. The tidal volume control terminates the inspiratory breath when the selected tidal volume has been reached. Tidal volumes of 20 to 760 ml are available for delivery.

The breath rate control offers 0 to 150 BPM in the volume-cycled mode.

When in the volume-cycled mode, the flow control is used to set the maximum flow delivered during mechanical breaths and the baseline flow delivered during the expiratory phase. Set flow is available from 3 to 100 L/min in the volume-cycled mode. The set flow rate does not affect the flow delivered during spontaneous or pressure supported breaths, which is available up to 120 L/min.

The high-pressure limit control serves as an alarm parameter in volume-cycled mode. The limit can be set from 3 to 120 cm H_2O. If the proximal pressure exceeds the set high-pressure limit, an audible alarm activates, the display flashes, flow ceases, and the ventilator enters the expiratory phase. This also occurs if the machine outlet pressure exceeds the alarm setting + 30 cm H_2O. If the pressure does not fail below the PEEP level + 3 cm H_2O within 3 seconds, the exhalation and safety valves are opened, allowing the patient to breathe room air. If the pressure does fall below the PEEP + 3 cm H_2O within 3 seconds, the ventilator resumes its normal operation.

The assist sensitivity control sets the amount of negative pressure that the patient must generate below the PEEP or CPAP level to trigger an assisted breath or to receive demand flow from the ventilator. Available settings are OFF and 1 to 20 cm H_2O.

Pressure support is available in the SIMV/CPAP mode and is used to set the pressure support level above PEEP/CPAP during spontaneous breaths. The pressure support breath is terminated when the flow rate decreases to 25% of the flow needed to achieve the support level. In the presence of a leak, the breath is terminated after 3 seconds or two breath periods, whichever comes first. The display flashes to alert the operator that the breath has been time limited.

The manual breath button delivers a single breath at the preset tidal volume when in the volume-cycled mode. The above-mentioned limitations apply to this mode as well.

Features. The V.I.P. ventilator contains a built-in monitoring package, which measures PIP, MAP, breath rate, inspiratory time, and I:E ratio.

The PIP is monitored from the proximal airway sensing line and measures the PIP of all breaths except spontaneous efforts without pressure support. The range is 0 to 120 cm H_2O.

MAP is measured and updated every 8 seconds. The measurement is based on a 40-second moving average and is displayed in all modes and breath types. The range for MAP is 0 to 80 cm H_2O.

The breath rate displays the average number of breaths per minute and includes all breaths detected by the ventilator. However, in the IMV/CPAP mode, only mandatory breaths are counted. The range is 0 to 150 BPM.

The inspiratory time monitor displays the operator defined inspiratory time. In volume cycle, the inspiratory time is defined by the set breath rate, tidal volume, and peak flow controls. In time cycle, inspiratory time is defined by the breath rate and inspiratory time controls. In the CPAP mode, the display exhibits three dashed lines. The range is 0.05 to 60 seconds.

All ventilators allow the patient to trigger a breath either by time, pressure, or flow. The V.I.P. is unique in that it allows the patient to trigger the end of inspiration. The feature *termination sensitivity* is another way of ending inspiration or triggering exhalation. Once the lungs become inflated with gas and inspiratory flow decreases, the breath is terminated. This point can be adjusted from 5% to 25% of peak inspiratory flow. For example, if we set a termination sensitivity of 5%, the breath will end or terminate when the inspiratory flow decreases 95%. Setting the termination sensitivity allows for total patient synchronization with the ventilator. However, the clinician must be careful to ensure that the set level of termination sensitivity ensures that the inspiratory time is adequate for the patient to maintain an optimal level of ventilation.

The I:E ratio monitor displays the ratio of inspiration to expiration with inspiratory time normalized to 1. It only measures ventilator breaths and exhibits three dashed lines in the CPAP mode. The I:E ratio is calculated as follows: I:E ratio = 1:(exhalation time/inspiratory time). If the I:E ratio becomes less than 1:1 (1:0.9 or less) the : on the display and the PE Ratio LED flash, alerting the operator of an inverse condition. The range is 1:0.1 to 1:60.

Additional features are a patient effort indicator and a demand indicator, which will be briefly discussed. The patient effort indicator lights when a spontaneous breath is detected that exceeds the assist sensitivity setting. In the assist/control and SIMV/CPAP modes, it indicates that a supported breath is being delivered. The demand indicator operates in the IMV/CPAP mode only and indicates that the demand system has been triggered by a spontaneous effort. The LED remains lit as long as the demand system is active.

The ventilator incorporates an overpressure relief control on the front of the ventilator. This safety valve opens at the set pressure and limits the amount of pressure that can build in the patient circuit, protecting the patient from excessive pressures.

Alarms. In addition to the previously mentioned high-pressure limit alarm, the V.I.P. ventilator has alarms for low peak pressure, low PEEP/CPAP, high/prolonged pressure, apnea, low inlet gas pressure, ventilator inoperative, and circuit fault. Each will be briefly examined.

The low peak pressure alarm is activated when the proximal pressure does not exceed the alarm setting during a mandatory breath. The range is 3 to 120 cm H_2O.

The low PEEP/CPAP alarm is activated when the proximal pressure falls below the alarm setting for more than 0.5 second during the ventilation cycle. The range is from –9 to 24 cm H_2O.

The high/prolonged pressure alarm is operative in both time-cycled and volume-cycled modes. In the time-cycled mode, the alarm is activated if the PIP exceeds the set level by 10 cm H_2) or more. As with the high-pressure limit control in the volume-cycled modes, the alarm causes the flow to cease, the expiratory and safety valves to open, and allows pressure to vent to ambient. If the pressure falls to a level of PEEP + 3 cm H_2O, the ventilator resets and resumes normal operation. In both time-cycled and volume-cycled modes, the alarm will activate if the proximal pressure exceeds PEEP + 6 cm H_2O for 250 msec, beginning 500 msec after the start of the expiratory phase. This function is an alarm only with no action taken by the ventilator.

The apnea alarm is activated whenever the interval between detected inspiratory efforts exceeds the set time interval. The alarm is inactivated in the IMV/CPAP mode. The range is 20, 40, and 60 seconds and is set internally.

The low inlet gas pressure alarm is activated whenever the system pressure falls below 22.5 PSIG (pounds per square inch gauge) or rises above 27.5 PSIG. If the pressure drops below 20 PSIG, or rises above 30 PSIG for more than 1 second, the ventilator enters an inoperative condition.

When activated, the ventilator inoperative alarm causes the ventilator to cease its normal function and allows the patient to breathe room air. Conditions that activate this alarm include power supply voltages that are out of range, system pressure fluctuations as mentioned above, and the detection by the software of an out-of-tolerance condition.

The circuit fault alarm alerts the clinician to a possible *transducer* or patient circuit malfunction. The ventilator compares the readings from the proximal and exhalation pressure transducers during inspiration and expiration, and the proximal and machine transducers during expiration. If the differences exceed the preset levels, the ventilator is forced into exhalation and the higher of the two pressures is fed to the exhalation valve to control the PEEP level. If the mismatch continues beyond 8 seconds, the flow ceases, the expiratory and safety valves open, and the patient is allowed to breathe room air. This alarm does not function during the inspiratory phase of a pressure-supported breath.

V.I.P. BIRD GOLD

The V.I.P. BIRD Gold ventilator is the next generation of the BIRD V.I.P. series of neonatal and pediatric ventilators.

In addition to those found on the V.I.P., the V.I.P. Gold offers several new features and new modes of ventilation, including *pressure support* in all (S)IMV/CPAP modes, *pressure control*, and *volume assured pressure support* (VAPS).

Pressure Support. When in the (S)IMV/CPAP mode (volume control, pressure control, TCPL, or VAPS), pressure support is available to augment all spontaneous respirations.

The range of pressure support is 1 to 50 cm H_2O above the PEEP/CPAP level, set using the pressure support control. Breaths may be either pressure or flow triggered. When a spontaneous breath is initiated, there is a rapid delivery of flow to achieve the preset level of pressure support. Flow is delivered using a decelerating waveform, with both flow rate and inspiratory time controlled by the patient. Pressure remains constant throughout the inspiratory phase. Termination sensitivity is automatically adjusted from 5% to 25%, depending on the internal measurement of tidal volume derived from the inspiratory time and flow—smaller tidal volumes at 5%, larger tidal volumes at 25%. In the event of a leak in the patient circuit, preventing the flow from decreasing to 25%, the breath will be terminated when the pressure support I-time limit has been reached. The pressure support I-time limit is set from 0.10 to 3.00 seconds.

Pressure Control. Pressure control is a time-cycled, pressure-limited mode of ventilation with a variable, decelerating flow delivery. It is the variable flow and termination sensitivity that distinguish pressure control from the time-cycled pressure-limited (TCPL) mode of ventilation on the V.I.P. Gold.

In pressure control, the operator has the option of (S)IMV/PS, assist/control, and CPAP. Tidal volume, flow, and termination sensitivity controls are disabled while in the pressure control mode. Inspiratory time is set with the inspiratory time control from 0.10 to 3.00 seconds. Inspiratory pressure is set using the inspiratory pressure control, with a range of 3 to 80 cm H_2O. This inspiratory pressure, in pressure control, is the pressure delivered above the PEEP/CPAP level (unlike TCPL, which sets the peak pressure). Total pressure should be verified by the clinician on the LED display. PEEP and CPAP are established with the PEEP/CPAP control at levels ranging from 0 to 2 cm H_2O. Breath rates from 0 to 150 BPM are available using the breath rate control.

Mechanical breaths may be pressure, flow, or time triggered (in the absence of spontaneous respirations). During inspiration, there is a rapid delivery of flow to the set inspiratory pressure level. As flow decelerates, a constant pressure is maintained throughout inspiration. Termination of the breath occurs when the set inspiratory time has been reached.

In the assist/control mode, all spontaneous respirations will be delivered as full mechanical breaths. In (S)IMV/PS any spontaneous respirations above the set rate will be delivered as the pressure support breaths described earlier.

VAPS. Volume assured pressure support is a mode of ventilation that combines the benefits of pressure support with those of volume ventilation. Breaths are delivered using a variable, decelerating waveform yet offer a guaranteed tidal volume delivery.

In VAPS, the operator has the option of (S)IMV/PS, assist/control, and CPAP. The target tidal volume has a range of 10 to 1200 ml and is set with the tidal volume control. The level of pressure support above PEEP/CPAP is available from 1 to 50 cm H_2O, and is applied to both mechanical and spontaneous breaths when in the (S)IMV/PS mode. Transition flow is set using the flow control with a range of 3 to 120 L/min. Breath rates from 0 to 150 BPM are available using the breath rate control.

Breaths may be either pressure, flow, or time triggered in VAPS. During inspiration of a control breath, there is a rapid delivery of flow to the set pressure support level. Flow decelerates as a constant pressure is maintained during the inspiratory phase. If the set tidal volume is delivered, then the breath will terminate as a pressure support breath. In the event of the set tidal volume not being delivered by the transition point (set by the flow control), flow will become constant until the tidal volume is delivered. Peak inspiratory pressure and inspiratory time may increase during a VAPS control breath. Pressure support I-time limit, 0.10 to 3.00 seconds, and the high-pressure alarm, 3 to 120 cm H_2O, are set as safety limits in VAPS.

Features. The V.I.P. Gold now includes the partner monitor integrated into the ventilator. The monitor displays measurements of PIP, MAP, PEEP, rate, Ti (sec), I:E ratio, Vt (inspiratory or expiratory), and inspiratory Ve.

The improved EPROM flow sensor is now autoclavable. The infant sensor is placed proximal to the patient airway, whereas the pediatric sensor is positioned distally, near the exhalation valve.

Flow triggering is available in all modes of ventilation on the V.I.P. Gold. The infant flow sensor provides a 3 L/min bias flow (except in TCPL) with a 0.2 to 3 L/min sensitivity adjustment. The pediatric flow sensor provides a 5 L/min bias flow and a sensitivity range of 1 to 5 L/min.

Inspiratory rise time is available in pressure control, pressure support, and VAPS. Rise time is set to adjust the delivery of inspiratory flow to the patient. A setting of 1 provides the fastest rise in peak flow delivery, whereas a 7 provides the slowest.

Set tidal volumes are now available from 10 to 1200 ml. The operator is also able to select between a square and a decelerating flow waveform in volume control.

Inspiratory and expiratory hold buttons are provided for static lung and auto-PEEP measurements.

Alarms. In addition to the alarms provided on the BIRD V.I.P., the V.I.P. Gold provides the aforementioned pressure support I-time limit. There is also high tidal volume alarm that may be set to OFF, or from 2 to 2000 ml. The low PEEP/CPAP pressure alarm is now fixed at 3 cm H_2O below the set PEEP/CPAP level.

BIO-MED MVP-10

Basic Mechanisms. The Bio-Med MPV-10 (Figure 16–5) is a pneumatically powered and controlled neonatal ventilator. Because of its small size and weight, it is used primarily as a transport ventilator and is MRI compatible.

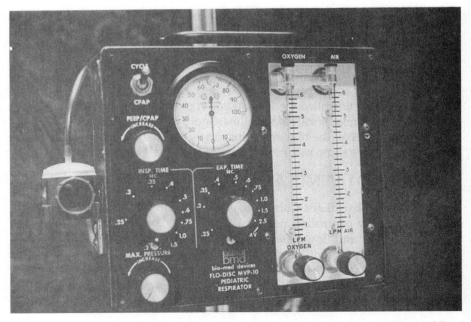

Figure 16–5 *The Bio-Med MVP-10 ventilator (Reproduced with permission from Bio-Med Devices Inc., Stamford, CT)*

Air and oxygen from 50 psi sources are connected to the rear of the ventilator and fed to respective flowmeters on the front of the ventilator. FiO_2 is determined by the ratio of air to oxygen, as set on the flowmeters. The formula for determining oxygen concentration is demonstrated in Table 16–1.

The gas that leaves the two flowmeters is combined and fed directly to the patient circuit, providing a continuous flow of mixed gas to the patient. A small tube is diverted off the inlet oxygen and fed to the ventilator control system, called the pneumatic logic circuit. This circuit provides operator controls for inspiratory time, expiratory time, PEEP and CPAP, the pressure limit, and the determination of IMV or CPAP ventilation.

Inspiration begins when the expiratory timer, set by the operator, diverts pressure from the pneumatic logic circuit to the maximum pressure control. Pressure is then diverted to a balloon or diaphragm type of expiratory valve, which inflates, closing the expiratory valve and diverting the continuous circuit flow to the patient airway.

Expiration occurs when the inspiratory time, set by the operator, stops the flow to the expiratory valve, opening up the valve and allowing gas to escape.

The ventilatory rate is determined by the setting of the inspiratory and expiratory time controls. Rates of less than 2 BPM and up to 120 BPM are possible on the MVP-10. The formula for calculating the expiratory time needed to achieve a desired rate is shown in Table 16–2.

The pressure limit is accomplished by the amount of pressure allowed to inflate the exhalation valve and is controlled by the maximum pressure control. The maximum pressure control is simply a needle valve that allows more or less flow to the expiratory valve. The more flow to the valve, the higher the inspiratory pressure and vice versa. PEEP and CPAP are adjusted in the same manner by the PEEP/CPAP control.

BEAR CUB BP 2001 VENTILATOR

Basic Mechanisms. The BEAR Cub ventilator, shown in Figure 16–6, is a pneumatically powered, electronically controlled neonatal ventilator. The BEAR Cub ventilator has a built-in oxygen blender and flowmeter, both of which are operator controlled.

TABLE 16–1 Calculation of FiO_2

To calculate the FiO_2 when the O_2 and airflow rates are known, the following formula is used:

$$FiO_2 = \frac{O_2 \text{ flow} + (0.21 \times \text{airflow})}{\text{Total flow}}$$

For example: What is the FiO_2 of the following?

$$O_2 \text{ flow} = 4.5 \text{ L/min}$$

$$\text{airflow} = 8 \text{ L/min}$$

$$FiO_2 = \frac{4.5 + (0.21 \times 8)}{12.5} = \frac{4.5 + 1.68}{12.5} = \frac{6.18}{12.5} = 0.49$$

TABLE 16–2   Calculating Expiratory Time in Order to Achieve a Desired Ventilator Rate

The desired rate is divided into 60 to determine the total breath time. This is followed by subtracting the desired inspiratory time from the total breath time. The remaining figure is expiratory time, which should be set to achieve the desired rate.

Example: What expiratory time is needed to achieve a rate of 40 with an inspiratory time of 0.5 second?

Total breath time = seconds per min/desired breath rate
Total breath time = 60/40
Total breath time = 1.5 seconds
Expiratory time = Total breath time − inspiratory time
Expiratory time = 1.5 seconds − 0.5 seconds
Expiratory time = 1 second

Rate is determined by a ventilator rate control located on the face of the ventilator. A toggle switch, located just below the rate control, allows rates of 76 to 150 when switched to the right.

Inspiration begins when the rate control signals a three-way solenoid, which diverts flow past the pressure limit control and out to a reference chamber in the exhalation valve. Pressurization of this chamber causes a plunger valve to close the outflow orifice, allowing pressure to build up in the patient circuit. The continuous gas flow is diverted into the patient's lungs, thus providing inspiration.

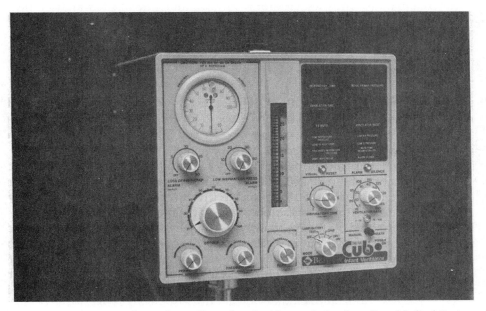

Figure 16–6 *The BEAR Cub ventilator. (Reproduced with permission from Bear Medical Systems, Inc., Riverside, CA)*

Inspiration is timed by the inspiratory time control and set by the operator. When the time limit is reached, the three-way solenoid is signaled and flow is diverted to the PEEP/CPAP control, which adjusts flow to the reference chamber in the expiratory valve. The amount of pressure allowed into the reference chamber during exhalation determines the level of PEEP.

Proper function of the BEAR Cub pneumatic control system requires that 3/16" tubing be used between the patient connection and the proximal airway pressure nipple on the back of the ventilator.

Unique Features. The BEAR Cub ventilator has a digital pressure monitor built into the face of the ventilator that measures and displays inspiratory time, mean airway pressure, exhalation time, I:E ratio, and ventilator rate.

Manual breaths can be delivered by the operator at the set inspiratory time and PIP by pressing the manual breath button found beneath the rate control. Older versions of the Cub only allow manual breaths while in the CPAP mode, whereas newer versions allow manual breaths in IMV or CPAP.

The Cub ventilator has two operator-set alarm limits: the loss of PEEP/CPAP and the low inspiratory pressure alarm. The loss of PEEP/CPAP alarm triggers an audiovisual alarm when the PEEP level falls below the set limit. The low inspiratory alarm also sets off an audiovisual alarm if the PIP does not reach the preset alarm level.

Other audiovisual alarms on the Cub include a prolonged inspiratory pressure, triggered when inspiratory pressure is 10 cm H_2O above the loss of PEEP/CPAP limit for 3.5 seconds, a ventilator inoperative alarm for electronic failures and low oxygen and air pressure alarms. Visual alerts include rate/time incompatibility and alarm silence.

HAMILTON VEOLAR VENTILATOR

Basic Mechanisms. The Hamilton Veolar ventilator is pneumatically powered and electronically controlled and offers pressure, time, and manual triggering; pressure, volume, and flow limiting; and pressure, flow, and time cycling (Figure 16–7). Modes of ventilation include (S)CMV, SIVM, Spontaneous, and MMV (minimum minute ventilation). The operator has the option of selecting the flow pattern and can choose between sine wave, decelerating flow, accelerating flow, and square wave.

In the spontaneous and MMV modes, the ventilator controls inspiratory pressure. In SIMV, control switches between pressure (during a spontaneous breath) and flow (during mandatory breaths). In the CMV mode, the ventilator controls flow.

The operator sets a trigger setting on the ventilator, which is adjustable between 1 and 15 cm H_2O below the baseline pressure. This feature may also be turned off. The patient triggers a mandatory breath when inspiratory flow is sufficient to drop baseline pressure below this point. Time triggering is adjustable from 5 to 60/min in the CMV mode, and 0.5 to 30/min in the SMIV mode. A mandatory breath can also be triggered by the operator.

When pressure support is not used, a demand flow system controls the inspiratory pressure by attempting to maintain the set PEEP/CPAP level (adjustable from 0 to 50 cm H_2O).

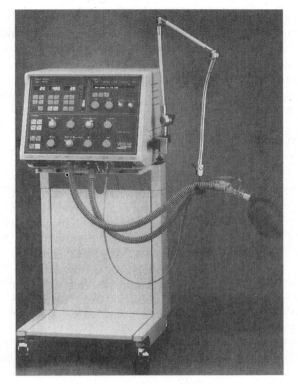

Figure 16–7 *The Hamilton Veolar ventilator. (Courtesy Hamilton Medical, Reno, NV)*

When pressure support is used, the pressure limit is adjustable from 0 to 50 cm H_2O above the PEEP/CPAP level. If inspiratory pause time is set to greater than zero, the inspiratory volume is limited. The inspiratory flow is limited for mandatory breaths. The peak flow is related to the tidal volume, percent cycle time, waveform and rate, and is available up to 180 L/min.

Termination of inspiration occurs when the set pressure limit is exceeded. The pressure limit is available to be set between 10 and 110 cm H_2O. While the Veolar ventilator cannot be volume cycled, a tidal volume of 20 to 2000 ml can be set when breaths are flow controlled. Inspiration can also be terminated with flow cycling when using pressure support. Inspiration is stopped when the inspiratory flow rate falls to 25% of the peak flow rate. Time cycling occurs when breaths are flow controlled when the inspiratory time reaches the valve determined by the frequency and the percent of cycle time setting. The percent of inspiration is adjustable from 20 to 80%.

MODES OF VENTILATION

CMV (Controlled Mechanical Ventilation). In this mode, breaths are pressure or time triggered, flow limited, and time cycled. During CMV, tidal volume remains relatively constant.

SIMV. During SIMV ventilation, mandatory breaths are synchronized to the patient's spontaneous effort. Mandatory breaths are flow controlled and pressure triggered, or time triggered if no spontaneous effort is detected. Mandatory breaths are either pressure cycled, or flow cycled if the pressure support (Pinsp) is set above zero. In this mode, a mandatory breath is given when a spontaneous effort is detected during the period determined by the set rate. If a breath is not detected, a mandatory breath is given at the beginning of the next period. The ventilator then maintains the set rate until a spontaneous breath is detected.

MMV. This mode is basically a spontaneous breathing mode with the addition of pressure support. When MMV is selected, the ventilator determines the level of pressure support based on the exhaled minute volume. The ventilator measures the tidal volume of the first eight breaths and compares that value to the preset MMV level. If the minute volume is less than desired, the ventilator begins to increase pressure support. Conversely, if the volume is higher than desired, pressure support is slowed.

The Veolar ventilator provides an emergency mode of ventilation if apnea is detected, or if the minute volume drops below 1 L/min in the MMV mode.

Features. Microprocessors in the ventilator receive information regarding airway pressure and inspiratory flow as well as control the variable settings and the output control signals. Airway pressure is measured by a transducer within the ventilator. This information is used to control the triggering, cycling, and alarms as well as to control the waveform.

Air and oxygen are mixed by an internal blender to the operator determined percentage. This mixed gas is then sent to a pressurized reservoir within the ventilator. This reservoir holds around 8 liters of gas at a pressure of 350 cm H_2O. As flow demands increase, a flow control solenoid opens and allows additional flow to enter the patient circuit, allowing a fast response time and a wide range of peak flow levels. A flush control on the front panel purges the reservoir and allows shorter response times when changing FiO_2.

Displays and Alarms. Available to the operator on the front of the ventilator are various displays, including spontaneous and total breaths/min; exhaled minute volume; delivered and exhaled tidal volumes; peak and mean airway pressures; PEEP/CPAP; and a bar graph of dynamic ventilatory pressure. The Veolar ventilator displays calculated system compliance and resistance. Compliance, resistance, spontaneous breathing rate, and expiratory minute volume can all be stored for later trend analysis.

The Veolar ventilator provides several alarms. An alarm is activated if power is interrupted or if the external gas source pressure drops below 29 PSIG. The ventilator also alarms if the pressure in the internal reservoir drops below 200 cm H_2O. A low PEEP/CPAP alarm is preset and nonadjustable. It is triggered if the pressure falls 3 cm H_2O below the set level. A high-pressure alarm is operator adjustable between 10 and 120 cm H_2O. Low and high exhaled minute volume alarms are adjustable from 1 to 40 L/min. A high-frequency alarm is adjustable from 0 to 70/min. An apnea alarm (nonadjustable) is triggered if the ventilator does not detect an exhaled breath for 15 seconds. When this alarm is triggered, the ventilator enters a back-up mode and delivers mandatory breaths. No inspiratory flow over a 20-second period triggers the fail to cycle alarm. High and low oxygen concentration alarms are operator set.

Several other alarms are triggered by the control circuit. If the desired peak flow rate is above the 180 L/min capability of the ventilator, a nonadjustable alarm is triggered. This often occurs if the percent inspiratory time is set too short. An alarm sounds if the operator attempts to activate SIMV, spontaneous, or MMV modes with the trigger set to the off position. The ventilator will switch to the desired mode at a trigger level of –5 cm H_2O; however, the alarm will continue until the operator sets the trigger level. Alarms are provided for both a ventilator disconnection and a patient disconnection. These are nonadjustable and are triggered when the ventilator measures a difference between the delivered volume and the measured volume. Two other nonadjustable alarms are the Vt insp and Vt exp (inspiratory and expiratory tidal volume) mismatch alarms. The inspiratory mismatch alarm is triggered when the measured inspiratory volume is more than twice the volume leaving the servo flow valve for three consecutive breaths. The expiratory mismatch is triggered when the measured volume is more than one-half the volume leaving the servo flow valve plus 25 ml, for two consecutive breaths. Finally, internal electronic failure results in a technical fault alarm.

DRAGER BABYLOG 8000 PLUS

Basic Mechanisms. The Babylog 8000 Plus is a dual microprocessor-controlled, pressure-limited, time-cycled, continuous-flow ventilator specifically designed for neonates and infants. Its available modes of ventilation are CPAP, assist/control, SIMV, pressure support, and volume guarantee, which uses a preset tidal volume on each supported breath regardless of patient effort or change in compliance. The breath rate can be set from 1 to 150 BPM. Inspiratory pressures can be set from 10 to 80 cm H_2O. Inspiratory time is set from 0.1 to 2 seconds and expiratory time can be set from 0.2 to 30 seconds. The range of tidal volume is 2 to 100 ml. PEEP can be set from 0 to 25 cm H_2O. Oxygen concentration can be set from 21% to 100%. Inspiratory and expiratory flow range from 1 to 30 L/min.

Features, Monitoring, and Alarms. Parameters on the Babylog 8000 Plus are measured at the patient wye with a heated wire anemometer. Peak pressure, PEEP, and mean pressure are measured from 0 to 99 cm H_2O. Tidal volume is measured from 0 to 999 ml and is displayed as expiratory volume. Minute ventilation is measured from 0 to 30 L/min. Leak is displayed from 0% to 100% and is calculated by the difference between inspiratory and expiratory tidal volumes. Breath rates are measured from 0 to 999 BPM. FiO_2 is measured from 18% to 100% using an internal oxygen analyzer.

The Babylog 8000 Plus also measures lung mechanics. Dynamic compliance, airway and endotracheal tube resistance, and lung overdistension are measured for each respiratory cycle. Rate-volume ratio (RVR) is also calculated and may be used as a tool for weaning.

The Babylog 8000 Plus features alarms that are automatically and manually set. High inspiratory pressure, high CPAP, low PEEP/CPAP, and disconnect alarms are automatically set. High and low minute ventilation, alarm delay, apnea, and tachypnea alarms are manually set.

INFANT STAR VENTILATOR 500/950

Basic Mechanisms. The Infant Star, depicted in Figure 16–8, is pneumatically powered and electronically controlled with dual microprocessors. The Infant Star offers both continuous flow and demand flow in both the CPAP and IMV modes. The ventilator has a built-in battery that will operate the electronics during a power failure or a transport.

The purpose of the dual microprocessors is to provide an added safety margin by running continual "health checks" between the two. One microprocessor controls the ventilator, whereas the other controls the display information. The microprocessors are easily updated with new enhancements as needed, making the ventilator versatile. The ventilator also has an interface connection that allows a computer to be attached for the collection of ventilator information used for trending and monitoring.

Unique Features. The availability of demand flow in both CPAP and IMV modes is a unique feature of the Infant Star. When demand flow is selected, the ventilator establishes 4 L/min of continuous flow to the circuit. As the patient begins an inhalation, the negative pressure created in the circuit opens a fast response demand valve that supplies additional flow to the circuit, relative to the negative pressure generated.

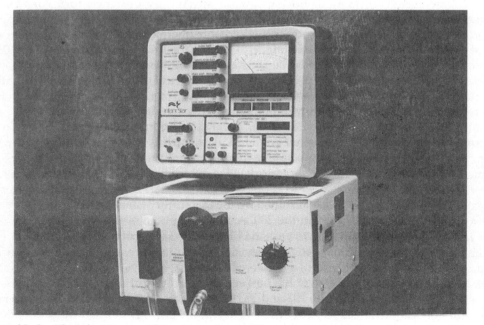

Figure 16–8 *The Infant Star ventilator. (Reproduced with permission from Infrasonics, Inc., San Diego, CA)*

Flow rate is adjustable from 4 to 40 L/min in 2 L/min increments with a background flow of 2 to 32 L/min. Ventilator rates of 1 to 150 BPM are available. Breaths from 1 to 60 are set in increments of 1 BPM, 2 breath increments from 60 to 130, and 5 breath increments from 130 to 150.

PIP is available from 5 to 90 cm H_2O and should always be set at least 5 cm H_2O above PEEP levels for proper function. The inspiratory timer allows a range of inspiratory time from 0.1 to 3.0 seconds. From 0.1 to 0.6 second, the increments are 0.01 second, increasing to 0.02-second increments from 0.6 to 1.0 second and in 0.1-second steps from 1.0 to 3.0 seconds.

The low inspiratory pressure control establishes the minimum pressure that must be reached during the mandatory inspiration. It is adjustable from 3 to 60 cm H_2O. Failure to reach the preset level activates an audiovisual alarm. A digital display is provided for each parameter located to the left of the respective control knob.

Manual ventilation is possible in all modes of ventilation with the manual breath button. PEEP and CPAP are available from 0 to 24 cm H_2O on the PEEP/CPAP control. The Infant Star provides direct continual digital readouts of PEEP/CPAP, mean airway pressure, and PIP. Displays of the PEEP/CPAP setting, I:E ratio, and expiratory time are available individually by the use of the display selector. The selected parameter is then digitally displayed to the right of the knob.

The Star-Sync interface provides triggered alternatives of synchronized intermittent mandatory ventilation (SIMV) and assist/control (A/C) to the patient.

High-frequency ventilation (HFV) and high-frequency ventilation combined with IMV are available on the Infant Star 950. High-frequency ventilation is discussed in Chapter 17. The 950 provides HFV rates of 2 to 22 Hz and amplitudes of 0 to 160 cm H_2O. A jet venturi enables the patient to actively exhale.

Alarm Systems. The Infant Star ventilator supplies a total of nine different alarm systems. In addition, an internal battery light indicates when the internal battery is being used. In addition to the low inspiratory pressure alarm previously discussed, the ventilator has the following alarms.

The low PEEP/CPAP alarm is set by the microprocessor depending on the set PEEP/CPAP level. With PEEP/CPAP levels of 0 to 5 cm H_2O, the alarm is set 2 cm H_2O below; levels of 6 to 8 cm H_2O, the alarm is 3 cm H_2O below; 9 to 12 cm H_2O, 4 cm H_2O below; and 13 to 24 cm H_2O, 5 cm H_2O below the set level.

The airway leak alarm is most effective in the demand flow modes but is also active in the continuous flow modes. The alarm activates when the demand flow exceeds the set flow rate by 8 L/min or more for 4 or more seconds.

The obstructed tube alarm is activated when one of five different violations occur. To differentiate between violations, the ventilator displays a message in the pressure and I:E ratio expiration time display areas when the alarm is activated. The messages are described next.

1. *A01*—High inspiratory alarm setting.
2. *A02*—The PIP was detected 5 cm H_2O above the PIP set point. The circuit pressure is immediately vented to ambient. This alarm usually indicates a blockage of the expiratory tubing or a nonfunctioning expiratory valve.

3. *A03*—This alarm indicates that the PIP did not drop to half of the difference between PIP and PEEP within 200 milliseconds, indicating a blocked expiratory tube. The circuit is immediately vented to ambient.
4. *A04*—This alarm is activated when the set PEEP/CPAP has been exceeded by 6 cm H_2O or more for up to 5 seconds. Again, when this alarm activates, the vent valve opens and drops the circuit pressure to ambient.
5. *A05*—This alarm triggers when the proximal pressure reaches 10 cm H_2O above the set peak pressure. It occurs when the proximal pressure line is blocked or when the inspiratory tubing is blocked.

The next alarm is the insufficient expiratory time. This alarm operates only during the IMV mode. On rates of up to 100/min, the alarm activates if expiratory time is less than 0.3 second and, on rates greater than 100, less than 0.2 second.

The low oxygen pressure alarm sounds when incoming PSIG drops below 45 PSIG. The low air pressure alarm sounds if incoming PSIG drops below 40 PSIG. When the internal battery is being utilized, the power loss signal lights up, alternating with the internal battery light, 5 to 10 minutes before the battery is fully discharged. Total discharge of the battery causes the ventilator inoperative and power loss indicators to light, the ventilator stops cycling, and the patient circuit is vented to ambient.

The ventilator is inoperative alarm also activates when the microprocessors have detected an unsafe condition. In this instance, the ventilator ceases to function and the circuit is vented to ambient.

NEWPORT BREEZE

Basic Mechanisms. The Breeze ventilator (Figure 16–9) is a new-generation ventilator that has the ability to ventilate neonates, pediatric, and adult patients. It is electronically controlled, pneumatically powered, and offers both volume-controlled, time-cycled, ventilation and pressure-controlled, time-cycled ventilation.

The control panel of the Breeze ventilator is arranged into five related panels: the digital flowmeter panel, the data display panel, the breath control panel, the alarm panel, and the pressure control panel. Additionally, the displays are color-coded: green for patient breath controls; red for alarm displays; and yellow for data and information.

A unique feature of the Breeze ventilator is the separation of a spontaneous flow system from the mandatory breath flow system. This concept is called the Duoflow® system. The spontaneous flow system functions as a free-standing CPAP system during the mandatory breath exhalation phase. While in the exhalation phase, the patient breathes from a separate flow of mixed gas, which includes either a reservoir bag or a reservoir bag cap at the base of the ventilator.

The flow rate during this phase is determined by the operator and set using the spontaneous flow control located on the digital flowmeter panel. During mandatory breath inspiration the spontaneous flow is turned off and the delivered flow is now determined by the flow control located on the breath control panel.

We will now compare the volume control and the pressure control capabilities of the ventilator.

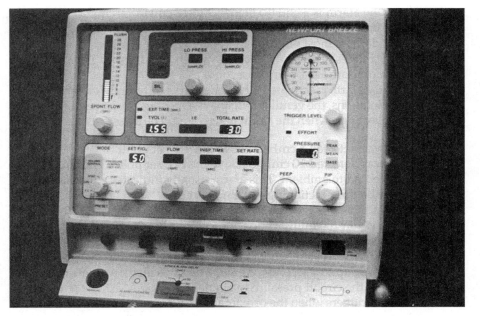

Figure 16–9 *The Newport Breeze E150 ventilator. (Reproduced with permission from Newport Medical Instruments, Inc., Newport Beach, CA)*

Volume Control. Volume control are selected with the mode selector knob located on the breath control. It offers the operator the choice of assist/control with sigh, assist/control, SIMV, and spontaneous breathing.

In the assist/control mode, a mandatory breath is delivered to the patient when a spontaneous effort is detected by the trigger level (see following discussion). The tidal volume is determined by the set flow and inspiratory time and is digitally displayed in the data display panel as SET TIDAL VOLUME. Mandatory breaths are delivered at the set rate when patient effort is not detected.

When the assist/control with sigh is selected, the ventilator delivers a sigh equal to 1.5 times the set inspiratory time (1.5 times the tidal volume) every 100 breaths.

In the SIMV mode, the patient breathes spontaneously from the spontaneous flow system and additionally receives breaths at the predetermined rate set by the operator. The mandatory breaths are synchronized with the patient's effort as long as the trigger level is correctly set. As with assist/control, the tidal volume is determined by the mandatory flow rate and the inspiratory time located on the breath control panel.

During the spontaneous mode, the patient draws all flow from the spontaneous flow system and the reservoir bag at the selected FiO_2.

The preset button, located below the mode selector knob, lights up the digital displays in the data display panel and allows the clinician to preset any of the ventilator parameters before changing the mode from spontaneous to an assisted mode.

The set rate control allows the operator to select a mandatory breath rate from 1 to 150 b/min.

Pressure Control. Pressure control modes are selected with the mode selector knob located on the breath control panel. It offers the operator the choice of assist/control, SIMV, and spontaneous modes of ventilation. Whenever pressure control is selected, the operator must set the PIP level located on the pressure control panel.

In the assist/control mode, a preset mandatory breath is delivered with each sensed patient effort (paient trigger). The inspiratory time control determines the length of the inspiration, the flow control determines the flow rate/pressure rise, and the PIP determines the target pressure. In the pressure control mode, expiratory time is displayed in place of the tidal volume on the data display panel. The machine delivers mandatory breaths at the set rate when a patient effort is not detected.

The SIMV mode allows the patient to breathe spontaneously from the spontaneous flow system and gives mandatory breaths at the set breath rate. The ventilator will synchronize the mandatory breaths with spontaneous breaths when a patient effort is detected.

The preset button can be used in the pressure control mode as described above.

Features. The ventilator has a built-in pressure display located on the pressure control panel. The pressure transducer monitors pressures from the proximal airway and displays MAP continuously. Peak pressure and base pressure are temporarily displayed for 30 seconds when the PEAK and BASE buttons are pushed. Pressure is measured 100 times per second by the transducer, and the average mean airway pressure is calculated with each patient or mandatory breath.

The ventilator face panel is equipped with an electronic pressure gauge, which is attached to the proximal pressure inlet and measures pressures from –10 to 120 cm H_2O. The trigger level, which is used to detect patient effort, is displayed as a lit segment on the gauge. The trigger level knob has two adjustment positions, coarse and fine. To adjust the trigger level in the coarse position, pull out on the trigger level knob, clicking it into position. To adjust the trigger level in the fine position, push in on the trigger level knob, clicking it into position. Rotate the knob until the lit trigger segment is set just below and as close as possible to the baseline pressure so that each time the patient begins a spontaneous breath, and proximal pressure drops the triggers detects the effort. The trigger allows the ventilator to provide assist/control and synchronized breaths in SIMV. In addition, it resets the apnea alarm delay in all modes.

The spontaneous flow is calibrated from minimum to 28 liters of flow. In the flush position, approximately 58 L/min of flow is delivered. The spontaneous flow is set by the operator to meet the patient's average spontaneous inspiratory demands during spontaneous breathing. This can be determined by observing the electronic pressure gauge for negative swings during inhalation or positive swings during exhalation.

The flow control, located on the breath control panel, is calibrated from 3 to 120 L/min and is graduated in increments of 1 L/min.

The inspiratory time control, also located on the breath control panel, is adjustable from 0.1 to 3.0 seconds and is graduated in increments of 0.01 second from 0.1 to 1 second and in increments of 0.1 second from 1 to 3 seconds.

As previously mentioned, the tidal volume is not set directly, but is a product of the flow and the inspiratory time settings.

A manual inflation control button, located behind the fold-down door at the bottom of the face panel, allows the delivery of a mandatory inflation in any mode. The operator is limited to a 2-second inspiratory time and cannot exceed a rate of 150 b/min. In the pressure control mode, the PIP setting will restrict the peak pressure to the set limit.

The Breeze ventilator is equipped with a nebulizer outlet to which a nebulizer can be attached. The nebulizer on/off switch is located behind the fold-down door at the base of the front panel. The flow is approximately 6 L/min and is delivered in addition to the set flow at the same FiO_2 set on the ventilator. Nebulizer outlet flow is only provided during mandatory inspiration. In the case of very low SIMV rates or very short inspiratory times, the auxiliary flowmeter, found on the left side of the Breeze, may be used to power the nebulizer. When the nebulizer outlet is used during volume-controlled ventilation, the ventilator automatically adds the approximate volume of nebulizer gas to the displayed tidal volume.

A pressure relief safety valve is located on the rear panel in the upper left corner. It can be set from 0 to 120 cm H_2O and is used to protect the patient from excessive circuit pressures.

The FiO_2 is set by the operator using the SET FiO_2 control knob located on the breath control panel. The set FiO_2 is displayed digitally above the control knob.

The Breeze has an internal battery which will provide backup power to run the ventilator for approximately 1 hour when fully charged.

Alarms. The alarms incorporated into the Breeze ventilator are located on the alarm panel. The alarm panel includes two operator-defined alarms, the high- and low-pressure alarms. A third operator-defined alarm, the apnea/low CPAP alarm, is located behind the fold-down door at the bottom of the front panel.

The low-pressure alarm is set by the operator to detect drops in pressure below the set level. The alarm is activated if the circuit pressure does not rise above the set level during the inspiratory time of a mandatory breath.

The high-pressure alarm is also set by the operator. The alarm is triggered if the circuit pressure reaches the set alarm level at any time. When the high pressure alarm is violated, the machine terminates any presurized inspiration in progress.

The apnea alarm senses the time between time triggered mandatory breaths or patient triggered mandatory or spontaneous breaths. The apnea alarm delay time is set by the operator to 10, 15, 30, or 60 seconds. If the trigger fails to detect a time or patient spontaneous trigger within the selected apnea delay time, the alarm is activated.

An additional alarm, available only in the spontaneous mode, is the low CPAP alarm. This alarm is activated by turning the apneal alarm delay knob to the first position, which in turn deactivates the apnea alarm. The total rate monitor on the panel will display "---" in place of a number and a number will appear in the low-presure alarm setting display. The low pressure alarm control and display, located on the data display panel, are now used to set the low CPAP alarm just below the CPAP level. When the low CPAP alarm is selected, the operator has the option of 0 to 99 cm H_2O instead of 3 to 99 cm H_2O on the low-pressure alarm. The low-pressure alarm is activated if the proximal airway pressure drops below the alarm limit for 4 seconds.

An alarm silence button, located on the data display panel, silences the audible portion of the alarms for 60 seconds.

The Breeze ventilator indicates when battery power is in use by both a visual alert and an audible alarm every 5 minutes. When the battery has approximately 20 minutes of remaining time, the audible alarm becomes continuous and the LO BATT visual alarm is activated.

SECHRIST IV-100 AND IV-100B

Basic Mechanisms. The Sechrist IV-100 and 100B (Figure 16–10) ventilators are pneumatically powered, controlled both electronically and with the use of fluidic valves.

The Sechrist ventilator is somewhat unique in that the delivered gas to the patient does not pass through the ventilator. The 50 psi source gases are connected directly to the oxygen blender located at the side of the ventilator. The blender reduces the pressure of the gases, blends them, and then directs the flow to an attached flowmeter, calibrated from 2 to 32 L/min. The gas flow then enters the patient circuit directly from the flowmeter.

All the functions of ventilation—rate, inspiratory time, PIP, and PEEP—are handled by the expiratory valve, which is controlled by the ventilator settings. A small portion of the inlet oxygen is diverted internally to the ventilator to power the exhalation valve.

The ventilator utilizes two *fluidic* valves, a back-pressure switch and an OR/NOR gate (Figure 16–11). The initiation of a breath is determined by an expiratory time control on the

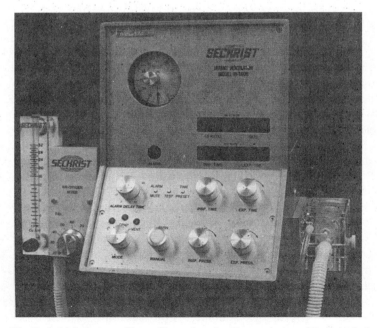

Figure 16–10   *The Sechrist Infant ventilator. (Reproduced with permission of Sechrist Industries, Inc.)*

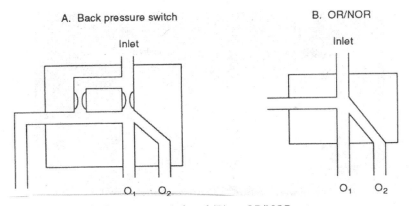

Figure 16–11   *(A) A back-pressure switch and (B) an OR/NOR gate.*

face of the ventilator. It is an electronic timer that signals the closure of a solenoid valve that is inline to the back-pressure switch-sensing line. The duration of the breath is determined by an inspiratory time control found to the left of the expiratory timer.

During the expiratory phase, the internally diverted gas flow is directed to both the back-pressure switch and the OR/NOR gate (Figure 16–12). Flow through both fluidic valves is directed through O1 during expiration.

The O1 outflow from the back-pressure switch is directed to a negative pressure jet, which enters a venturi in the exhalation valve and eliminates inadvertent PEEP. Outflow from O1 of the back-pressure switch is also diverted through the proximal airway pressure line to help reduce condensation. Flow through the back-pressure switch-sensing line passes the manual breath control and then a solenoid valve before venting into the atmosphere.

The O1 output from the OR/NOR gate during exhalation is directed past the expiratory pressure control to the exhalation valve diaphragm. The expiratory pressure control is a needle valve that directs more or less flow of gas to reach the expiratory diaphragm. More flow results in higher levels of PEEP and CPAP, and less flow results in lower PEEP and CPAP levels.

A mechanical breath occurs when the expiratory timer signals the closure of the solenoid valve, closing the back-pressure switch-sensing line. Occlusion of this line forces the gas to reverse through the back-pressure switch and divert the outflow to O_2. The flow from the back-pressure switch enters the OR/NOR side gate and diverts its outflow to O_2 also. This outflow is then directed to the inspiratory pressure control and to the expiratory diaphragm (Figure 16–13). Like the expiratory pressure control, the inspiratory pressure control is a needle valve that allows varied levels of flow to reach the expiratory diaphragm. The higher the flow from the inspiratory pressure control, the higher the PIP. Exhaled gases entering the exhalation valve block must overcome the pressure being exerted on the diaphragm to be vented to the atmosphere.

Unique Features. The Sechrist has the ability to mimic a *sine-wave* flow pattern, or a square-wave flow pattern. The sine-wave pattern is achieved by turning a small allen screw, located

Expiratory phase

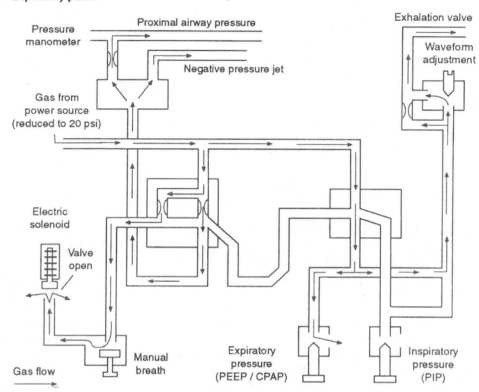

Figure 16–12 *Flow through the back-pressure switch and OR/NOR gate during expiration.*

just above the expiratory block. As the screw is tightened, the normal pathway of flow to the expiratory diaphragm is cut off, forcing the flow of gas from the fluidic valve to pass through a restricted orifice before reaching the expiratory diaphragm (Figure 16–14). The result is a slowing of the flow to the diaphragm, a slow closure of the expiratory valve, and a slow build-up of pressure in the circuit. Flow to the patient begins slowly, and then reaches its preset level when the valve is occluded, creating a rounded flow, or sine-wave pattern.

The manual breath button is placed inline with the flow from the back-pressure switch before reaching the solenoid valve. Physically pressing the button occludes the flow, resulting in the switching to the inspiratory phase. The inspiration lasts as long as the button is held in, so care must be taken to monitor the inspiratory time closely.

The Sechrist ventilator has a built-in digital display of I:E ratio, inspiratory time, and expiratory time. Rate is easily determined as the expiratory timer is adjusted by reading the rate display.

Alarm System. The main alarm system for the Sechrist is a pressure monitor that is located on the pressure manometer. It utilizes an infrared sensor to detect movement of the

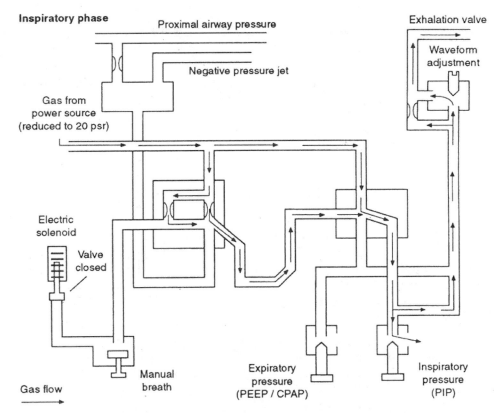

Figure 16–13 *Flow through the back-presure switch and OR/NOR gate during inspiration.*

manometer needle. A delay timer on the face of the ventilator sets the amount of time that needle movement is undetected and the triggering of the alarm.

The monitor uses a thin red line on the face of the manometer to set the pressure limit. If the needle does not cross the red line during the time delay limit, the audiovisual alarm is triggered. The alarm, therefore, can detect low inspiratory pressures from circuit leaks, circuit disconnects, failures to cycle, apnea, and excessive inspiratory time. Other alarms include a low source gas pressure and electrical power failure.

SECHRIST IV-200 SAVI

Basic Mechanisms. The IV-200 ventilator comes with or without the SAVI system (Synchronized Assisted Ventilation of Infants) (Figure 16–15). With this system, the ventilator synchronizes both inspiration and expiration with the patient's breathing. Asynchrony of ventilation theoretically results in a higher risk of barotrauma, and may predispose the patient to chronic lung disease, pneumothoraces, air leak, and IVH.[1]

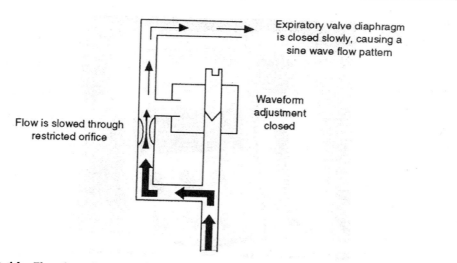

Figure 16–14 *Flow through a restricted orifice causes a slow closure of the expiratory valve and results in a sine-wave flow pattern to the patient.*

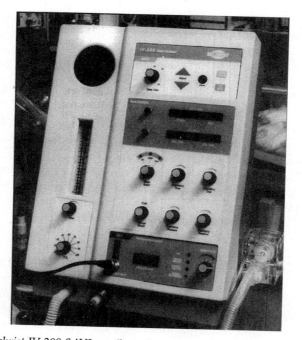

Figure 16–15 *The Sechrist IV-200 SAVI ventilator. (Courtesy Sechrist Industries, Anaheim, CA)*

The ventilator achieves synchronization by connecting to a cardiorespiratory monitor that has a real-time analog respiratory waveform output. The ventilator analyzes this signal and initiates the inspiratory phase when an inspiratory phase is detected. The time from detection of the inspiratory effort until a mandatory breath begins is 15 milliseconds. Exhalation is also synchronized so that the inspiratory phase is terminated when patient exhalation is detected. If the ventilator does not detect a patient inspiratory effort, the ventilator delivers mandatory breaths at the operator determined back-up rate.

The IV-200 has similar controls to the original Sechrist infant ventilator. Modes of ventilation include *CPAP*, which allows spontaneous breathing by the patient, and VENT, which provides IMV, CMV, and Pressure Assist (only with SAVI). Flow rates of 0 to 32 L/min, up to 40 L/min when flush, are selected via a thorpe tube flowmeter incorporated into the front of the ventilator. An inspiratory timer provides inspiratory times between 0.10 to 2.90 seconds. Rate is controlled by an expiratory timer, allowing expiratory times of 0.30 to 60 seconds. Inspiratory pressures of 5 to 70 cm H_2O are available, with a range of –2 to 20 cm H_2O available as expiratory pressure. A manual breath button on the ventilator allows the operator to deliver manual breaths above the set rate of the ventilator.

Displayed in the Vent Control area are I:E ratio, rate, inspiratory time, expiratory time, and a red LED indicating an inspiratory phase. A test button checks microprocessor function, the displays, and alarm functions, when pressed. While in the CPAP mode, a time preset button allows the operator to select and preview inspiratory and expiratory times before switching to the vent mode. An LCD pressure gauge, incorporated into the ventilator above the flowmeter, displays peak inspiratory pressure, PEEP/CPAP, mean airway pressure, and the high- and low-pressure alarm limit settings.

Alarms. The IV-200 ventilator incorporates several alarm systems. The Alarm area is located at the top of the ventilator. An alarm mute is available to silence all alarms for approximately 30 seconds. This is represented as a bell with a diagonal line passing through it. Alarm settings include high- and low-inspiratory pressure limits. These alarms detect excessive, or prolonged inspiratory pressures, circuit leaks, patient disconnects, failure-to-cycle, and apnea. The delay timer can be set from 3 to 60 seconds. This delays activation of the low-pressure alarm for the desired time internal. Both high- and low-pressure alarms are set by using the adjust arrows on the ventilator face. The user selects which to adjust by using the select (reset) button. This button also cancels the high-limit alarm, when activated. Finally, the ventilator alarms if there is a source gas failure, or a power failure.

SAVI Controls and Displays. The SAVI module, when present, is located at the bottom of the ventilator. It displays the trigger rate (from 1 to 300 BPM) and also shows the impedance signal by way of a bar graph. Synchronization is achieved by use of the sensitivity control, which offers an off position, and minimum to maximum settings. The sensitivity control is used to calibrate the response of the ventilator to the patient's effort. This is done by setting the sensitivity control to begin inspiration at the instant the patient initiates a breath. Also displayed on the SAVI module are an indicate light for triggered and controlled breaths, and an alarm when no trigger is detected.

SIEMENS SERVO 900C VENTILATOR

Basic Mechanisms. The Siemens Servo 900C ventilator (Figure 16–16) us unlike any of the previously mentioned ventilators. It is a complex machine that has the ability to ventilate in a wide variety of modes and is applicable on patients from newborn to adult. The Siemens ventilator is pneumatically powered and electronically controlled.

Use on Neonatal Patients. The mode of ventilation that is closest to that provided by the neonatal ventilators is the pressure control mode. In this mode, the inspiratory gas is delivered at a constant pressure until the time limit stops the breath. The desired pressure to be delivered is set on the inspiratory pressure level (above PEEP). The set pressure is added to the PEEP level to determine the pressure level. For example, if an inspiratory pressure of 20 cm H_2O were desired and the ventilator were set to deliver a PEEP of 4 cm H_2O, the inspiratory pressure level would be set at 16 cm H_2O to achieve the desired inspiratory pressure.

Three controls, located on the upper right portion of the ventilator face, control the breaths per minute, percent of inspiratory time, and percent of pause time. Inspiratory time, instead of being an actual set time limit as on other neonatal ventilators, is set as a percent of the total cycle time. Thus, if the ventilator were set at 30 BPM and inspiratory time set at 33%, the inspiratory time is calculated by dividing 30 into 60, or a 2-second cycle time, and multiplying the result by the percent of inspiratory time. In this case, the inspiratory time

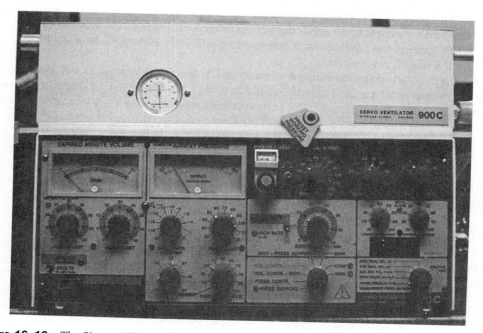

Figure 16–16 *The Siemens-Elema Servo 900C ventilator. (Courtesy Siemens Medical Systems, Danvers, MA)*

would be 0.66 second, which is 33% of 2 seconds. If a pause time is present, it must be added to the inspiratory time percent before dividing into the cycle time.

A breath is initiated by either a patient effort (assist) or by the rate timer (control). Flow rates and tidal volumes are determined by the difference in the working pressure, set on the ventilator, and the patient airway. It may be advantageous when using the ventilator on small newborns to lower the working pressure to a level just above the set pressure limit. This will allow for lower flow rates and possibly help prevent barotrauma.

Use on Pediatric Patients. For the pediatric patient, the 900C ventilator offers diverse modes, including pressure support, volume control, SIMV, and CPAP. In addition, there is a choice of volume control with sigh and SIMV with pressure support.

Tidal volume is set with the preset inspiratory minute volume control divided by the breath rate control. For example, if a tidal volume of 300 ml is desired and a rate of 30 BPM is used, the minute volume control would be set at 9.0 liters and the breath rate control set at 30. If the SIMV mode is to be used, the breath rate control should be set above the anticipated SIMV rate as the SIMV breath rate control will only provide a rate up to but not exceeding the breath rate control.

Flow is a product of the set minute volume and % inspiratory time. The % inspiratory time determines what percent of the ventilatory cycle is dedicated to inspiration. It is adjustable at 20, 25, 33, 50, 67, and 80% of the ventilatory cycle. The ventilator also has five inspiratory pause times: zero, 5, 10, 20 and 30%.

To calculate the delivered flow rate, the following formula is used:

$$\text{flow rate} = \frac{\text{set minute volume}}{\text{insp. time\%}}$$

For example, assuming a set minute volume of 9.0 liters and an inspiratory time % of 25%, the flow would be calculated:

$$\text{flow rate} = \frac{9.0}{0.25} = 36 \text{ L/min}$$

Features. The 900C displays both expired minute volume and airway pressure on analog displays. A trigger sensitivity control is used to set the amount of negative pressure below PEEP that must be generated to initiate an assisted breath.

PEEP is set using the PEEP control, which is adjustable from 0 to 50 cm H_2O. In the SIMV mode, the desired rate is set on the SIMV BPM control, which is below the breath rate control. It is adjustable in a low range from 0.4 to 4 BPM and in a high range from 4 to 40 BPM. The desired range is selected by a toggle switch located to the side of the control knob.

Alarms. Alarms that are adjustable by the operator include high minute volume, low minute volume, high oxygen percent, low oxygen percent, and high airway pressure. One nonadjustable alarm is the apnea alarm, which is activated if the ventilator does not sense flow through the expiratory flow sensor for 15 seconds.

The high and low minute volume alarms are adjustable in an infant range from 0 to 4

L/min and in an adult range from 0 to 40 L/min. The alarm is triggered whenever the high or low alarm limits are violated.

The high and low oxygen percents are adjustable from 0.20 to 1.0 and are used to warn of changes in the delivered FiO_2.

The upper pressure limit is set above the peak inspiratory pressure. The alarm is activated if the pressure limit is exceeded during inspiration and the ventilator immediately enters an expiratory phase.

SIEMENS SERVO 300/300A VENTILATOR

Basic Mechanisms. The Servo 300 ventilator is designed to ventilate adults, pediatric, and neonatal patients. An addition to the Servo 300 ventilator, is the integrated oxygen blender, which previous Servo ventilators have not had (Figure 16–17). The Servo 300 can be triggered manually, flow, or by time or pressure. Inspiration is limited by volume, pressure, or flow. The inspiratory phase is cycled off by pressure, flow, or time.

There are several operator selected variables on the Servo 300 ventilator. The patient type switch (adult, pediatric, neonatal) determines the range of available pressures and/or volumes that can be selected. The Servo 300 offers eight modes of ventilation; three for controlled ventilation, and five for supported ventilation. Six parameters must be set for each mode: the patient range (adult, pediatric, neonatal); the upper pressure limit; upper and lower minute volume alarm limits; trigger sensitivity; percent inspiratory rise time; and the oxygen percent. The other parameters vary, depending on which mode is being used. In each mode, the active controls are indicated by a yellow light.

The mode of ventilation choices include pressure control, volume control, *pressure regulated volume control* (PRVC), *volume support, SIMV* (volume control) + pressure support, SIMV (pressure control) + pressure support, and pressure support/CPAP. The operator

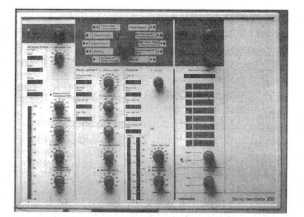

Figure 16–17   *The Siemens Servo 300 ventilator. (Courtesy Siemens Medical Systems, Danvers, MA).*

may also determine pressure or flow triggering, percent inspiratory time, percent inspiratory pause time, percent of inspiratory rise time, pressure limit, PEEP/CPAP, minute volume, rate and FiO_2.

The percent of inspiratory rise time is a unique control. It determines how quickly the pressure or flow reaches the preset level, at the start of a breath. It is adjustable from 0 to 10% of the entire ventilatory period. The higher the percentage, the longer it takes to reach the preset level, resulting in a tapering of the pattern. Low values cause a rapid rise to the preset level and result in a more square wave pattern.

The Servo 300 controls inspiratory flow or pressure, depending on which mode is selected. Flow is controlled in volume control and SIMV (volume control) plus pressure support (when pressure support is not used). Inspiratory pressure is controlled in pressure control, pressure support, SIMV (pressure control) plus pressure support, PRVC, volume support, and CPAP.

In the pressure control mode, an assisted breath is triggered by the patient as determined by the set sensitivity level. Triggering can also be timed, as determined by the CMV Frequency knob. Pressure is limited by the Pressure Control Level Above PEEP knob. The breath is time cycled off, as determined by the frequency and % Insp. Time knob.

In volume control mode, the flow is controlled, time or patient triggered and time cycled (determined by the % Insp. Time, % Pause Time, and the CMV frequency. In this mode, the inspiratory time is limited to no more than 80% of the ventilatory period. If more flow is required by the patient during inspiration, as determined by reducing the pressure below the PEEP level, the ventilator switches to pressure control and provides flow to maintain PEEP. If this occurs, the breath cycles off when the delivered tidal volume exceeds 125% of the set tidal volume. The set tidal volume is determined by dividing the set minute volume by the frequency.

Pressure-regulated volume control is a unique mode of ventilation. In this mode, each inspiration is time triggered (according to the CMV frequency setting), pressure limited and controlled, and time cycled. In this mode, the first breath is delivered at 10 cm H_2O. The ventilator then measures the volume delivered at this pressure and calculates compliance. The next three breaths are then delivered at 75% of the pressure calculated to deliver the preset tidal volume. The inspiratory pressure for each successive breath is then regulated, based on the compliance calculated from the previous breath. While inspiratory pressure may change from breath to breath, it is limited to change no more than 3 cm H_2O from one breath to the next.

Volume support may be used in weaning, or in the patient whose own breathing effort is not sufficient. The controls that are set in volume support are the same as those set in PRVC. This is important, because if apnea occurs, the ventilator automatically switches from volume support to PRVC. Once the initial values have been set, the ventilator initiates a test sequence. The level of pressure support is then regulated based on the calculated compliance from the previous breath, compared to the set tidal volume. The support ends when flow has decreased to 5% of the peak flow or upon reaching 80% of the set breath cycle time. If the patient breathes above the preset tidal volume, the inspiratory pressure level lowers in steps to maintain. If the patient breathes above or below the set frequency, pressure is again altered to maintain the desired tidal volume.

Two SIMV plus pressure support modes are offered: one with volume control, and one with pressure control. The main difference is that in volume control, mandatory breaths are flow controlled, whereas they are pressure controlled in pressure control.

In the pressure support/CPAP mode, spontaneous breaths are supported at a user determined pressure level. Breaths are triggered by pressure or flow, depending on the sensitivity control and the patient's spontaneous breathing effort. The supported breath cycles off if the pressure exceeds the preset level by 20 cm H_2O, when the flow reaches 5% of the peak flow, or at 80% of the SIMV period.

Alarms and Displays. The Servo 300 has an alphanumeric window that displays Alarms and Messages. Under the window are eight touchpad/light strips. If an alarm level is reached, an audible alarm sounds, a red LED flashes on the appropriate alarm strip, and a message is displayed in the window. A yellow LED indicates that the alarm has been overridden, or that a high priority alarm situation was corrected.

Alarms include: a battery alarm, indicating a power failure with a resultant switch to battery power; a gas supply alarm, triggered when inlet gas pressure is outside of the 29 to 94 psig range; the airway pressure alarm, which activates if the upper pressure limit is exceeded, or the airway pressure exceeds the set PEEP level plus 15 cm H_2O for more than 15 seconds; the oxygen concentration alarm, which activates if the measured FiO_2 falls above or below 6% of the set alarm value, or if the fuel cell is disconnected; the expiratory minute volume alarm, activated if the measured minute volume exceeds the set value, of if it falls below the default values (0.3 L/min for adults and children, 0.06 L/min for neonates); the apnea alarm, which is triggered if the time between spontaneous breaths exceeds 10 seconds for adults, 15 seconds for children, or 20 seconds for neonates; and the technical alarm, which usually indicates the need for servicing.

Other displays on the ventilator include: peak, mean, pause, and end expiratory pressures; frequency in breaths/min, breath cycle time in seconds, inspiratory period in seconds, and inspiratory flow in liters/second; tidal volume in milliliters, minute volume in liters/min; inspiratory tidal volume in milliliters, expiratory tidal volume in milliliters, and expiratory minute volume in liters/min; and oxygen concentration.

The Servo 300A is the same ventilator as the 300 except for one feature called *automode.* Automode is featured when two consecutive triggering efforts from the patient will shift the ventilator from a control mode to a support mode. The goal of automode is to increase patient comfort by decreasing the amount that the patient "fights" the ventilator. Another goal of automode is to accelerate weaning. To activate this feature, the clinician must turn the automode switch located in the upper right part of the control panel to the on position. When automode is activated, the pressure-regulated volume control mode will switch over to volume support. Pressure control will switch over to pressure support. Volume control will switch to volume support. Apnea time in automode is different when automode is activated. The patient range select knob defines apnea time. If the patient does not breathe spontaneously, the ventilator will audibly alarm and switch back to the control mode. The switch will be made after 12 secondes of apnea for adults, 8 seconds for pediatric patients, and 5 seconds for neonates.

VENTILATOR MONITORS

BEAR NVM-1 NEONATAL VOLUME MONITOR

Basic Mechanisms. The BEAR NVM-1 volume monitor (Figure 16–18) is a compact microprocessor controlled monitor of neonatal tidal volumes. The monitor utilizes a double hot wire *anemometer* for the sensor, which is placed inline between the endotracheal tube adapter and the ventilator connection.

The sensor head is available as a 4 cc deadspace universal adapter or as a 1.5 to 2.1 cc deadspace endotracheal tube adapter. The 1.5 cc deadspace is for the size 2.0 tube, and the 2.1 cc deadspace is for the 5.0 tube.

The monitor continuously displays the expiratory tidal volume, expiratory minute volume, and the respiratory frequency. Additional parameters that can be optionally selected and displayed are inspiratory tidal volume and percent tube leakage.

Alarms. The lower-limit minute ventilation alarm is enabled when the expired minute volume drops below the lower limit minute volume set limit. The upper-limit minute volume alarm triggers when the expired minute volume exceeds the set value.

The disconnection alarm indicates a disconnection of the sensor, extubation, or occlusion

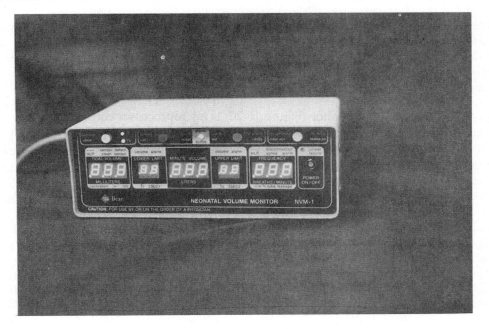

Figure 16–18 *The BEAR NVM-1 volume monitor. (Reproduced with permission from Bear Medical Systems, Inc., Riverside, CA)*

of the endotracheal tube. The sensor defect alarm detects damage to the sensor heating wires or sensor cable, or when the sensor head becomes disconnected from the sensor cable, or the sensor cable from the unit.

The clean sensor alarm indicates an excessive amount of water or contaminants on the sensor wires, requiring a recalibration and possible cleaning. The apnea alarm triggers when the monitor does not detect flow through the sensor for 8 to 20 seconds. The % tube leakage alarm indicates a possible increase in the amount of tube leakage, as determined by a change in expiratory minute volume and an increase in the % of tube leakage detected.

Whenever an alarm is violated, an audible alarm sounds, the green "alarm active" LED flashes, the breath average LED flashes, and all of the displayed parameters being blinking.

Calibration. The NVM-1 monitor is calibrated by occluding both ends of the sensor adapter while holding in the red calibration button. When calibration is complete, a beep is heard and the number 100 is displayed in the tidal volume window.

BIRD PARTNER VOLUME MONITOR

Basic Mechanisms. The Partner volume monitor (Figure 16–19) is designed to measure the exhaled volumes of neonatal, pediatric, and adult patients who are being mechanically ventilated. For each patient group, the monitor provides a sensor that is specifically designed to match the characteristics of the age group.

The Partner is microprocessor controlled and measures flows through a variable orifice differential pressure flow sensor. As the gas progresses through the sensor, it passes a variable flow element, which is located between two chambers in the sensor. A pressure difference is created between the two chambers by the flow element. The pressure differences in the chambers are measured and an *analog* signal is sent to the microprocessor, which then translates the flow into a volume. The expired volume is then displayed on the face of the monitor.

Because continuous flow through the sensor, which is present in many neonatal and pediatric applications, may affect the volume measurement, the monitor provides a continuous flow button which zeroes the flow measurement to the existing flow at the time the button is pushed. The monitor then measures only flows above the zero level as volumes.

The monitor continuously displays the tidal volume in ml, with the value being updated at the beginning of each breath. The monitor can display volumes from 0 to 9999 ml.

Inspiratory volumes can be measured when the infant sensor is used by placing it between the patient connection and the endotracheal tube. A button on the face of the monitor is then pressed to display the inspired volume in tidal volume display.

The breath rate is displayed continuously and is updated at the beginning of each breath. It is calculated on an eight-breath average. The range of breath rate is from 0 to 999 BPM.

Minute volume is continuously displayed and is calculated by multiplying the breath rate by the average tidal volume of the previous eight breaths. It is updated each breath and ranges from 0 to 99.9 liters.

When flow is detected by the monitor, a small LED is illuminated on the lower right cor-

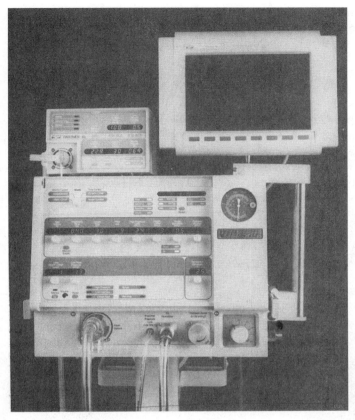

Figure 16–19 *The BIRD Partner volume monitor (seen on the left top of the V.I.P. ventilator). (Courtesy Bird Products Corporation, Palm Springs, CA)*

ner of the monitor. The minimum detectable flow for infants is 0.2 L/min, 2.0 L/min for pediatric patients, and 4.0 L/min for adults.

Alarms. The high breath alarm is set by the operator using the arrow keys below the display. The alarm is activated when the total breath rate exceeds the alarm setting. The range offered is from 0 to 999 BPM.

The low minute volume alarm is also set by the operator using the arrow keys below the display. The alarm is activated if the total minute volume does not exceed the alarm setting. The operator can select any minute volume between 0 and 99 L/min.

The silence/reset button deactivates the alarms for a period of 60 seconds. It is also used to reset the flashing displays of violated alarm settings.

An apnea interval alarm is located on the back panel of the monitor. When the switch is depressed, the current setting is displayed in the breath rate window. Depressing the switch increases the value by 5 seconds, from 10 seconds to a maximum of 60 seconds. The alarm is activated if the monitor fails to sense an inspiratory effort within the selected time interval.

A monitor inoperative alarm is activated in the event of a power failure or if a fault is detected during the power up self-test. A sensor alarm is activated if the monitor detects that the flow sensor is improperly installed.

SECHRIST AIRWAY PRESSURE MONITOR MODEL 400

Basic Mechanics. The Sechrist airway pressure monitor (Figure 16–20) is an electronic monitor that measures and displays several parameters. One window displays the parameter that is selected by the control knob.

The monitor can measure both mechanical breaths and spontaneous breaths. A mechanical breath is counted if it reaches 5 cm H_2O above the baseline pressure. In the CPAP mode, spontaneous breaths are counted if the patient creates at least a 1.5 cm H_2O deflection from baseline pressure.

The following parameters are also measured and can be selected for display: inspiratory time, duration of positive pressure, mean airway pressure, peak pressure (PIP), and baseline pressure (PEEP).

Alarms. The peak alarm limit is selected by the operator to be 5, 10, 15, or 20 cm H_2O above the PIP. The monitor automatically sets the desired alarm limit when it is armed. The mean alarm limit is set by the operator to be ±2 or ±5 and automatically fixed when the monitor

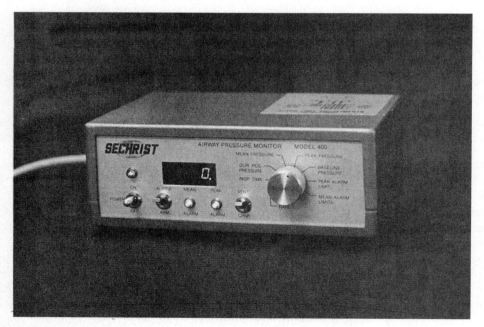

Figure 16–20 *The Sechrist airway pressure monitor, model 400. (Courtesy Sechrist Industries, Inc.)*

is armed. A disconnect alarm is also available and is activated if the monitor fails to detect a ventilator breath during four normal cycles.

Upon placement inline with a ventilator circuit, the operator arms the monitor by depressing the "arm" toggle switch. The monitor then analyzes the ventilatory pattern for 30 seconds, at which point it determines the "normal" pressure and sets the appropriate alarm limits. The alarm limits are set by the operator using a series of toggle switches on the back of the monitor.

SECHRIST AIRWAY PRESSURE MONITOR MODEL 600

Basic Mechanics. The Sechrist model 600 (Figure 16–21) is an advanced pressure monitor designed to be used with the Sechrist IV-100B ventilator. The monitor measures and displays the breath rate up to 2000 BPM, I:E ratio, duration of positive pressure, rise time (the slope of the inspiratory pressure curve), PIP, MAP, and base pressure (PEEP/CPAP).

The measurement of rise time by the model 600 alerts the operator to changes in patient compliance and resistance by measuring the slope of the upward inspiratory curve. As compliance and resistance change, the upward slope of the curve changes and is detected by the monitor. The operator sets the rest time between ±10% to ±90% in ±5% increments. If the rest time changes beyond the set limit, the alarm is activated.

The monitor also integrates with the IV-100B ventilator to provide a vent to ambient pres-

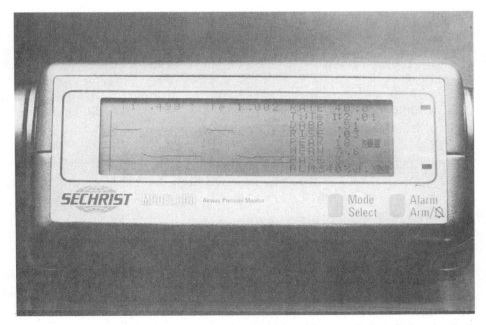

Figure 16–21 *The Sechrist airway pressure monitor, model 600. (Courtesy Sechrist Industries, Inc.)*

sure in the event of an accidental overpressure. A computer interface allows the data from the monitor to be fed to a computer to generate continuous data collection.

The monitor automatically sets several alarm limits. The peak pressure limit is set 10 cm H_2O above the recorded PIP. Low inspiratory pressure is set at a level of 5 cm H_2O below the PIP. A fail-to-cycle alarm is activated if the pressure difference between PIP and PEEP decreases to 0 cm H_2O.

SUMMARY

As technology develops, new ventilators have also been developed incorporating modes of ventilation that have greatly improved the ability to ventilate with less risk and side effects. The advent of microtechnology has allowed neonatal ventilators to enter the realm of synchronization, which may reduce the risk of barotrauma and "fighting" the ventilator.

New ventilators enter the market with new ventilatory modes and advances, requiring a sound understanding of basic ventilatory techniques by the practitioner. Before working with any ventilator, the practitioner must become familiar with all aspects of the ventilator before applying it to a patient. Many of the new generation ventilators were preceded by earlier versions and maintain many of the characteristics of the original. Examples include the BEAR Cub ventilator and the BP 200, the Sechrist IV-200 and the IV-100, and the Siemens Servo 300 and the Servo 900. Other new generation ventilators are relative newcomers to the market and include the Infant Star and the Hamilton Veolar. Others, like the V.I.P. Bird, had predecessors, but have few of the original characteristics.

The use of fluidic valves, as seen in the Bio-Med MVP-10, and Sechrist ventilators, demonstrates the incorporation of physics into ventilator design, making them more reliable and less likely to break down.

The advent of microprocessors has also brought about the ability to closely and accurately measure and display airway pressures, inspiratory and expiratory times, and flow patterns. This allows the practitioner to fine-tune the ventilator settings to the specific needs of the patient. Additionally, the risk of barotrauma and other deleterious side effects is reduced.

References

1. Visveshware, N. et al., "Patient-triggered synchronized assisted ventilation of newborns: Report of a preliminary study and three years' experience" *J. Perinatol* 11(4):347 54 (1991).

2. Donn, S. M., Sinha, S. K., *Manual of Neonatal Respiratory Care.* Armonk, NY: Futura, 2000.

Bibliography and Suggested Readings

BEAR Cub Infant Ventilator instruction manual. Bear Medical Systems, Inc., Riverside, CA.

Bio-Med MVP-10 Pediatric/Neonatal Ventilator instruction manual. Bio-Med Devices Inc., Stamford, CT.

Branson, R. D., Hess, D. R., and Chatburn, R. L. *Respiratory Care Equipment.* Philadelphia: J. B. Lippincott Co., 1999.

Infant Star Neonatal Ventilator operating instructions. Nellcor-Puritan Bennkt, Pleasanton, CA. 1997.

Newport Breeze Ventilator operating manual. Newport Medical Instruments, Inc., Newport Beach, CA. 1991.

Partner Volume Monitor instruction manual. Bird Products Corporation, Palm Springs, CA. 1990.

Sechrist Airway Pressure Monitor, Models 400 and 600 operational instructions. Sechrist Industries, Inc., Anaheim, CA.

V.I.P. Bird Infant-Pediatric Ventilator instruction manual. Bird Products Corporation, Palm Springs, CA. 1990.

Posttest

1. The PEEP adjustment on the Babybird ventilator is located:
   a. on the face of the ventilator
   b. on the rear of the ventilator
   c. on the inspiratory line
   d. on the expiratory valve.
2. Which of the following is TRUE regarding the Babybird 2 ventilator?
   a. The patient can be ventilated in the event of a power failure using the manual inspiration button.
   b. The ventilator is both pneumatically powered and controlled.
   c. The ventilator is capable of delivering rates only up to 120/min.
   d. The ventilator has a built-in power backup.
3. While using the V.I.P. Bird ventilator, the "vent inop" alarm is activated. Which of the problems is a possible cause of the alarm?
   a. The respiratory rate has exceeded the set limit.
   b. The incoming oxygen pressure has dropped below 22.5 PSIG.
   c. The high-pressure setting has been violated.
   d. The ventilator has detected a leak in the system.
4. Of the following, which would make the best transport ventilator?
   a. BEAR Cub
   b. Bio-Med MVP-10
   c. Siemens Servo 900C
5. When using the Bio-Med MVP-10 at an oaygen flow of 6 L/min and an airflow of 7 L/min, which of the following represents the correct FiO_2.
   a. 0.26

    b. 0.38

    c. 0.57

    d. 0.77

6. Proper function of the BEAR Cub pneumatic control system requires which of the following?

    a. calibration at least every 24 hours

    b. an I:E ratio of at least 1:1

    c. the use of 3/16″ proximal airway pressure tubing

    d. proper setting of the pneumatic limits

7. Which of the following *best* describes the MMV mode of ventilation when using the Hamilton Veolar ventilator?

    a. MMV is basically spontaneous breathing with the addition of pressure support.

    b. MMV is not available on the Veolar ventilator.

    c. MMV is another term for controlled ventilation.

    d. MMV is only available with the addition of the MMV module.

8. When using the Infant Star ventilator, which of the following alarms would indicate a blocked inspiratory tube?

    a. A02

    b. A03

    c. A04

    d. A05

9. While monitoring a patient on a Newport Breeze ventilator, the practitioner notices the pressure manometer is pulled below 0 on each spontaneous breath. This indicates which of the following?

    a. The FLOW setting is too high.

    b. The tidal volume is too high.

    c. The PEEP level is not adjusted properly.

    d. The trigger level is set inappropriately.

10. Which of the following ventilators has the option of providing a sine-wave inspiratory flow pattern?

    a. BEAR Cub

    b. BabyBird 2

    c. Sechrist IV-100

    d. Healthdyne 105.

11. While using the Sechrist IV-200 SAVI system, the practitioner notes that while the patient is breathing spontaneously, the ventilator is not synchronized to the patient's breaths. Which of the following is the most likely source of the problem?

    a. The mode selector has not been switched to SAVI.

    b. The PEEP/CPAP level is too high.

    c. The PIP is set too low.

    d. The sensitivity is improperly set.

12. While working with a patient on a Servo 900C ventilator, the physician asks for the actual flow rate. The settings are:

set minute volume = 3.6 liters

set breath rate = 15
Inspiratory time % = 33%
Pause time % = 5%
The actual flow rate for this patient is:
  a. 11 L/min
  b. 13 L/min
  c. 15 L/min
  d. 17 L/min
13. A patient is being ventilated on a Servo 300 ventilator. While doing a ventilator check, you are asked to provide the set tidal volume. Which of the following formulas would you use?
  a. Minute volume/inspiratory time
  b. Minute volume/CMV frequency
  c. Inspiratory time × % pause time
  d. Inspiratory rise time/total breath cycle time
14. Which of the following monitors is able to measure tidal volumes?
  a. Novametric Pneumogard 1230A
  b. BEAR PM 200
  c. Sechrist Airway Pressure Monitor Model 400
  d. BEAR NVM-1
15. Which of the following statements *best* describes the function of the continuous flow button on the Partner volume monitor?
  a. It allows the monitor to measure volumes even when continuous flow is present.
  b. It allows the measurement of inspiratory volumes.
  c. It prevents a backward flow of gas through the sensor.
  d. It provides a continuous flow of gas through the sensor to eliminate moisture buildup.
16. An increase in the rise time, as displayed on a Sechrist Model 600 airway pressure monitor, indicates which of the following?
  a. The flow rate is inappropriate set.
  b. The breath rate is incompatible with the inspiratory rate.
  c. The compliance or resistance has changed.
  d. The PEEP level is set too low.
17. In the V.I.P. BIRD Gold, what rest time setting will result in the fastest delivery of flow?
  a. 1
  b. 7
  c. 5
  d. 3
18. What differentiates pressure control ventilation from TCPL in the V.I.P. BIRD Gold?
  a. variable flow rate
  b. no termination sensitivity
  c. both a and b
  d. none of the above

19. Rate-volume ratio, a measurement used for weaning, is calculated by which ventilator?
    a. Servo 300A
    b. Infant Star 950
    c. Drager Babylog 8000-Plus
    d. Bird V.I.P. Gold

20. In the Pressure Regulated Volume Control mode on Servo 300/300A, the initial test breath is delivered at how many cm H_2O.
    a. 5
    b. 10
    c. 7
    d. PRVC mode does not deliver a test breath.

CHAPTER SEVENTEEN

SPECIAL PROCEDURES AND NONCONVENTIONAL VENTILATORY TECHNIQUES

OBJECTIVES

Upon completion of this chapter, the reader should be able to:

1. Describe each of the following, as they relate to surfactant replacement therapy.
   a. History
   b. Indications
   c. Administration techniques
   d. Outcomes
2. Identify the major advantage of HFV.
3. Describe, for each of the three types of HFV, the following:
   a. Rates of ventilation
   b. Indications
   c. Clinical uses
   d. Hazards
4. Explain why a conventional ventilator is used in conjunction with HFJV and HFO.
5. Discuss the two theories of gas flow characteristics that are associated with HFJV and HFO.
6. Describe the mechanisms of action of inhaled nitric oxide and its role in treatment of the newborn and pediatric patient in respiratory failure.
7. Describe the basic components of inhaled nitric oxide delivery.
8. Discuss the safety of inhaled nitric oxide and possible adverse effects of its use.
9. Discuss the use of heliox for pediatric patients with airflow obstruction.
10. Describe each of the following as they relate to ECLS:
    a. History
    b. Venoarterial vs. venovenuous bypass
    c. Components of the ECLS circuit
    d. Use of mechanical ventilation during ECLS
11. Identify methods used for selecting patients for ECLS and recognize those for which ECLS is contraindicated.

12. Describe how ECLS is initiated, the indications for termination, and the complications associated with its use.
13. Discuss each of the following, as they relate to negative pressure ventilation:
    a. History
    b. Methods of delivery
    c. Current uses
    d. Advantages and disadvantages
14. Briefly describe the history and use of partial liquid ventilation.

KEY TERMS

air leak syndrome	methemoglobinemia	thrombocytopenia
amplitude	necrotizing tracheobronchitis	venoarterial
DPPC	phospholipid	venovenous
frequency		

INTRODUCTION

In addition to conventional methods of treating the critically ill newborn or pediatric patient, adjunct therapy may involve nontraditional methods of resuscitation and ventilation. These special procedures include surfactant replacement therapy (SRT), high-frequency ventilation (HFV), special medical gas administration, extracorporeal life support (ECLS), partial liquid ventilation (PLV), and negative pressure ventilation. Although considered nontraditional, these special procedures are playing a role in neonatal and pediatric care in the critical care unit and are becoming increasingly routine.

SURFACTANT REPLACEMENT THERAPY

It has long been understood that primary dysfunction in RDS is abnormal alveolar surface forces resulting from a lack of surfactant. It therefore became an item of major interest in the scientific community to develop a surfactant that could be administered to an infant, to replace that which was lacking. Naturally occurring surfactant is composed of several phospholipids and lipids, and four or more specific apoproteins. It appears as though each component may have its own distinct characteristics with regard to production, secretion, and removal.[1] These factors have made it difficult to produce an ideal replacement surfactant.

Approximately 90% of surfactant is phospholipid, with phosphatidylcholine (PC) comprising 85% of the total. Roughly 60% of the PC is dipalmitoyl phosphatidylcholine (DPPC). It is the DPPC that allows surfactant to lower surface tension.[2] The remaining phospholipids are phosphatidylglycerol (PG) and phosphatidylinositol (PI). Cholesterol is the predominant neutral lipid in surfactant. The four proteins found in surfactant, given the names of surfactant proteins A, B, C, and D (SP-A, etc.), make up 5 to 10% of the total. Although small in quantity, their presence is essential for proper activity of pulmonary surfactant.[2]

Early studies were discouraging because researchers could not find the right combination of components that formed a useful surfactant. Dosages and method of delivery also inhibited the usefulness of surfactant replacement.

Early surfactants were made with DPPC and were nebulized into the trachea. This type of surfactant alone and method of delivery did not produce the desired results. Continued research and later studies of surfactant and its biochemical and biophysical properties illustrated the important role of the other proteins and lipids. New surfactants were developed that included the additional lipids and proteins. Delivery was changed from nebulization to direct instillation of the surfactant into the patient trachea at higher dosages than had previously been used.

The release of surfactant for use in the United States in 1990 has had a dramatic effect on perinatal mortality and morbidity; its use in the treatment of lung injury beyond the neonatal period, now being studied, holds similar promise.[3]

INDICATIONS

There are currently two protocols for the administration of surfactant during the neonatal period. Prophylactic administration of surfactant is indicated for those infants who are at a high risk of developing RDS. Included are those infants born before 32 weeks, weigh less than 1300 grams, those with an L/S ratio less than 2:1, or the absence of PG in the amniotic fluid. Under this protocol, the infant receives the surfactant as quickly as possible, following delivery. Therapeutic administration (also called rescue) is not given until the patient develops signs of RDS. Indications include those infants who require ventilatory assistance due to an increased work of breathing (grunting, nasal flaring, retractions), increasing oxygen requirements, and have chest x-ray evidence of RDS.[4] SRT has also been effective in other causes of respiratory failure in the newborn, such as pneumonia and meconium aspiration syndrome.[5]

The indications for surfactant use for the pediatric patient in respiratory failure are not as well established. Unlike RDS in infants where surfactant is lacking, the role that surfactant deficiency or inactivation plays in the child with acute lung injury is unclear. SRT for the child with acute hypoxemic respiratory failure may therefore be indicated when current therapy, which includes mechanical ventilator support and treatment of the underlying cause, has failed to yield positive results. Although SRT may not reverse the lung injury, it has been shown to improve lung volumes by stabilizing alveoli and increasing compliance and oxygenation.[6]

TYPES OF SURFACTANT

Currently used surfactants fall into two categories: those obtained from mammalian lungs and those that are synthetically produced. Mammalian preparations typically contain all surfactant proteins, but the proportions of their active ingredients are different. Varying the amount of cholesterol, free fatty acids and total phospholipids has been shown to vary the biophysical activity of these surfactant preparations.[7] Additionally, the absorption of lung surfactant is largely controlled by surfactant proteins. Synthetically produced preparations that are protein free contain detergent-like substances that act as spreading agents to enhance disbursement and thus absorption. The difference in relative components of lipids and proteins in exogenous surfactants varies the amount of surface activity from each commercially marketed surfactant.[8] (Refer to Table 17–1).

OUTCOMES

There are several reported adverse reactions associated with dosing procedures during SRT. The most common are usually transient with full recovery. Adverse effects can include bradycardia, oxygen desaturation, and ETT reflux. The infant must be monitored during the dosing procedure and appropriate action taken should any of these adverse effects occur. Because SRT can significantly affect oxygenation and lung compliance, the infant must be closely monitored after administration. Improvement in oxygenation may require reduction in the oxygen concentration, and improvement in lung compliance may require a reduction in ventilator pressures.[9]

On the positive side, SRT has been shown to reduce the severity of RDS, pulmonary air leaks, and the development of BPD.[7] When used in conjunction with other special procedures such as high-frequency oscillatory ventilation[10] and inhaled nitric oxide,[11] SRT has shown significant clinical improvement. SRT in the pediatric population has been shown to improve pulmonary dynamic compliance and stabilize gas exchange[12] and reduce the length of ventilatory support and lead to earlier PICU discharge.[13]

Since coming of age, SRT has dramatically decreased mortality and morbidity rates in RDS[3] and has become the standard of care for neonates with RDS.

HIGH-FREQUENCY VENTILATION (HFV)

The normally held understanding of ventilation is that the tidal volume must exceed the amount of physiologic dead space for alveolar ventilation to occur. Conventional ventilation utilizes this principle by inflating the patient's lungs with a tidal volume that exceeds dead space and inflates the alveoli. Expiration then occurs by the passive recoil of the thorax and lung.

HFV is a technique of ventilation that delivers small tidal volumes at very high respiratory rates. According to the FDA, HFV is any form of mechanical ventilation that delivers

TABLE 17–1 COMPARISON OF EXOGENOUS SURFACTANTS

	EXOSURF	SURVANTA	INFASURF	CUROSURF
Source	Synthetic	Calf lung	Calf lung	Pig lung
Proteins	—	SP-B, C	SP-B, C	SP-B, C
Phospholipids	13 mg/ml	25 mg/ml	35 mg/ml	80 mg/ml
Dosage/birth wt.	5 ml/kg	4 ml/kg	3 ml/kg	2.5 ml/kg

respiratory rates that are greater than 150 per minute. High-frequency rates are expressed in hertz (Hz), where 1 Hz is equal to 60 cycles per minute or one cycle per second. Amplitude refers to peak-to-peak pressures or the difference between peak inspiratory pressure (PIP) and positive end-expiratory pressure (PEEP). Oxygenation is primarily controlled by adjusting the mean airway pressure, whereas carbon dioxide removal is a result of the amplitude pressure.

Conventional ventilation that depends on the bulk movement of gas in and out of the lungs may require high pressures and volumes in order to achieve adequate oxygenation and ventilation. These high pressures and volumes have been known to contribute to barotrauma and the development of BPD in neonates. Early studies involving HFV showed that adequate ventilation occurred even when tidal volumes far below dead space were used.[14]

The major advantage of delivering small tidal volumes is that it can be done at relatively low pressures, greatly reducing the risk of barotrauma.

INDICATIONS

The indications for any type of HFV in the neonatal population are primarily linked to respiratory failure that does not respond to conventional methods of mechanical ventilation. These infants usually have further complications such as pulmonary air leaks or persistent pulmonary hypertension that would be exacerbated by positive pressure ventilation.[15] High-frequency oscillatory ventilation (HFOV) has been shown to be a safe and effective rescue technique in treating patients who have failed conventional ventilation,[16] in newborns with congenital diaphragmatic hernia,[17] and in neonates with RDS or air leak syndrome.[18]

The benefits of HFV for the pediatric population are becoming more apparent. A study by Arnold demonstrated that HFOV offered rapid and sustained improvements in oxygenation without adverse effects on ventilation in patients with diffuse alveolar disease or air leak syndrome.[19] Other studies have reported decreased mortality in pediatric patients with ARDS as a result of HFV.[20]

HAZARDS

As with any method of mechanical ventilation, there are problems associated with HFV as well. HFV has been known to cause gas trapping, hyperinflation, obstruction of the airway with secretions, hypotension, and necrotizing tracheobronchitis.[21,22] Furthermore, chest assessment of patients on HFV is difficult. Assessment for adequate ventilation is based on chest wall vibration rather than chest rise and fall. A decrease in chest wall vibration with an increased $PaCO_2$ without a decrease in PaO_2 may indicate an obstruction or malposition of the ETT. Decreased lung compliance and pneumothoraces are observed by a decrease in chest wall vibration, increase in $PaCO_2$ and a decrease in PaO_2. The infant should be assessed for signs of pallor, cyanosis, bradycardia, hypotension, and increased respiratory effort, all of which indicate a worsening of status.

TYPES OF HIGH-FREQUENCY VENTILATORS

High-frequency ventilators deliver rates between 150 and 3000 BPM. The major types of HFV are categorized by the frequency of ventilation and the method with which the tidal volume is delivered. The four categories examined here are high-frequency positive pressure ventilation (HFPPV), high flow jet ventilation (HFJV), high-frequency flow interruption (HFFI), and high-frequency oscillatory ventilation (HFOV) (Table 17–2).

High-Frequency Positive Pressure Ventilation (HFPPV). HFPPV is simply conventional ventilatory breaths delivered at rates between 60 and 150 BPM (1 to 2.5 Hz). The delivery of tidal volume during HFPPV occurs via convective air movement, in which tidal volume exceeds dead space. Studies have shown a reduction in $PaCO_2$ and in FiO_2 when HFPPV was used. These studies additionally showed a lower rate of pneumothoraces in the neonates ventilated with HFPPV when compared to those receiving conventional ventilation.[15] Other studies have shown that fighting the ventilator by the neonate may be eliminated at ventilatory rates of 100 to 120 BPM.

High-Frequency Flow Interruption. High-frequency flow interruption (HFFI) can deliver frequencies as high as 15 Hz. In this type of HFV a control mechanism, usually a rotating ball with a gas pathway, interrupts a high-pressure gas source in order to deliver rapid rates. As with HFPPV and HFJV, exhalation occurs passively.

High-Frequency Jet Ventilation (HFJV). High-frequency jet ventilators generally operate in the range of 4 to 11 Hz. The high-frequency jet ventilator delivers a high-pressure pulse of gas to the patient airway. This is done through a special adaptor attached to the endotracheal tube, or through a specially designed endotracheal tube that allows the pulsed gas to exit inside the endotracheal tube, depicted in Figure 17–1.

HFJV is used in tandem with conventional ventilators. The purpose of the conventional ventilator is threefold. First, it provides occasional sighs, which help stimulate the production of surfactant and prevent microatelectasis. Second, the conventional ventilator provides PEEP to the patient airway. Third, it makes a continuous flow of gas available at the endotracheal tube for entrainment by the jet ventilation.[21]

High-Frequency Oscillatory Ventilation (HFOV). HFOV utilizes the highest of rates, usually in the range of 8 to 30 Hz. The oscillatory waves that deliver the gas to the lungs are produced by either an electromagnetically driven piston pump (Figure 17–2) or a loudspeaker. These oscillatory waves produce a vibration or shaking motion of the infant's chest

TABLE 17–2 Classification of High-Frequency Ventilation

MODE	FREQUENCY
HFPPV	1–2.5 Hz
HFJV	4–11 Hz
HFFI	15 Hz
HFOV	8–30 Hz

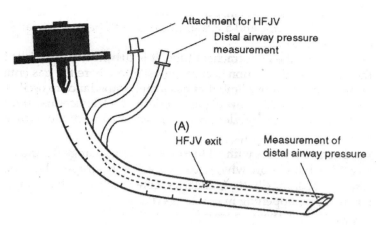

Figure 17-1 *Endotracheal tube adapted for use with high-frequency jet ventilation. The pulsed jet flow exits into the endotracheal tube at point A.*

that should be observed to verify adequate amplitude and thus gas delivery. HFOV is the most widely used method of HFV. It does not require a specialized endotracheal tube or conventional ventilation in tandem with the oscillator.

A unique feature of HFOV is that it produces a positive as well as a negative stroke, which assists both inspiration and exhalation. During exhalation gas is actively "pulled-out" of the lungs; there is active exhalation. Other forms of HFV simply rely on recoil of the lungs and the chest wall to eliminate the gas; exhalation in this case is therefore passive.

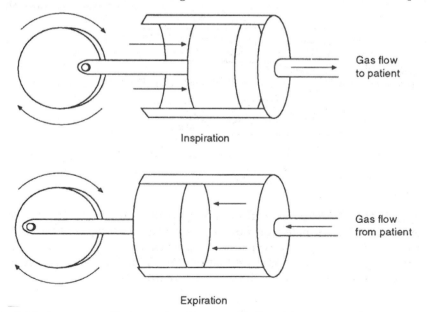

Figure 17-2 *High-frequency oscillation produced by an oscillating piston.*

The HFOV device is placed inline with the endotracheal tube, and a gas source is passed perpendicular to the tube, as illustrated in Figure 17–3. As the fresh gas enters the endotracheal tube, it is driven to the patient by the waves coming from the oscillator. Expiration occurs opposite to where the gas enters the endotracheal tube through an expiratory limb that has a high impedance to oscillations, but low impedance when there is a steady flow of gas. Marked swings in pressure between inspiration and expiration to reopen alveoli do not occur during HFOV because the alveoli remain open continuously.

SPECIALTY MEDICAL GASES

In addition to oxygen, the administration of other medical gases such as nitric oxide and helium are becoming more popular in respiratory care. Nitric oxide has shown great promise in the treatment of neonates with pulmonary hypertension, while helium has proven its value in severe airway obstructions.

INHALED NITRIC OXIDE (I-NO)

Nitric oxide (NO) is a colorless gas that is produced in endothelial cells of the body. In 1987 Palmer and colleagues discovered that NO diffuses from the endothelium into smooth muscle cells that form the vascular walls and is responsible for vascular dilation.[24] NO relaxes vascular smooth muscle by activating guanylate cyclase and increasing the levels of cyclic guanosine 3', 5'-monophosphate (cGMP), which causes vasodilation. In 1991 Frostell and coworkers gave experimental proof that when inhaled, NO mimics the effect of naturally released NO and selectively produces pulmonary vasodilation.[25] The pharmacological effect is an increase in oxygenation tension due to dilation of pulmonary vessels in better ventilated areas of the lung.[26]

NO for inhalation is supplied as a gaseous blend of 0.8% NO and 99.2% nitrogen (N_2).

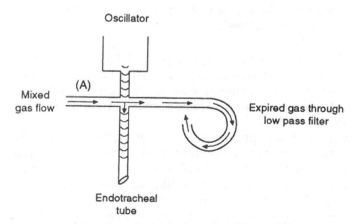

Oscillator

(A)

Mixed
gas flow

Expired gas through
low pass filter

Endotracheal
tube

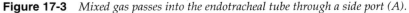

Figure 17-3 *Mixed gas passes into the endotracheal tube through a side port (A).*

The recommended does of I-NO is 20 ppm (parts per million) in conjunction with oxygen. Administration of I-NO through a system, such as the INOvent Delivery System provides consistent concentrations of NO throughout the respiration cycle with continuous monitoring of NO, nitric oxide (NO_2), and oxygen concentrations.[27]

Indications. I-NO is indicated when a deficiency occurs in the body's ability to produce its own NO. This can be a direct result of illness or injury, which causes hypoxic respiratory failure. Conditions such as PPHN, RDS, MAS, pneumonia, sepsis, and congenital diaphragmatic hernia have been shown to respond favorably to I-NO, by either reduction in the incidence of death or reduction in the need for extracorporeal membrane oxygenation.[28] In a study by Kinsella, it was found that the greatest improvement in oxygenation occurred when I-NO was combined with HFOV.[29] It was speculated that improved lung inflation during HFOV may augment the response to I-NO by decreasing intrapulmonary shunting and improving I-NO delivery to the pulmonary circulation.[29]

The use of NO for the pediatric population is currently being evaluated. Several studies have indicated that I-NO may be a therapeutic alternative for bronchodilation.[30, 31] Other studies are investigating the role of NO in pediatric ARDS with promising results.[32] I-NO in pediatric ARDS appears to improve oxygenation and lower mechanical ventilation support and lessen complications.[31]

Outcomes. Positive outcomes require that the patient be monitored for methemoglobinemia and nitrogen dioxide (NO_2). Methemoglobinemia results when NO comes into contact with blood and binds with the hemoglobin to form nitrosylhemoglobin (NOHb). The presence of oxygen causes nitrosylhemoglobin to become oxidized, forming methemoglobin and NO_2. Once the NO_2 is excreted in the urine, methemoglobin is enzymatically reduced to hemoglobin again. NO_2 levels should not exceed 5 ppm by Occupational Safety and Health Administration (OSHA) standards. Clinically, the goal is to maintain NO_2 levels below 2 ppm during NO administration. This requires accurate and continuous monitoring of NO_2 production. Without accurate monitoring of delivered I-NO and NO_2 production, the patient may develop pulmonary edema, injury, and death.[33]

Care must be taken in the withdrawal of I-NO. A sudden withdrawal of I-NO may cause a rebound effect, resulting in pulmonary hypertension and hypoxemia.[34] Recommended guidelines are that, first, the lowest effective I-NO dose, often less than 10 ppm, be used. Withdrawal should not be considered until the patient shows marked clinical improvement; the patient should be hemodynamically stable on an FiO_2 less than .40 with a PEEP of 5 cm H_2O or less. If the patient meets these criteria the next recommended step is to increase the FiO_2 to .60 to .70 before withdrawal of I-NO and prepare to support the patient hemodynamically if necessary. I-NO withdrawal has been well tolerated when these guidelines are followed.[34]

HELIOX THERAPY

Helium (He) and oxygen (O_2) mixtures have been used therapeutically since as early as the 1930s. Because of helium's known low density and its inert property, it makes it an ideal gas to mix with oxygen to reduce both turbulence in airflow and resistive pressure in the airways. The therapeutic result is reduction in airway resistance and respiratory muscle work. Delivery of O_2 as well as medicated aerosols can therefore be enhanced when He is used in place of nitrogen.

Indications. The primary indication for heliox therapy is during any clinical situation where airway obstruction prevents or significantly impedes the delivery of gas flow throughout the airways. Clinically, this can be seen during severe bronchospasm or upper airway obstruction due to infection or foreign body aspiration. This may include infants and children with severe asthma, laryngotracheobronchitis, or postextubation stridor.

Heliox can be delivered in 60:40 to 75:25 blends of He and O_2, depending on the patient's FiO_2 needs. However, as the amount of O_2 increases in the mixture, above 30%, the less the benefit in reducing airway resistance.[35] Heliox can be delivered by a nonrebreather face mask to nonintubated patients or directly to a mechanical ventilator in cases requiring intubation and ventilatory support. Heliox can also be used to power pneumatic nebulizers when aerosolized medication delivery is indicated.

Outcomes. Patients treated with heliox therapy during severe asthma showed improvement in $PaCO_2$, pH, increased peak expiratory flow rates, and reduction in the work of breathing. Intubated and mechanically ventilated patients with severe bronchospasm showed reduction in peak inspiratory pressures and $PaCO_2$. All patients on heliox therapy should be monitored for oxygenation either by pulse oximetry or arterial blood gas analysis.

EXTRACORPOREAL LIFE SUPPORT (ECLS)

Oxygenation of blood outside the body, through a membrane oxygenator, was first developed for use in open heart surgery in the 1950s. The technology continued to improve and modifications allowed the long-term use of the technique in the 1960s.[14]

The first use of the extracorporeal membrane oxygenator on an infant was described in 1971.[36] This paved the way for science to perfect and refine the technique used today in many institutions across the country.

Because of the potential risks associated with ELCS, selection is based on strict criteria and only those infants who are at an 80% or greater risk of mortality should be treated with ECLS. Several authors have proposed the use of the alveolar-arterial oxygen difference $P(A-a)O_2$ or the oxygen index (OI) to determine selection of infants for ECLS. Furthermore, it is recommended that infants at a gestational age less than 35 weeks and those with pre-existing intraventricular hemorrhage (IVH) be excluded. ECLS candidates are also excluded in some institutions if they have been managed with conventional mechanical ventilation (CMV) for as little as 7 days. Bower and Petit report success of these long-term CMV infants diagnosed with bronchopulmonary dysplasia (BPD).[18] (See Table 17–3.)

MECHANISMS OF BYPASS

There are two types of ECLS procedures: venoarterial and venovenous.

TABLE 17–3   RECOMMENDED CRITERIA FOR ECLS

Include infants with:
    A-a difference: >620 torr for 6–12 hours
    Oxygen Index: >40 for 1–6 hours
Exclude infants with:
    Gestational Age: <35 weeks
    Pre-existing Conditions: Intraventricular hemorrhage
                        Conventional ventilaton >7 days

Venoarterial. In the venoarterial route, blood is drawn from the right atrium via the internal jugular vein. The oxygenated blood is returned to the aortic arch via the right common carotid artery, as shown in Figure 17–4. Venoarterial ECLS not only oxygenates the blood, but also supports the cardiac function of the patient.

Venovenous. In the venovenous route, blood is removed from the right atrium via a catheter inserted in the right internal jugular vein. The oxygenated blood is returned to the right atrium through a catheter inserted via the femoral vein. This method oxygenates the blood, but does not support cardiac output.

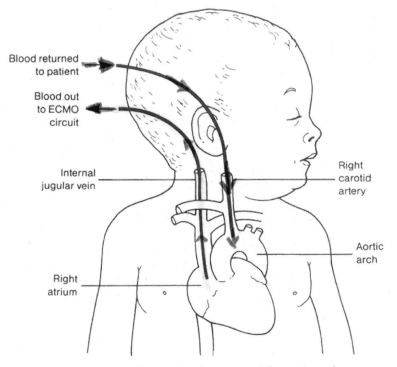

Figure 17-4   *Placement of ECLS catheter when the venoarterial route is used.*

ECLS Circuit. The ECLS circuit utilizes a modified heart-lung bypass machine consisting of a venous-blood drainage reservoir, a blood pump, the membrane oxygenator where the exchange of O_2 and CO_2 takes place, and a heat exchanger to maintain temperature. Figure 17–5 depicts a typical ECLS circuit.

COMPLICATIONS

Complications of ECLS are both technical and physiologic. Common physiologic complications of ECLS are those related to bleeding, secondary to the high level of heparin required for anticoagulation.[37] Cardiovascular complications arise from hypo- and hypervolemia leading to hypo- and hypertension in the infant. Anemia, leukopenia, and thrombocytopenia are all possible hematologic complications caused by the consumption of blood components by the membrane oxygenator.[14] Due to the invasive nature of ECLS, there is also an increased risk of infection.

Technical complications that may arise during ECLS include failure of the pump, rupture of the tubing, failure of the membrane, and difficulties with the cannuls.[38]

Outcomes. The use of ECLS has added an important tool in the care of patients who previously had no hope. As of October 1994, 9663 neonates had been treated with ECLS with an overall survival rate of 81%, while 845 pediatric patients were treated with a survival rate of 51%.[18] The survival rate appears to be related to the severity of lung disease and to the occurrence of ECLS complications, not the length of time on ECLS.[39]

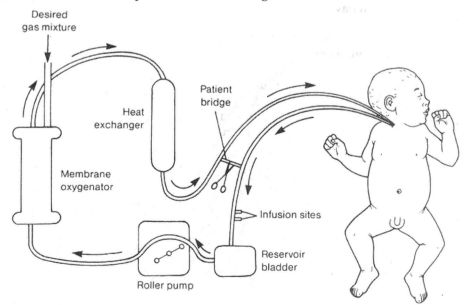

Figure 17-5 *A typical ECLS circuit.*

Due to the invasive nature of the procedure and severity of disease, the outcome of surviving patients may involve serious, long-term problems. Problems such as cerebral palsy, visual and hearing loss, seizures, and severe cognitive disabilities were seen in a higher percentage of ECLS patients than those treated conventionally.[40] Impairment of renal function and marked fluid retention appear to be unique complications when the venovenous route of ECLS is used.[41]

The need for ECLS has declined in patients managed with SRT and HFOV. Furthermore, the use of I-NO may also reduce the use of ECLS in patients with PPHN. Despite this decline, ECLS remains an important life support option for a very select group of critically ill infants.

PARTIAL LIQUID VENTILATION (PLV)

An exciting technology in the area of neonatal ventilation is partial liquid ventilation (PLV). Although not a new concept, the ability to successfully utilize this technology has only recently been developed. The concept behind liquid ventilation is to obliterate the air/liquid interface at the alveoli and thus substantially lower surface tension. Mechanical inflation could then occur at pressures low enough to not damage lung tissues.

Many substances have been used through the years. In the first experiments, saline was used. It proved, however, to be a poor carrier of oxygen and was too viscous and dense when compared to gas. Other substances, such as oils and silicone, which have a high capacity to carry gases, proved to be toxic to the lungs. Perfluorochemical (PFC) liquids are the first substances that have been shown to support respiration while remaining relatively nontoxic to the lungs.

PFCs have a very high solubility for oxygen and carbon dioxide, and minimize pulmonary surface tension. They are inert, odorless, clear liquids derived from common organic compounds.[42]

PLV with perfluorocarbon liquid occurs by using the liquid to recruit atelectatic lung and reduce surface tension in the alveolar lining. During exhalation the liquid acts as a reservoir of oxygen, preventing alveolar collapse and intrapulmonary shunting. With the next inspiration, tidal volume gas removes carbon dioxide from the liquid and replenishes it with a new supply of dissolved oxygen.

USES

PLV has potential application for use in several diseases that traditionally have been difficult to treat. Included are RDS, aspiration syndromes, persistent pulmonary hypertension of the newborn, and pneumonia.[42] PLV has been shown to improve pulmonary gas exchange, lung compliance, and reduce lung injury.[43] PLV has been shown to be compatible with surfactant administration, and may even be superior to surfactant.[44]

Clinical trials with perflubron (LiquiVent) in infants with RDS have shown a decrease in mortality rates as well as physiologic improvements in gas exchange and lung compliance.

While the potential of a favorable impact on the treatment of neonates is nearer, more research is still necessary before PLV takes its place among current treatment modalities.

NEGATIVE PRESSURE VENTILATION (NPV)

Although not technically a "new" concept in ventilation, NPV continues to draw interest as a method of ventilation. NPV utilized the application of negative pressure to the external thorax, causing the thorax to expand. The negative pressure generated within the thorax then causes air to enter the lungs (Figure 17–6). Because it mimics normal spontaneous breathing patterns, cardiopulmonary complications that result from positive pressure are not seen.

The concept of NPV was the primary factor that led to the development of the Drinker iron lung in 1928. Researchers have subsequently scaled the iron lung down to allow the technique to be used on infants. Even with some initial success, NPV was never accepted as an alternative to PPV, possibly due to the inconvenience created by limited access to the infant as well as limited success on the infant with severe IRDS.

CURRENT USE

Current research is focusing on an application of NPV that involves the use of high-frequency technology. In one such technology, termed transthoracic oscillation, a chest shell is placed on the infant and pressure is generated external to the thorax at high frequencies.

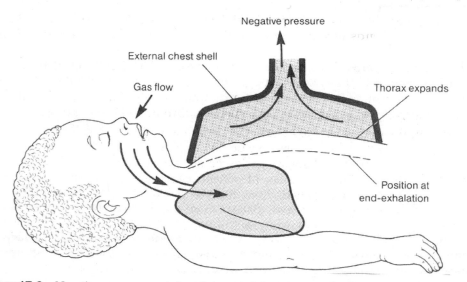

Figure 17-6 *Negative pressure exerted on the external thorax causes the thorax to expand, allowing gas to enter the lungs.*

This external pressure causes a forced exhalation, with inhalation occurring passively from chest recoil. A study using this technology showed an improvement in gas exchange and a significant reduction in respiratory rate.[45]

ADVANTAGES AND DISADVANTAGES

The major advantage to the use of NPV is that ventilation can be accomplished with little risk of barotrauma and the complications of invasive positive pressure ventilation.[46] Additionally, the cardiac system is not compromised as it is during positive pressure ventilation. Disadvantages include poor access to the patient, pressure sores at contact points, and air leaks.

SUMMARY

The advent of new, nonconventional ventilatory techniques and procedures in neonatal and pediatric care has changed the way these patients are treated in a dramatic way. Nothing has had quite as profound an effect as surfactant replacement therapy. While the need for replacement has been understood for many years, only fairly recently has the ability to produce useful surfactants and a method to deliver them, been developed. It is well understood that prematurity predisposes a newborn's lungs to surfactant deficiency, leading to decreased compliance and RDS. Surfactant replacement therapy appears to reduce the severity of RDS and its consequences. Continuing research will undoubtedly uncover further uses for surfactant allowing successful use in all patients.

High-frequency ventilation has been investigated for many years. Early researchers noted that hummingbirds breathe in synchrony with their wing beats, in excess of 2000 times per minute. Observation of a dog on a hot day reveals panting breaths that may approach 200 breaths per minute. The traditional idea of ventilation is that the inhaled tidal volume must be greater than the dead space. It is obvious that at respiratory rates of several hundred to thousands of breaths per minute, the tidal volume is not exceeding dead space. Although the exact mechanism of gas movement with high-frequency ventilation is not fully understood, it appears as though a continuous flow of gas is created. This allows gas exchange to take place continuously and at lower pressures than those required with conventional ventilation.

The four types of high-frequency ventilation are: high-frequency positive pressure ventilation (HFPPV); high-frequency flow interruption (HFFI); high-frequency jet ventilation (HFJV); and high-frequency oscillation (HFO). Each mode delivers its breaths by a different modality. Additionally, each mode operates within a certain frequency: HFPPV between 60 and 150 BPM; HFJV between 250 and 640 BPM; and HFOV between 500 and 2000 BPM.

Another nonconventional therapy that has gained renewed interest in recent years, is extracorporeal life support (ECLS). With ECLS, blood is removed from the patient, passed through a membrane oxygenator, and returned to the patient. Routes of blood removal and return are either venoarterial, in which the blood is removed from the right atrium and returned to the aortic arch, or venovenous, in which the blood is removed and returned to the right atrium. Because of its invasive nature, it is only used on those patients at an 80% or greater risk of mortality. Methods used to determine candidates include the A-a gradient and the oxygen index.

Speciality medical gases have gained popularity in the care of the infant and pediatric patient in recent years. Nitric oxides use as a potent pulmonary vasodilator has proven to be successful in the treatment of PPHN and illness that cause pulmonary hypertension. Heliox has shown success when used in the treatment of severe airway obstruction such as asthma and upper airway inflammation.

Partial liquid ventilation is an exciting new ventilatory technique that has the potential of ventilating at low pressures. The liquids, perfluorochemicals, have been shown to be relatively nontoxic to the lungs, and able to support respiration. As the liquid enters the alveoli, surface tension is obliterated by removing the air-gas interface. Expansion can then take place with minimal pressure.

Finally, the use of negative pressure ventilation has given rise to less invasive ventilation of the infant and pediatric patient, minimizing the complications of invasive conventional mechanical ventilation.

References

1. Jobe, A.H., and Ikegami, M. "Surfactant metabolism." *Clin Perinat* 20(4):65–73 (1993).

2. Holm, B.A., and Waring, A.J. "Designer surfactants: The next generation in surfactant replacement." *Clin Perinat* 20(4):813–29 (1993).

3. Willson D. Surfactant in Pediatric Respiratory Failure. *Respiratory Care* 1998; 43(12):1070–1086.

4. AARC Clinical Practice Guideline: Surfactant Replacement Therapy. *Respiratory Care* 1994; 39(8):824–829.

5. Jobe, A., Ikegami M. The Future of Surfactant Replacement Therapy. *Neonatal Respiratory Diseases* 1997; 7(4):2–10.

6. Willson, D., et al. Calf's Lung Surfactant Extract in Acute Hypoxemic Respiratory Failure in Children. *Critical Care Medicine* 1996; 24(8):1316–1322.

7. Bloom, B., et al. Comparison of Infasurf (Calf Lund Surfacant Extract) to Survanta (Beractant) in the Treatment and Prevention of Respiratory Distress Syndrome. *Pediatrics* 1997; 100(1):31–38.

8. Forest Pharmaceuticals.

9. GlaxoWellcome.

10. Jackson, J.C., et al. "Reduction in lung injury after combined surfactant and high-frequency ventilation." *Am J Resp Crit Care Med* 150(2):534–9 (1994).

11. Colburn, S., et al. Nitric Oxide and Surfactant Replacement in Pediatric ARDS. RT The Journal for Respiratory Care Practitioners 2000; 13(4):84–87.

12. Perez-Benavides, F., et al. Adult Respiratory Distress Syndrome and Artificial Surfactant Replacement in the Pediatric Patient. Pediatric Emergency Care 1994; 11(3):153–155.

13. Wilson 1999.

14. Carlo, W.A., and Chatburn, R.L. *Neonatal Respiratory Care,* 2d ed. Chicago: Year Book Medical Publishers Inc., 1988.

15. Boynton, B.R. "High-frequency ventilation in newborn infants." *Resp Care* 31(6):480–87 (1986).

16. Clark, R.H., et al. "Prospective, randomized comparison of high-frequency oscillation and conventional ventilation in candidates for extracorporeal membrane oxygenation" *J Pediatr* 124(3):447–54 (1994).

17. Miguet, D., et al. "Preoperative stabilization using high-frequency oscillatory ventilation in the management of congenital diaphragmatic hernia." *Crit Care Med* 22(9 suppl):s77–82 (1994).

18. Bower L, Betit P. Extracorporeal Life Support and High Frequency Oscillatory Ventilation: Alternatives for the Neonate in Severe Respiratory Failure. Respiratory Care 1994; 40(1) 61–73.

19. Arnold 1998.

20. Hewlitt 1998.

21. Gordin, P. "High-frequency jet ventilation for severe respiratory failure." *Pediatr Nurs* 15(6):625–9 (1989).

22. Richardson, C. "Hyaline membrane disease: future treatment modalities." *J Perinat Neonat Nurs* 2(1):78–88 (1988).

23. Milner, A.D., and Hoskins, E.W. "High-frequency positive pressure ventilation in neonates." *Arch Dis Child* 64(1) (Feta Neonatal ed)::1–3 (1989).

24. Palmer RMJ, et al. Nitric Oxide Release Accounts for Biological Activity of Endothelium Derived Relaxing Factor. Nature 1987; 327:524–526.

25. Frostell CG, et al. Inhaled Nitric Oxide: A Selective Pulmonary Vasodilator Reversing Hypoxic Pulmonary Vasoconstriction. Circulation 1991;83. 2038–2047.

26. Kazufumi, 1998.

27. Branson 1999.

28. NIHOS, 1997.

29. Kinsella, 1997.

30. Pfeffer, 1996.

31. Thompson J, et al. Pediatric Application of Inhaled Nitric Oxide. Respiratory Care 1999; 44(2) 177–182.

32. Okamoto K, et al. Efficacy of Inhaled Nitric Oxide in Children with ARDS. Chest 1998; 114(3) 827–833.

33. Roberts J. Inhaled Nitric Oxide for Hypoxemic Respiratory Failure of the Newborn. Respiratory Care 1999; 44(2) 169–173.

34. Hess D. Adverse Effects and Toxicity of Inhaled Nitric Oxide. Respiratory Care 1999; 44(3) 315–328.

35. Manthous C, et al. Heliox in the Treatment of Airflow Obstruction: A Critical Review of the Literature. Respiratory Care 1997; 42(11) 1034–1042.

36. Zwishchengerger, J.B., et al. "The role of extracorporeal membrane oxygenation in the management of respiratory failure in the newborn." *Resp Care* 31 (6):491–5 (1986).

37. Wilson B. Extracorporeal and Intracorporeal Techniques for the Treatment of Severe Respiratory Failure. Respiratory Care 1996; 41(4) 306–317.

38. Donn, S.M. "ECMO indications and complications." *Hosp Practice* 25(6):143–6 (1990).

39. Green, T.P., et al. "Probability of survival after prolonged extracorporeal membrane oxygenation in pediatric patients with acute respiratory failure." *Crit Care Med* 23(6):1132 (1995).

40. Robertson, C.M., et al. "Neurodevelopmental outcome after neonatal extracorporeal membrane oxygenation." *Can Med Assoc* 152(12):1981–8 (1995).

41. Roy, B.J., et al. "Venovenous extracorporeal membrane oxygenation affects renal function." *Pediatrics* 95(4):573 (1995).

42. Greenspan, J.S. "Liquid ventilation: A developing technology." *Neonatal Network* 12(4):23–8 (1993).

43. Hirschl, R.B., et al. "Liquid ventilation improves pulmonary function, gas exchange, and lung injury in a model of respiratory failure." *Ann Surg* 221(1):79–88 (1995).

44. Leach, C.L., et al. "Partial liquid ventilation in premature lambs with respiratory distress syndrome: Efficacy and compatibility with exogenous surfactant." *J Pediatr* 126(3): 412–20 (1995).

45. Hardinge, F.M., et al. "Effects of short term high frequency negative pressure ventilation on gas exchange using the hayet oscillator in normal subjects." *Thorax* 50(1):44–9 (1995).

46. Klonin H, et al. Negative Pressure Ventilation via Chest Cuirass to Decrease Ventilator-Associated Complications in Infants with Acute Respiratory Failure: A Case Series. Respiratory Care 2000; 45(5) 486–493.

Bibliography and Suggested Readings

Clark, R.H. "High-frequency ventilation in acute pediatric respiratory failure" editorial *Chest* 105(3):98 (1994).

Fuhrman B, et al. Partial Liquid Ventilation and the Challenges of Randomized, Controlled Trials in Acute Respiratory Distress Syndrome. Respiratory Care 1998; 43(12) 1086–1091.

Gross, G.W., et al. "Use of liquid ventilation with perflubron during extracorporeal membrane oxygenation: Chest radiographic appearances." *Radiology* 194(3):717–20 (1995).

Jobe, A. "Surfactant treatment for respiratory distress syndrome." *Resp Care* 31(6):467–76 (1986).

Short, B.L. "Extracorporeal membrane oxygenation" in G.B. Avery et al. eds *Neonatology: Pathophysiology and Management of the Newborn* 4th ed. Philadelphia: J.B. Lippincott Co. 1994.

Posttest

1. Rescue surfactant is given:
   a. as quickly as possible following delivery
   b. to any patient less than 32 weeks' gestation

    c. before the onset of RDS symptoms

    d. after the onset of RDS symptoms

2. Artificial surfactant is best administered:

    a. directly instilled into the endotracheal tube

    b. nebulized into the endotracheal tube

    c. through a peripheral IV site

    d. adding it to the ventilator circuitry

3. The major advantage to HFV is:

    a. improved oxygenation

    b. improved ventilation

    c. reduced barotrauma

    d. reduced cost

4. The convective movement of a tidal volume that is larger than dead space is achieved with:

    a. HFPPV

    b. HFJV

    c. HFOV

    d. HFV

5. All of the following are hazards of HFV except:

    a. air trapping

    b. hypertension

    c. hyperinflation

    d. necrotizing tracheobronchitis

6. While managing a patient receiving HFOV the respiratory care practitioner notices that the PaO_2 is decreased. This can be corrected by all of the following except:

    a. increasing the PEEP

    b. increasing the frequency

    c. increasing the amplitude

    d. increasing the PIP

7. Which of the following HFV methods requires the use of an adapted ETT?

    a. HFFI

    b. HFPPV

    c. HFJV

    d. HFOV

8. Which of the following describes the venoarterial route of ECLS?

    a. blood is taken from the subclavian vein and returned to the subclavian artery

    b. blood is taken from the femoral vein and returned to the femoral artery

    c. blood is taken from the right atrium and returned to the aortic arch

    d. blood is taken from the pulmonary vein and returned to the pulmonary artery

9. Two criteria used to determine potential ECLS patients are:

    a. patient age and weight

    b. level of $PaCO_2$ and pH

    c. level of hypoxemia and ventilatory support

    d. A-a gradient and the oxygen index

10. The most common complication of ECLS is:
    a. infection
    b. bleeding
    c. barotrauma
    d. machine failure
11. An advantage to the use of negative pressure ventilation is:
    a. better access to the patient
    b. less cost to the patient
    c. allows the use of lower FiO_2
    d. reduced cardiopulmonary complications
12. Which of the following is not true regarding partial liquid ventilation?
    a. reduces infection
    b. improves pulmonary gas exchange
    c. improves lung compliance
    d. reduces lung injury

TRANSPORT, HOME CARE, AND CARE OF THE PARENTS

CHAPTER EIGHTEEN

PERINATAL TRANSPORT

OBJECTIVES

Upon completion of this chapter, the reader should be able to:

1. Define regionalization and the role of transport.
2. Compare and contrast the types of transport, with regard to distances covered, advantages, and disadvantages.
3. Discuss the effects of altitude on PaO_2 and discuss the changes required in FiO_2 as altitude increases to maintain PaO_2.
4. Describe the effects of altitude on closed air spaces.
5. Describe the skills required by transport personnel.
6. List the equipment needed for transport and describe the modifications required for use during transport.
7. Calculate the duration of oxygen flow with an E and H cylinder when given necessary data.
8. Discuss the preparation required before transporting an infant.
9. Describe four methods to help thermoregulate an infant during transport.
10. Describe the care and transport of the following disorders:
    a. Diaphragmatic hernia
    b. Tracheoesophageal fistula
    c. Omphalocele
    d. Gastroschisis
    e. Meningomyelocele
    f. Cyanotic heart disease

KEY TERMS

Dalton's law	hypobaric	omphalocele
DeLee suction	Kling gauze	regionalization
gastroschisis	meningomyelocele	thyrotoxicosis

HISTORY

As neonatal medicine grew increasingly more sophisticated, it became apparent that not every hospital could afford the necessary equipment and personnel or had sufficient births to justify having an NICU. All hospitals that deliver babies, however, must have access to a NICU for those times when a compromised neonate is born.

The solution to this problem was a widespread regionalization of neonatal care, with one hospital in a specified geographic region providing a level II or level III NICU. The designation of level I, II, and III NICUs is outlined in Table 18–1. *Regionalization* allows for a localization of equipment, resources, and experts and avoids costly duplications.

One key element in a successful regionalization effort is a method to transport mothers and neonates from outlying hospitals to the regional center to receive care. Transport allows expert personnel and sophisticated equipment needed to provide the appropriate level of care for the high-risk mother or compromised neonate. Transport, therefore, is the vital link that connects the rural and smaller hospitals to the advanced care that is found in the NICU.

The major goal of transport is to bring a high-risk mother or a distressed neonate to a tertiary care center in stable condition where advanced care can then be given. Possible indications for transport are listed in Table 18–2.

TABLE 18–1   Responsibilities of Differing Levels of NICUs

Level I
- Care for uncomplicated maternity and neonatal cases
- Competent emergency care for unanticipated obstetric or neonatal complications
- Early identification of high-risk maternal and neonatal patients
- Provision of social services and other preventative assistance

Level II
- Total care of uncomplicated maternal and neonatal cases and 75–90% high-risk patients
- Ability to perform cesarean deliveries with a short start-up time (usually less than 15 minutes)
- In-house obstetric anesthesia with 24-hour coverage
- Ability to provide short-term mechanical ventilation of newborns and therapeutic respiratory care with 24-hour coverage
- 24-hour laboratory, radiology, and blood bank services
- Ability to provide fetal monitoring
- Special nursery for providing care

Level III
- Total care of all maternal and neonatal cases, including all high-risk patients
- 24-hour consultation assistance for hospitals within the region
- Methods and personnel to transport patients from any hospital within region to the level III nursery
- Provisions and personnel to coordinate educational program for the region
- Provides data analysis for the region

TABLE 18–2   Common Problems That May Require Transport

---

1. Obstetric problems
   a. Premature rupture of the amniotic membranes
   b. Premature labor
   c. Bleeding during the third trimester
   d. Rh incompatibility
   e. Twins, triplets, etc.
   f. Severe maternal eclampsia or preeclampsia
   g. Premature dilation of the cervix
   h. Presence of intrauterine growth retardation with signs of fetal distress
2. Surgical problems
   a. Congenital heart defect
   b. Diaphragmatic hernia
   c. Neural tube defects
   d. Abdominal defects (gastroschisis, etc.)
   e. Hydrocephalus
   f. Maternal problems
      I. Any trauma requiring intensive care
      II. Abdominal or thoracic surgery
3. Medical problems
   a. Severe maternal infection or maternal infection that may affect the fetus or cause premature delivery
   b. Maternal drug overdose
   c. Worsening maternal renal disease
   d. *Thyrotoxicosis*
   e. Class 3 to 4 organic heart disease
   f. Persistent pulmonary hypertension (PPH)

TYPES OF TRANSPORT

MATERNAL TRANSPORT

The ideal method of transporting a neonate is while it is still in utero, called *maternal transport*. While sophisticated neonatal transport techniques have improved the safety of transporting infants, research shows that in utero transports are safer than post-birth neonatal transports. Morbidity, mortality, and length of hospital intervention remain lower for maternal in utero transportation.[1] The identification of high-risk mothers, using the criteria outlined in Chapter 2, makes it possible to transport the mother still carrying the fetus to the regional center, where both can receive the necessary care.

Unfortunately, not all sick neonates are identified before birth. Many are born in a compromised condition with no indication of their status before birth. This problem necessitates a mechanism of transport that allows the NICU team to be taken to the referring hospital to care for the neonate and then transport the patient back to the NICU. This "portable

NICU" is accomplished either by ground, in an ambulance or a customized van, or by air, in a helicopter or fixed-wing aircraft. The means of transport used depends on the location of the NICU and the distances and terrain that need to be covered to access each of the hospitals within the region (Table 18–3).

GROUND TRANSPORT

Under normal circumstances, transports of less than 100 miles are best handled by ground via an ambulance.[2] The advantages of ground transport are that it can be done in more diverse weather conditions, and if difficulties arise during transport that require invasive procedures, the vehicle can be stopped, quieting the vibrations that may hinder the procedure.

The main disadvantage to ground transport is that it is relatively slow, and it may be limited by obstacles such as traffic jams, and natural boundaries.

AIR TRANSPORT

Helicopter. Air transport by helicopter is normally indicated for distances from 100 to 250 miles.[2] It is also the preferred method of transport where difficult terrain makes ground transport too time consuming or even impossible.

The major disadvantage to helicopter transport is the noise level and the vibrations that accompany the ride. The speed of the helicopter, however, makes up for these inconveniences. The main advantage over fixed-wing aircraft is the ability to land at or near the hospital, saving valuable time.

Fixed-Wing Aircraft. Fixed-wing aircraft are utilized for transports of over 250 miles.[2] These aircraft range from single engine planes to small jets, depending on the distance to be covered. Although the noise level is usually less in a fixed-wing aircraft, the vibrations and turbulence are similar to that found in a helicopter.

Obviously, the main advantage to fixed-wing transport is the speed and the distance that can be covered in a short time.

A major disadvantage to air transport is that it is usually confined to acceptable weather conditions. Severe weather, either at the departure point, en route, or at the destination, may make air transport unavailable. Another disadvantage is the lack of space in the aircraft. With two adult personnel, equipment, and the incubator, space is at a premium.

The use of fixed-wing aircraft requires some type of general aviation facility nearby. In some instances, the distance factor may need to be disregarded to allow a helicopter closer access to the hospital.

Considerations for Air Transport. Transport in an aircraft requires special attention to the effects of altitude. In particular, one aspect that requires special attention is the effect of altitude on gas pressures.

TABLE 18–3   Modes of Maternal and Neonatal Transport

Ground

Most efficient within a 100-mile radius of referring hospital.

Advantages:
    a. Can be used when there is unavailability of landing sites for a helicopter or fixed-wing aircraft.
    b. Can be used when inclement weather prevents air travel.
    c. Usually provides more work area.
    d. Less vibration and noise than helicopter.

Disadvantages:
    a. Obstacles on the ground and difficult terrain may tremendously slow the transport.
    b. Too slow for distances beyond 100 miles.

Helicopter

Most efficient when distances are greater than 100 miles but less than 250 miles.

Advantages:
    a. Faster mode of transport than ground methods.
    b. May be faster for shorter distances if ground conditions or terrain make ground transport impractical.
    c. Does not require a landing strip, can land at or near the hospital.

Disadvantages:
    a. High noise and vibration levels make assessment and monitoring difficult.
    b. May become grounded during inclement weather.
    c. Small work area.
    d. Lighting in the patient area after nightfall may interfere with the pilot's vision.
    e. Requires highly trained crew.
    f. Expensive to operate and maintain helicopter.
    g. Hypobaric effects on patient and equipment.

Fixed-wing Aircraft

Most efficient for distances of greater than 250 miles.

Advantages:
    a. Able to travel long distances in a short time.
    b. Less vibration and noise than helicopter.
    c. Able to travel at higher altitudes, possibly flying over areas of inclement weather or other obstacles.

Disadvantages:
    a. Must land at an airport, requiring ground transport of the patient between the hospital and aircraft.
    b. May be grounded in inclement weather.
    c. Small work area.
    d. Crew must understand the effects of altitude on the patient.
    e. Expensive to operate and maintain aircraft.
    f. Hypobaric effects on patient and equipment.

Dalton's law states that the total pressure of a mixture of gases is the sum of each of the pressures exerted by the individual gases. Thus we can determine the partial pressure of any gas by knowing what percent it is of the total mixture and by knowing the total pressure of the gas mixture.

The percentage of oxygen is always 20.9% of the total atmospheric gas (21% is used for ease of calculation). Therefore, at any barometric pressure, we can determine the pressure that oxygen is exerting simply by multiplying the barometric pressure by 0.21. As one rises in altitude, the total pressure of the atmosphere decreases, known as *hypobaric* conditions. The percent of the gases, however, always remains the same.

At sea level with an average barometric pressure of 760 mm Hg, oxygen exerts a pressure of approximately 160 mm Hg ($760 \times 0.21 = 160$). At 5000 feet elevation, with an approximate barometric pressure of 640 mm Hg, oxygen exerts a pressure of 134 mm Hg ($640 \times 0.21 = 134$). It is apparent that as altitude is increased, the partial pressure of oxygen decreases. The relationship between altitude and PO_2 is demonstrated in Table 18–4.

As altitude is increased, it is necessary to increase the percent of oxygen delivered to the patient to maintain the same arterial PO_2. The chart presented in Table 18–5 shows the FiO_2 required to maintain a constant PaO_2 at increasing altitudes. The value of a transcutaneous monitor or pulse oximeter during transport is apparent, as the FiO_2 can be titrated up or down as needed to maintain a level PaO_2 or saturation.

A second factor that must be considered regarding hypobaric conditions during air transport is that gas in a closed space expands as the barometric pressure decreases. This is an expression of Boyle's law, where volume varies inversely with pressure. Applying this to the patient, any enclosed volume of gas will expand as altitude is increased. An untreated pneumothorax will expand in the thorax as altitude is increased. Gas that is trapped in the stomach or bowel will also distend and create potential problems. Proper drainage of this free air before lifting off will alleviate most problems.

Seen as insignificant by adults, the effects of acceleration and deceleration need to be con-

---

TABLE 18–4   The Relationship Between Altitude and PO$_2$

ALTITUDE	PO$_2$
Sea level	160 mm Hg
1000 ft.	155 mm Hg
2000 ft.	150 mm Hg
3000 ft.	145 mm Hg
4000 ft.	140 mm Hg
5000 ft.	134 mm Hg
6000 ft.	129 mm Hg
7000 ft.	124 mm Hg
8000 ft.	119 mm Hg
9000 ft.	114 mm Hg
10,000 ft.	109 mm Hg
15,000 ft.	85 mm Hg
20,000 ft.	59 mm Hg
30,000 ft.	8 mm Hg

TABLE 18–5 FiO$_2$ Required to Maintain a Constant PaO$_2$ at Increasing Altitude

	SEA LEVEL	ALTITUDE (FT.)									
		2000	4000	6000	8000	10,000	12,000	14,000	16,000	18,000	20,000
	0.21	0.23	0.24	0.27	0.29	0.31	0.34	0.37	0.41	0.45	0.49
	0.30	0.32	0.35	0.38	0.41	0.45	0.49	0.53	0.59	0.64	0.71
	0.40	0.43	0.47	0.51	0.55	0.60	0.65	0.71	0.78	0.85	0.94
FiO$_2$	0.50	0.54	0.58	0.63	0.69	0.75	0.81	0.89	0.98		
	0.60	0.65	0.70	0.76	0.83	0.89	0.98				
	0.70	0.76	0.82	0.89	0.96						
	0.80	0.86	0.94								
	0.90	0.97									
	1.00										

Source: Cloherty JP, Stark AR, eds. Manual of Neonatal Care. 4th ed. Philadelphia: Lippincott; 1998. Reproduced with permission.

sidered when transporting any patient, especially the neonatal patient. With the patient lying inline with the aircraft, the forces of acceleration and deceleration may cause significant changes in blood flow. For example, if the head is toward the front of the craft, acceleration may cause blood to be pulled to the lower extremities, reducing blood flow to the brain and cardiopulmonary systems. Conversely, if the head is toward the tail of the craft, acceleration forces may move blood to the head, possibly causing intracranial hemorrhage. One recommendation, is to place the patient parallel to the wings. This may be impractical owing to the limited space and design of the aircraft.[3] In addition, research suggests that the use of specially designed equipment such as pneumatic lifts can reduce acceleration forces.[4]

Other Stressors. Transporting patients, especially pediatric and neonatal patients, has a number of other potential stressors that should be recognized and minimized. Stress may induce bradycardia, apnea, and a decrease in oxygen saturation. These stressors include vibration, excessive motion, noise, and possibly hypothermia. While there are practical limitations on what can be done about vibration and noise during transport, such levels inside transport incubators often exceed recommended levels. Furthermore, these and others stressors have been shown to increase morbidity in such patients. Consequently, ways of reducing noise and vibration levels during transportation, such as novel incubator designs and optimal ways to secure such patients, are being investigated.[5] Additionally, it is important to not leave any unsecured equipment inside the incubator that may cause injury during turbulence or while traveling bumpy roads. If noise levels are excessive (60 to 90 dB), hearing protection devices should be provided for the patient. During air transport, outside air temperature drops as altitude is increased. With the change in external temperature, cabin temperature may also fall and create hypothermia in the patient. Constant monitoring of environmental and patient temperatures help in preventing this stressor. The importance of thermoregulation is discussed later in this chapter.

There are some differing philosophies regarding whether parents should be allowed to accompany the sick neonate or pediatric patient during transport. Often, modes of ground and air transportation have extra seating for passengers but policies on parent-passengers vary widely within the health care transportation environment. The benefits of emotional support for the family and patient, availability of parents for history and consent, and good public relations should be weighed against the potential drawbacks of increased parent and crew anxiety and space limitations.[6]

PERSONNEL

The need for highly skilled, trained personnel on the transport team is obvious. Team members vary from institution to institution and may consist of physicians, respiratory care practitioners, nurses, paramedics, and emergency medical technicians.

Regardless of which personnel are assigned to the transport team, each must be highly trained to treat and stabilize the sick neonate (Table 18–6). Skills must include placement of IVs, placement of umbilical artery and vein catheters, intubation, and chest tube placement.[7] A thorough understanding of thermoregulation, oxygenation, ventilation, and management of glucose is also vital.

Transport team members are usually those who have extensive experience in the NICU and are familiar with the treatment of a wide variety of disorders in neonates and high-risk mothers. Extensive training is then done to familiarize each member of the team with the equipment and the special skills that will be required.

EQUIPMENT

NECESSARY EQUIPMENT

Every piece of equipment that is available in the NICU must be available during a transport. The equipment needed for transport is listed in Table 18–7.

TABLE 18–6   Skills of the Transport Team

1. Able to identify maternal and neonatal high-risk factors.
2. Trained in all aspects of neonatal resuscitation.
3. Trained in speciality skills:
   a. Intubation
   b. Starting IVs
   c. Thermoregulation
   d. Needle aspiration
   e. Mechanical ventilation
4. Able to perform a complete physical assessment and determine gestational age.
5. Capable of identifying and treating all types of respiratory distress and its complications.
6. Understands and is able to provide emotional and psychosocial support to parents and families.
7. Ability to recognize and respond to physiologic effects of transport, particularly hypobaric conditions, noise, and vibration.

TABLE 18–7   Equipment and Supplies Needed for Transport

Transport incubator
Transport ventilator(s)
Heart rate, blood pressure, and transcutaneous monitors
IV equipment:
    Assorted needles and syringes
    One-half normal saline
    5% D_5W
    Ringer's lactate
    25 and 50% dextrose
    Blood administration set
Suction equipment:
    5, 6, 8, and 10 Fr. catheters
    Bulb syringe
    DeLee suction
    Suction tubing
Thermometer and equipment
Full oxygen and air cylinders
Blood pressure cuff and Doppler device
Stethoscope
Oxygen analyzer
Resuscitation bag and pressure manometer
Intubation equipment:
    Laryngoscope handle
    No. 0 and 1 blade
    Extra light bulbs
    Extra batteries, fully charged
    Magill forceps
    Endotracheal tubes sizes 2.5, 3.0, 3.5, 4.0, 4.5
    Tape
CPAP Nasal prongs
Ventilator circuits
Umbilical artery catheterization tray
Blood gas equipment:
    Blood gas syringes
    Glass pipettes for collecting capillary samples
    Stopcocks
    Heparin flush solution
    Lancets
Laboratory equipment:
    Tubes for blood specimens
    Collection bags for urine
    Blood culture tubes
Miscellaneous equipment:
    Appropriate batteries
    Sterile gloves and floor exam gloves

(*continued*)

TABLE 18–7   (continued)

Miscellaneous equipment (continued):
    Lubricating ointment
    Suture materials
    Scalpels and blades
    Sterile gowns
    Oxygen tubing, masks, and cannulas
    Alcohol swabs
    Iodophor skin prep solution
    Kelly clamps
    Dextrostix
    Scissors
    Portable light source
    Various sizes of gauze sponges
    Feeding tubes, 5 and 8 Fr.
    Instant camera and film
Drugs:
    25% albumin
    Dexamethasone
    Naloxone
    Diazepam
    Morphine
    Atropine
    Phenobarbital
    Sodium bicarbonate
    Tolazoline
    Dopamine
    Furosemide
    Epinephrine
    Ampicillin
    Gentamicin
    Kanmycin
    Oxycillin
    Penicillin
    Magnesium sulfate
    Heparin
    Calcium gluconate
    Lidocaine
    Pancuronium
    Phytonadione (Aquamephyton)
    Prostaglandin E
    Albuterol
    Indomethasin
    Racemic Epinephrine
    Surfactant

This equipment must be carried in a box or bag that is portable and relatively small. Larger equipment, such as the ventilator and tanks, are normally incorporated into the transport incubator.

SELF-SUPPORTING EQUIPMENT

Any equipment used during a transport must be self-supporting. Thus, it must be battery operated or otherwise able to operate without direct electrical current. Battery-operated equipment should be able to last at least 30 to 45 minutes beyond the expected length of the transport. The ventilator and manual resuscitator should be run from the medical gas cylinders, which requires enough cylinders to provide at least 50% more gas than expected use.

The rationale for the excess battery life and gas requirement is that the unexpected must always be anticipated. There could be nothing worse than to have the oxygen run out on a critically ill neonate as the tire to the ambulance is being replaced. Anticipation of potential difficulties will prevent dreaded outcomes.

DETERMINING THE DURATION OF CYLINDER GASES

The amount of time left in a medical gas cylinder can be determined. Each cylinder has a known factor that converts the gauge pressure into the liters of gas remaining in the cylinder. By dividing the total liters of gas in the cylinder by the gas flow, the duration of time in minutes can be determined. The equation and cylinder factors are outlined in Table 18–8.

TABLE 18-8   Calculation of Cylinder Duration

CYLINDER SIZE	FACTOR
D	0.16
E	0.28
G	2.41
H	3.14

To calculate the duration of gas flow, use the following equation:

$$\text{duration of flow (minutes)} = \frac{\text{factor} \times \text{gauge pressure (psi)}}{\text{flow rate (L/min)}}$$

For example, an E cylinder with 2000 psi running at 3 LPM:

$$\frac{\text{factor (0.28)} \times \text{gauge pressure (2000)}}{\text{flow rate (3 LPM)}}$$

$$\frac{0.28 \times 2000}{3} = \frac{560}{3} = 186.7 \text{ minutes} \Rightarrow 3 \text{ hrs } 7 \text{ min.}$$

VOLTAGE CONVERTERS

Some transport vehicles have voltage inverters that allow the equipment to be plugged into a 120-volt source during the transport, saving battery power. It is also possible to run some equipment from the 12- or 24-volt vehicle system, in which case the internal battery source could also be saved.

EQUIPMENT USED DURING AIR TRANSPORT

Of special consideration during air transport is that certain monitors may interfere with the aircraft instrumentation. This equipment should be identified and not used during air transport.

MEDICATIONS

In addition to equipment, there is a host of medications that are commonly administered during neonatal and pediatric transports. Over two thirds of neonatal and pediatric patients are administered some form of medication while being transported. More than one third of such transport patients receive antibiotics, approximately one fourth receive morphine, with about the same number given anticonvulsants. Other classes of medications given during transport include neuromuscular blocking agents, respiratory drugs, inotropes, and sedatives.

The use of different classes of drugs varies by age group. Anticonvulsants are most commonly given to children, sedatives and respiratory medications to infants, and antibiotics to newborns.[8]

INFANT PREPARATION AND TRANSPORTATION

To achieve the goal of transporting the patient to a tertiary center in stable condition, the patient should be stable before being transported. This is accomplished by personnel skilled in resuscitation and stabilization techniques who are present at the delivery. This emphasizes the importance of having personnel trained in resuscitative skills present at every delivery.

STABILIZATION

Proper stabilization of the neonate includes appropriate medication administration, thermoregulation, oxygenation, ventilation, acid-base balance, proper vascular volume and glucose levels, and stable vital signs.[2] Once stabilization is achieved, the neonate is placed in the transport incubator and connected to the necessary monitors and equipment. The destination hospital is then contacted and advised of the status of the patient.

FOLLOWING STABILIZATION

Before leaving, the transport team should have a copy of the patient's chart with all lab data and copies of any x-rays that were taken. The patient is then taken to the mother's room, where the parents are allowed to touch and see their neonate. The procedures for the transport are explained and the parents assured that their neonate will receive the required medical attention. Often a photograph of the infant is taken and left with the parents.

The parents are then asked to sign a release form, consenting to the transport of the neonate. This interaction with the parents is important to help alleviate their fears and concerns. They must be assured that a member of the team will contact them on arrival at the destination and that they are free to call whenever they desire.

The transport team must be sensitive to the parents' needs at this point, because they will often be very frightened and worried.

TRANSPORTATION PROCEDURES

Following the visit with the parents, the patient is taken to the transport vehicle and secured. During the transport the patient is constantly monitored for changes in status. Appropriate care is provided during the transport to maintain stability.

Upon arrival at the regional hospital, the patient is admitted and care is continued as required. A blood gas should be drawn soon after arrival to ensure appropriate oxygenation and ventilation. The parents are then notified of the arrival and the baby's condition.

SPECIAL NEEDS

A majority of neonates requiring transport suffer from lung disease secondary to prematurity and other factors. Besides having lung problems, a premature neonate can be very difficult to thermoregulate, and special attention may be required.

THERMOREGULATION

To assist with thermoregulation, incubators, warmed IV bags wrapped in a blanket, a cap over the head, a warming blanket, and commercially produced chemical heating pads may all be used.[9] Extreme caution must be exercised on patients with poor perfusion. Burns can develop at even moderate temperatures on these neonates, requiring close attention to temperatures.

In addition, plastic shields and wraps and aluminum foil can be used to reduce radiant and convective heat losses. Minimal handling and opening of incubator doors will also help with the maintenance of a neutral thermal environment.

In recent years, there has been significant improvement in the avoidance of hypothermia and cold stress in infants requiring emergency transport. Research has shown that the rate of hypothermia, defined as body temperature of less than 36˚C, in such patients has decreased from 22% in 1977 to 1979 to 7% in 1995–1996. Adjunct measures, such as continual monitoring of temperature, staff education, and equipment enhancements are largely credited with this improvement. Infants weighing less than 1000 grams account for the largest number of patients experiencing hypothermia.[10]

DIAPHRAGMATIC HERNIA

Patients requiring surgical intervention will require special attention during transport. The patient with a *diaphragmatic hernia* should be positioned on his or her side with the head elevated and the affected side of the thorax down, as demonstrated in Figure 18–1.[11] A nasogastric (NG) tube must be in place to evacuate any air that enters the stomach.

The patient should never be bag and mask ventilated, but intubated and ventilated through the ET tube. These procedures help minimize the amount of gastric air distention that further compromises ventilation.

TRACHEOESOPHAGEAL FISTULA

Patients with a *tracheoesophageal fistula* are transported with their head elevated, a feeding tube placed in the esophageal pouch, which is evacuated regularly to remove the buildup of secretions. If possible, mechanical ventilation should be avoided to avoid distention of the gastrointestinal tract.

OMPHALOCELE AND GASTROSCHISIS

Another group of patients who may be difficult to thermoregulate are those with an

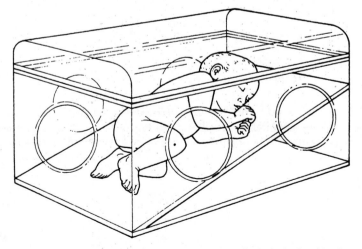

Figure 18-1 *When transporting a neonate with a diaphragmatic hernia, the head is elevated and the patient is placed with the affected side down (usually the left side).*

omphalocele or *gastroschisis*. Omphalocele involves the herniation of the intestines directly into the base of the umbilical cord. The organs are covered by a transparent sac. In gastroschisis, the organs herniate through the abdominal wall, typically to the right of an intact umbilicus. The organs in this defect are not covered by a sac.

The primary goals in transporting these patients are to maintain an aseptic environment for the herniated organs, prevent pulmonary aspiration of abdominal contents, prevent excess loss of heat through evaporation, provide respiratory support, and prevent vascular compromise of the organs.[9]

Preparation of the omphalocele patient before transport requires special precautions. An NG tube is placed and regularly evacuated. The herniated bowel is carefully covered with a layer of warm, sterile, saline-soaked gauze. Antiseptics such as povidone iodine may be added to the gauze. The sac is then wrapped with a layer of dry *Kling gauze* in a figure-eight fashion. No attempt should be made to reduce the defect back into the abdomen. This may damage the intestinal loops, cause an interruption of venous return, and compromise the respiratory status.[9]

Continual monitoring of patient temperature helps maintain thermoregulation. Both evaporative and radiant heat loss from the herniated organs create a major problem. Temperature is maintained by placing the entire lower half of the body in a sterile plastic bag or wraping the abdomen with clear plastic wrap.[7] The environmental temperature of the incubator is recommended to be kept between 36.5 and 37.0˚C.[9]

Extensive fluid losses, hypovolemic shock, and poor tissue perfusion are seen in many of these patients. To counter these problems, an IV is started in an upper extremity, and fluid replacement is started and kept at two to four times the maintenance range.[9] The upper regions are used for the IV because of the risk of impaired venous return from the lower extremities following dressing and positioning the defect. Broad-spectrum antibiotics such as ampicillin and gentamicin are then started to avert the onset of sepsis.[7]

The patient is then transported with the head elevated. Extreme care must be taken to prevent contamination of the defect and to prevent kinking the intestine.

MENINGOMYELOCELE

In the patient with *meningomyelocele*, or *spina bifida*, extreme care must be taken to avoid contamination of the defect with stool or the environment. If the covering membranes are intact, extreme care must be taken to avoid rupturing them. Covering with sterile saline-soaked gauze and a plastic shield will help protect the defect and maintain thermoregulation.[7] The patient is then transported in the supine position.[12]

CYANOTIC HEART DISEASE

Patients with cyanotic heart diseases may need to be treated with prostaglandin E_1 to maintain the patency of the ductus arteriosus during transport.

SUMMARY

Of all the types of transport, the most desirable is maternal transport, where the high-risk mother is transported before delivery to a tertiary center. Ground transport via an ambulance or specially equipped vehicle is often used when the distance is less than 100 miles, or if weather or other obstacles prevent air transport. Air transport is done via helicopter, usually for distances between 100 and 250 miles, and fixed-wing aircraft for distances greater than 250 miles.

Special considerations are required for air transport. The effect of hypobaric conditions relating to altitude on gas pressures can make a significant impact on patients with air leaks, or air pockets within closed spaces. Additionally, the pressure of oxygen decreases as altitude increases, requiring constant monitoring and adjustment to ensure the patient does not become hypoxemic. Gravitational forces during takeoff and landing may cause alterations in blood flow to the head or vital organs.

Stressors associated with all forms of transport include vibration, excessive movement, noise, and hypothermia. Careful monitoring and securing can help reduce these potential problems.

Personnel on the transport team must be well versed in all aspects of neonatal and maternal care, and able to manage any problem that may arise. These individuals are often highly crosstrained and knowledgeable of the effects of transport on the patient and how to minimize those effects.

All equipment found in the NICU should be available during transport and must be checked for proper function and secured before leaving. Special attention should be afforded the amount of oxygen, to ensure adequate supplies. The possibility of delays and unforeseen problems should be taken into account when determining the necessary supply.

Preparing the patient for transport requires stabilization of vital signs, temperature, blood sugar, acid-base balance, oxygenation, and blood volume. Also, any air leak or trapped air must be treated if a change in altitude is anticipated. All necessary documents must be in order and a visit to the family members must be done prior to departure. The presence of certain defects such as diaphragmatic hernia, tracheoesophageal fistula, omphalocele, meningomyelocele, and cyanotic heart disease require special preparation and handling prior to and during the transport.

The transportation of the high-risk mother or the distressed neonate to a regional center has become a vital part of the health care system. Proper advanced planning, strong communication, and cooperation between hospitals greatly enhances the regionalization concept. With proper coordination, skilled personnel, and appropriate equipment, any neonate should be able to receive the care provided by the modern NICU.

References

1. Shlossman PA, et al. An analysis of neonatal morbidity in maternal (in utero) and neonatal transports at 24–34 weeks' gestation. *Am J Perinatol*. 1997;14:449–456.

2. Merenstein GB, Gardner SL. *Handbook of Neonatal Care*. 4th ed. St. Louis: CV Mosby Co; 1998.

3. Miller C. The physiologic effects of air transport on the neonate. *Neonatal Network*. 1994;13:7–10.

4. Peters C, et al. Measuring vibrations of transport stress in premature and newborn infants during incubator transport. *Clin Pediatr* (in German). 1997;209:315–320.

5. Macnab A, et al. Vibration and noise in pediatric emergency transport vehicles: a potential cause of morbidity. *Aviat Space Environ Med*. 1995;66:212–219.

6. Lewis MM, et al. Parents as passengers during pediatric transport. *Air Medicine Journal*. 1997;16:38–42.

7. Cloherty JP, Stark AR, eds. *Manual of Neonatal Care*. 4th ed. Philadelphia: Lippincott; 1998.

8. Kronick JB, et al. Pediatric and neonatal critical care transport: a comparison of therapeutic interventions. *Pediatr Emerg Care*. 1996;12:23–26.

9. Richey DA. Transporting the infant with an abdominal wall defect. *Neonatal Network*. 1990;9:53–56.

10. Bowman ED, Roy RN. Control of temperature during newborn transport: an old problem with new difficulties. *J. Paediatr Child Health*. 1997;33:398–401.

11. Koff PB, Eitzman DV, Nev J. *Neonatal and Pediatric Respiratory Care*. 2nd ed. St. Louis: CV Mosby Co; 1993.

12. Avery GB, Fletcher MA, MacDonald MG. *Pathophysiology and Management of the Newborn*. 5th ed. Philadelphia: JB Lippincott Co; 1999.

Bibliography and Suggested Readings

Brann AW, Cefalo RC, eds. *Guidelines for Perinatal Care*. Evanston, Ill: American Academy of Pediatrics/American College of Obstetrics and Gynecology; 1983.

Carlo WA, Chatburn RL. *Neonatal Respiratory Care*. 2nd ed. Chicago: Year-Book Medical Publishers Inc; 1998.

Korones SB. *High-Risk Newborn Infants*. 4th ed. St. Louis: CV Mosby Co; 1986.

Posttest

1. Air transport by helicopter is indicated for distances of:
   a. over 300 miles
   b. 150 to 300 miles
   c. 80 to 150 miles
   d. 60 to 80 miles
2. Before departure on a helicopter transport, a neonate's PaO\IN{2} is 65 mm Hg. During the flight, the PaO_2 will most likely:
   a. remain the same
   b. decrease
   c. increase
   d. rise initially, then return to baseline.

3. Which of the following statements regarding air transport is true?
   a. Trapped air will expand as altitude increases.
   b. Trapped air will decrease in size as altitude increases.
   c. Trapped air in the stomach must not be removed before transport.
   d. As altitude increases, barometric pressure increases.
4. Which of the following skills are needed by a transport team member?
   I. placement of IVs
   II. placement of UAC catheters
   III. chest tube placement
   IV. intubation
   V. placement of UVC catheters
      a. I, III, V
      b. I, II, IV
      c. II, III, IV
      d. I, II, III, IV, V
5. Batteries used to power equipment during a transport should last:
   a. 30 to 45 minutes beyond the expected length of the transport
   b. 10 to 15 minutes beyond the expected length of the transport
   c. 3 to 4 hours
   d. 24 hours
6. How long will an E cylinder of oxygen last with a gauge pressure of 1900 psi running at 5 lpm?
   a. 106 hours
   b. 1 hour 46 minutes
   c. 2 hours 17 minutes
   d. 3 hours
7. Before transporting the neonate to the NICU, the transport team should:
   a. stabilize the infant
   b. contact and advise the NICU
   c. collect all patient chart data
   d. all of the above.
8. Of the following, which can help thermoregulate the infant during transport?
   a. warmed IV bags wrapped in a blanket
   b. sprinkle the baby with warm water
   c. blow warmed oxygen over the baby
   d. place a small 12-volt heater in the transport incubator
9. Which of the following disorders present the greatest potential thermoregulation problem during transport?
   a. diaphragmatic hernia
   b. gastroschisis
   c. intraventricular hemorrhage
   d. cardiac anomaly.

10. To maintain the same PaO_2 for a patient during air transport, hypobaric conditions would generally require what adjustment to the FiO_2?
    a. decrease
    b. increase
    c. no change
    d. initial decrease then increase

CHAPTER NINETEEN

HOME CARE

OBJECTIVES

Upon completion of this chapter, the reader should be able to:

1. Describe the history of modern home care.
2. Identify those factors that make home care preferable over hospital care.
3. Compare and contrast hospital-based, community-based, and bureaucratic home care models.
4. Describe steps in selecting a home care patient.
5. With regard to home ventilator patients, describe each of the following:
   a. Selection of candidates
   b. Preparation for home ventilator care
   c. Selection of a home care ventilator
   d. Training parents and family
6. Describe the equipment and techniques for administering aerosols in the home.
7. Discuss the family training for providing chest physiotherapy and suctioning at home.
8. Define ALTE.
9. Regarding home apnea monitoring, describe each of the following:
   a. Identification of patients for monitoring.
   b. Problems associated with home monitoring.
10. List the equipment necessary to provide oxygen in the home.
11. Compare and contrast the three methods of home oxygen delivery, including advantages and disadvantages of each.
12. Discuss the role of each of the following in discharge planning:
    a. Case manager
    b. Physician
    c. Respiratory care practitioner
    d. Nursing
    e. Social worker
    f. Dietician
    g. Physical, occupational, and speech therapists
    h. Home care company
13. Describe the events and necessary supports involved at the time of discharge.

14. Discuss the effects of home care on the family.
15. Describe why home care sometimes fails and what the practitioner can do to prevent failure.

KEY TERMS

cognitive

metered dose inhaler

spacer

diaphragmatic pacers

sieve

turfism

OVERVIEW

It is interesting that as health care has improved in quality over the last century, emphasis is beginning to be placed on care of the patient at home, where it originally started. When dealing with home care of the infant, improved technology and equipment have improved patient survival, resulting in many infant patients requiring long-term chronic care. With a shortage of long-term care facilities, a natural choice for this care is the home.

HISTORY OF MODERN HOME CARE

A major advance in home care occurred in the early 1980s when an Iowa parent wanted to take her chronically ill child home. She soon discovered there were no mechanisms in place for the reimbursement of home care. She appealed to then President Reagan for help. The president, seeing the merits of home care, arranged for Iowa authorities to waive Medicaid rules to cover the home care of this patient.

From this case, interest in the care of technology-assisted children surged and was in part responsible for the U.S. Surgeon General's Workshop on Children with Handicaps and Their Families.[1] From this original conference, the groundwork was laid, which resulted in the funding of programs and reports that have given us current models of home care.

An additional concern, further supporting the need for home care, is the effect of the hospital environment on the chronically ill child. It is obvious that the hospital environment does not allow the normal development of family bonds or allow for normal social interactions with siblings, or other children. The long-term effects of this lack of interaction remain unknown, but undoubtedly there are some detrimental aspects. The advantages of home care are outlined in Table 19–1.

TABLE 19–1   Advantages of Home Care

1. Normalization of family activities
2. Development of normal parent-sibling and other social relationships
3. Normalization of sleeping, eating, and activity habits for the patient
4. Cost effective
5. Enhanced cognitive development

Home care allows for more normal family activities to occur. The patient, being in the home environment, is in the constant companionship of those who care for him or her the most. The environment is much more low key than that in the hospital with its constant noise, alarms, bright lights, and constantly changing personnel. Families are encouraged to send older children to school and even infants should attend special out-of-home programs. The current trend of mainstreaming in school classrooms provides the opportunity for these patients to attend school with "normal" children. The benefits of this are enhanced *cognitive* skills and normal psychosocial development.

CONTROVERSIES SURROUNDING HOME CARE

Despite the changes in legislation and the increase in interest in home care, several questions remain unanswered. These include: Which patients are candidates for home care? How is the decision for home care made, and who makes it? Who will help the family and the patient during the transition, and how long will help be provided? These are not easy questions to answer because many complex issues are involved. Possibly the most difficult question to answer is the first, deciding who is a candidate for home care. This is discussed in more detail later in this chapter. While this chapter does not pretend to answer all questions, it does present some rationale on which to base decisions.

HOME CARE MODELS

There are three basic models for pediatric home care described by Aitken: the hospital-based, community-based, and bureaucratic models.[1] We will briefly examine each.

Hospital-based. As is apparent from the name, this model is located in the hospital, with personnel, financial planning, and care provided by the hospital. The hospital provides all training for those who will be caring for the patient.

The major advantage of this model is the ability of the discharge planning group to maintain some control over the discharge plan. Additionally, the hospital has plenty of human resources in each specialty group to provide support and training.

The major disadvantage to this model is that if outside funding cannot be obtained, the child may remain in the hospital longer, increasing the cost of the hospital stay. The longer hospital stay may also cause the hospital to lose money.

Community-based. This model is designed to provide all necessary elements of a home care program, using community resources. The organization must hire its own personnel and a board of directors to oversee policies and procedures. Funding is solicited by the board from private sources to ease the burden on families. The community-based model acts as a coordinator between the patient and the hospital in planning the home care.

There are two main advantages to this system. First, the community-based model is better able to determine which available agencies are best suited to handle the needs of the patient and help the parents in their decision. They have the ability to draw from many sources and are not tied to their own resources. Also, by not being supported by a particular hospital, there is less *turfism* between hospitals.

The main disadvantage to this model is the expense involved. In areas of limited human and financial resources, this model may be impractical to operate. There may also be reluctance on the part of the primary care physician to turn over care to another. Finally, personnel involved in this model may have little, if any, control over the discharge planning for the patient.

Bureaucratic. This model integrates home care into an existing public support organization. Structurally, it is similar to the community-based model, but has been absorbed by an established agency to survive financially.

Being a part of an established government agency, this model may be more readily accepted by health care providers. Another advantage is that these agencies often have in place necessary ancillary services, such as nursing, physical, speech, and occupational therapy. Access to financial resources may be facilitated in this model also.

The main disadvantage to this type of model is that eligibility may be limited to families who are eligible for Medicaid. There also may be a tendency not to use the agency because of a dislike for government bureaucracies. Case managers may be overburdened with the addition of a technology-assisted patient to their heavy load of regular patients.

PATIENT SELECTION

The first step in home care is the selection of appropriate patients who will benefit from home care.

COMMON DISORDERS ALLOWING HOME CARE

Survivors of respiratory distress syndrome who have developed bronchopulmonary dysplasia probably constitute a majority of ventilator-dependent children. The second category consists of the congenital anomalies, such as diaphragmatic hernia, tracheoesophageal fistula, and esophageal atresia. The third category is the neuromuscular and neurologic diseases. These include myopathies, myelomeningocele, encephalopathy, and infantile botulism. The fourth category consists of patients who have suffered traumatic injuries.

HOME ENVIRONMENT

Another factor in patient selection is the home environment and the confidence in the parents to provide the necessary care. The decision to provide home care must be made by the parents. The decision should only be made after the parents have had an extended stay in the hospital.[2]

The parents and all others who will be involved in the care of the infant or child must be willing to sacrifice their time and be willing to dedicate themselves to the care of the infant or child. They should not only be willing, but eager to learn. They must understand the stresses that will come into the family and learn how to deal with them. Parents who do not have these traits may end up not being able to cope with the various situations that arise.

It is the responsibility of the health care team to assist the family in making an informed, responsible decision by reviewing all the alternatives. Home care may not be the best option for every child. It is therefore important to examine all the variables and options before deciding.

HOME CARE OF THE VENTILATOR-DEPENDENT CHILD

Providing home care for the ventilator-dependent patient has become more prevalent. The overall goal should be to select those patients who have the best chance of recovery, or at least who can have an adequate quality of life with home care. The overall objective is to provide an environment that promotes, protects, and supports the physical, cognitive, and social growth and development of the patient.

PATIENT SELECTION FOR HOME VENTILATOR CARE

The most difficult patients to select for home care are those requiring long-term mechanical ventilation. Home care of the ventilator-dependent patient presents one of the most gratifying, as well as difficult, situations. On the one hand, the child can leave the confines of the hospital and enjoy the environment of home and family. On the other hand, the care of the patient places a major stress on the family and they must learn the coping skills needed to deal with their situation.

An assessment of need should be conducted when considering any patient for home mechanical ventilation. The American Association for Respiratory Care's (AARC) clinical practice guideline (CPG) on long-term invasive mechanical ventilation mandates four primary areas be met:

1. Indications are present and contraindications are absent.
2. The goals of home mechanical ventilation can be met.
3. No continued need for higher level of services exists.
4. Frequent changes in the plan of care will not be needed.

The success of home mechanical ventilation depends largely on the underlying disease. Conditions often linked with long-term ventilator care include neuromuscular disorders and injuries, such as trauma, polio, and muscular dystrophies, thoracic cage deformities such as kyphosis, and pulmonary disorders, such as bronchopulmonary dysplasia (BPD). Typically, the candidate for home ventilator care is one who meets the following criteria outlined by Gilmartin.[3] First, the patient can make no spontaneous effort to breath, or the effort is seriously impaired. Second, the patient has failed several attempts to wean following an acute respiratory failure. Third, the patient's disease causes chronic respiratory failure in which repeated hospital admissions are required, or which severely limits his or her ability to function. Gilmartin also points out that patients with a primary diagnosis of skeletal disease, and/or neuromuscular disease, are better candidates for long-term home ventilator care.

Often, the primary disorder is compounded by an underlying disease or disorder, such as chronic cardiopulmonary disease or infection. These secondary conditions must also be considered when home care is contemplated.

Additionally, as cited by the AARC's CPG, indications for ventilation in the home include a progression of disease etiology that requires increasing ventilatory support. Contraindications to home ventilation include the presence of a physiologically unstable medical condition requiring higher levels of care than are available in the home. Examples of medical conditions too unstable for home care are outlined in Table 19–2.

PREPARATION FOR HOME VENTILATOR CARE

The preparation to provide home care is initiated when the patient is first admitted to the intensive care unit. From the beginning, parents and family members are familiarized with equipment and the care provided for their infant or child. This initial familiarization paves the way for the family to assume more and more of the care.

Besides being familiar with the machinery, the family must also know how to care for the tracheostomy tube. This can be a frightening and challenging experience for parents and caregivers. An uncuffed tube is preferred for use in the home care setting, to avoid laryngeal and tracheal damage. The patient is also able to vocalize as a small amount of gas is allowed to leak past the tube. Care of the tracheostomy tube, stoma, and secretion removal, must be thoroughly taught to the family and caregivers. Excellent guides for caregivers are available through Shiley Division of Mallinckrodt Corporation, as well as the Pennsylvania Society for Respiratory Care's *Home Care Procedure Manual*, 2nd ed.

Ideally, the use of monitors should be kept to a minimum in the home. Excessive monitors may reduce the observation of the patient by the parents, which is critical in taking care of these patients. Additionally, excess monitors may perpetuate the feeling of having a NICU in the home, taking away the home-like environment. The home should be organized to create a developmentally appropriate atmosphere. The equipment should be organized

---

TABLE 19–2 Unstable Medical Conditions

FiO_2 requirements > 0.40
PEEP > 10 cm H_2O
Lack of mature tracheostomy
Need for continuous invasive monitoring
Inadequate nutritional intake

---

and arranged in an accessible, safe, and workable manner. The basic equipment required for ventilator home care is listed in Table 19–3.

SELECTION OF A HOME CARE VENTILATOR

The selection of a ventilator is made by the discharge team and determined by patient need and availability of equipment. Ideally, the home ventilator should be small, mobile, fairly simple to understand and operate, with built-in alarms to detect disconnects and other possible hazardous situations. In addition, it should have a battery backup, in case of a power outage.

Due to the choice of ventilators available, the following factors should be considered when making a selection:

1. Simplicity, ease of operation, and reliability
2. Wide range of respiratory rates
3. Accurate delivery of VT over a wide range of values
4. All modes of ventilation such as assist, assist-control, SIMV, CPAP, and pressure support
5. Adequate humidification
6. Variable or constant flow rates
7. Variety of audible and visual alarms
8. Adjustable pressure relief valve/limit
9. Maximum and minimum pressure capabilities

Pediatric and infant patients present with additional problems that must be considered when making a selection. They require a sensitivity setting that is more sensitive to patient effort. Because infant and pediatric patients have smaller tidal volumes and faster respiratory rates, ventilators must have the ability to deliver these set values. The ventilator must have a quick response time as well as a low internal compliance.[4]

Common home ventilators are listed in Table 19–4, and one is shown in Figure 19–1. Other options for ventilation include *diaphragmatic pacers* and negative pressure chest shells.

TABLE 19–3   Equipment Needed for Home Ventilator Care

Oxygen source (if applicable) with back-up cylinder and regulator
Ventilators with patient circuits and humidification device
Alternate power source (i.e., generator or battery with charger)
Self-inflating resuscitation bag
Stationary and AC/DC suction machine
Tracheostomy tube and tracheostomy care items
Pulse oximeter (if indicated)
Sterile water and sterile saline
All necessary disposable items

TABLE 19–4   Common Home Ventilators

1. Mallinckrodt Corp. LP10 and Achieva X, Achieva PS, Achieva PSX
2. Respironics PLV 100, PLV 102
3. Bear Medical Systems Bear 33
4. Pulmonetic Systems LTV 900, LTV 950

Back-up ventilation must be made available in the event of a power outage or equipment failure. This is best accomplished with the use of a manual resuscitator attached to an oxygen tank. In addition, additional ventilator allows the patient to be moved from room to room and prevents the child from being confined to one area in the home.

TRAINING OR PARENTS AND FAMILY

Training of the parents and caregivers in the use of the home ventilator should begin well before the child is ready for discharge. A checklist is often helpful in determining the level of understanding and comprehension of the parents and caregivers. A sample checklist, outlining the training needed to care for the ventilator-dependent child, is shown in Table 19–5. Before discharge can take place, the parents or caregivers must demonstrate competency in these areas by way of return demonstration. The hospital and home care agencies must have documentation attesting to this.

HOME AEROSOL THERAPY

Children may require continuous aerosol therapy to wet and mobilize secretions or may only require intermittent use to reverse bronchospasm. Those who require continuous aerosol are often those with tracheostomy tubes who need supplemental moisture to over-

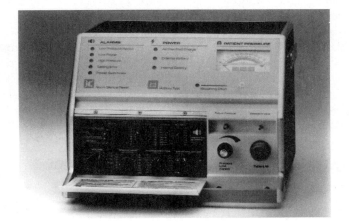

Figure 19–1   *Mallinckrodt Inc., LP10 mechanical ventilator.*

TABLE 19–5 Family Education Plan Checklist

The family, extended family, and any others planning on caring for the patient should be able to demonstrate the following:
  Performance of routine daily care activities
  Ability to adequately provide nutrition to the patient
  Ability to assess the patient's respiratory function
  Performance of correct suctioning, CPT, manual ventilation, and tracheostomy care skills
  Ability to describe signs and symptoms of infection, extubation or decannulation, airway obstruction, hypoxia, and the appropriate intervention for each
  Ability to describe signs of cardiopulmonary arrest and the proper procedure for performing CPR
  Knowledge of the function of the home ventilator and all associated equipment
  Ability to correctly care for, clean, and store equipment
  Understand the dosages, side effects, and demonstrate the ability to administer all medications

---

come the effects of dry gas delivery. These aerosols are often heated to provide maximal humidity to the airway.

Two precautions must be observed closely when continuous aerosols are given to a young patient. First, smaller infants and especially those with cardiac defects are at a risk of fluid overload. Second, there is a possibility that the airway may become burned if the gas temperature is not monitored closely.

ADMINISTRATION OF AEROSOLIZED MEDICATIONS

The administration of aerosolized medications using a hand-held nebulizer may require a compressed gas source. This is provided either by a small electrically powered air compressor or by an air or oxygen cylinder. Another method of medication delivery is by the use of an ultrasonic nebulizer, specifically made for medication delivery.

The patient, family, and caregivers should all be trained in the proper delivery of aerosolized medications. In addition, they should be taught to recognize medication side effects and when to alter the therapy accordingly.

Another method of delivering aerosolized medications at home is through *metered dose inhalers (MDI)*. MDIs are often most effective when delivered using a *spacer* device. Spacers usually require less coordination and may result in better compliance by the patient. Smaller children may be given the medication from an MDI by attaching a mask to the outlet of the spacer, as shown in Figure 19–2, or by using a commercially available spacer supplied with a preattached mask.

CHEST PHYSIOTHERAPY AND SUCTIONING

Many infant patients with chronic lung disorders require chest physiotherapy and suctioning on a long-term basis. Both may be done routinely on patients with a tracheostomy tube to mobilize and remove airway secretions.

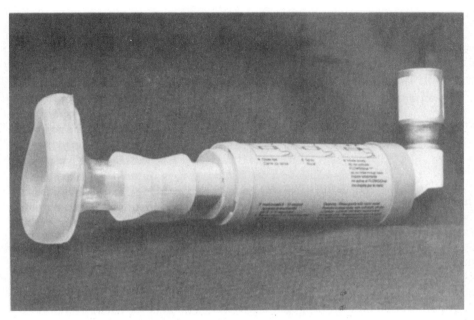

Figure 19–2   *An MDI spacer adapted for use with children using a face mask.*

FAMILY INSTRUCTION

Family and caregivers should be instructed in proper techniques and positioning, and all hazards and potential problems should be covered. Alternative devices to percuss and vibrate the patient should be explained to the family. For example, a small paper cup may be used for percussion and a padded electric toothbrush handle makes an effective vibrator.[5] Percussor cups or palm cups, made of soft vinyl, are available in sizes appropriate for neonatal and pediatric use.

When teaching the family about the pulmonary care of their infant, the practitioner should emphasize the importance of detecting changes in the infant's status that may indicate infection or heart failure. This is best accomplished by establishing a baseline of normal patient status. Once the family is able to identify this baseline information, they can better identify those changes that may indicate infection or heart problems. The family should be instructed to report any changes in status as quickly as possible.

APNEA MONITORING

The use of apnea monitors at home continues to be controversial. With the increased visibility of sudden infant death syndrome (SIDS), home apnea monitoring became very common, with thousands of home monitors placed in the last two decades. The facts, however, show that the presence of these monitors has not lowered the incidence of SIDS.[6]

IDENTIFICATION OF HOME APNEA MONITORING PATIENTS

To work out some of the controversy surrounding the use of these monitors, the National Institutes of Health (NIH) sponsored the Consensus Development Conference on Infantile Apnea and Home Monitoring in 1986. An important term was defined in this conference, Apparent Life-Threatening Event (ALTE). The conference defined this term as an episode that is frightening to the observer and that is characterized by some combination of apnea (central or occasionally obstructive), color change (usually cyanotic or pallid but occasionally erythematous or plethoric), marked change in muscle tone (usually marked limpness), choking, or "gagging." The conference further recommended that the term ALTE be used instead of "near-miss SIDS."

Several important statements regarding the relationship between apnea and morbidity and mortality are summarized in Table 19–6.

The consensus conference additionally identified a number of features deemed to be desirable for a home apnea monitor. Included are: the ability to store events for later analysis; the ability to detect hypoxemia in addition to detecting hypoventilation; the estimation of tidal volume; and the identification of heart patterns and arrhythmias.[7]

Recommendations made by the conference participants regarding the use of home apnea monitors are listed in Table 19–7.

An important outcome of the conference was a statement that in any circumstances, the use of an apnea monitor cannot guarantee survival.[6]

PROBLEMS ASSOCIATED WITH HOME APNEA MONITORING

A common problem associated with apnea monitors is frequent false alarms that can either keep the family and caregivers continually unsettled or lull them into the "cry wolf" mode where the alarm is either ignored or turned off completely. False alarms may be caused by loose, misapplied, or broken electrodes.

Another potential problem is a lack of compliance in the use of the equipment, especially by teenaged mothers and those in low socioeconomic groups.[6]

OXYGEN THERAPY

The selection of the patient for chronic oxygen therapy is usually based on the inability of the patient to maintain a normal PaO_2 on room air. Documentation of room air PaO_2 is often necessary before third-party payers will pay for home oxygen.

TABLE 19-6 Relationship of Apnea to Morbidity and Mortality

1. Apnea of prematurity is not a risk factor of SIDS.
2. An ALTE is a risk factor for sudden death.
3. Apnea of prematurity does not per se cause morbidity.
4. An ALTE may be associated with increased morbidity.
5. Infants with a history of ALTE or apnea of prematurity make up only a small portion of SIDS cases.

TABLE 19–7   Recommendations Regarding the Use of Home Apnea Monitors

---

1. Monitoring is indicated for infants at high risk for sudden death.
   a. Infants with one or more severe ALTE
   b. Symptomatic preterm infants
   c. Siblings of two or more SIDS victims
   d. Infants with conditions such as central hypoventilation
2. Home monitoring is *not* indicated for normal infants.
3. Routine monitoring of asymptomatic preterm infants is not warranted.
4. Pneumograms should not be used to screen for SIDS.
5. The decision to discontinue home monitoring is based on clinical criteria.
   a. Two to three months without significant numbers of alarms or episodes of apnea
   b. Ability to tolerate stress (immunizations, illnesses)
6. The decision-making process with regard to home monitoring is a collaborative enterprise.
7. There should be an adequate support system (medical, technical, psychosocial, and community support).

The candidate for home oxygen therapy should be in stable condition with no other major problems at the time of discharge. Home oxygen therapy requires the regular monitoring of PaO_2 or SaO_2 to ensure adequate oxygenation, prevent hyperoxia, and determine possible weaning from the oxygen. This is facilitated by the use of pulse oximeters and transcutaneous monitors.

Family members and all caregivers of the patient on oxygen must be instructed regarding the potential fire hazard associated with its use. The patient should never be near lit cigarettes or any open flame or spark. The parents must understand that, while not explosive, combustion is extremely enhanced in an oxygen-enriched environment.

OXYGEN ADMINISTRATION EQUIPMENT

The equipment used for delivery of oxygen at home includes a nasal cannula, extension tubing, an oxyhood, flowmeter, and humidifier. In most cases, the infant patient will require low-flow oxygen, which is easily provided by a nasal cannula. An oxygen source that can deliver flows of less than 1 L/min should be available because many patients require only fractional amounts of oxygen. This is accomplished by the use of special regulators and flowmeters that deliver $\frac{1}{16}$ to $\frac{3}{4}$ L/min. During naps and at nighttime, an oxyhood may be used to relieve the constant pressure and presence of the cannula on the patient's face. Some type of portable tank should be available to allow movement outside the home. In addition, a full oxygen cylinder should always be available in case of an emergency.

OXYGEN SOURCES

Oxygen Cylinders. Oxygen cylinders come in a variety of sizes. The most common sizes for home use are the H or K cylinders for the home, and D or E sizes for travel, shown in Figure 19–3.

Cylinders are advantageous for use on the patient with intermittent oxygen requirements. There are, however, several disadvantages to cylinders, which make them a poor

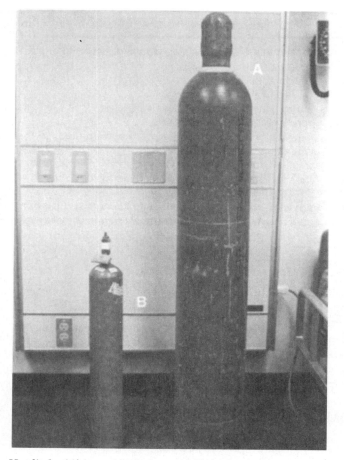

Figure 19–3 *The H cylinder (A) is used in the home while the E cylinder (B) is used for travel.*

choice in most instances. Because of their size and weight, they pose a hazard if they were to fall. They are also relatively expensive for continuous use. A full H cylinder, running at 2 L/min, will only last roughly 2.5 days. A full E cylinder, running at 2 L/min, will only last 5.5 hours.

The amount of time left in a cylinder of gas at any liter flow can be calculated by knowing the cylinder factor, gauge-pressure, and flow rate. (The various cylinder factors and a sample calculation are shown in Table 19–8.)

Obviously, higher flows cause the tank to run out sooner, and lower flows allow a longer use of the tank. Either way, the frequent replacement of tanks becomes expensive and is an ineffective method of delivering continuous home oxygen.

Liquid Systems. Liquid oxygen systems (Figure 19–4) use an insulated tank to hold the extremely cold liquid oxygen. Liquid home systems allow the liquid oxygen to be siphoned

TABLE 19–8   Calculation of Cylinder Duration

For each size cylinder there is a factor. Duration is calculated by multiplying the factor by the pressure in the tank, then dividing the product by the rate of flow.

$$\frac{Factor \times Pressure}{Flow\ Rate}$$

Cylinder Size	Cylinder Factor
D	0.16
E	0.28
H/K	3.14

For example, an E cylinder running at 2 L/min with 1200 psi left in the tank, would be calculated as follows: 0.28 × 1200 psi = 336. Dividing 336 by a flow rate of 2 L/min = 168 minutes. Dividing by 60 minutes will give you 2 hours and 48 minutes of flow left in the tank.

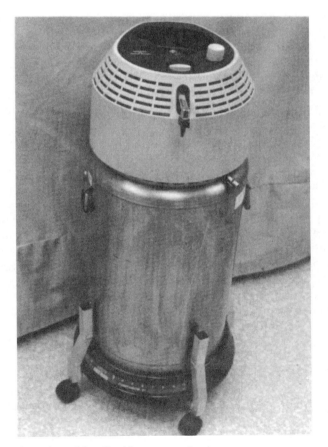

Figure 19–4   *The main tank used in a liquid oxygen system.*

TABLE 19-9   Calculation of Liquid Oxygen Duration

Liquid oxygen weighs 1 pound for every 342 gaseous liters. Therefore, duration of flow in minutes is calculated by multiplying the weight by 342, then dividing the product by the liter flow. A typical liquid oxygen reservoir weighs 70 pounds and at any given flow, the duration can be calculated:

For example, at 2 L/min of flow, the duration of a full reservoir would be calculated as follows:

$70 \times 342 = 23,940$ liters of oxygen

Dividing 23,940 liters by a flow rate of 2 L/min = 11,970 minutes of flow. 11,970 divided by 60 minutes results in 199.5 hours of total flow, which is a little over 8 days.

If the tank is $^3/_4$ full, simply multiply the full weight by 0.75 to find the amount of oxygen left in the reservoir. The duration can then be determined following the above calculation. The same procedure is followed for any reservoir level.

---

to fill a portable tank or allow the liquid to pass through vaporizer coils, becoming a gas that can then be used by the patient.

The main advantage to a liquid system is that it holds a fairly large quantity of gas. Each liter of liquid oxygen is the equivalent of 860 liters of gas. A 30-liter liquid oxygen tank, running at a constant 2 L/min, will last almost 9 days.

The calculation of time left with a liquid system is based on weight instead of pressure. To calculate the time remaining, one must know the capacity of the system and the gauge reading of how much liquid is left. Most liquid oxygen tanks are supplied with a gauge that measures the liquid as being $^3/_4$, $^1/_2$, or $^1/_4$ gone. An example of how to calculate the remaining time in a liquid system is shown in Table 19–9.

Portable liquid oxygen tanks that are filled from the large tank are used for added mobility. With the small tank, the patient is able to be transported away from the home for short periods.

A disadvantage associated with the use of liquid systems is that the liquid oxygen is continuously evaporating and must be vented to the atmosphere. An unused liquid oxygen tank will eventually lose all of its oxygen through evaporation. Because of this, the vented oxygen will create an oxygen-enriched environment, especially if it is in an enclosed space. Continual evaporation also makes it inappropriate when only intermittent oxygen is required. An additional concern is the possibility of frostbite if the unit tips over and liquid oxygen comes into contact with the skin. The modern home liquid oxygen system, however, has very little risk of spilling the liquid oxygen.

When compared to oxygen cylinders, liquid systems are much more cost effective when oxygen must be used continuously.

OXYGEN CONCENTRATORS

Another method of delivering home oxygen is by an oxygen concentrator (Figure 19–5). The concentrator utilizes a nitrogen *sieve*, which filters the nitrogen out of atmospheric air and typically produces 95% oxygen at 1 to 2 L/min. The highest liter flow available on a concentrator today is 6 L/min.[8]

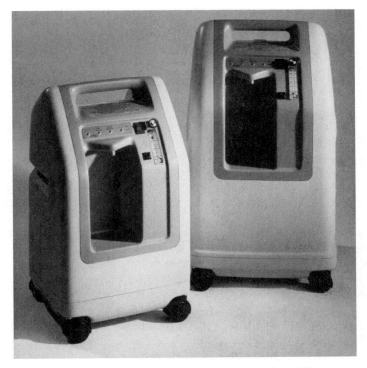

Figure 19–5 (left) Devilbiss SolAiris series 3-liter and (right) 5-liter oxygen concentrators. *(Courtesty of Sunrise Medical Inc., Somerset, PA)*

The percentage of oxygen depends on the liter flow desired, with flows of 1 to 2 L/min delivering the highest oxygen percentage and flows above 2 L/min having a progressively lower oxygen percentage. Oxygen concentrators require electricity to operate and must have a cylinder as a backup in case of a power failure.

Concentrators are generally leased or rented on a monthly basis at a cost far below that of liquid or gas cylinders. For patients requiring low oxygen flows on a continuous basis, the oxygen concentrator is the most cost-effective method of delivering home oxygen.[9] D or E cylinders are used when the patient needs to travel, because the concentrator is restricted to use in the home environment.

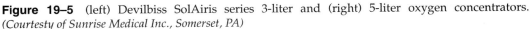

DISCHARGE PLANNING

Once the patient has met the criteria for potential home care, planning begins for the discharge of the infant or child. Planning must begin well before the actual discharge date to allow adequate time for parent training and preparedness. Discharge planning involves many disciplines, each contributing their expertise to the home care plan of the patient.

PERSONNEL INVOLVED IN DISCHARGE PLANNING

Case Manager. The case manager is usually a certified public health nurse or a certified case management nurse who assesses the patient, family, and home environment and develops a plan of care. The care plan includes all medically necessary services, patient and family strengths and weaknesses, services to be provided by the family, and available community resources.

The case manager coordinates the multitude of services required for the patient and acts as a liaison for the family. Additionally, the case manager monitors and evaluates the quality of care being provided.

Physician. The home care physician is a pediatrician experienced in the home management of children. The physician oversees the entire medical care of the infant or child and evaluates the appropriateness and quality of care.

The physician receives information from each of the disciplines and from that determines the time of discharge and the follow-up that will be necessary. The physician should be on call 24 hours a day. As care continues, the physician establishes and then reviews a written home care plan, which specifies the necessary medical care.[10]

The physician should receive reports from the health care providers to assess the ongoing care of the infant or child.

Respiratory Care Practitioner. The involvement of the respiratory care practitioner in discharge planning is to determine the respiratory needs of the patient and to train the parents to perform the necessary procedures. If the patient will be on a ventilator, the practitioner helps in the selection of an appropriate ventilator and then teaches the parents the necessary skills to provide ventilator care.

Close attention should be paid to teaching the parents the signs of respiratory distress and infection. The parents should also be taught how to perform CPT, suction, and tracheostomy care.

The parents must gain the confidence to ventilate their baby manually if the need arises, so adequate time must be allowed for practice. If a pulse oximeter is to be used, the parents are instructed in care and placement of the sensor and the setting of alarm limits. They must also be instructed in appropriate measures to take if the alarm limits are violated.

During the training period the parents are gradually allowed to assume the responsibilities that they will be doing at home. The respiratory care practitioner also develops a plan for eventual weaning off the ventilator, if appropriate, and establish goals for that accomplishment. For the patient requiring continuous oxygen therapy, the practitioner helps determine the best mode of delivery and then provides the appropriate documentation for the writing of the prescription by the physician.

The parents are taught the signs of hypoxia and how to check for disconnects or blockage in the tubing. They must also be instructed when to order more oxygen so they do not run out.

For patients requiring an apnea monitor, the practitioner helps select an appropriate monitor and then instructs the parents in its use. Of utmost priority is teaching CPR skills to parents, grandparents, and potential babysitters before the infant is discharged. Care must be taken not to frighten the parents into thinking that something disastrous will happen. They must understand that the purpose of all of this training is to prepare them in case the need arises.

Nursing. The role of the nurse in the discharge planning is to map out the nursing care that will be required. The nurse teaches the family proper skills in delivering medications, providing hygiene, feeding, dressing changes, and skin care. The nurse also teaches the family assessment skills as required. Home care visits are arranged as needed by the nurse.

The nurse who is involved in discharge planning works very closely with the case manager in follow-up and evaluation of care. Once the infant or child is discharged, the nurse is often the one who actually moves in with the family during the transition to home care.

The home care nurse must be trained in all aspects of the care of the infant or child to handle any emergency that arises.

Social Worker. The role of the social worker is to assist the discharge planning by identifying environmental, social, and emotional factors that are of significance. The social worker determines the appropriateness of admission into the home care program and helps develop the child/family psychosocial plan.

Through visits to the family, the social worker provides support and assistance to the family regarding psychosocial and developmental issues. The social worker provides valuable assistance to the family in obtaining financial aid and also serves as the ombudsman for the family.

Dietician. The dietician maps out a strategy for the nutritional needs of the infant. Any special diets or supplements are planned and the parents instructed in their use. The dietician closely follows the infant's growth and development and upgrades the diet as needed to meet the ongoing needs of the infant. Close attention is also paid to the caloric intake of the infant. The dietician should be experienced in working with ventilator-dependent infants and understand their special caloric, fluid, and electrolyte needs.

Physical, Occupational, and Speech Therapy. Occupational therapy, speech therapy, and physical therapy are involved in the developmental and physical growth of the infant or child. During discharge planning, their plans center around the appropriate social and physical development that should be taking place. Plans are developed that will allow the infant or child learn skills that are appropriate for his or her age and hopefully prevent an underdevelopment in these skills.

Physical therapy is planned around the needs of the infant or child to gain muscular strength and coordination and reduce the effects of inactivity.

Home Care Company. A decision by the discharge planning group regarding the appropriate home care company should be made well before the infant or child is to be discharged. The decision should be based on the needs of the infant or child, the ability of the company to respond quickly to calls, and expert personnel who know and understand the equipment that will be used. The home care company that is chosen should have an on-call respiratory therapist, available 24 hours a day, 7 days a week for any questions or service that may be needed.

The company and their personnel should be involved in the discharge planning as early as possible to assess potential needs and understand the level of care the infant or child will require.

Before the infant or child is discharged, the home care provider assesses the home environment. The home assessment should determine whether there are an appropriate number of properly grounded electrical outlets, appropriate doorway clearance and accessibility, the presence of any hazards such as open flames or sparks, and the presence of a functioning telephone. The room that the patient will be in must have proper ventilation and lighting and be in close proximity to the parents' room. Any recommended changes can then be made prior to discharge of the child. Letters notifying the electric company, telephone company, and local emergency services of life support equipment in the home are sent to establish priority service.

DISCHARGE

The actual day that the patient is discharged will be an emotional day for the parents and family. The health care team must be sure that all the parents' emotional needs will be met. The team informs the parents of support group meeting times and places, possible religious counseling, and counseling for the siblings.

PERSONNEL NEEDS

The first few days with the child at home may require 24-hour presence of a nurse to provide support as the family becomes accustomed to the new situation. The presence of the health care worker is gradually withdrawn as the family becomes more comfortable with caring for the child. Eventually, the family is left alone to care entirely for their child.

Some patients, because of the nature of their illness or other circumstances, will require regular home visits by a health care worker. The family must understand that they can call for assistance at any time and must be provided with the appropriate telephone numbers. The family will require a lot of support, manifest by frequent phone calls, regular visits, and words of encouragement. They should be invited to participate in family-to-family support groups.

THE EFFECTS OF HOME CARE ON THE FAMILY

A study by McKim indicated that almost half of the mothers of premature infants found the first week to be difficult, even though they were well supported by family and friends.[11]

The effects of home care on the family are numerous. The presence of a sick infant in the home causes major disruptions of family life. The family may feel like they live in an NCIU, with frequent changes of personnel, alarms, and doctor appointments. The sick child becomes the center of the family's life, and attempts to continue with normal activities are often unsuccessful.

The necessity of a live-in nurse brings with it a potential loss of normal interactions and intimacy. The family may be grateful for the care being rendered to their child, but the challenge of having someone live in the home may become a major stumbling block.

The family may become consumed with the care of the infant and the siblings may feel left out and neglected. The relationships among all family members often need to be gradually redefined. The siblings should be included in the care of the infant and made to feel like their brother or sister needs them.

The family may have problems dealing with the health care and financial establishments, adding more stress to the situation. A good case manager and social worker can be of invaluable assistance in these circumstances by providing help to the family in dealing with these establishments.

Another source of potential stress is the impact home care has on the careers of the parents. There may be two opposing feelings: one of guilt for leaving the child home versus one of need for the additional income.[12]

Despite all of the stress that comes from the home care of an infant, most families grow and develop through the experience and handle the stress admirably. Many find that the extraordinary giving and selflessness that is required enhances their love for their child and for the family. The family is bonded tighter by the experience, with family members relying on each other for support and comfort.

Any family who provides home care must receive plenty of empathy and encouragement from the health care team. The success of the home care effort is dependent on a group effort and the combined efforts of all involved.

FAILURE OF HOME CARE

Even with the most well-thought-out and anticipated home care plan, not all home care cases are successful. The most common causes of home care failure should be understood by the health care team in an attempt to avoid them, if possible. A good overview of the reasons for home care failure can be found in Harris.[13]

The most common cause of home care failure is a lack of community and family resources. Signs that the plan is failing include weight loss by the patient, developing skin breakdown and infections, depression of the family, failure to perform treatments, and frequent visits to the emergency department.

Another source of failure is the depiction of the family's financial resources. The consequences of financial depiction include lack of food and transportation and loss of telephone service. The patient may suffer because of the house being too hot in the summer or too cold in the winter.

The emotional depletion of the family occurs when they become financially stressed and physically exhausted. Clues that signal emotional depletion include loss of hope, spirituality, and humor.

Lack of communication among family members, between family and health care workers, and among health care workers may lead to incongruent priorities in the care of the infant. Each participant may have his or her own ideas as to what should be done for the patient. Any mismatch of ideas or priorities should be quickly rendered by opening communication between all involved. In all cases, the opinions and priorities of the family should be preference, with the health care team providing second opinions as necessary.

Although an understanding of these mechanisms for failure may not avert all breakdowns in home care, it may allow the health care team to avoid the most common problems.

SUMMARY

Home care has blossomed in recent years as a viable and often better option to hospitalization. Despite this, questions still remain regarding how to select candidates, how the decision for home care is made, who will help the parents and family, and how long help will be provided.

There are three basic models to providing pediatric home care: 1) hospital based; 2) community based; 3) bureaucratic. Patient selection should be based on the type of patient, the type and severity of the illness, and the home environment. Home ventilator care is possible, assuming certain conditions are in place. They include a mature tracheostomy, FiO_2 requirements less than .40, no need for invasive monitoring, and an adequate nutritional intake. Several home ventilators are available that are fairly simple to operate, have back-up power mechanisms, and alarms to indicate disconnects or ventilator problems.

Home aerosol therapy is often necessary during the home care of respiratory patients. Several companies offer medical compressors that power small volume nebulizers. Portable ultrasonic nebulizers are also available for home use. MDIs are a popular method of delivering aerosolized medicines, but require training and coordination to be effective. Patients and their families can also be trained to provide CPT and suctioning at home. Percussors are available for home use, or the patient and family may feel comfortable using hand cupping.

Home apnea monitors have gone from immense popularity to far fewer uses currently. The main reason for the decline in home use is that, despite their use, the incidence of SIDS did not decline. There are, however, a group of patients who stand to benefit from the use of a home apnea monitor. These are patients who have a history of apnea and ALTEs.

Oxygen therapy is becoming more acceptable as a home care treatment. The arrival of oxygen concentrators and liquid oxygen tanks greatly reduced the overall cost and risk associated with long-term oxygen use. Small portable tanks have also made short trips possible.

Discharge planning is a group process and requires the skills of several health care workers. Included in the process are a case manager, physician, respiratory care practitioner, nurse, social worker, dietician, physical therapy, occupational therapy, speech therapy, and the home care company.

Of great concern with home care is the stress that comes to the family. Proper planning and solid follow-up and support help ease the stress. Because the system is not perfect, home care failures occur. The most common cause of failure is a lack of resources. Other factors include emotional depletion and lack of communication.

Home care of a pediatric or infant patient has many positive aspects and should be encouraged where possible. It is not, however, without some negative aspects. The negative aspects can be minimized by proper preparation of the patient and family. The involvement of many disciplines helps create a successful environment. Anticipation of future problems and needs will help alleviate negative outcomes by allowing proper preparation.

As the role of medicine in our society continues to change, home health care will undoubtedly continue to play a major part.

References

1. Aitken MJ. Matching models to environments: a planning guide to the selection of pediatric home care models. *Home Healthc Nurse.* 1989;7:13–21.

2. Donar ME. Community care: pediatric home mechanical ventilation. *Holistic Nurs Pract.* 1988;2:68–80.

3. Gilmartin M. Transition from the intensive care unit to home: patient selection and discharge planning. *Resp Care.* 1994;39:456–480.

4. *Respiratory Home Care Procedure Manual.* 2d ed.: Pennsylvania Society for Respiratory Care Inc; 1997.

5. Lynch M. Bronchopulmonary dysplasia: management after discharge. *Home Healthc Nurs.* 1989;7:34–40.

6. Lott D. Home apnea monitoring: an update. *Perinat/Neonat.* 1988;12:223-237.

7. Consensus Statement: National Institute of Health Consensus Development Conference on Infantile Apnea and Home Monitoring, Sept. 29 to Oct. 1, 1986. *Pediatrics* 1987;79:292–299.

8. Wyka K. *Respiratory Care in Alternate Sites.* Albany, NY: Delmar Thomson Learning; 1998.

9. Koff PB, Eitzman DV, Nev J. *Neonatal and Pediatric Respiratory Care.* St. Louis: CV Mosby Co; 1993.

10. Bedore B, Leighton L. Ventilator-dependent children: comprehensive home management. *Caring.* 1989;8:50–52, 54–55.

11. McKim EM. The difficult first week at home with a premature infant. *Neonatal Network.* 1993;12:72.

12. Feinberg EA. Family stress in pediatric home care. *Caring.* 1985;4:38, 40–41.

13. Harris PJ. Sometimes pediatric home care doesn't work. *Am J Nurs.* 1988;88:851–854.

Bibliography and Suggested Readings

American Association for Respiratory Care. AARC Clinical Practice Guideline: discharge planning for the respiratory care patient. *Respiratory Care.* 1995a;40:1308–1312.

American Association for Respiratory Care. AARC Clinical Practice Guideline: long-term invasive mechanical ventilation in the home. *Respiratory Care.* 1995b;40:1313–1320.

Burton GG, et al. *Respiratory Care. A Guide to Clinical Practice.* 4th ed. Philadelphia: JB Lippincott Co; 1997.

Pierson DJ. Controversies in home respiratory care: conference summary. *Resp Care.* 1994;39:294–308.

White G. *Equipment Theory for Respiratory Care.* 2nd ed. Albany, NY: Delmar Thomson Learning; 1996.

Posttest

1. Which of the following are advantages of home care?
   I. allows more normal family interaction
   II. patients get infections less frequently
   III. cost savings
   IV. faster recovery from the disease process
      a. I, III, IV
      b. I, II, III
      c. II, II, IV
      d. III only

2. Which of the following is *not* true regarding the bureaucratic type of home care?
   a. available to all families
   b. may be more readily accepted by health care providers
   c. many ancillary services are already in place
   d. financial resources may be facilitated

3. Of the following disorders, which is most likely to produce candidates for ventilator home care?
   a. cardiogenic anomalies
   b. esophageal atresia
   c. BPD
   d. infantile botulism

4. Regarding tracheostomy tubes, which of the following is best suited for home care?
   a. fenestrated, cuffed tube
   b. uncuffed, slightly smaller than the trachea
   c. cuffed, slightly larger than the trachea
   d. uncuffed, larger than the trachea

5. Which of the following are possible hazards of home aerosol therapy?
   I. tracheal irritation
   II. fluid overload
   III. excessive secretions
   IV. burns
      a. I, II
      b. I, III, IV
      c. III, IV
      d. II, IV

6. Detecting clinical changes that may indicate infection or heart failure requires:
   a. outpatient blood work
   b. frequent examinations by a physician
   c. in-depth training of parents and caregivers
   d. establishing a baseline of normal patient status
7. Which of the following is a common cause of problems with home apnea monitoring?
   a. unfamiliarity with the equipment
   b. interference from radio and television signals
   c. frequent false alarms
   d. the equipment is not indicated
8. The main advantage to liquid oxygen sysstems is:
   a. they are very inexpensive
   b. they are very lightweight
   c. they hold a large quantity of gas
   d. the delivered oxygen is of a higher purity
9. Which of the following people coordinates home care services and acts as a liaison to the family?
   a. case manager
   b. physician
   c. nurse
   d. social worker
10. Of the following, which is the *least* likely to cause parental stress during home care?
    a. disruption of the family life
    b. the presence of a live-in caretaker
    c. the visual appearance of the infant
    d. constant noise and alarms
11. Which of the following is the *most* common cause of home care failure?
    a. family stress
    b. depiction of family resources
    c. lack of community and family resources
    d. physical exhaustion

CHAPTER TWENTY

CARE OF THE PARENTS

OBJECTIVES

Upon completion of this chapter, the reader should be able to:

1. Describe the bonding that takes place during each of the following periods:
   a. Pregnancy
   b. Labor and delivery
   c. Home
2. List the factors that cause stress to the parents following delivery of a sick neonate.
3. Describe the following environmental factors and their role in creating stress in the parents:
   a. Appearance of the neonate
   b. Staff communications
   c. Alteration of parental roles
4. Compare and contrast maternal and paternal stress as it relates to the above factors.
5. Describe how the practitioner can reduce stress factors for the parents.
6. Define grief.
7. Describe each stage of grief and its accompanying clinical signs and symptoms.
8. Describe how the practitioner can help the parents through each stage of grief.

KEY TERMS

anticipatory grief	lethargy	pessimism
bonding	optimism	psychosocial
empathetic		

OVERVIEW

One very important area of concern that has risen from the rapid advance of neonatology, and one that is frequently overlooked, is caring for the family of the sick neonate. An essential part of the work of any neonatal practitioner is addressing the psychologic needs of each family member. Although not intended to be all-inclusive, this chapter takes a brief look at the bonding process, the grieving process, and how the practitioner can help the family cope.

BONDING

BONDING DURING PREGNANCY

The *bonding* of parent to child begins with the anticipation of the child (Table 20–1). Upon discovering that pregnancy has begun the family begins preparations for the new addition. The nursery is prepared, furniture and bedding are purchased. The family begins to imagine what the child will look like, guessing its sex and thinking of potential names. They dream of the future and the happiness the newborn will bring to them. The first sounds of the heartbeat and the first signs of movement further increase expectations and heighten the excitement, because the baby is now an individual, no longer an imagined being.

As pregnancy continues, the mother is made continuously aware of the fetus's presence, as the physical discomfort of the pregnancy begins to weigh on her. The father, although not physically involved in the pregnancy, may find himself worrying about his wife and the baby. As the pregnancy advances, the lifestyle of the family changes. The mother is not able to do those things that she could previously do, and plans may be altered and changed.

Even though not present, the fetus is making a significant impact on the life of the family. It is already developing a personality, and the family finds itself laughing at the internal gyrations, hiccoughs, and limb stretches.

BONDING DURING LABOR AND DELIVERY

The onset of labor presents an emotional and psychologic crisis for the family. The long-awaited time has finally arrived. All the difficulties encountered during the pregnancy and the anticipation are rewarded by the birth of a healthy infant. Everyone present is in an excited and anticipatory state; however, labor is also a time of physiologic crisis for the mother. She must endure tremendous pain and discomfort, for the most part, alone.

TABLE 20–1   Steps of Bonding and Attachment

1. Planning of the pregnancy
2. Confirmation of the pregnancy
3. Acceptance of the pregnancy
4. Feeling the first fetal movements
5. Acceptance of the fetus as an individual
6. Labor and subsequent birth of the infant
7. Seeing the infant for the first time
8. Touching the infant
9. Taking care of the infant

Birth of the infant brings tears, kisses, and joy to the family. The sound of a healthy cry and the presence of all fingers and toes and no defects bring a sigh of relief. Bonding now begins at an advanced level. The neonate, before now only seen in the imagination, is now held by the family. The initial touching and eye contact is an important part of the bonding process. The parents spend the first hours encouraging their neonate to look at them and having the newborn grasp their fingers. In addition to the psychological benefits of skin-to-skin contact between the parent and the infant, research suggests that physiological improvements in respiratory rates and pattern, heart rate, and oxyhemoglobin may also be promoted.[1]

During this time shortly following the delivery, the neonate is identified as having characteristics similar to the parents and other family members. This inspection is important and serves to allow the parents and family to accept the infant as a part of the family.

BONDING AT HOME

Arrival at home brings a new lifestyle to the family. The first few months are filled with frequent awakenings at night and other adaptations. The infant is totally dependent on the parents for his or her welfare. This is a time of tremendous growth in the maturity of the family and in their love for the new infant. The love and bonding that develop continue to increase as the infant grows.

Thus, bonding has taken place from the moment that the pregnancy was planned and continues throughout the life of the child. Any disruption of these normal bonding events can cause an emotional and psychological crisis for the family. It is during these times that the health care worker must be aware of the needs of the family and be able to address those needs appropriately.

CAUSES OF PARENTAL STRESS

The premature delivery of a neonate produces many stressors on the family. The sudden disruption of the pregnancy is a grief-producing occurrence that must be dealt with by the family. Additionally, several environmental stressors have been identified with which the family must also deal.

In the event of a premature delivery or other birth crisis, what should have been a happy, joyful time has become a major stress-inducing experience for the family. It is during this time and in the days and weeks to follow that the NICU team must be aware of the emotional and psychological needs of the family. By understanding the factors that create stress and individually assessing each neonate and their family with regard to such stress, the practitioner can help reduce those factors through an individualized approach to care and family dynamics. Following a discussion of stress factors, we will examine the stages of grief, which the family commonly passes through following a birth crisis.

IDENTIFYING STRESS FACTORS

Three sources of stress have been identified: 1) *personal and family background factors;* 2) *situational conditions,* and 3) *environmental stimuli.*[2] Personal and family background factors are the past and present experiences, beliefs, and attitudes that the family brings to the crisis. Situational conditions are threats to normal family behavior and interaction that occur following the birth of an ill neonate. The final factors, environmental stimuli, arisen from both the *psychosocial* and physical environment of the NICU.[2] Our focus will be on these environmental factors.

ENVIRONMENTAL STRESS FACTORS

The entire environment of the NICU creates varying degrees of stress on the family. The physical separation from the newborn, the heat, noise and alarms, abundance of high-tech equipment, crowds of medical personnel, and the sight of other critically ill neonates may overwhelm the parents. In fact, research has shown that parental anxiety levels can reach near-panic levels initially.[3] Other research has found that 28% of the mothers of critically ill neonates reported clinically significant psychological distress compared to 10% of the general population.[4]

Appearance of the Neonate. The appearance and behavior of the neonate are another source of stress for the parents and family. Their newborn does not look like they had imagined.

The shock produced by the visual appearance of the newborn is often difficult to get over. In addition, the tangle of wires and tubing attached to their newborn furthers the shock. The preemie may have gelatinous skin with numerous bruises and abrasions from delivery. Neonates may also be subject to potentially painful procedures. Preparation of the parents for these sights will help reduce the visual shock.

High-Tech/Impersonal Environment. An additional source of stress can be the high-tech, impersonal appearance of the NICU. Initially, many parents find the NICU appearance shocking and intimidating. Equipment with wiring, tubing, and blinking lights looks frightening. These factors combined with audible alarms can be unnerving to parents, who themselves may be adversely affected by sensory overload and a sense of alienation.[5]

Staff Communication. Another source of environmental stress is the communication, or lack thereof, between staff and family. As much as possible, the parents should be involved in the care of the neonate. They should be involved in decision making and not simply told what will happen next.

Alteration of Parental Role. A final source of environmental stress is the alteration of the parental role in the care of the neonate. The family takes on a subordinate role, and often may feel as though they are spectators only, without any control over outcomes. This is often magnified by the thoughtless treatment of parents by practitioners as though they are outsiders.

Maternal versus Paternal Stress. Research has shown that the mothers of critically ill neonates have a more adverse reaction to the NICU environment than the fathers.

An interesting study done by Perehudoff sampled the reactions of fathers and mothers to various NICU environmental stressors.[2] The study indicates that mothers and fathers perceived environmental stress differently, and that overall the mother was more stressed than the father. Mothers indicated that parental role alteration was the highest source of stress, followed by NICU sights and sounds, the neonate's appearance and behaviors, and, finally, staff communications and relations.

In contrast, fathers indicated that the highest degree of stress was caused by the sights and sounds, followed by parental role alteration. The final two stressors were the same in fathers as in the mothers.

Another study performed by Shields-Poe and colleagues supported some of the findings described above and found that other factors also affected parental stress levels such as where and when the parents first saw their infant.[6]

Other Stressors. In addition to the environmental stressors, other factors have been shown to contribute to parental stress. Increased tendency toward trait-anxiety and a strong desire for the pregnancy resulted in higher stress levels for parents of NICU patients.[6] Other research indicates that additional parental stressors may be related to siblings' reaction to the NICU experience and disruption from the daily family routine.[7]

IMPLICATIONS FOR THE PRACTITIONER

An understanding of the environmental stress factors will aid the practitioner in helping the parents and family cope with the multitude of stressors. Allowing the parents opportunities to care for their neonate may help reduce the alteration of their parental role.

The shock of the sights and sounds of the NICU can be lessened by explaining to the parents in advance what they will see and what to expect. Pictures of premature infants will allow the parents and family to prepare for what their neonate will look like. It is important to emphasize that their baby looks perfectly normal for its gestational age. The parents must be assured that their baby looks exactly like it should. Cultural and religious considerations should also be identified early and respected to avoid additional stress for the family.

Finally, good communication between staff members and family will greatly lessen stress by instilling in the parents some degree of participation and control. The parents must feel comfortable to call whenever they desire to get an update on their baby's status. The staff should avoid phrases such as "he's stable" or "there's no change in her status." Instead, the parents should be informed of current ventilator settings, weight gains or losses, and the rationale for any change in medications or treatments should be explained to the parents. The staff should encourage the parents to share their feelings and frustrations openly, always being *empathetic* toward their difficult situation. Support-group participation by parents should also be encouraged.

UNDERSTANDING GRIEF

Grief has been defined as "an abiding and pervasive sense of sadness that overwhelms us when we are separated from a person, place, or object important to our emotional life.[8] Unless one has experienced grief, it is unlikely that person truly understands what a grieving person is feeling. An unfortunate consequence of this lack of understanding is the tendency to ignore the symptoms and needs of one who is grieving.

The birth of an ill neonate is a situation that produces grief in the parents and family members. Critical illness or death of an infant or child is one of the greatest stresses that a parent can experience. The anticipation that the baby may not survive further enhances the grief.[9] An understanding of what occurs during the grieving period will help practitioners provide the necessary support and will enable them to better empathize with and tolerate the behavior of the family. It is also important for the practitioner to recognize individual differences in each person's grieving process. The practitioner should try to empathize and not get defensive if parents manifest feelings of anger, frustration, and self-pity toward them.

ANTICIPATORY GRIEF

Death does not necessarily have to occur for grief to be present. *Anticipatory grief* occurs when the death of a love one appears likely.[8] This is often the type of grief that parents and family members of a critically ill neonate experience. A person undergoing anticipatory grief passes through the same stages as if death had actually occurred. They require the same amount of support and assistance as any other grieving person.[8]

STAGES OF GRIEF

A pioneer in the development of grief stages was Elisabeth Kübler-Ross.[10] Studies done on the dying revealed that grieving is a process that occurs in an inexact pattern. Each phase represents the dominant feelings or processes that are occurring. The phases are not limited to any time frame, nor does every grieving person pass through each stage to the same degree. These are merely presented to allow some insight into what the parents of an ill infant may be experiencing. The stages presented here follow the pattern offered by Weizman and Kamm.[11]

Shock: The First Stage of Grief. The initial emotion felt by the parents is one of shock, denial, and disbelief. No matter how prepared the family may think they are for the delivery, no one is ever totally ready for the shock that accompanies a premature delivery. It often occurs during the time in the pregnancy when the mother is still bonding with the infant. The mother is in the process of undergoing not only a physical change, but also a psychological change as the pregnancy advances. The pregnancy has usually progressed far enough to allow the family to accept the infant as an individual, but not to the point where they are emotionally ready for the delivery.

The premature delivery causes a type of psychological dislocation to take place. As previously mentioned, the initial shock is intensified by several environmental factors, such as the sight of the neonate and the high-tech environment of the NICU.

Confusion. Included in the feeling of shock is an overwhelming sense of confusion. There is a feeling of not knowing what to do or who to turn to. Time may become distorted, and memory of the events surrounding the birth of the neonate may be cloudy.

Denial. Another phase of shock is denial. Denial is an attempt to shield oneself from the pain and impact of the event. Denial may present itself subtly or openly by the parents. They may refuse to believe what is told them by the physician and may even go so far as to look for another "specialist" to take care of their infant.

Denial may take one of two contrasting patterns. Some parents may feel that, regardless of what they are being told, their infant will be all right. On the other extreme, they may believe that the situation is hopeless, regardless of what they are told. In these instances, parents may exhibit a reluctance to see, touch, or hold their infant (Lundquist, et al, 1998).

Parents often tend to be more *pessimistic* or *optimistic* about their infant. This pessimism may be fostered by overly pessimistic reports from the health care team. Whereas it is never justified to give unrealistic hope to the family, it is equally damaging to be overly pessimistic in the prognosis. The odds are weighed heavily in the infant's favor in most NICUs, so a cautious optimism may be more helpful to the parents than a continual negative outlook.

The NICU team must work together when talking to the family. It is not uncommon for one team member to report that the infant is doing better, only to have another claim that the infant is the same or worse than before. Such mixed signals cause the parents to lose faith in the team and possibly wonder if anyone really knows what they are talking about. Discussions with the family regarding the overall status of their infant may best be handled by the attending neonatologist.

Bargaining. Bargaining is an attempt to find a magical solution by promising anything in return for a healthy infant. Promises such as "I will be the perfect parent" and "I'll never do anything wrong again" are common pleas.

Bargaining often had deep religious overtones. Promises are made to God that the person will do whatever is required, if God will only heal their child. Bargaining is like denial, in that it is a temporary release from reality that allows the person to feel like they have some control over what is happening. It allows the person more time to acquire the needed strength to face the problem.

Isolation. An attempt to become isolated from the entire situation is often seen next in grieving people. The isolation may be an attempt to be protected from further emotional damage. The person may feel that no one understands, causing them to withdraw from the situation.

The health care team should make every effort to close the gap of isolation, to stay in contact with the family, encourage their presence in the NICU, and consider support-group referral.

Undoing: The Second Stage of Grief. During this stage, the person attempts to undo what has happened so life can return to what it was. There may be thoughts of what should have or could have been done to prevent the premature birth. Thoughts such as these are an attempt to undo what has happened in the mind of the parent.

Guilt. A common feeling during the undoing stage is that of guilt. In an attempt to undo the situation, the mother may become obsessed with the idea that something she did, or did not do, caused the premature birth. The parents may feel that they have some sort of physical defect that caused the birth. The mother often feels that she is at fault for the crisis.

The NICU team must be careful to in no way reinforce this idea. The family, and especially the mother, must understand that nothing she did, or did not do, caused the premature delivery. Some may feel that the early birth is a punishment for something they did. The fixation of blame is a natural human tendency, even if it is upon oneself. Positive reinforcement by the NICU team will help to minimize the guilt that may be present.

Anger: The Third Stage of Grief. Many families undergoing a crisis may at some point become angry. Anger is directed in many ways and toward many people. Anger may be directed at the health care team, whom the parents may see as ghouls whose only desire is to inflict further pain on their infant. They may vent their anger on anyone who is present. The expression of anger is an attempt to affix blame for the crisis on someone or something.

Threats of lawsuits may be directed at the nurse for starting an IV or at the respiratory care practitioner for obtaining a heel stick blood gas. Anger is often directed toward God, with the family wondering why He would allow such a thing to happen to them. The mother may be angry at those who have normal babies, or at every pregnant woman.

Parents and families may even blame each other for the premature birth. The father may blame the mother for not quitting work or for some other action that he views as causing the premature birth. The family may even express anger toward the infant for being born early. The in-laws may accuse the son-in-law of not earning enough money to allow their daughter to quit work while pregnant.

Regardless of where the anger is directed, the practitioner must understand that it is a natural part of the grieving process and must be patient with the family. One must always keep in mind that the expression of anger is essential in the grieving process.

Sadness: The Fourth Stage of Grief. When the reality of the event finally begins to sink in, an overwhelming feeling of sadness occurs. Parents may feel like life is not worth living without their baby. They express extreme disappointment and hopelessness in their situation. This stage is possibly the most painful stage of grief, one in which the family requires much love and support.

Avoidance of Sadness. To avoid the profound sadness of this stage, the parents may being a bustle of activity so they will not have time to feel sad. They may withhold and suppress feelings of sadness by refusing to cry or talk about the situation. During this time, the health care worker must encourage the parents to express their sadness and talk openly about their disappointment. Suppressing the feeling only brings anger and a prolongation of the sadness. Only when the feelings of anger and sadness are relieved are the parents able to continue their emotional recovery.

Depression. Continued feelings of guilt and the inability to express anger may lead to depression. Depression is often characterized by a loss of appetite, lack of sleep, and overall *lethargy*. The person becomes withdrawn and unresponsive. In addition, the mother may suffer a normal postpartum depression, which is heaped on the previous depression.

Physical exhaustion from lack of sleep further complicates the depression. The person suffering from severe depression may need to be treated with medications to induce sleep and help with the feelings of hopelessness. As always, continual support by the NICU team is invaluable. The mother must understand that she is not a failure. Severe extended depression requires immediate attention and should never be passed off as being just a part of the grieving process.

Integration: The Fifth Stage of Grief. As a person slowly passes through each stage of grief, there is a gradual accomplishment of integration.

Acceptance. An important milestone in integration is acceptance. The time will finally arrive when the parents accept the crisis and begin to handle it in a constructive way. It may arrive quickly, or may be delayed, but eventually comes. Acceptance comes when the family becomes familiar with the surroundings in the NICU.

The parents have adapted to the dramatic change in their lifestyle, and visiting their sick baby is now a part of their routine. They know and trust the health care team and understand what is happening to their infant. They are involved in the care of the infant and hold it as often as possible. Once acceptance occurs, the parents of infants with a favourable NICU outcome can now look forward to the day the baby is released with anticipation and happiness.

In situations where the infant dies, it will take a considerable amount of time before acceptance occurs. Often in such situations, pictures are taken of the baby to aid in the grieving and acceptance process. Professional counseling and bereavement support groups often benefit the parents and family of the deceased infant.

Grieving and the Practitioner. Death is a reality in the NICU setting and can significantly add to practitioners' job stress. Research reveals that practitioners often experience feelings of helplessness, intense sorrow, chronic fatigue, and irritability when an infant dies. It is important for practitioners to first acknowledge such feelings. Communication with coworkers, counseling professionals, and friends and family is often helpful in this grieving process.[12]

SUMMARY

An understanding of the stages of grief will help the practitioner to accept and be empathetic toward parental behaviors. With this enhanced understanding in hand, the practitioner can help address parental grief by appropriately sharing information with parents to avoid a sense of abandonment. Additionally, they can also assist parents in the grieving process by being sensitive to cultural and religious issues and taking an overall empathetic approach to family interaction and patient care.[13] Grieving often involves feelings of shock, denial, anger, and bargaining, which are necessary in that they allow time to accept the crisis in small, manageable doses. The stages discussed may not occur in order, and some may not occur at all.

Members of the family may go through stages at different speeds and be at different levels of understanding, making communication among them difficult. The mother, because of her deeper feelings toward the infant, often suffers more severely than the father during the various stages.

The intensity of emotions will vary among family members. Some persons may accept the crisis from the beginning, while others withdraw and want nothing to do with the neonate. Although the parents have reached acceptance of the initial crisis, they may go through each stage again with each new setback.

The parents should be encouraged to have frequent contact with their infant. This tends to hasten the acceptance of the child. The family must be informed of the various equipment being used and why it is being used. Daily updates are vital and help the family to adapt to the situation. Counselors who are experts in dealing with crisis should be involved with the family from the beginning.

Parents should be encouraged to express emotions and seek help in dealing with those emotions. Positive reinforcement by members of the health care team is vital in supporting the parents during these difficult trials. Programs may also be developed for the siblings to help them understand what is happening to their brother or sister.

Even with an understanding of the grief process, it is still impossible to know how the family is feeling at any one moment. It is at those times that a hug or a shoulder to cry on are the best things that the health care worker can offer.

References

1. Cleary GM, et al. Skin-to-skin parental contact with fragile preterm infants. *J Am Osteopath Assoc*. 1997;97:457–460.

2. Perehudoff B. Parents' perceptions of environmental stressors in the special care nursery. *Neonatal Network* 1990;9:39–44.

3. Huckabay LM, Tilem-Kessler D. Patterns of parental stress in PICU emergency admission. *Dimensions in Critical Care Nursing*. 1999;18:36–42.

4. Meyer EC, et al. Psychological distress in mothers of pre-term infants. *J Dev Behav Pediatr*. 1995;16:412–417.

5. Jamsa K, Jamsa T. Technology in neonatal intensive care—a study on parents' experiences. *Technol Health Care*. 1998;6:225–230.

6. Shields-Poe D, Pinelli J. Varibles associated with parental stress in neonatal intensive care units. *Neonatal Network*. 1997;16:29–37.

7. Haines C, et al. A comparison of the stressors experienced by parents of intubated and non-intubated children. *J Adv Nurs*. 1995;21:350–355.

8. Doyle P. *Grief Counseling and Sudden Death: A Manual and Guide.* Sprinfield, Ill: Charles C Thomas; 1980.

9. Kenner C, Lott JW. Parent transition after discharge from the NICU. *Neonatal Network.* 1990;9:31–37.

10. Kübler-Ross E. *On Death and Dying.* New York: The Macmillan Co; 1969.

11. Weizman SG, Kamm P. *About Mourning: Support and Guidance for the Bereaved.* New York: Human Sciences Press Inc; 1985.

12. Downey V, et al. Dying babies and associated stress in NICU nurses. *Neonatal Network.* 1995;14:41–46.

13. Sahler OJ, et al. Medical education about end-of-life care in the pediatric setting: principles, challenges, and opportunities. *Pediatrics 105.* 2000;3(pt 1):575–584.

Bibliography and Suggested Readings

Catlett AT, et al. Maternal perception of illness severity in premature infants. *Neonatal Network.* 1994;13:45–49.

Harrigan R, et al. Perinatal grief: response to the loss of an infant. *Neonatal Network.* 1993;12:25–31.

Lundqvist A, Nilstun N. Neonatal death and parents' grief. Experience, behaviour and attitudes of Swedish nurses. *Scandinavian Journal of Caring Sciences.* 1998;12:246–250.

Merenstein GB, Gardner SL. *Handbook of Neonatal Intensive Care.* 4th ed. St. Louis: CV Mosby Co; 1998.

Posttest

1. Parent-to-child bonding begins:
   a. with the anticipation of the child
   b. at the first signs of life
   c. during the last trimester of pregnancy
   d. during delivery
2. Which of the following are potential sources of stress for the parents of sick neonates?
   I. personal and fmaily background
   II. physiological compromise
   III. ethical judgments
   IV. situational conditions
   V. enviornmental stimuli
      a. I, III, IV
      b. II, III
      c. III only
      d. I, IV, V
3. Studies have shown that the highest source of stress in mothers of sick neonates is:
   a. the appearance of the neonate
   b. alteration of the parental role

    c. NICU sights and sounds

    d. staff communications

4. When the death of a loved one appears likely, grief felt by the family is termed:

    a. contemplatory

    b. expectant

    c. anticipatory

    d. envisioning

5. The first stage of grief includes which of the following?

    I. shock

    II. confusion

    III. denial

    IV. guilt

    V. isolation

        a. I, III, IV

        b. I, V

        c. I, II, III, IV, V

        d. I, II, III, V

6. Sadness and its avoidance are found in which stage of grief?

    a. stage I

    b. stage II

    c. stage III

    d. stage IV

7. A visit to the NICU prior to delivery of a high-risk infant may reduce which of the following stages of grief?

    a. denial

    b. anger

    c. guilt

    d. shock

8. The human tendency to affix blame on someone or something generally produces:

    a. anger

    b. guilt

    c. shock

    d. acceptance

9. The family member who begins making promises is in the phase of:

    a. denial

    b. acceptance

    c. bargaining

    d. anger

10. When the family becomes familiar with the NICU surroundings and personnel and begins involving themselves in the care of the infant, they have entered the stage of:

    a. denial

    b. bargaining

    c. anger

    d. acceptance.

11. Parents and family members may best be helped through grief by which of the following?
    I. constant encouragement
    II. explanations of the care being given
    III. allowing involvement in the care of the infant
    IV. leaving them alone
    V. recommending professional help
        a. II, III, V
        b. I, II, III
        c. I, II, III, V
        d. I, III, V

12. The practitioner can help reduce the stress level of parents of critically ill neonates by doing all of the following *except*:
    a. displaying empathy toward the family
    b. communicating as openly as practical with the parents
    c. support-group referral
    d. being pessimistic so as not to get the parents' hopes up

CHAPTER TWENTY-ONE

CLINICAL CASE STUDIES

CLINICAL CASE STUDY 1

SUBJECTIVE HISTORY

JJ is a newborn male, delivered vaginally following an uneventful pregnancy. Labor began approximately 12 hours prior to delivery. Fetal heart rate was monitored throughout the labor with approximately 5 early decelerations noted. Mother was given epidural anesthesia at approximately 6 cm of dilation and 100 effacement.

Spontaneous crying occurred within 20 seconds of delivery, following vigorous wiping and stimulation. JJ was cyanotic and had a heart rate of approximately 150/min. An Apgar score of 7 was recorded at 1 minute with 1 point taken away for muscle tone, respiratory effort, and cyanosis. Blow-by oxygen was provided and quickly followed with mask CPAP at 5 cm H_2O when the cyanosis did not resolve. Arterial catheterization was accomplished via an umbilical artery.

1. What are the pertinent positive findings in the history?
2. On physical examination, what organ systems should be closely examined?
3. What laboratory tests and exams should be ordered?

OBJECTIVE DATA

Physical Examination. Weight: 2200 g. Temp (Axillary): 36.6 (97.8 F) Systolic BP: 40 mm Hg. Despite mask CPAP and 100% oxygen, central cyanosis persisted. An SPO_2 monitor was placed on the foot and showed an arterial blood saturation of 78 to 80%. Breath sounds were diminished with some basilar crackles noted in both lung fields. Auscultation of the heart sounds revealed a III/VI systolic murmur with some variation of intensity at the pulmonic area. S2 was particularly loud and no gallup rhythm was audible. GI, GU, and neurological examination were within normal limits.

Laboratory Data. An arterial blood gas sample was drawn approximately 15 minutes post delivery through the umbilical atery catheter, with the patient on mask CPAP at 5 cm H_2O and 100% oxygen.

pH: 7.25
$PaCO_2$: 53 mm Hg
PaO_2: 55 mm Hg
HCO_3: 19 mEq/1

A chest radiograph showed hazy infiltrates in both lung fields with a normal sized heart. An electrocardiogram was performed and demonstrated enlargement of the right ventricle and an irregular rhythm with a slight tachycardia of 165 beats/min. Due to the evidence of right ventricular enlargement, an echocardiogram was performed with color flow mapping of the blood flow. The echocardiogram showed right ventricle outflow obstruction, an enlarged right ventricle, and a large ventricular septal defect (VSD). The aorta was also mal-positioned across the VSD.

Over the next several hours, the patient had 3 spells that consisted of increased cyanosis, irritability, pallor, tachypnea, and flaccidity. He was intubated and placed on mechanical ventilation at the following settings:

Mode: IMV
Rate: 40 breaths/min
PIP: 28 cm H_2O
PEEP: 5 cm H_2O
FiO_2: 100%

He remained cyanotic despite the mechanical ventilation. Arterial blood gases 20 minutes later were:

pH: 7.28
$PaCO_2$: 50 mm Hg
PaO_2: 59 mm Hg
HCO_3: 21 mEq/1

1. From the history and objective data given, develop a list of possible differential diagnoses.

   JJ was transported to a level III hospital at 7 hours of age. Cardiac catheterization done at the receiving hospital revealed the presence of a large ventricular septal defect, malpositioned aorta, and severe pulmonary valve stenosis. The patient was started on propranolol and prostaglandin E1 until surgical invention could be undertaken.
2. With this new information, what is the most likely diagnosis?

ASSESSMENT

The history of persistent cyanosis in the face of 100% oxygenation and adequate lung aeration indicates the presence of a right-to-left shunt. A systolic murmur along with changing intensity at the pulmonic area raises the suspicion of some type of pulmonic obstruction. The chest radiograph did not raise suspicion of an enlarged right ventricle; however, the ECG did show right ventricular enlargement with dysrhythmia, further supporting the presence of pulmonary obstruction. The most likely differential diagnoses are pulmonary atresia and tetralogy of Fallot (TOF). The presence of spells of increased symptoms further raised the suspicion of TOF. This suspicion was confirmed with echocardiogram and cardiac catheterization, which demonstrated the ventricular septal defect, malpositioned aorta, and pulmonary atresia (one of many types of right ventricle outflow obstruction). Along with the right ventricular hypertrophy, these make up the four components of TOF.

1. With the diagnosis of TOF, what respiratory care measures will likely be needed?
2. Describe the care of the patient with TOF, in particular, what are the potential problems that must be closely monitored?
3. What is the treatment for TOF?

PLAN

The treatment for TOF is surgical correction of the defects. Propranolol, morphine, and prostaglandin E1 are used to reduce arterial vascular resistance and to keep the ductus arteriosus open, allowing more unoxygenated blood to pass into the pulmonary tree to reduce the right-to-left shunt. Hypercyanotic spells, or TET spells, usually respond to the knee-chest position because this decreases venous return and reduces the shunt. Surgical repair of TOF involves a patch closure of the septal defect and relief of the pulmonary valve obstruction.

DISCUSSION

Tetralogy of Fallot is is so named because of the 4 elements of the disorder; it occurs in 40 out of 100,000 live births. Persistent cyanosis is the result of a serious right-to-left shunt. The shunt results from high right-sided heart pressures due to the right ventricle outflow obstruction, which pushes unoxygenated blood from the right side of the heart to the left through the ventricular septal defect. The aorta then carries this unoxygenated blood to the body. Despite 100% oxygen and adequate aeration of the lungs, the patient remains cyanotic unless blood flow to the lungs can be increased. Often this is only accomplished by keeping the ductus arteriosus open with prostaglandin E1.

Complications seen with this disorder include right bundle branch block, third-degree heart block, residual shunt, pulmonary insufficiency, polycythemia, and bacterial endocarditis. Overall mortality is roughly 10%, but worsens if surgical correction is not done. The earlier the surgery is done, the more favorable the prognosis because it protects the right ventricle.

CLINICAL CASE STUDY 2

SUBJECTIVE HISTORY

Mrs. Barbara Dunkley, age 28, arrived at the emergency department in active labor on February 16. The due date for the baby is March 30. She states that she has had some vaginal bleeding for the past 2 weeks following a fall on an icy sidewalk; otherwise the pregnancy has been unremarkable. Her obstetric history is 4-1-0-3. She has had no drug or alcohol intake during the pregnancy. She states that on her last visit to the obstetrician, approximately 3 weeks ago, the fetal heart tones were normal and that growth and weight gain were on schedule.

1. What are the pertinent positive findings in the history?
2. What other historical information, if any, would you obtain?

Further questioning about the patient's obstetric history reveals that her last baby was born 6 weeks prematurely and subsequently died following a 3-week hospitalization for RDS complicated by sepsis. This occurred nearly 6 years ago. She states that she could not go through that again.

1. From the history, list the possible maternal and fetal risks associated with this pregnancy.
2. What are some possible causes of the vaginal bleeding and premature labor?

OBJECTIVE DATA

BP: 110/75
Pulse: 85
Respirations: 23
Oral temperature: 37.3°C (99.2°F)

The patient does not appear to be in any acute distress. There is a small amount of clotted blood visible at the vaginal opening. External palpation of the uterus shows it to be tense and the patient states that the palpation is painful. Fetal heart tones and rate are normal. Breath sounds are clear and equal bilaterally. The uterine fundus measures 34 cm from the symphysis pubis.

Laboratory Data. CBC was as follows:

Hct: 35%
Hgb: 13 g/100 ml

RBC: 3.8 million/mm^3
WBC: 8,000/mm^3 with a normal differential

1. What aspects of the physical examination are pertinent?
2. From the physical exam and lab data information, can it be determined whether there is any immediate risk to either the fetus or the mother? Explain your answer.

ASSESSMENT

There are several aspects of the history and physical examination that are vital in assessing this situation. The most critical information is the presence of vaginal bleeding, especially with the history of a fall. This late in the pregnancy, the possibility of placental abruption (separation of the placenta from the uterine wall) should be the primary concern. Additionally, the fact that she has had one prior premature delivery that resulted in death places her in a high-risk category for subsequent premature deliveries. Of concern also is the psychological risk to the mother, should this baby be delivered prematurely and have medical complications.

Physical examination revealed a tense, tender uterus. When considered along with the presence of vaginal blood, the diagnosis of abruptio placenta is strongly suspected.

With the diagnosis made by ultrasound, it is important to assess the condition of both mother and fetus. When placental separation is suspected, maternal hypotension and/or tachycardia and tachypnea are ominous signs, indicating severe blood loss. This patient has normal vital signs, indicating that blood volume is probably at an acceptable level for now. This is confirmed by the CBC, showing Hct and Hgb in normal ranges. The fact that fetal heart rate and tones are normal indicates little, if any, fetal distress is present.

1. What is the treatment for abruptio placenta?

PLAN

Mrs. Dunkley was immediately hospitalized and placed on strict bed rest, lying in a left lateral position. An IV was started and maintenance crystalloids given. Monitoring of vital signs was done every 4 hours for the first 24 hours, then every 8 hours. A nasal cannula was inserted and set at 3 L/min to maximize fetal oxygenation. Fetal heart rate was monitored constantly with an external monitor. Those caring for the patient were advised to prepare for an emergency delivery or cesarean section should signs of maternal or fetal distress develop.

DISCUSSION

Abruptio placenta is a premature separation of the placenta from the uterine wall. It is often the result of trauma, but may occur spontaneously. Separation can be partial or complete and the resultant hemorrhage may be visible (apparent hemorrhage), or not (concealed hemorrhage). Abruptio placenta frequently causes labor to start. The main risk to the mother is blood loss with resultant shock. The fetus may suffer hypoxia, asphyxia, or blood loss. Abruptio placenta is graded from 0 to 3. The presence of vaginal bleeding, tetany, and tenderness of the uterus, and the absence of maternal shock or fetal distress, place this as a grade 1 abruption.

Treatment is focused on the careful assessment and management of maternal blood volume, maintaining a Hct of at least 30%. Strict bed rest is enforced, and the mother is instructed to lie in a left lateral position to maximize placental circulation. Preparations are made for emergency delivery by cesarean section should maternal shock or fetal distress manifest.

CLINICAL CASE STUDY 3

SUBJECTIVE HISTORY

Carlin is a 3-year-old female who is brought to the emergency department by her father at 2:30 am. Her father states that she awoke about 11:00 pm wheezing and coughing, and that it has been getting progressively worse. He has not noted any blueness of her lips or nail beds. She has had a "cold" for the past 3 days, with a stuffy nose, cough, and slight fever. Treatment has been with diphenhydramine and cough suppressants. She is allergic to penicillin, with no other known allergies. She has not received any antibiotics recently. The father has not noted any drooling and the patient has not complained of a sore throat. No one else in the family has been sick.

1. What are the pertinent positive findings in the history?
2. What are the pertinent negative findings in the history?
3. On physical examination, what organ systems should be closely examined?
4. What laboratory data should be obtained?

OBJECTIVE DATA

The patient appears to be in moderate distress by inspection; however, no cyanosis is noted.

BP: 95/65
Pulse: 135
Respirations: 40
Temperature: 36.6°C (97.9°F)

Further examination reveals no deviation of the trachea. She has moderate suprasternal retractions with bilateral intercostal retractions. Breath sounds are diminished and equal bilaterally. No crackles are heard in the lung periphery. Stridor is heard over the trachea. Heart sounds are rapid with a normal S1 or S2. She has tender cervical adenopathy.

Laboratory Data. An aerterial blood gas was obtained on room air with the following results:

pH: 7.35
PCO_2: 45 mm Hg
PO_2: 55 mm Hg
HCO_3: 23 mEq/1

A lateral and A-P neck radiograph were obtained. The lateral appeared normal, with moderate narrowing of the trachea seen at the level of the larynx on the A-P view.

1. From the history and objective data given, develop a list of possible differential diagnoses.
2. From the list, describe which diagnosis is the most likely and why.
3. Interpret the arterial blood gas.

ASSESSMENT

The initial history of the patient indicates several pertinent positives. First is the history of waking at night with a tight cough following several days of URI symptoms. It is important to determine whether this is an acute problem, and this history helps rule that out. An additional pertinent positive is that she is allergic to penicillin. Pertinent negatives include no drooling, no sore throat, no one else in the family has been sick, she has no other known allergies, and has not received any antibiotics.

The arterial blood gas shows mild respiratory acidosis and hypoxemia. The neck radiograph indicates a narrowing of the trachea in the area of the larynx. With all symptoms taken together, the diagnosis of croup was made.

1. What respiratory care measures are needed by this patient? Describe specific therapies, drugs, and dosages.
2. Describe the care of the patient with croup; in particular, what are the potential problems that must be closely monitored?

PLAN

The patient was started on oxygen via blow-by at 4 L/min and immediately given a small volume nebulizer treatment with 0.5 ml of racemic epinephrine mixed with normal saline. She was also given a weight-based loading dose of liquid oral corticosteroids. Following the treatment, her status improved slightly but started worsening 20 minutes after the treatment. She was admitted to the pediatric unit for careful observation. Nebulizer therapy with 0.5 ml racemic epinephrine was ordered Q2 hours. The patient was also started on a decelerating dose of weight-based liquid oral corticosteroids and cool, continuous mist at FiO_2 0.40. She was able to drink PO fluids and had no vomiting.

1. Why is it important to closely monitor croup patients?
2. Discuss why racemic epinephrine and corticosteroids are used to treat coup.

DISCUSSION

Croup is one of the most common reasons pediatric patients are brought to the emergency department with breathing problems. Because it can mimic other causes of upper airway distress, such as epiglottitis, foreign body aspiration, and anaphylaxis, it is crucial to obtain a thorough history and physical examination. It typically affects children between 6 months and 3 years old.

Because it is caused by a virus (75% by parainfluenza), the treatment is mostly aimed at symptoms. Oxygen is usually indicated, because hypoxemia may be missed by physical examination alone. Ideally, an arterial blood gas is obtained, but the value of the arterial blood gas results must be weighed against the trauma of the needlestick, which can significantly worsen respiratory distress. A pulse oximeter is ideal to monitor oxygenation status. Treatment of the symptoms is aimed at reducing the inflammation of laryngeal tissues. Racemic epinephrine is beneficial due to its vasoconstrictive properties. As the drug settles on the inflamed tissues, resultant vasoconstriction reduces swelling and improves airflow. Additionally, systemic corticosteroids are given to reduce inflammation.

Vasoconstriction is also achieved by the use of cool aerosols, which may be given with or without oxygen, based on SPO_2 values.

When caring for children, it is important to approach them with treatments that are appropriate for their developmental age. A 3-year-old like Carlin may be frightened by a mask used to deliver aerosol treatments or cool mist therapy. It is often more successful to use a paper cup that is familiar to the child, poke a hole in the bottom, and thread the tubing through the hole. The child is less likely to be frightened by holding a paper cup up to her face. In addition, stickers placed on the inside of the cup can encourage the child to hold the cup up to her face to see the stickers. Parents are usually happy to participate in their child's care by holding the child on their lap and holding the cup up to the child's face.

CLINICAL CASE STUDY 4

SUBJECTIVE HISTORY

PV is a newborn infant who was delivered 5 minutes ago. She is reportedly full term as assessed by dates. The pregnancy was uneventful and the mother received good prenatal care. The mother has no history of drug or alcohol use during the pregnancy. The mother is 28 years old, 5'8" in height and weighs 155 pounds. She gained 28 pounds during the pregnancy. Her obstetrical history is 2-0-0-2. The labor and delivery were also unremarkable with stage I of labor lasting 4 hours, and stage II lasting 25 minutes. The fetus did have some mild heart decelerations with uterine contractions for the last 20 minutes of stage I. The obstetrician observed possible polyhydramnios upon rupture of the amniotic membrane.

1. Describe the pertinent positives and pertinent negatives of the history.

OBJECTIVE DATA

Five minutes after delivery, baby PV is cyanotic and in severe respiratory distress. Expiratory grunting, nasal flaring, and retractions are present. No breath sounds are heard in the left chest, and they are minimally heard in the right. Heart sounds and PMI are shifted to the right but appear normal. The abdomen is noted to be flat.

1. From the history and objective data given, develop a list of possible differential diagnoses.

Laboratory Data. An abdominal/chest radiograph shows the presence of bowel loops in the left hemithorax.

ASSESSMENT

There are two pertinent positives found in the history. First is that of heart decelerations, and second is that of polyhydramnios. Polyhydramnios is an excessive amount of amniotic fluid. It is seen with CNS malformations, orogastric disturbances, and congenital heart disease. Pertinent negatives include no high-risk factors (term baby, no drug use, good obstetric care, favorable obstetric history, unremarkable pregnancy, patient height, weight, and weight gain during pregnancy), and an unremarkable labor and delivery. The negatives help rule out prematurity, pregnancy, or labor/delivery problems.

Physical examination findings of the newborn are remarkable. Pertinent findings include severe respiratory distress, cyanosis, absent breath sounds on the left, shift of heart sounds to the right, and a flat abdomen. These findings suggest pneumothorax, or congenital diaphragmatic hernia. The presence of polyhydramnios further points toward the diagnosis of diaphragmatic hernia. This diagnosis is then verified by the radiograph.

1. With the diagnosis of diaphragmatic hernia, what respiratory care measures will likely be needed?
2. Describe why a diaphragmatic hernia would cause polyhydramnios.
3. Describe the treatment for this condition.

PLAN

The patient was immediately intubated and a nasogastric tube placed. Ventilation was done at a rate of 120/min at a PIP of 18 mm Hg and a PEET of 2 mm Hg. An umbilical artery catheter was placed. The patient was then transported to a level III referral hospital for surgical correction of the defect.

1. Discuss the necessity of intubation and placement of an NG tube.
2. Describe why ventilation should be done at high rates and low pressures.

DISCUSSION

Congenital diaphragmatic hernia is the result of an incomplete embryological formation of the diaphragm. It most often occurs on the left through the foramen of Bochdalek. In this case, the herniation was on the left, which allowed the stomach and intestines to enter into the thoracic cavity. The absence of bowel in the abdomen makes it flat or sunken. This movement of bowel severely hampers development of the left lung and causes the mediastinum to shift to the right, resulting in severe restriction of the right lung. Ventilation is further hampered if any air enters the stomach by causing additional compression of the lungs. This is why intubation and the placement of an NG tube are vital. Intubation reduces the risk of air entering the stomach during bag-valve-mask ventilation or gasping, and the NG tube allows for the escape of any air that may make it to the stomach. Owing to the low compliance of the lungs in this condition, the risk of pneumothorax is high. Ventilation should therefore be done at high rates and low pressures to avoid causing a pneumothorax.

The definitive treatment is placement of the bowel back into the abdomen and surgical correction of the opening in the diaphragm.

Depending on fetal developmental factors, the left lung may be hypoplastic. The combination of one hypoplastic lung (typically on the left) and one atelectatic lung (typically on the right) often leads to increased pulmonary vascular pressures and may lead to persistent pulmonary hypertension (PPH) that may ultimately require maximal support with nitric oxide, high-frequency ventilation, and ECMO preoperatively. Infants with a hypoplastic lung and PPH have a high mortality rate despite surgery and maximal medical support.

CLINICAL CASE STUDY 5

SUBJECTIVE HISTORY

BJ is a 3-week-old neonate in the NICU. She was born at 28 weeks' gestation, and despite rescue surfactant, developed RDS. She has been on mechanical ventilation since 5 hours of age. Weaning has been slow.

Current ventilator settings are as follows:

Rate: 45 breaths per minute
PIP: 24 cm H_2O
PEEP: 4 cm H_2O
FiO_2: 0.57
IT: 0.5 sec

Her last blood gas results are:

pH: 7.34
PCO_2: 55 cm H_2O
PaO_2: 57 cm H_2O
HCO_3: 27 mEq/1

Following a diaper change, the baby developed increasing respiratory distress with retractions and tachypnea. Bradycardia followed with broad cyanosis.

1. What are the pertinent positive findings in the history?
2. From the history, develop a list of possible diagnoses.
3. Describe the areas of examination that will most help establish the diagnosis.

OBJECTIVE DATA

On examination, there is mottling and diffuse cyanosis present. HR is 70 and falling. Oxygen saturation per pulse oximeter is 68%. Ventilator parameters are not changed. A quick examination of the ventilator circuit reveals no obvious disconnection or occlusion. Chest excursion is greatly diminished bilaterally. Breath sounds are decreased on the right side. Heart sounds are muffled and the PMI has shifted slightly left.

1. What tests should now be performed?

The patient was transilluminated and a large atypical light reflection was seen on the right superior thoracic area.

1. From the original list of diagnoses, discuss how the further objective information has helped to focus on one diagnosis.

ASSESSMENT

Pertinent positive from the history include a diagnosis of RDS, mechanical ventilation, and a sudden change in status with respiratory distress, cyanosis, and bradycardia. Physical examination reveals mottling, cyanosis, bradycardia, decreased breath sounds on the right, and a shift of the PMI to the left. Positive transillumination in the right thoracic area confirms the diagnosis of pneumothorax.

1. With the above information, develop a treatment plan for this patient.

PLAN

The right thorax was quickly cleansed with iodophor, and needle thoracentesis was performed in the second intercostal space in the mid-clavicular line. A large amount of air was vented from the right thorax. The heart rate immediately began improving and color improved dramatically. The needle was left in place and evacuation of free air continued until a chest tube was placed. A subsequent chest radiograph showed the right lung to be fully expanded and the chest tube to be in good position.

DISCUSSION

Pneumothorax is the most common of the air leak syndromes. The initial history of sudden worsening of status on a neonate being mechanically ventilated should raise several initial suspicions. First, one must consider the possibility of accidental extubation. Other concerns include occlusion of the endotracheal tube with secretions, or occlusion or disconnection of the ventilator circuit, and barotrauma. Although less likely, the possibility of accidental changes of ventilator settings must also be considered.

To focus in on the diagnosis, a quick visual examination of the patient, endotracheal tube, and ventilator circuit is done. The fact that there were slight chest excursions, no obvious disconnections, extubation, or blockages, and intact ventilator settings, help to rule them out as the cause. To exclude the ventilator as the source, simply disconnect and use a manual resuscitation bag for ventilation during this assessment phase. The physical examination is probably the most crucial part of the diagnosis and must be done rapidly and expertly. The absence of breath sounds on the right, along with a shift of the PMI to the left, indicate a probable right-sided pneumothorax. This is confirmed with the positive transillumination.

In the presence of a pneumothorax, patient symptoms may occur rapidly or slowly, depending on how quickly gas is accumulating in the thorax. As pressure builds, lung compliance drops, and cardiac output is compromised, resulting in widespread $\dot{V}/\dot{Q}$ mismatching in the lungs and peripheral hypoperfusion. The result is cyanosis and mottling of the skin. Prompt evacuation of the trapped air is the only method of reversing the downward spiral. Precious time is wasted by ordering a chest radiograph; therefore, the decision to perform needle venting is made by history and physical examination alone. Once the patient is stable, a chest tube is then inserted and a radiograph obtained to ensure proper tube placement. The chest tube is then left in place until the air leak is sealed.

CLINICAL CASE STUDY 6

SUBJECTIVE HISTORY

Chad is a 6-year-old boy who comes to the respiratory clinic with his mother with a chief complaint of difficulty breathing, which is coming with increasing frequency. The symptoms first appeared about 1 year before this visit following a viral URI. At first, the patient only had a dry hacking cough, but in the past few months, this has changed to include dyspnea and wheezing. The last episode occurred 3 days ago while the patient was running with a friend in the yard. He is currently on no medications and has no known allergies.

1. What are the pertinent positive findings in the history taken thus far?
2. Describe any other historical data that may help with the diagnosis.
3. Make a list of differential diagnoses.

Further questioning revealed that Chad has had frequent URIs since he was a baby. He has two older siblings; neither has had similar symptoms. There is a history of asthma in the patient's paternal grandfather; otherwise, no other family members are afflicted. Neither parents are smokers. The patient is otherwise well, has a normal appetite, and has always been near the 50th percentile for growth.

1. What pertinent information is obtained from this further questioning? List positives and negatives.
2. Describe the organ system(s) that should be carefully examined on this patient and which examinations should be done.
3. Should any laboratory studies be ordered? If so, which ones and why?

OBJECTIVE DATA

Patient is quiet, well nourished and appears slightly thin for his height. He is no acute distress. Breathing pattern is regular with no use of accessory muscles. The patient's thoracic AP diameter appears slightly increased. No cyanosis is noted.

BP: 87/55
Pulse: 90
Respirations: 22
Temperature: 37.3°C (99.1°F)

Oral examination is normal, with no enlargement of the tonsils. No palpable adenopathy in the cervical chain. Trachea is midline. Heart sounds, normal S1, S2 with a regular rhythm.

Percussion of the chest reveals moderate tympany bilaterally. Breath sounds are equal bilaterally, decreased, with expiratory wheezing.

Laboratory Data. Arterial blood gases on room air as follows:

pH: 7.36
PCO_2: 47 mm Hg
PaO_2: 62 mm Hg
HCO_3: 26 mEq/1

An A-P and lateral chest radiograph show slight flattening of both diaphragms, hyperlucency throughout the lung fields and increased A-P diameter. Heart size is normal.

Basic spirometry was done, including peak flow, forced vital capacity (FVC), and FEV_1. Peak flow was 75% of predicted, FVC was 98% of predicted, and FEV_1/FVC ratio was 80%.

1. Discuss the importance of the laboratory data in establishing a diagnosis.
2. How is the lab data used to determine the severity of the disease?
3. Discuss your diagnosis and classify its severity.

ASSESSMENT

There are several pertinent positives in the history. First is difficulty breathing, which is coming with increasing frequency. Others include a dry hacking cough, dyspnea, and wheezing, which occur following exercise. Further questioning revealed other pertinent positives, including frequent URIs since infancy and a history of asthma in the patient's paternal grandfather. Pertinent negatives include no medications, no known allergies, two older siblings without similar symptoms, parents are nonsmokers, patient otherwise well, and growth is normal.

Inspection reveals that the patient is not in acute distress and that he is slightly barrel chested. Other pertinent findings on examination are tympany with percussion, decreased breath sounds, and wheezing. Blood gases reveal a compensated respiratory acidosis with mild hypoxemia. The chest radiograph shows signs of air-trapping, which is consistent with the apparent barrel chest and tympany. Spirometry results are consistent with obstructive lung disease, with decreased flows and normal volumes. All of these findings are consistent with the diagnosis of asthma, triggered by exercise and possibly other factors.

1. With the diagnosis of asthma, discuss which respiratory care measures will likely be needed.
2. Describe the care of the patient with asthma. In particular, what are the potential problems that must be closely monitored?
3. Describe the treatment of asthma. Included drugs and dosages.

PLAN

Significant time was spent with the patient and his parents regarding asthma and its care. They were instructed how to monitor for an acute attack and how to assess the severity using a peak flowmeter. They were strongly encouraged to take the patient to the emergency department if the attack was severe. The patient was started on an aerosolized beta-adrenergic drug delivered via MDI to be used when he has symptoms or when his peak flow drops below 80% of normal. Instruction regarding the use of the MDI was provided. He will use the MDI 1 hour before any exercise and prn as guided by peak flow rates during an acute attack. He was also given an inhaled steroid for prophylaxis to be used daily. The possible need to meet with an allergist to determine other triggers of symptoms was discussed.

1. Would you add anything to the plan? If so, what and why?
2. How often should follow-up be planned?
3. Discuss strategies that could be used to help ensure patient compliance with the prescribed use of the MDI.

DISCUSSION

Asthma is the most common cause of obstructive airway disease in children. It ranges in severity from the occasional mild cough to severe airway obstruction, which requires mechanical ventilation. The key to the treatment of asthma is prompt and accurate diagnosis. Identification and avoidance of triggering factors can help prevent attacks. Patient understanding of the disease and its treatment are vital. Mortality and morbidity are increased when the patient does not understand how and when to treat. Follow-up should be planned at least monthly, until you are sure that the patient has good control of the disease. It is also vital that the patient knows when to go to the emergency department. Waiting too long when the home treatment is ineffective may prove fatal.

CLINICAL CASE STUDY 7

SUBJECTIVE HISTORY

Tina is a 13-year-old figure skater with a chief complaint of rapid onset shortness of breath after she was taken to the local ice rink to practice. Shortly after she started to skate the symptoms of shortness of breath and difficulty breathing came on. Paramedics were called to the scene. She was given oxygen via a mask. The paramedics reportedly heard mild stridor on auscultation; her vital signs were BP 110/70, HR 125, RR 28. They also found her color to be "ashen." She has hives on her torso, and her lips and eyelids are slightly swollen. The paramedics transported the patient to the emergency department.

1. From this history, list possible differential diagnoses.
2. What further information would you elicit from the patient?

OBJECTIVE DATA

In the ED:

BP: 110/70
Respirations: 24
Pulse: 102
Temperature: 36.8°C (98.2°F)

Currently, the patient appears to be in minimal distress. Her breathing is slightly labored. No cyanosis is present. Oxygen saturation via pulse oximeter is 93% on RA. Oral examination is unremarkable except for slightly swollen lips. Trachea is midline. No palpable adenopathy. Slight suprasternal retractions are noted. Heart sounds are within normal limits with a regular rhythm. The patient is mildly tachycardic. Breath sounds are equal bilaterally with no crackles or rhonchi. Inspiratory and expiratory stridor are present over the trachea. Chest expansion and percussion are both normal. Hives are present on the torso.

1. Are any other tests or examinations indicated? If so, which ones and why?
2. From the history and objective data given, discuss the most likely diagnosis.

ASSESSMENT

The history of this patient initially raised several possible diagnoses. Initial differential diagnoses included asthma, pneumonia, croup, hyperventilation, laryngeal obstruction, endobronchial foreign body, and anxiety attack. With no past history of asthma, normal spirometry, oximetry, and a lack of physical findings such as wheezing, the likelihood of asthma is diminished. Pneumonia and croup are unlikely due to the sudden onset without previous symptoms or illness. Further, at 13 years of age, croup is very uncommon. Foreign body aspiration is remote due to the negative history of anything in the patient's mouth when the symptoms started. Anxiety attack is unlikely due to the persistence of symptoms, especially stridor and hives. The most likely diagnosis is that of laryngeal edema, probably secondary to an allergic reaction to something she had for lunch.

1. Discuss the pathogenesis of laryngeal edema caused by an allergic response.
2. Describe the possible dangers associated with anaphylaxis.
3. Develop a treatment plan for this patient based on the history, physical, and lab data.

PLAN

Tina was initially treated with an IM dose of diphenhydramine and a weight-based loading dose of liquid corticosteroids. She was carefully monitored. Within 90 minutes, her hives and stridor were gone. She was observed for another 90 minutes and discharged with a prescription for corticosteroids and instructions to continue diphenhydramine for 24 hours. She and her parents were advised to follow up with an allergist in an attempt to discover the offending allergen. The danger of total airway occlusion was discussed and they were instructed to immediately call 911 to return to the emergency department if the patient's breathing became more difficult, or if any symptoms returned, particularly hives.

DISCUSSION

Allergic reactions occur when the IgE antibody becomes sensitized to an antigen. When the antigen contacts the IgE on basophils and mast cells, mediators such as histamine, leukotrienes, and anaphylactic mediators are released. These mediators lead to diffuse vasodilation with resultant plasma leakage and edema, and bronchoconstriction. The larynx frequently becomes edematous and partially occludes the airway. In children, this is more dangerous due to the smaller diameter of the airway. Of greatest concern is the possibility of total occlusion of the trachea. Treatment in severe cases is with epinephrine delivered subcutaneously, and possible intubation to bypass the occlusion and maintain a patent airway.

CLINICAL CASE STUDY 8

SUBJECTIVE HISTORY

Beth is a 36-week gestation newborn admitted to the NICU from the general newborn nursery at 24 hours of age due to tachypnea, tachycardia, a hyperdynamic precordium, and bounding peripheral pulses.

Maternal obstetric history is essentially uneventful with good prenatal care and normal labor and delivery, with the exception of possible exposure to rubella during the first trimester. Apgar scores were 8 and 9.

1. Discuss the pertinent positive findings.
2. Are any other subjective data required at this point? If so, which data and why?
3. From the information provided thus far, develop a list of differential diagnoses.
4. Describe any additional physical, laboratory, or medical imaging exams that should be done to help establish the diagnosis.

OBJECTIVE HISTORY

On admission to the NICU, vital signs are:

Heart rate: 140
Respirations: 72
Temperature: 36.1°C axillary (97°F)

Physical examination reveals signs noted in the general newborn nursery. There is a continuous heart murmur with a humming quality heard best at the second left interspace.

Beth continues to be tachypneic but is not retracting or showing other signs of respiratory distress. Breath sounds have scattered end-inspiratory crackles. ECG is normal; chest radiograph shows no evidence of cardiomegaly but slightly increased pulmonary vascular markings. SpO_2 with the probe placed on the left foot is 93% on room air.

Examination of other body systems, neurologic, GI, and GU, are completely normal.

1. Discuss the pertinent findings on further workup.
2. Are any other diagnostic tests appropriate at this point?

Beth has a bedside echocardiogram. Results show a moderately sized patent ductus arteriosus with a left-to-right shunt.

ASSESSMENT

The presence of tachypnea, tachycardia, a hyperdynamic precordium, and bounding peripheral pulses indicate some problem in the cardiorespiratory system that requires additional workup. In this case, pulmonary findings were essentially normal, which placed the focus on a cardiac examination and workup.

The maternal history is significant for a possible exposure to rubella in the first trimester. The mother's rubella immunization and titer should be checked to see if that exposure could have resulted in maternal infection, or if the mother was adequately protected before the exposure. A number of congenital anomalies can occur as a result of a rubella infection during the first trimester of pregnancy.

There are several significant findings on the physical examination. First are the cardiac signs: tachycardia, a hyperdynamic precordium and bounding peripheral pulses. All of these can indicate a left-to-right shunt. Conditions causing a left-to-right shunt without cyanosis in an infant include:

- Ventricular septal defect
- Patent ductus arteriosus
- Atrial septal defect
- Atrioventricular septal defect
- Endocardial cushion defect (common in trisomy 21)

In addition, Beth had a continuous heart murmur with a humming quality, which is characteristic of a patent ductus arteriosus. Pertinent negative findings were a normal ECG, absence of cardiomegaly, and adequate oxygenation. The echocardiographic exam confirmed the diagnosis of patent ductus arteriosus.

PLAN

Beth will be observed in the NICU to see if she stabilizes or if her condition worsens. She will be monitored for increasing signs and symptoms of heart failure. If indicated, she can be treated with fluid restriction, and if she develops pulmonary symptoms, she may require mechanical ventilation.

Infants with no other cardiac defects should have the ductus arteriosus closed. If Beth's symptoms subside, she can be watched for a couple of months to see if the vessel closes on its own. If not, it can be ligated through a surgical procedure, or it can be plugged during a cardiac catheterization. It is important that the vessel be closed. If the vessel remains open for an extended period of time, the volume of blood shunted into the lungs can increase pulmonary vascular pressures and result in chronic pulmonary vascular disease.

DISCUSSION

Patent ductus arteriosus (PDA) is common in premature infants and occurs in 8/1000 live births in the United States. It is much less common in full-term infants, and in infants with no other cardiac defects, it is due to a defect in the wall of the ductus arteriosus. The defect can be associated with maternal rubella infection during the first trimester.

It is not common for infants to show symptoms so early in life; the babies typically go home and subsequently develop trouble, with recurrent respiratory infections, easy fatigability, dyspnea on exertion, and failure to grow at the expected rate. A small PDA may remain asymptomatic but provides a potential site for infection, which requires antibiotic prophylaxis, similar to that for an abnormal valve.

Spontaneous closure after three months of age is rare. Closure in premature infants is about 75%, and in term infants, about 40%.

If there is a condition of high pulmonary vascular pressure in addition to PDA, the shunt may reverse and become right-to-left. In this situation, the child will have cyanosis unresponsive to oxygen administration. The child will need cardiac catheterization to fully assess the cardiopulmonary structure of vascular defects present.

CLINICAL CASE STUDY 9

SUBJECTIVE HISTORY

Baby Anna is 12 hours post delivery. She was delivered to a 15-year-old single mother, who had received no prenatal care. The mother does not know her due date and guesses that she is maybe 7 months pregnant. Fetal heart rates were extremely variable during the short labor. Emergency cesarean delivery was performed due to prolonged fetal bradycardia. Vigorous resuscitation was performed on the baby. The baby was intubated and manually ventilated because of prolonged apnea. Blood gases showed severe respiratory acidosis and hypoxemia, despite rapid ventilation and high FiO_2.

1. List the pertinent positive findings in the history.
2. Develop a list of possible diagnoses.
3. Is any other history needed? If so, what history and why?

OBJECTIVE DATA

Weight: 870 grams
Heart rate: 154
Respirations: 83 and labored
Temperature: 36.1°C axillary (97°F)

Anna is intubated with a 2.5 ETT and currently being manually ventilated at a rate of 50 pbm, PIP 25 cm H_2O, 1.0 FiO_2. Pulse oximetry 84% with the probe on the left foot. Patient has moderate intercostal retractions. Gestational age is assessed at 28 weeks. Heart sounds are within normal limits. Breath sounds very diminished with poor aeration.

1. What other objective information should be obtained to help with the diagnosis?

A chest radiograph showed both lungs to have poor aeration with a ground glass appearance. A few air bronchograms are seen peripherally. Heart appears normally sized. The endotracheal tube is in good position.

1. Discuss the radiograph findings in context with the history and physical examination.
2. Describe the most likely diagnosis and how you came to that conclusion.

ASSESSMENT

The history of a 15-year-old single mother with no prenatal care places this infant in a high-risk group. The variable heart rate during labor, along with the need for vigorous resuscitation following delivery all point toward significant intrauterine asphyxia. Prolonged apnea requiring intubation and ventilation supports this.

At 28 weeks' gestation, lung immaturity is almost ensured and RDS is the primary concern. The presence of RDS is confirmed through physical examination (decreased breath sounds with poor aeration), and chest radiograph (ground glass appearance).

1. With the diagnosis of RDS, what respiratory care measures will likely be needed?
2. Describe the care of the patient with RDS. In particular, what are the potential problems that must be closely monitored?
3. Discuss the treatment for RDS.

PLAN

The patient was placed on mechanical ventilation at the following settings: PIP: titrate to achieve good chest excursion. Rate: 60 bpm, PEEP: 4 cm H_2O, FiO_2: 1.0. Blood gases ordered 20 minutes following initiation of support via the umbilical artery catheter placed earlier. An initial dose of rescue surfactant was given via the endotracheal tube. Strict monitoring of intake and output will be carried out. Continuous monitoring of heart and respiratory rate, SpO_2, and transcutaneous CO_2 will be done. Chest radiographs are ordered daily for the first 3 days.

DISCUSSION

RDS is one of the most common complications of premature birth. Immaturity of the lungs results in a lack of endogenous surfactant. The lungs become stiff, and ventilation and oxygenation become difficult. Surfactant replacement is the treatment of choice in an attempt to improve lung function by correcting the deficit resulting in the pulmonary changes, and to reduce the possibility of injury secondary to mechanical ventilation. Repeat doses may be given as indicated by the infant's condition and response to therapy. Mechanical ventilation is maintained at minimal levels of support to provide adequate oxygenation and ventilation while attempting to minimize iatrogenic lung damage. Maintenance of thermoregulation is an absolute necessity in these patients. Fluid and electrolyte balance is tricky but an essential part of the care for these patients. Continuous monitoring of transcutaneous PCO_2 and oxygen saturation is vital to allow titration of ventilatory support and reduce the need for blood gas analysis, which can result in significant blood volume loss.

CLINICAL CASE STUDY 10

SUBJECTIVE HISTORY

Sammy is a 3-week-old male patient admitted to the emergency department. The history is obtained from his mother. She states that 2 days ago, Sammy developed a cough, nasal congestion, and slight fever. Over the past 24 hours, he has become lethargic and pale. His appetite has dropped significantly. She feels that his breathing has become more labored.

1. What are the pertinent positive findings in the history?

OBJECTIVE DATA

HR: 127
Respirations: 70
Temperature: 38.1°C (100.6°F) rectally

On visual examination, the patient is seen to have retractions and nasal flaring. Breath sounds are decreased with diffuse inspiratory crackles throughout the lung fields. Heart sounds are normal. Chest radiograph shows slight hyperinflation with diffuse patchy infiltrates.

1. From the history and objective data given, develop a list of possible differential diagnoses.
2. What further tests would help establish the diagnosis?

656 · CHAPTER TWENTY-ONE

ASSESSMENT

Pertinent positive findings from the history include URI symptoms consisting of cough, nasal congestion, and slight fever, leading to the patient becoming lethargic and pale with increasingly labored breathing over the last 24 hours. His lack of appetite is also pertinent.

Pertinent physical exam findings include crackles diffusely scattered throughout the lung fields and diffuse patchy infiltrates as seen on the chest radiograph. The most likely diagnosis based on the history and physical is bronchiiolitis.

1. With the diagnosis of bronchiolitis, what respiratory care measures will likely be needed?
2. Describe the care of the patient with bronchiolitis. In particular, what are the potential problems that must be closely monitored?
3. Describe the treatment for bronchiolitis.

PLAN

The patient was admitted to the hospital and placed in a headbox at 40% oxygen. Continuous pulse oximetry was ordered. An RSV culture was also ordered. Vital signs will be monitored regularly, with the frequency determined by the patient's condition. Treatment with ribavirin will be considered if the RSV culture turns out to be positive.

DISCUSSION

Bronchiolitis is a viral infection of the bronchioles, with the main causative agent being RSV. It typically occurs in the winter months and affects patients younger than 2 years of age, particularly those between newborn and 5 months. Of particular concern are those patients with underlying cardiopulmonary disorders, in whom RSV is a particular danger. The treatment is mainly supportive, with supplemental oxygen as needed. Ribavirin may be given to those patients at high risk, or with particularly severe symptoms. The disease usually runs its course in 7 to 10 days.

Bibliography and Suggested Readings

Beers MH, and Berkow R, eds. *The Merck Manual of Diagnosis and Therapy*. West Point, PA: Merck & Co; 1999.

Behrman RE, Kliegman RM, Jenson HB. *Nelson Textbook of Pediatrics*. 16th ed. Philadelphia: WB Saunders Co.; 2000.

Curley MAQ, Smith JB, Moloney-Harmon PA. *Critical Care Nursing of Infants and Children*. Philadelphia: WB Saunders Co.; 1996.

Dambro MR, Griffith JA. *Griffith's 5 Minute Clinical Consult*. 3rd ed. Philadelphia: Lippincott Williams and Wilkins; 1999.

Siberry GK, Iannone R, eds. *Johns Hopkins: The Harriet Lane Handbook*. 15th ed. St. Louis: Mosby, Inc. 2000.

LABORATORY AND CLINICAL PROFICIENCY CHECK-OFFS

OXYGEN THERAPY

OBJECTIVE

The student will be able to correctly assemble the necessary equipment and apply the following oxygen administration devices in a laboratory and clinical setting. This will be done following aseptic guidelines and in a competent manner as determined by lab and clinical instructors.

TASK A: Review the Chart. The administration of oxygen begins with a review of the patient's chart. The order for oxygen therapy should include a documented need for the oxygen, the liter flow, or FiO$_2$, and the type of administration device desired. During the chart review, the student will note any orders or indications for patient isolation techniques.

TASK B: Wash Hands. The student should now wash, following standard procedures as outlined by the instructor.

TASK C: Gather Equipment. Depending on the type of device to be used, you will need one or more flowmeters, an oxygen blender, a humidifier or nebulizer, sterile water, oxygen or aerosol tubing, a cannula, an appropriate size oxygen mask, an oxygen hood, T connector, oxygen analyzer, water trap, and no smoking signs.

TASK D: Confirm Patient Identity. Before performing any patient procedure, confirm that you have the correct patient by looking at the name bracelet attached to a patient limb.

TASK E: Perform Procedure; Oxygen Cannula or Mask. First, attach the oxygen flowmeter to the wall outlet. If applicable, fill the humidifier with the appropriate amount of sterile water. Attach the humidifier to the flowmeter and check the pop-off valve by occluding the outlet and turning on a flow of oxygen. This should activate the pop-off valve. If the pop-off valve does not activate, determine and correct the cause of the problem before continuing. A humidifier should not be used unless it has a functioning pop-off valve.

Next, attach the cannula, or mask tubing, to the humidifier and place it on the patient's face. A mask should fit over the mouth and nose, without extending over the eyes.

Set the flow rate on the flowmeter. The desired flow rate may be determined by adjusting the flow until the desires SpO_2 is achieved. A cannula is generally used at flows of less than 2 L/min on newborns and at flows up to 6 L/min on older pediatric patients. Simple oxygen masks are normally used at flows of 3 to 5 L/min on neonates and at flows of 6 L/min or greater on older pediatric patients. Check the entire system to be certain it is functioning appropriately by checking for bubbling in the humidifier and listening for gas flow from the device. Apply the device to the patient.

TASK F: Perform Procedure; Oxygen Hood. Whenever an oxygen hood is used, FiO_2 must be regulated by using an oxygen blender or a nebulizer with adjustable oxygen concentrations. A heated humidifier is preferable for neonates, to help with thermoregulation and to minimize noise levels inside the hood. The first step is to attach the blender to the wall gas outlets and set the desired FiO_2 on the blender dial. The next step is to attach the oxygen flow to the humidifier. This is done by attaching a small-bore, high-pressure tube to the blended gas flowmeter and attaching the opposite end to the humidifier inlet. The tubing is often attached to the humidifier inlet by a small nipple, which fits over the inlet orifice. If a nebulizer is used, it is appropriately assembled and attached to the flowmeter. If an oxygen blender is not used, the nebulizer should be set to the appropriate FiO_2.

The oxygen hood is now placed in the incubator or warmer but not covering the patient at this point. The flow from the humidifier/nebulizer is connected to the oxygen hood by a length of large-bore aerosol tubing. Between the humidifier/nebulizer and oxyhood, there should be a water trap to collect the water that rains out in the tubing.

A thermometer or temperature probe attached to the humidifier is placed in-line with the aerosol tubing before the entry into the oxyhood. Add water to the humidifier or nebulizer and turn it on to begin heating. Set the flow rate as necessary to maintain FiO_2, usually 7 to 10 L/min. With flow running to the hood, you can now place the hood over the patient's head.

Analyze the FiO_2 at the same level as the patient's head inside the hood to ensure the patient is receiving the desired concentration. Finally, after a few minutes, check the temperature and make whatever adjustments are necessary to achieve the desired temperature.

TASK G: Assess Vital Signs. Assess the patient's breath sounds, pulse rate, respiratory rate and effort, presence of cyanosis, and oxygen saturation, if available. This evaluation will serve as a baseline for subsequent patient evaluation.

TASK H: No-Smoking Sign Placement. Place no-smoking signs on the wall near the patient and at the room entrance.

TASK I: Document Results in Chart. Document all of the pertinent data in the patient's chart.

TASK J: Monitoring. Monitor the patient and equipment based on any orders, written department standards, and patient condition.

PERFORMANCE EVALUATION 1
OXYGEN THERAPY, VIA CANNULA OR MASK

Date: Lab _____   Clinical _____   Hospital _____

Lab: Pass _____ Fail _____   Clinical: Pass _____   Fail _____

Student name _____   Instructor name _____

Number of required observations: Lab _____   Clinical _____

Number of times observed: Lab _____   Clinical _____

Number of required practices: Lab _____   Clinical _____

Number of times practice: Lab _____   Clinical _____

PASSING CRITERIA:

Obtain 90 percent or better on the procedure. Tasks indicated by an asterisk (*) must receive at least 1 point or the evaluation is terminated. The procedure must be performed within the designated time or the performance receives a failing grade.

SCORING:

2 points—Task performed satisfactorily without prompting.
1 point—Task performed satisfactorily with self-initiated correction.
0 points—Task performed incorrectly or with prompting required.
NA—Task not applicable to the patient care situation.

TASKS:	PEER	LAB	CLINICAL
A. Review chart			
* 1. document need for oxygen	☐	☐	☐
* 2. liter flow or FiO_2	☐	☐	☐
* 3. determine type of device to administer the oxygen	☐	☐	☐
* 4. orders or indications for isolation	☐	☐	☐
B. Wash hands	☐	☐	☐
C. Gather equipment			
* 1. flowmeter	☐	☐	☐
* 2. oxygen blender	☐	☐	☐
* 3. humidifier and sterile water	☐	☐	☐
* 4. connecting tubing	☐	☐	☐
* 5. cannula or mask	☐	☐	☐
* 6. no-smoking signs	☐	☐	☐
D. Confirm patient identity	☐	☐	☐
E. Perform procedure	☐	☐	☐
* 1. wash hands	☐	☐	☐
* 2. attach flowmeter to wall outlet	☐	☐	☐

TASKS:	PEER	LAB	CLINICAL
* 3. fill humidifier, as appropriate	☐	☐	☐
* 4. attach humidifier to flowmeter	☐	☐	☐
* 5. check pop-off valve	☐	☐	☐
* 6. attach tubing to the flowmeter or humidifier (if used)	☐	☐	☐
* 7. set desired flow rate	☐	☐	☐
* 8. check the system	☐	☐	☐
* 9. apply device to patient	☐	☐	☐
F. Assess vital signs			
* 1. breath sounds	☐	☐	☐
* 2. pulse rate	☐	☐	☐
* 3. respiratory rate and effort	☐	☐	☐
* 4. color	☐	☐	☐
* G. Place no-smoking signs at bedside and room entrance	☐	☐	☐
* H. Document pertinent data in patient chart	☐	☐	☐
* I. Monitor appropriately	☐	☐	☐

SCORE:

Peer: _____   points out of _____ (56) _____ %

Lab: _____   points out of _____ (56) _____ %

Clinical: _____ points out of _____ (56) _____ %

TIME: _____ out of possible 10 minutes.

STUDENT SIGNATURES   **INSTRUCTOR SIGNATURES**

PEER: _____   LAB: _____

STUDENT: _____   CLINICAL: _____

PERFORMANCE EVALUATION 2
OXYGEN HOOD THERAPY

Date: Lab _____   Clinical _____   Hospital _____

Lab: Pass _____ Fail _____   Clinical: Pass _____   Fail _____

Student name _____   Instructor name _____

Number of required observations: Lab _____   Clinical _____

Number of times observed: Lab _____   Clinical _____

Number of required practices: Lab _____   Clinical _____

Number of times practice: Lab _____   Clinical _____

PASSING CRITERIA:

Obtain 90 percent or better on the procedure. Tasks indicated by an asterisk (*) must receive at least 1 point or the evaluation is terminated. The procedure must be performed within the designated time or the performance receives a failing grade.

SCORING:

2 points—Task performed satisfactorily without prompting.
1 point—Task performed satisfactorily with self-initiated correction.
0 points—Task performed incorrectly or with prompting required.
NA—Task not applicable to the patient care situation

TASKS:	PEER	LAB	CLINICAL
A. Review chart			
* 1. document need for oxygen	☐	☐	☐
* 2. FiO$_2$	☐	☐	☐
* 3. orders or indications for isolation	☐	☐	☐
* B. Wash hands	☐	☐	☐
C. Gather equipment			
* 1. flowmeter	☐	☐	☐
* 2. oxygen blender	☐	☐	☐
* 3. humidifier/nebulizer and sterile water	☐	☐	☐
* 4. connecting tubing	☐	☐	☐
* 5. appropriate sized hood	☐	☐	☐
* 6. oxygen analyzer	☐	☐	☐
* 7. water trap	☐	☐	☐
* 8. no-smoking signs	☐	☐	☐
* 9. thermometer or temperature probe	☐	☐	☐
* D. Confirm patient identity	☐	☐	☐

TASKS:	PEER	LAB	CLINICAL
* E. Perform procedure	☐	☐	☐
* 1. wash hands	☐	☐	☐
* 2. connect blender to gas outlets	☐	☐	☐
* 3. set desired FiO_2	☐	☐	☐
* 4. connect the blender flow to the humidifier, or attach the nebulizer to flowmeter	☐	☐	☐
* 5. position hood next to patient	☐	☐	☐
* 6. connect aerosol tubing from the humidifier or nebulizer to the hood	☐	☐	☐
* 7. attach T connector to the end of the tubing, if needed	☐	☐	☐
* 8. place water trap in line			
* 9. insert thermometer or temperature probe	☐	☐	☐
* 10. add sterile water to humidifier or nebulizer	☐	☐	☐
* 11. turn on heater	☐	☐	☐
* 12. set desired flow rate	☐	☐	☐
* 13. place infant in hood	☐	☐	☐
* 14. analyze the FiO_2	☐	☐	☐
* 15. check the temperature	☐	☐	☐
F. Assess vital signs	☐	☐	☐
* 1. breath sounds	☐	☐	☐
* 2. pulse rate	☐	☐	☐
* 3. respiratory rate and effort	☐	☐	☐
* 4. color	☐	☐	☐
* G. Place no-smoking signs at bedside and room entrance	☐	☐	☐
* H. Document pertinent data in patient chart	☐	☐	☐
* I. Monitor appropriately	☐	☐	☐

SCORE:

Peer: _____ points out of _____ (68) _____ %

Lab: _____ points out of _____ (68) _____ %

Clinical: _____ points out of _____ (68) _____ %

TIME: _____ out of possible 15 minutes.

STUDENT SIGNATURES

PEER: _____

STUDENT: _____

INSTRUCTOR SIGNATURES

LAB: _____

CLINICAL: _____

MEDICATION NEBULIZER

OBJECTIVE

The student will be able to correctly assemble the necessary equipment and administer a medication nebulizer in a laboratory and clinical setting. This will be done following aseptic guidelines and in a competent manner as determined by lab and clinical instructors.

TASK A: Review the Chart. Before proceeding with this procedure, the patient chart should be reviewed. The student should first check the order to ensure that the prescribed medication and dosage are being followed. Evaluate the presence of any contraindications to the therapy and the patient's current condition as noted in the progress and nursing notes. This will help the student prepare for interaction with the patient and any potential changes that may be warranted in the therapy.

The patient's past response to previous therapy should be reviewed for possible adverse side effects or other problems encountered. These notes should serve as a follow-up and reminder of the report received on the patient. During the chart review, the student will note any orders or indications for patient isolation techniques.

TASK B: Obtain Equipment. Obtain the medication nebulizer. If not included with the nebulizer, you will also need a mouthpiece, T adapter, reservoir tube, and connecting tubing. Nose clips may be needed for patients unable to coordinate mouth breathing. For infants and toddlers, you will need an appropriate size aerosol mask to be used in place of the mouthpiece.

Next, obtain a flowmeter or compressor to power the nebulizer. Under normal circumstances, the nebulizer will be powered by an oxygen flowmeter.

Now get the prescribed medication. Make sure that the concentration is correct and that the expiration date has not been passed. You will also need to obtain sterile saline or other diluent for the medication at this time.

A stethoscope is necessary to evaluate the breath sounds both before and after the treatment. The bell should be appropriately sized for the patient. For patients old enough to perform the maneuver, generally older than 5 years of age, peak flow measurements should be done before and after bronchodilator administration to evaluate the effectiveness of the therapy. You will therefore require a peak flowmeter for these patients.

Finally, because of the probability of contact with secretions, the student should obtain a pair of exam gloves before continuing with this procedure.

TASK C: Wash Hands. After gathering the equipment, the student should perform a thorough hand washing followed by placement of the gloves.

TASK D: Confirm Patient. Before administering any drug to a patient, confirm that you have the correct patient by looking at the name bracelet attached to a patient limb.

TASK E: Assess Patient. Before administering the therapy, auscultate the patient's lungs and determine breath sounds. Careful auscultation is invaluable at this point in determining a baseline for comparison following the therapy. The student should also obtain the pulse rate, respiratory rate and effort, and peak flow.

TASK F: Position Patient. To achieve the best expansion of the lung bases, the patient should be elevated to an upright position for the treatment. For patients who are unable to be elevated, the therapy may be modified as needed.

TASK G: Administer the Therapy. First, assemble the nebulizer by placing the T piece on the nebulizer, inserting the mouthpiece into the T piece, and placing the reservoir tubing opposite the mouthpiece on the T piece. Now add the prescribed medication and diluent to the nebulizer. Depending on the type of nebulizer, this is done by either unscrewing the nebulizer and adding the liquids to the lower reservoir or by removing the T piece and adding the liquids through the nebulizer outlet.

Connect the nebulizer to the flowmeter or compressor with the connecting tube. Turn on the flow and assure proper function of the nebulizer. Most nebulizers require flows of 5 to 6 L/min to achieve the desired particle size, but in all cases, follow the manufacturer's recommended flow rate for the nebulizer being used.

The nebulizer is now ready for the patient. Place the mouthpiece between the teeth and the lips and have the patient close the lips to provide a seal around the mouthpiece. The patient is then coached in the proper breathing technique of slow deep inhalations through the mouth followed by a slight breath hold before exhalation. Patients who have trouble breathing through the mouth may require the use of nose clips. If the patient is unable to use the mouthpiece, an appropriate size of aerosol mask may be used.

TASK H: Monitor the Patient. During the treatment, the patient is monitored for pulse rate, respiratory rate and pattern, and any adverse side effects. Blood pressure is monitored on unstable patients. The treatment is terminated if any of the following occur:

1. Increase of 20 beats per minute of the heart rate.
2. Sudden chest pain.
3. A decrease in the blood pressure.

TASK I: Conclude the Procedure. The treatment is terminated normally when the medication in the nebulizer has run out. Remove the nebulizer from the patient's mouth and clean it by opening the nebulizer and shaking any remaining medication from the nebulizer vial. At this point, the nebulizer may be rinsed with sterile water. The nebulizer, T piece, mouthpiece, and reservoir tubing should then be placed in a clean location and allowed to air dry.

Now ask the patient to cough. Any secretions coughed up should be placed in a tissue or other appropriate receptacle.

Repeat the evaluation of breath sounds, pulse rate, respiratory rate and effort, and peak expiratory flow rate.

Return the patient to the previous or other desired position.

TASK J: Record in Patient Chart. Chart the appropriate information in the patient record. These data should include before and after parameters, vital signs, breath sounds, description of patient toleration, sputum production, and any adverse effects.

TASK K: Hand Washing. Wash hands again.

PERFORMANCE EVALUATION 3
MEDICATION NEBULIZER

Date: Lab _____   Clinical _____   Hospital _____

Lab: Pass _____ Fail _____   Clinical: Pass _____   Fail _____

Student name _____   Instructor name _____

Number of required observations: Lab _____   Clinical _____

Number of times observed: Lab _____   Clinical _____

Number of required practices: Lab _____   Clinical _____

Number of times practice: Lab _____   Clinical _____

PASSING CRITERIA:

Obtain 90 percent or better on the procedure. Tasks indicated by an asterisk (*) must receive at least 1 point or the evaluation is terminated. The procedure must be performed within the designated time or the performance receives a failing grade.

SCORING:

2 points—Task performed satisfactorily without prompting.
1 point—Task performed satisfactorily with self-initiated correction.
0 points—Task performed incorrectly or with prompting required.
NA—Task not applicable to the patient care situation

TASKS:	PEER	LAB	CLINICAL
A. Review chart			
* 1. check order	☐	☐	☐
* 2. contraindications	☐	☐	☐
3. patient condition	☐	☐	☐
* 4. past response to therapy	☐	☐	☐
* 5. orders or indications for isolation	☐	☐	☐
B. Obtain equipment			
* 1. medication nebulizer (to include T piece, mouthpiece, reservoir tubing, and connecting tubing), mask	☐	☐	☐

TASKS:	PEER	LAB	CLINICAL
* 2. flowmeter or compressor	☐	☐	☐
* 3. prescribed medication			
a. correct concentration	☐	☐	☐
b. check expiration date	☐	☐	☐
* 4. sterile normal saline	☐	☐	☐
* 5. nose clips	☐	☐	☐
* 6. stethoscope	☐	☐	☐
* 7. peak flowmeter	☐	☐	☐
* 8. exam gloves	☐	☐	☐
* C. Wash hands; put on gloves	☐	☐	☐
* D. Confirm and identify patient	☐	☐	☐
E. Assess patient			
* 1. breath sounds	☐	☐	☐
* 2. pulse rate	☐	☐	☐
* 3. respiratory rate and effort	☐	☐	☐
* 4. peak flow	☐	☐	☐
* F. Place patient in upright position (as possible)	☐	☐	☐
G. Administer therapy			
1. assemble nebulizer			
* a. T piece on nebulizer	☐	☐	☐
* b. mouthpiece inserted into T	☐	☐	☐
* c. reservoir tubing into T	☐	☐	☐
* 2. place medication and diluent into nebulizer	☐	☐	☐
* 3. connect nebulizer to flowmeter or compressor	☐	☐	☐
* 4. turn on flow to ensure proper function (usually 5 to 6 L/min)	☐	☐	☐
* 5. place mouthpiece in patient's mouth or mask over mouth and nose	☐	☐	☐
* 6. place nose clips (as necessary)			
7. coach patient in proper breathing technique			
* a. slow deep inhalation through mouth	☐	☐	☐
* b. small breath hold before exhalation	☐	☐	☐
H. Monitor patient during therapy			
* 1. pulse rate	☐	☐	☐
* 2. respiratory rate and pattern	☐	☐	☐
* 3. adverse side effects	☐	☐	☐
I. Conclude procedure			
1. remove nebulizer and clean			
* a. open nebulizer vial and sanitarily dispose of remaining medication	☐	☐	☐
* b. place nebulizer in appropriate location to air dry	☐	☐	☐

TASKS:		PEER	LAB	CLINICAL
*	2. have patient cough	☐	☐	☐
	3. reevaluate patient's vital signs' parameters			
*	a. breath sounds	☐	☐	☐
*	b. pulse rate	☐	☐	☐
*	c. respiratory rate and effort	☐	☐	☐
*	d. peak flow	☐	☐	☐
*	4. return patient to desired position			
*	J. Record results and observations	☐	☐	☐
	K. Wash hands	☐	☐	☐

SCORE:

Peer: _____ points out of _____ (104) _____ %

Lab: _____ points out of _____ (104) _____ %

Clinical: _____ points out of _____ (104) _____ %

TIME: _____ out of possible 25 minutes.

STUDENT SIGNATURES

PEER: _____

STUDENT: _____

INSTRUCTOR SIGNATURES

LAB: _____

CLINICAL: _____

POSTURAL DRAINAGE AND CHEST PERCUSSION

OBJECTIVE

The student will be able to properly position a patient and perform chest physiotherapy (CPT) in a laboratory and clinical setting. This will be done following aseptic guidelines and in a competent manner as determined by lab and clinical instructors.

TASK A: Review the Chart. When initiating chest physiotherapy, it is important to verify that the order has been written, along with the frequency and goals of the therapy.
If this is the first time that CPT will be performed, any contraindications or hazards should be determined, in addition to the following: the volume and nature of the lung secretions, pathophysiology of the lung disease, and current clinical conditions.

If the patient has been receiving CPT, the response to past CPT treatments and indications to modify the positions used to drain the affected lung regions should be evaluated. A review of the latest chest radiograph will help evaluate any lung areas that need special attention. Note any orders or indications for patient isolation techniques.

TASK B: Obtain Equipment. Now obtain any equipment that will be used during the CPT treatment. This will include a stethoscope, the equipment or device to be used to perform the percussion and vibration, a resuscitation bag and mask, and suction equipment.

TASK C: Hand Washing. A thorough hand washing should now be done. Observe universal precautions.

TASK D: Confirm Patient. Proceed to patient room or bed and confirm that it is the correct patient by looking at the patient's identification.

TASK E: Obtain Baseline Data. Before starting the treatment, assess the patient's breath sounds, pulse rate, respiratory rate, and color. A transcutaneous monitor or pulse oximeter may be used to monitor the oxygenation status during the treatment.

TASK F: Position Patient. The patient should be positioned according to the lung area that is to be drained. Determining the correct position is done by an understanding of the disease and the goal of the CPT. If there is a specific lung segment involved, the position used would drain the segment. CPT done for prophylaxis, or to help remove thick secretions, may best be done by percussing over all lung fields. Correct positioning of the patient will facilitate drainage and enhance the vibration or percussion of the desired area. After determining the appropriate position, place the patient accordingly. Infants may be held on the lap, and positioning may be assisted with the use of pillows.

These positions may need to be modified in certain instances. For example, the critically ill neonate may require too great an increase in FiO_2 when positioned. Neonates with chest tubes, endotracheal tubes, and IV lines require cautious handling and may not tolerate changes in position. Care must also be taken with patients who have a history of recent surgery, head injury, or hemodynamic instability.

Positions for Postural Drainage. Positions used to drain specific lung segments are primarily used on the older patient. On the neonate, positioning is mainly done by placing the patient on one side. The side that is elevated is then percussed, or vibrated. The patient is then turned on the opposite side, and the procedure is repeated.

For patients in whom a specific lung segment is to be percussed and drained, a description of the proper positions follows. Each position is shown accompanying the descriptive text.

Upper Lobes, Posterior Segments. (Figure A–1). Lean the patient over at a 30-degree angle from a sitting position and percuss or vibrate over upper back on both sides. Percussion and vibration are then done on the upper back of the affected side.

Upper Lobes, Anterior Segments. (Figure A–2). This positioning is accomplished by placing the patient on the back, with the head of the bed elevated. Percussion is then done between the nipples and clavicles over the affected side.

Upper Lobe, Apical Segment. (Figure A–2). Lean the patient backwards about 30 degrees from a sitting position. Percuss or vibrate above the clavicle over the involved area. The patient may also be positioned on his or her back, with the head of the bed elevated. Percussion or vibration is then done above the clavicles.

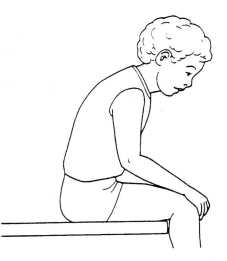

Figure A–1

Right Middle Lobe. (FIgure A–3). The patient is positioned on the left side, elevating the hips about 5 inches higher than the head. The patient is then rolled backwards 1/4 turn. The patient is percussed over the area of the right nipple.

Lingular Segments of the Left Upper Lobe. (Figure A–4). Place the patient in the same position, only with the left side up. Percussion is then done over the area of the left nipple.

Right Lower Lobe, Lateral Basal Segment. (Figure A–5). Position the patient on his or her left side with the hips about 8 inches higher than the head. The shoulders are then rolled forward $\frac{1}{4}$ turn. Percussion is done over the lower ribs.

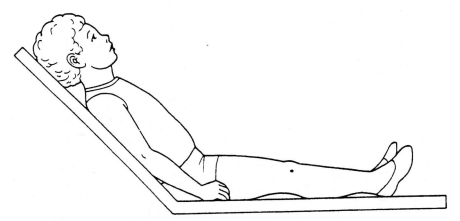

Figure A–2

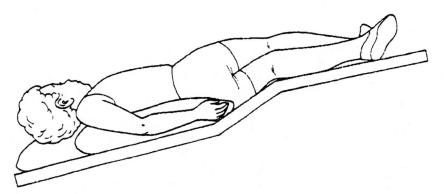

Figure A–3

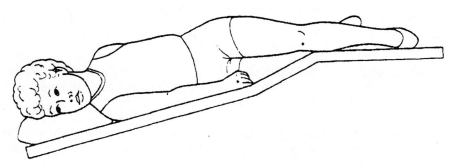

Figure A–4

Left Lower Lobe, Lateral Basal Segment. Drainage of this segment is identical to that described for the right lower lobe, except that the patient is placed on the right side.

Lower Lobes, Superior Segments. (Figure A–6). The patient is positioned face down, with the bed flat. Percussion is then done at the top of the scapula over the involved area.

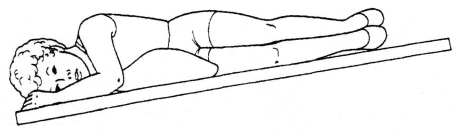

Figure A–5

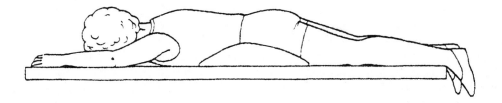

Figure A–6

Lower Lobes, Posterior Basal Segments. (Figure A–7). The patient is placed face done, with the hips 8 inches higher than the head. Percuss or vibrate on the involved side, over the lower ribs close to the spine.

Lower Lobes, Anterior Basal Segment. (Figure A–8). Place the patient on the side opposite the involved area, with the hips about 8 inches higher than the head. Percuss or vibrate just beneath the axilla.

TASK G: Percuss Patient. Whichever type of percussor is used, it should be small enough to cover the area involved and not extend beyond the ribs onto the abdomen. It should be done at a relaxed but vigorous rhythmic rate and should never be painful or stressful to the patient. On larger patients, cupped hands may be used in place of a mechanical percussor.

Excessive force when percussing does not increase the mobilization of secretions and is

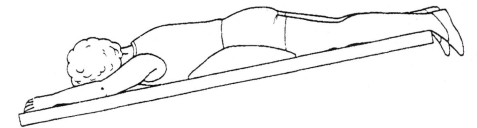

Figure A–7

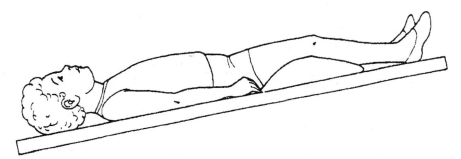

Figure A–8

never indicated. Percussion may produce skin erythema, a reddening of the skin, or bruising. Avoid percussing over bony areas, such as the clavicles, sternum, and vertebrae, to prevent bruising and potential fractures.

Extreme care must be taken not to percuss over the abdomen or outside the boundaries of the thorax. Failure to do this may cause damage to internal organs and tissues.

The duration of the CPT depends on who well the patient tolerates the treatment and on the patient's condition. CPT done to the small neonate should be limited to 5 minutes per side. This reduces the stress on the neonate and the accompanying changes in oxygenation and vital signs. For older patients, percussion may be done for 3 to 5 minutes in each position, as tolerated.

If CPT must be done on the critically ill or unstable patient, 2 or 3 minutes per side may be all that is tolerated.

When doing CPT on the pediatric patient, perform CPT first to the lobes most affected, allowing 3 to 5 minutes per area. CPT is then done to other involved segments as needed. The total treatment should not last longer than 10 to 20 minutes. Longer treatments may tire the patient excessively and usually do not increase mucus removal.

TASK H: Vibration. Vibration can be done via mechanical vibrator or by hand. It is done following percussion or in place of it, when indicated. Vibration is indicated over percussion on neonates weighing less than 900 grams, those with chest tubes, and patients who are postoperative.

Vibration is applied to the chest well, above the desired area. This facilitates the movement of the secretions from that lung area. Hand vibration is done by producing a quivering motion similar to that during isometic exercises. Battery-operated vibrators offer an easier and superior method of vibration. Many newly developed vibrators are designed specifically for the neonate and concentrate the vibration to small areas.

In substitution for percussion, vibration is done for approximately 5 minutes per area, for a total of 10 to 15 minutes' duration. When done following percussion, vibration should be limited to 2 to 3 minutes on each area.

TASK I: Monitor Patient. Throughout the treatment, the patient must be monitored for signs of distress. The heart rate is most easily monitored by the ECG. Respiratory rate and pattern should be assessed every 3 to 5 minutes. The treatment should be stopped if the patient becomes tachycardic or bradycardic.

Signs of increasing respiratory distress are indications for stopping the treatment and further evaluating the patient. The patient's oxygenation status should be monitored as well. Small decreases in PaO_2 or saturation can be treated by increasing the FiO_2 to achieve the desired level. Prolonged or profound drops in PaO_2, however, require that the treatment be stopped and the patient further evaluated and treated.

Evaluate the need for suctioning. If secretions are heard in the large airways and the patient is unable to generate an effective cough, suctioning should be done.

TASK J: Conclude Procedure. Following completion of the procedure, the patient is returned to the desired position. The vital signs are reevaluated and compared to beginning vital signs.

TASK K: Documenting Procedure. The procedure is completed by documenting all pertinent information in the patient chart. This should include the positions used, duration of therapy, how the patient tolerated the procedure, vital signs, breath sounds, and sputum production.

PERFORMANCE EVALUATION 4
POSTURAL DRAINAGE AND CHEST PERCUSSION

Date: Lab _____ Clinical _____ Hospital _____

Lab: Pass _____ Fail _____ Clinical: Pass _____ Fail _____

Student name _____ Instructor name _____

Number of required observations: Lab _____ Clinical _____

Number of times observed: Lab _____ Clinical _____

Number of required practices: Lab _____ Clinical _____

Number of times practice: Lab _____ Clinical _____

PASSING CRITERIA:

Obtain 90 percent or better on the procedure. Tasks indicated by an asterisk (*) must receive at least 1 point or the evaluation is terminated. The procedure must be performed within the designated time or the performance receives a failing grade.

SCORING:

2 points—Task performed satisfactorily without prompting.
1 point—Task performed satisfactorily with self-initiated correction.
0 points—Task performed incorrectly or with prompting required.
NA—Task not applicable to the patient care situation

TASKS:	PEER	LAB	CLINICAL
A. Review chart			
* 1. check order	☐	☐	☐
* 2. contraindications	☐	☐	☐
3. secretions	☐	☐	☐
4. pathophysiology of lung disease	☐	☐	☐
5. patient condition	☐	☐	☐
6. past response to therapy	☐	☐	☐
* 7. current chest x-ray	☐	☐	☐
* 8. orders or indications for isolation	☐	☐	☐
B. Obtain equipment			
* 1. stethoscope	☐	☐	☐
* 2. percussor	☐	☐	☐

TASKS:	**PEER**	**LAB**	**CLINICAL**
* 3. resuscitation bag and mask	☐	☐	☐
* 4. suction equipment	☐	☐	☐
* C. Wash hands and maintain asepsis	☐	☐	☐
* D. Confirm and identify patient	☐	☐	☐
E. Obtain baseline and vital signs			
* 1. breath sounds	☐	☐	☐
* 2. heart rate	☐	☐	☐
* 3. respiratory rate and effort	☐	☐	☐
* 4. color	☐	☐	☐
* 5. oxygenation status, if available	☐	☐	☐
* F. Place patient in upright positions	☐	☐	☐
G. Appropriately percuss patient			
* 1. correct equipment	☐	☐	☐
* 2. acceptable rate and rhythm	☐	☐	☐
* 3. appropriate striking force	☐	☐	☐
* 4. performed within boundaries	☐	☐	☐
* 5. appropriate duration	☐	☐	☐
H. Vibration			
* 1. Indications	☐	☐	☐
2. proper equipment	☐	☐	☐
3. appropriate duration	☐	☐	☐
I. Monitor patient			
* 1. heart and respiratory rate	☐	☐	☐
2. observe			
* a. respiratory pattern	☐	☐	☐
* b. patient appearance	☐	☐	☐
J. Conclude procedure			
1. return patient to desired position	☐	☐	☐
* 2. reassess vital signs	☐	☐	☐
* 3. appropriately suction patient	☐	☐	☐
* K. Record results and observations	☐	☐	☐

SCORE:

        Peer: _____ points out of _____ (72) _____ %

        Lab: _____ points out of _____ (72) _____ %

        Clinical: _____ points out of _____ (72) _____ %

TIME: _____ out of possible 25 minutes.

STUDENT SIGNATURES   **INSTRUCTOR SIGNATURES**

PEER: _____   LAB: _____

STUDENT: _____   CLINICAL: _____

SUCTIONING: ENDOTRACHEAL, OROPHARYNGEAL, AND NASOPHARYNGEAL

OBJECTIVE

The student will be able to properly suction a patient through the endotracheal tube, orally and nasally, in a laboratory and clinical setting. This will be done following aseptic guidelines under universal precaution procedures and in a competent manner as determined by lab and clinical instructors.

Suctioning is the technique of inserting a catheter into the airway, applying a negative pressure, and removing secretions through the catheter. It is recommended that it always be done with two people, one to perform the suctioning procedure and the other to monitor the patient and provide support as needed.

TASK A: Prepare Equipment. The first task in preparing for suctioning the airway is the preparation of the equipment. You will need a vacuum source with a reservoir and adjustable regulator, sterile catheter kit, resuscitation bag and appropriate size mask, and eye protection.

The appropriately sized suction catheter should be selected for the patient. The suction catheter used should be ≤ $\frac{1}{2}$ the inner diameter of the airway. Approximate sizes are as follows:

Suction Catheter sizes (intubated patient)

Endotracheal Tube (mm I.D.)	Suction Catheter (French)
2.5	5, 6
3.0	5, 6
3.5	6 to 8
4.0	8

Suction Catheter Sizes (nonintubated patient)

Age	Suction Catheter (French)
Preemie	5, 6
Term Newborn	6 to 8
Newborn to 6 months	8

The next step, determining catheter insertion distance, applies only to endotracheal suctioning. The proper catheter insertion distance is determined by noting the centimeter mark on the exterior ETT that corresponds to the level of the adapter, as illustrated in Figure A–9.

The adapter length, which is approximately 4 cm, is added to the centimeter mark on the ETT. This represents the distance from the tip of the ETT to the opening of the adapter and can then be used to determine the appropriate depth of catheter insertion.

Once the insertion distance is determined, it should be noted and placed on a card near

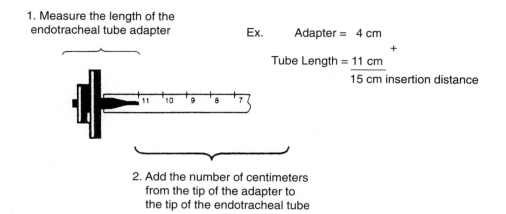

1. Measure the length of the endotracheal tube adapter

Ex.   Adapter =   4 cm

Tube Length = 11 cm

    +

15 cm insertion distance

2. Add the number of centimeters from the tip of the adapter to the tip of the endotracheal tube

Figure A–9   *The method of determining proper insertion of a suction catheter.*

the patient's bedside. The vacuum pressure should be adjusted next. Occlude the opening of the suction line and adjust the vacuum to –50 to –120 mm Hg. Use the lowest pressure that will provide effective airway clearance.

Observe Universal precautions.

TASK B: Prepare Patient. The patient should now be prepared for the procedure. As always, before touching the patient, you must perform an adequate hand washing. The chest should now be ausculated for the presence of mucus in the airways. Suctioning is indicated if there is evidence of audible secretions in the large airways or visible secretions in the endotracheal tube. The patient is then hyperoxygenated by the assistant. This should be done for 30 seconds to 1 minute before the procedure by using a resuscitation bag connected to oxygen or by increasing the FiO_2 of the ventilator. Observe and note the vital signs at this point, to include pulse rate, respiratory rate, blood pressure (on unstable patients), and oxygenation status.

TASK C: Perform Procedure; Endotracheal Tube. First, place eye protection. Aseptically open the suction kit, making certain not to contaminate the catheter or gloves. Put the sterile gloves on, using sterile technique. Using the dominant hand, carefully remove the catheter from the protective package. If the patient is inside an incubator, the catheter should be wrapped around the hand or inside the clenched hand to protect it from being contaminated as the hand is inserted into the porthole.

The next step is to attach the suction catheter to the suction tubing, carefully maintaining sterility. By holding the thumb port between the thumb and index fingers of the gloved hand, the catheter tubing connection can be pushed into the secretion tubing without resulting contamination.

The ventilator connector is removed and the suction catheter is inserted into the endotracheal tube, without applied suction, to the previously determined depth. The thumb port is then occluded and the catheter is withdrawn. Some recommend the intermittent application of suction. The entire duration of the suction procedure should not exceed 15 seconds.

The patient is immediately reattached to the ventilator or bag, monitored, and treated for bradycardia and hypoxemia. If secretions are thick and difficult to remove, normal saline lavage may be used. This is accomplished by instilling a small amount of sterile saline into the endotracheal tube. Premature infants should receive less than 0.5 ml of sterile saline. Older patients may require several milliliters to sufficiently loosen secretions. The suctioning is repeated as necessary until all secretions are removed. The patient must be monitored for bradycardia and hypoxemia throughout the procedure. Severe bradycardia (< 100 beats per minute in neonates) requires immediate cessation of the procedure. When the patient is stable, the FiO_2 must be returned to its presuction level.

TASK C: Perform Procedure; Oropharyngeal. Although not a sterile procedure, it is recommended that the person performing the oral suctioning wear exam gloves and eye protection during the procedure. You may use the catheter previously used to suction the nasopharynx or endotracheal tube. If using a catheter that does not contain gloves, the student should obtain them and put them on at this point.

The catheter is next removed from the package and connected to the suction tubing. Insert the catheter tip into the patient's mouth and carefully follow the surface of the tongue to the oropharynx. Suction is now applied, and the catheter withdrawn. As with endotracheal suctioning, some advise the use of intermittent suction.

Bradycardia and hypoxia are treated by the administration of oxygen. The technique is repeated as necessary to remove all secretions.

TASK C: Perform Procedure; Nasopharyngeal. Nasopharyngeal suctioning is accomplished in a manner similar to oropharyngeal suctioning. Gloves and eye protection should be worn. It may be helpful to add a water-soluble jelly to the catheter to ease insertion into the nose and reduce injury.

The catheter is inserted in a slightly upward direction and toward the back of the head until it enters the nasopharynx. Suction is applied and the catheter is withdrawn. As with the other suction procedures, some advocate the use of intermittent suction. The patient is monitored and treated for any hypoxia and bradycardia. The procedure is repeated as needed.

NOTE: The duration of the actual suction procedure should not be more than 15 seconds for any of the techniques.

TASK D: Document Procedure. The final step in suctioning the patient is documentation in the patient chart. This should include how well the patient tolerated the procedure, amount and color of sputum, vital signs, and breath sounds.

TASK E: Monitoring. The appropriate timing and method of monitoring the equipment and the patient should be determined. This is based on any orders, written department standards, and patient condition.

PERFORMANCE EVALUATION 5
ENDOTRACHEAL SUCTIONING

Date: Lab _____   Clinical _____   Hospital _____

Lab: Pass ____ Fail _____   Clinical: Pass _____   Fail _____

Student name _____   Instructor name _____

Number of required observations: Lab _____   Clinical _____

Number of times observed: Lab _____   Clinical _____

Number of required practices: Lab _____   Clinical _____

Number of times practice: Lab _____   Clinical _____

PASSING CRITERIA:

Obtain 90 percent or better on the procedure. Tasks indicated by an asterisk (*) must receive at least 1 point or the evaluation is terminated. The procedure must be performed within the designated time or the performance receives a failing grade.

SCORING:

2 points—Task performed satisfactorily without prompting.
1 point—Task performed satisfactorily with self-initiated correction.
0 points—Task performed incorrectly or with prompting required.
NA—Task not applicable to the patient care situation

TASKS:

	PEER	LAB	CLINICAL
A. Prepare equipment			
* 1. select appropriately sized catheter	☐	☐	☐
* 2. determine catheter insertion distance (when suctioning the endotracheal tube)	☐	☐	☐
* 3. adjust vacuum pressure (–50 to –120 mm Hg)	☐	☐	☐
* 4. prepare ventilator/manual resuscitation bag	☐	☐	☐
B. Prepare patient			
* 1. wash hands	☐	☐	☐
2. auscultate chest and determine breath sounds	☐	☐	☐
* 3. hyperoxygenate as needed	☐	☐	☐
* 4. observe baseline vital signs	☐	☐	☐

TASKS:	PEER	LAB	CLINICAL
C. Perform procedure: Endotracheal tube			
* 1. place eye protection	☐	☐	☐
* 2. aseptically open suction kit	☐	☐	☐
* 3. aseptically place gloves	☐	☐	☐
* 4. remove catheter from package	☐	☐	☐
* 5. attach catheter to suction tubing (do not contaminate sterile hand)	☐	☐	☐
* 6. disconnect patient from ventilator	☐	☐	☐
* 7. insert catheter into ET tube without suction and advance to predetermined depth	☐	☐	☐
* 8. apply suction and withdraw catheter	☐	☐	☐
* 9. reconnect ventilator (or manually ventilate) for 4 to 5 breaths. Total time patient is disconnected from ventilator should not exceed 15 seconds	☐	☐	☐
* 10. observe vital signs; treat patient for any bradycardia or hypoxia	☐	☐	☐
* 11. instill appropriate amount of sterile saline, if indicated	☐	☐	☐
* 12. repeat suction as needed	☐	☐	☐
* 13. resume ventilation of patient	☐	☐	☐
* 14. return FiO_2 to presuction level when clinically indicated	☐	☐	☐
* D. Document the procedure and pertinent information in the patient chart	☐	☐	☐
* E. Monitor appropriately	☐	☐	☐

SCORE:

Peer: _____ points out of _____ (48) _____ %

Lab: _____ points out of _____ (48) _____ %

Clinical: _____ points out of _____ (48) _____ %

TIME: _____ out of possible 30 minutes.

STUDENT SIGNATURES

PEER: _____

STUDENT: _____

INSTRUCTOR SIGNATURES

LAB: _____

CLINICAL: _____

PERFORMANCE EVALUATION 6
OROPHARYNGEAL SUCTIONING

Date: Lab _____   Clinical _____   Hospital _____

Lab: Pass _____   Fail _____   Clinical: Pass _____   Fail _____

Student name _____   Instructor name _____

Number of required observations:	Lab _____	Clinical _____
Number of times observed:	Lab _____	Clinical _____
Number of required practices:	Lab _____	Clinical _____
Number of times practice:	Lab _____	Clinical _____

PASSING CRITERIA:

Obtain 90 percent or better on the procedure. Tasks indicated by an asterisk (*) must receive at least 1 point or the evaluation is terminated. The procedure must be performed within the designated time or the performance receives a failing grade.

SCORING:

2 points—Task performed satisfactorily without prompting.
1 point—Task performed satisfactorily with self-initiated correction.
0 points—Task performed incorrectly or with prompting required.
NA—Task not applicable to the patient care situation

TASKS:	PEER	LAB	CLINICAL
A. Prepare equipment			
* 1. select appropriately sized catheter	☐	☐	☐
* 2. adjust vacuum pressure (−50 to −120 mm Hg)	☐	☐	☐
* 3. prepare ventilator/manual restriction bag	☐	☐	☐
B. Prepare patient			
* 1. wash hands	☐	☐	☐
2. auscultate chest and determine breath sounds	☐	☐	☐
* 3. hyperoxygenate as needed	☐	☐	☐
* 4. observe baseline vital signs	☐	☐	☐
C. Perform procedure			
* 1. place eye protection	☐	☐	☐
* 2. open suction kit	☐	☐	☐
* 3. place gloves	☐	☐	☐
* 4. remove catheter from package	☐	☐	☐

TASKS:	PEER	LAB	CLINICAL
* 5. attach catheter to suction tubing	☐	☐	☐
* 6. insert catheter into mouth until the oropharynx is reached	☐	☐	☐
* 7. apply (intermittent) suction and withdraw catheter	☐	☐	☐
* 8. monitor and treat bradycardia and hypoxia	☐	☐	☐
9. repeat as necessary	☐	☐	☐
* D. Document the procedure and pertinent information in the patient chart	☐	☐	☐
* E. Monitor appropriately	☐	☐	☐

SCORE:

Peer: _____ points out of _____ (36) _____ %

Lab: _____ points out of _____ (36) _____ %

Clinical: _____ points out of _____ (36) _____ %

TIME: _____ out of possible 30 minutes.

STUDENT SIGNATURES

PEER: _____

STUDENT: _____

INSTRUCTOR SIGNATURES

LAB: _____

CLINICAL: _____

PERFORMANCE EVALUATION 7
NASOPHARYNGEAL SUCTIONING

Date: Lab _____ Clinical _____ Hospital _____

Lab: Pass _____ Fail _____ Clinical: Pass _____ Fail _____

Student name _____ Instructor name _____

Number of required observations: Lab _____ Clinical _____

Number of times observed: Lab _____ Clinical _____

Number of required practices: Lab _____ Clinical _____

Number of times practice: Lab _____ Clinical _____

PASSING CRITERIA:

Obtain 90 percent or better on the procedure. Tasks indicated by an asterisk (*) must receive at least 1 point or the evaluation is terminated. The procedure must be performed within the designated time or the performance receives a failing grade.

SCORING:

2 points—Task performed satisfactorily without prompting.
1 point—Task performed satisfactorily with self-initiated correction.
0 points—Task performed incorrectly or with prompting required.
NA—Task not applicable to the patient care situation

TASKS:	PEER	LAB	CLINICAL
A. Prepare equipment			
* 1. select appropriately sized catheter	☐	☐	☐
* 2. adjust vacuum pressure (−50 to −120 mm Hg)	☐	☐	☐
* 3. prepare ventilator/manual resuscitation bag	☐	☐	☐
B. Prepare patient			
* 1. wash hands	☐	☐	☐
2. auscultate chest and determine breath sounds	☐	☐	☐
* 3. hyperoxygenate as needed	☐	☐	☐
* 4. observe baseline vital signs	☐	☐	☐
C. Perform procedure			
* 1. place eye protection	☐	☐	☐
* 2. open suction kit	☐	☐	☐
* 3. place gloves	☐	☐	☐
* 4. remove catheter from package	☐	☐	☐
* 5. attach catheter to suction tubing	☐	☐	☐
* 6. apply water-soluble jelly as needed	☐	☐	☐
* 7. insert catheter into nares, applying gentle upward, backward pressure until the nasopharynx is reached	☐	☐	☐
* 8. apply (intermittent) suction and withdraw the catheter	☐	☐	☐
* 9. monitor and treat bradycardia and hypoxia	☐	☐	☐
* 10. repeat as necessary			
* D. Document the procedure and pertinent information in the patient chart	☐	☐	☐
* E. Monitor appropriately	☐	☐	☐

SCORE:

Peer: _____ points out of _____ (38) _____ %

Lab: _____ points out of _____ (38) _____ %

Clinical: _____ points out of _____ (38) _____ %

TIME: _____ out of possible 30 minutes.

STUDENT SIGNATURES

PEER: _____

STUDENT: _____

INSTRUCTOR SIGNATURES

LAB: _____

CLINICAL: _____

NEONATAL BAG AND MASK VENTILATION

OBJECTIVE

The student will be able to properly oxygenate and ventilate a patient using a bag and mask in a laboratory and clinical setting. This will be done following aseptic guidelines and in a competent manner as determined by lab and clinical instructors.

TASK A: Hand Washing. Before performing bag and mask ventilation on a patient, proper hand washing is required.

TASK B: Obtain Equipment. Next, obtain the necessary equipment that will be used. Get a resuscitation bag that is designed for use on neonates. If the bag is self-inflating, it must have a reservoir attached to provide an adequate FiO_2. A pressure manometer and necessary tubing should be procured for both self-inflating and flow-inflating bags. The mask should be the correct size for the patient. It should cover the nose and mouth, allowing for a good seal without extending over the eyes. An oral airway may also be obtained, if its use is indicated. Obtain gloves.

TASK C: Check Bag for Proper Function. Attach the resuscitation bag tubing to the oxygen source to check it for proper function. This is done by turning on a flow of gas to the bag and occluding the bag outlet with the palm of the hand. When using a flow-inflating bag, the bag itself should fill. Adjust the flowmeter and control valve to allow the bag to inflate without excessive buildup of PEEP. The bag is now gently squeezed and checked for any leaks. The generated pressure should reach 30 to 40 cm H_2O. When the self-inflating bag is squeezed, the pop-off valve should open and release the excess pressure.

If the flow-inflating bag decompresses, or the pop-off valve does not open on the self-inflating bag, check for missing parts or leaks.

TASK D: Put on Gloves. Before bagging the patient, put on the exam gloves. Observe universal precautions.

TASK E: Position the Patient. With a properly functioning bag, position the patient and prepare to ventilate by properly extending the head to open the airway. The head should be slightly tilted. Be careful not to hyperextend the head because that will close the airway and prevent ventilation from occurring.

TASK F: Place Mask on Patient. The mask is placed over the mouth and nose and is held in place with the fingers of one hand. The thumb is placed over the nose with the index and middle fingers wrapping around the mask over the chin. The ring and little fingers are placed under the patient's chin to maintain the necessary head tilt.

TASK G: Ventilate the Patient. The bag is now squeezed with the fingertips of the opposite hand until chest expansion occurs. Keep in mind that the lungs of a neonate are very small. Resuscitation bags may hold from 240 to 1000 cc, so a slight squeeze will ventilate the lungs. Oxygen flow to the bag should be set appropriately to allow filling after each breath.

The initial rate of ventilation should be 40 to 60 breaths per minute. The initial pressure required depends on whether the patient has already taken a breath. If you will be delivering the initial breath to the neonate, a pressure of 30 to 40 cm H_2O may be required. Succeeding breaths require pressures of 15 to 20 cm H_2O to maintain ventilation. Neonates suffering from RDS may require pressures of 20 to 40 cm H_2O to achieve a good chest expansion.

Because these ranges are only offered as guidelines, the rule of thumb when providing manual ventilation is to use only the pressure that is required to get good chest excursion.

TASK H: Insert Nasogastric Tube. If the patient is to be bagged for more than 2 minutes, a nasogastric tube should be passed to evacuate air that enters the stomach. Air in the stomach, called gastric distention, pushes up on the diaphragm and impedes lung expansion. It also greatly increases the chance of vomiting and aspiration.

TASK I: Auscultate. The chest is now auscultated bilaterally with the stethoscope to ensure proper aeration of both lungs.

TASK J: Monitor Oxygenation and Ventilation. Monitor and document the patient's oxygenation and ventilation status with the use of blood gases, transcutaneous monitors and/or a pulse oximeter. Proper ventilation and oxygenation are also assessed by the patient's color and heart rate.

TASK K: Continue Ventilation. Continue ventilating until the patient is sustaining spontaneous respirations or the patient is intubated and placed on a ventilator.

PERFORMANCE EVALUATION 8
BAG AND MASK VENTILATION

Date: Lab _____   Clinical _____   Hospital _____

Lab: Pass _____ Fail _____   Clinical: Pass _____   Fail _____

Student name _____   Instructor name _____

Number of required observations: Lab _____   Clinical _____

Number of times observed: Lab _____   Clinical _____

Number of required practices: Lab _____   Clinical _____

Number of times practice: Lab _____   Clinical _____

PASSING CRITERIA:

Obtain 90 percent or better on the procedure. Tasks indicated by an asterisk (*) must receive at least 1 point or the evaluation is terminated. The procedure must be performed within the designated time or the performance receives a failing grade.

SCORING:

2 points—Task performed satisfactorily without prompting.
1 point—Task performed satisfactorily with self-initiated correction.
0 points—Task performed incorrectly or with prompting required.
NA—Task not applicable to the patient care situation

TASKS:	PEER	LAB	CLINICAL
A. Wash hands	☐	☐	☐
B. Obtain equipment			
* 1. resuscitation bag, with reservoir if self-inflating	☐	☐	☐
* 2. pressure manometer and tubing	☐	☐	☐
* 3. properly fitting mask	☐	☐	☐
* 4. exam gloves	☐	☐	☐
C. Check bag for proper function			
* 1. occlude bag opening	☐	☐	☐
* 2. fill bag with gas	☐	☐	☐
* 3. compress bag	☐	☐	☐
* 4. check for leaks	☐	☐	☐
* 5. attain 30 to 40 cm H_2O pressure	☐	☐	☐
6. check function of pop-off valve (if present)	☐	☐	☐
* D. Put on gloves	☐	☐	☐
* E. Position the patient: head slightly tilted	☐	☐	☐
* F. Position the mask on the patient: proper seal on face	☐	☐	☐
G. Ventilate the patient			
* 1. watch for chest rise	☐	☐	☐
* 2. rate of 40 to 60 breaths per minute	☐	☐	☐
* 3. appropriate inspiratory pressures	☐	☐	☐
* H. Insert nasogastric tube if ventilations are longer than 2 minutes	☐	☐	☐
* I. Auscultate lungs	☐	☐	☐

* J. Monitor and document oxygenation and ventilation ☐ ☐ ☐

  K. Continue ventilation until

*   1. spontaneous effort is adequate ☐ ☐ ☐

*   2. patient is intubated and placed on ventilator ☐ ☐ ☐

SCORE:

Peer: _____ points out of _____ (46) _____ %

Lab: _____ points out of _____ (46) _____ %

Clinical: _____ points out of _____ (46) _____ %

TIME: _____ out of possible 15 minutes.

STUDENT SIGNATURES   **INSTRUCTOR SIGNATURES**

PEER: _____   LAB: _____

STUDENT: _____   CLINICAL: _____

CHEST COMPRESSIONS (NEONATE)

OBJECTIVE

The student will be able to perform chest compressions using the correct hand or finger placement and the correct rate and depth in a laboratory and clinical setting. This will be done following aseptic guidelines and in a competent manner as determined by lab and clinical instructors.

TASK A: Wash Hands. Because of the emergency nature of this procedure, it may not be possible to wash the hands before the procedure unless compressions were anticipated. As possible, hand washing should be done before performing compressions.

TASK B: Put on Gloves. If the compressions are done on a newly delivered neonate, wearing gloves is a mandatory. Observe universal precautions.

TASK C: Identify Indications. If, after 15 to 30 seconds of bag-mask ventilating using 100% oxygen, the heart rate is less than 60, or if it is between 60 and 80 and not rising, chest compressions are indicated.

TASK D: Position the Patient. Position the patient for the initiation of compressions. Chest compressions are accomplished by either the two-finger method or the thumb method.

The two-finger method is done by placing the tips of the middle and ring fingers over the lower third of the sternum above the xiphoid process and below the nipple line. The other hand should be used to support the infant's back.

The thumb method is preferred. With this method, both thumbs are placed side by side over the middle third of the sternum, with the fingers wrapped around the thorax and supporting the back. When performing compressions, position yourself so as not to interfere with other personnel.

TASK E: Perform Compressions. To compress the chest, enough pressure is applied to the sternum to depress it 0.5 to 0.75 inch at a rate of 120 per minute, with a 0.5-second pause following every third compression. This pause is to allow time for a breath, and will result in the delivery of 90 compressions per minute. Counting aloud helps to compress at an appropriate rate. To prevent trauma, it is very important not to allow the fingers or the thumbs to come off the sternum or to move while doing compressions. The compressions must be done consistently to be effective.

TASK F: Discontinue Compressions. Continue with compressions until the heart rate is 80 or above.

TASK G: Document in Patient Chart. Complete the procedure by documenting in the patient chart. Documentation should include the length of time compressions were performed, patient response, and any side effects noted.

PERFORMANCE EVALUATION 9
CHEST COMPRESSIONS (NEONATE)

Date: Lab _____   Clinical _____   Hospital _____

Lab: Pass ____ Fail _____   Clinical: Pass _____   Fail _____

Student name _____   Instructor name _____

Number of required observations: Lab _____   Clinical _____

Number of times observed: Lab _____   Clinical _____

Number of required practices: Lab _____   Clinical _____

Number of times practice: Lab _____   Clinical _____

PASSING CRITERIA:
Obtain 90 percent or better on the procedure. Tasks indicated by an asterisk (*) must receive at least 1 point or the evaluation is terminated. The procedure must be performed within the designated time or the performance receives a failing grade.

SCORING:

2 points—Task performed satisfactorily without prompting.
1 point—Task performed satisfactorily with self-initiated correction.
0 points—Task performed incorrectly or with prompting required.
NA—Task not applicable to the patient care situation

TASKS:	PEER	LAB	CLINICAL
A. Wash hands (as appropriate)	☐	☐	☐
B. Put on exam gloves (as appropriate)	☐	☐	☐
C. Identify the indications for compressions (following 15 to 30 seconds of PPV with 10% oxygen)	☐	☐	☐
* 1. heart rate less than 60	☐	☐	☐
* 2. heart rate between 60 and 80 and not rising	☐	☐	☐
D. Position patient for compressions			
* 1. two-finger method	☐	☐	☐
* 2. thumb method	☐	☐	☐
* 3. proper location on chest	☐	☐	☐
E. Perform compressions			
* 1. proper depth	☐	☐	☐
* 2. proper rate	☐	☐	☐
* 3. consistent performance	☐	☐	☐
* F. Discontinue compressions when indicated	☐	☐	☐
* G. Document pertinent information in patient chart	☐	☐	☐

SCORE:

Peer: _____ points out of _____ (24) _____ %

Lab: _____ points out of _____ (24) _____ %

Clinical: _____ points out of _____ (24) _____ %

TIME: _____ out of possible 15 minutes.

STUDENT SIGNATURES   **INSTRUCTOR SIGNATURES**

PEER: _____   LAB: _____

STUDENT: _____   CLINICAL: _____

ENDOTRACHEAL INTUBATION

OBJECTIVE

The student will be able to demonstrate proper intubation technique to include selection of appropriately sized equipment in a laboratory and clinical setting. This will be done following aseptic guidelines and in a competent manner as determined by lab and clinical instructors.

It is assumed that the student is either anticipating a required intubation (such as with an expected premature delivery) or that the patient is being manually ventilated while the student obtains equipment and washes his or her hands.

TASK A: State Indications. It is important to understand and commit to memory the indications for intubation. The four indications are (1) prolonged PPV is required; (2) ineffective bag/mask ventilation; (3) tracheal suctioning is necessary (short or long term); and (4) the patient has a suspected diaphragmatic hernia.

TASK B: Obtain and Prepare Equipment. When it is determined that the patient needs intubation, gather the necessary equipment. First, select an appropriately sized endotracheal tube (ETT):

Guidelines for Selection of an Endotracheal Tube

<1100 g	2.5 ETT
1000–2000 g	3.0 ETT
2000–3000 g	3.5 ETT
>3000 g	4.0 ETT

After selecting an appropriate ETT, obtain a wire stylet. The stylet may be inserted into the ETT to make it rigid, facilitating intubation. Be certain that the tip of the stylet does not extend beyond the tip of the ETT because it may cause trauma.

Now gather the appropriate suction equipment and assemble as necessary. Obtain a laryngoscope and an appropriately sized blade. Use a size 0 blade for premature neonates and a size 1 blade for term neonates. Attach the blade to the laryngoscope to ensure proper function of the light.

Next, a shoulder roll should be obtained to help hyperextend the neck. Obtain a roll of $\frac{1}{2}$- or $\frac{1}{4}$-inch tape or some other device to secure the ETT. A pair of scissors are invaluable and should be found at this time.

A properly functioning resuscitation bag and mask must be set up and ready for use at the bedside. For this intubation, eye protection and exam gloves should be obtained. Finally, solicit the help of another person who will monitor the patient and assist as required during the procedure.

TASK C: Wash Hands. Washing hands before performing an intubation will greatly reduce the risk of contaminating the endotracheal tube and introducing organisms to the trachea.

TASK D: Place Gloves and Eye Protection. Because of the invasive nature of tracheal intubation, eye protection and gloves are required. Put them on at this time.

TASK E: Position the Patient. Place the patient in the supine position, the head straight, and the neck extended slightly. Placing the shoulder roll under the shoulders helps to maintain the desired head position.

TASK F: Hyperoxygenate the Patient. Just before performing the intubation, hyperoxygenate the patient with 1.0 FiO_2 using a manual resuscitation bag.

TASK G: Perform the Procedure. You are now ready to intubate the patient. The laryngoscope is picked up in the left hand and the blade locked in place so that the light illuminates. The blade is inserted into the mouth along the right side until the tip of the blade reaches the approximate level of the base of the tongue. Sweep the handle of the laryngoscope to midline in the mouth to displace the tongue. Gently lift the laryngoscope to visualize the epiglottis. Secretions should be suctioned at this point, if necessary, to improve visibility. Gentle lifting of the laryngoscope raises the epiglottis and exposes the vocal cords and the trachea. When lifting the laryngoscope to visualize the trachea, lift up and away from the root of the mouth. Never use the upper gums as a fulcrum to pry the laryngoscope handle downward while raising the blade tip.

Using the right hand, the endotracheal tube is inserted into the trachea, the tip going just beyond the vocal cords. The endotracheal tube is now held in place with the right hand, and the laryngoscope blade is gently removed. The stylet is then removed from the ETT. The tube must be securely held while removing the stylet to prevent accidental extubation.

TASK H: Hyperoxygenate and Auscultate. PPV is immediately initiated and the lungs auscultated for breath sounds. Good aeration in both lungs with adequate chest excursion indicates good tube position. Auscultation above the stomach will also help to rule out an esophageal intubation. The practitioner must be cautious, however, because breath sounds may be transmitted and heard over the stomach.

TASK I: Secure the Tube. Before securing the tube, the centimeter marking on the tube that is at the level of the gumline should be noted for future reference. When the chest x-ray is returned, this information facilitates any necessary movement of the tube to achieve proper placement. The tube is then taped securely to the patient's face.

TASK J: Obtain Chest X-Ray. A chest x-ray is then obtained to verify proper placement of the ETT above the carina. Ideally, the tip of the tube should be midway between the carina and the clavicles.

TASK K: Record Results. Following completion of the intubation, the procedure is documented in the patient chart. Charting should include the size of endotracheal tube, tube placement on chest x-ray, tube marking at patient lip, oxygenation status, breath sounds, pulse rate, and patient toleration of procedure.

TASK L: Monitoring. The appropriate timing and method of monitoring the equipment and the patient should be determined. This is based on any orders, written department standards, and patient condition.

PERFORMANCE EVALUATION 10
INTUBATION

Date: Lab _____   Clinical _____   Hospital _____

Lab: Pass _____ Fail _____   Clinical: Pass _____ Fail _____

Student name _____   Instructor name _____

Number of required observations: Lab _____ Clinical _____

Number of times observed: Lab _____ Clinical _____

Number of required practices: Lab _____ Clinical _____

Number of times practice: Lab _____ Clinical _____

PASSING CRITERIA:

Obtain 90 percent or better on the procedure. Tasks indicated by an asterisk (*) must receive at least 1 point or the evaluation is terminated. The procedure must be performed within the designated time or the performance receives a failing grade.

SCORING:

2 points—Task performed satisfactorily without prompting.
1 point—Task performed satisfactorily with self-initiated correction.
0 points—Task performed incorrectly or with prompting required.
NA—Task not applicable to the patient care situation

TASKS:	PEER	LAB	CLINICAL
* A. State indications for intubation	☐	☐	☐
B. Obtain equipment	☐	☐	☐
* 1. appropriately sized endotracheal tubes and stylet	☐	☐	☐
* 2. suction equipment	☐	☐	☐
* 3. laryngoscope and appropriately sized blade; check for proper function	☐	☐	☐
4. shoulder roll	☐	☐	☐
* 5. tape or other securing advice	☐	☐	☐
6 scissors	☐	☐	☐
* 7. resuscitation bag and mask attached to 100% oxygen source	☐	☐	☐

TASKS:	PEER	LAB	CLINICAL
* 8. eye protection and gloves	☐	☐	☐
* 9. another person to monitor vital signs and assist	☐	☐	☐
* C. Wash hands	☐	☐	☐
* D. Put on eye protection and gloves	☐	☐	☐
* E. Position the patient	☐	☐	☐
* F. Hyperoxygenate the patient	☐	☐	☐
G. Perform the procedure			
1. insert blade into mouth with laryngoscope in left hand	☐	☐	☐
* 2. insert blade to base of tongue	☐	☐	☐
* 3. lift the blade up and away from the roof of mouth	☐	☐	☐
4. suction as needed	☐	☐	☐
* 5. visualize epiglottis	☐	☐	☐
* 6. gently lift to open the epiglottis and insert ETT into trachea to proper depth	☐	☐	☐
* 7. secure tube and remove blades and stylet	☐	☐	☐
* H. Hyperoxygenate and auscultate	☐	☐	☐
* I. Secure the tube with tape or device	☐	☐	☐
* J. Obtain chest x-ray for tube placement	☐	☐	☐
* K. Record results and observations	☐	☐	☐
* L. Monitor appropriately	☐	☐	☐

SCORE:

Peer: _____ points out of _____ (52) _____ %

Lab: _____ points out of _____ (52) _____ %

Clinical: _____ points out of _____ (52) _____ %

TIME: _____ out of possible 15 minutes.

STUDENT SIGNATURES   **INSTRUCTOR SIGNATURES**

PEER: _____   LAB: _____

STUDENT: _____   CLINICAL: _____

NEONATAL RESUSCITATION

OBJECTIVE

The student will be able to perform the steps of a resuscitation following the appropriate sequence in a laboratory and clinical setting. This will be done following aseptic guidelines and in a competent manner as determined by lab and clinical instructors.

TASK A: Wash Hands. If the resuscitation is anticipated, such as with a premature delivery, the hands should be washed thoroughly before the arrival of the patient. An in-hospital emergency may not allow hand washing before the procedure. Observe universal precautions.

TASK B: Obtain and Prepare Equipment. After washing hands, obtain and prepare the equipment that will be used to ensure it is present and functioning correctly. The importance of checking resuscitation equipment on an ongoing basis should be apparent because the practitioner will not always have the time to check equipment before a resuscitation.

Check the resuscitation bag and mask for proper function and size. Check the laryngoscope for the appropriately sized blade and to assure the light functions. The suction equipment should be set up and ready, with a variety of sizes of suction catheters nearby. You should also obtain a bulb syringe, appropriate size endotracheal tubes, and warm dry towels. Turn on the radiant warmer so that it will be warm when the patient arrives. The final but equally important step is to obtain and put on exam gloves.

TASK C: Perform Initial Steps. Now perform the initial steps of the resuscitation. Place the patient under the radiant warmer to help maintain thermoregulation. Additionally, thoroughly dry the neonate with a warm, dry towel and remove the wet linen. This greatly reduces evaporative heat loss. Position the infant on its back with the head in a neutral position to open the airway. After opening the airway, suction the mouth and then the nose with the bulb syringe or a suction catheter.

It is important to suction the mouth first, to remove any debris that may be aspirated if the patient gasps during nasal suctioning. In the presence of thick meconium, intubate the patient and suction the trachea until clear.

The patient is then stimulated to help initiate breathing by slapping or flicking the soles of the feet or rubbing the patient's back.

TASK D: Evaluate the Respirations. If spontaneous respirations are present, evaluate the heart rate. If no respirations are present, immediately start PPV at a rate of 40 to 60 per minute using 100% oxygen. Monitor chest excursions.

TASK E: Evaluate Heart Rate (Spontaneous Respirations). If the patient is breathing spontaneously and the heart rate is above 100 beats/min, move on to evaluate the patient's color. If the heart rate is below 100 beats/min, begin PPV using 100% oxygen.

TASK F: Evaluate Heart Rate (Following PPV). Following 15 to 30 seconds of PPV with a FiO_2 of 1.0, reevaluate the heart rate. If it is less than 60 beats/min, continue the PPV and initiate chest compressions. If the heart rate is 60 to 80 beats/min and not increasing, continue PPV and initiate chest compressions. If the heart rate is between 60 and 100 beats/min and rising, continue PPV. Once the heart rate is greater than 100 beats/min, watch for the return of spontaneous ventilations, when PPV may be discontinued. Medications are given if the heart rate remains less than 80 beats/min, despite PPV with 100% oxygen and chest compressions.

TASK G: Evaluate Color. With respirations present and heart rate above 100 beats/min, evaluate the patient's color. If the patient is pink, or has acrocyanosis, which is blueness of the extremities, observe and monitor the patient.

TASK H: Intubation. If bag and mask ventilation is ineffective, tracheal suctioning is necessary, or prolonged assisted ventilation is anticipated, endotracheal intubation should be performed.

TASK I: Continue Assessment. Continue to monitor and evaluate the respirations, heart rate, and color throughout the resuscitation.

TASK J: Assign Apgar Score. Assign an Apgar score at 1 and 5 minutes using the following scale:

APGAR SCORE

	0	1	2
Heart rate	Absent	<100	>100
Respiratory effort	Absent	Slow	Good
Muscle tone	Limp	Flexion	Active
Reflex irritability	None	Grimace	Cough
Color	Blue	Acrocyanosis	Pink

TASK K: Transport to NICU. When stable, transport the patient to the NICU for further treatment and monitoring.

TASK L: Document Procedure. Finally, document all pertinent information in the patient chart. This should include all steps taking during the resuscitation; medications used; FiO_2, pressures, and rates while bagging; APGAR scores; and all vital signs during resuscitation.

PERFORMANCE EVALUATION 11
NEONATAL RESUSCITATION

Date: Lab _____   Clinical _____   Hospital _____

Lab: Pass _____ Fail _____   Clinical: Pass _____   Fail _____

Student name _____   Instructor name _____

Number of required observations: Lab _____   Clinical _____

Number of times observed: Lab _____   Clinical _____

Number of required practices: Lab _____   Clinical _____

Number of times practice: Lab _____   Clinical _____

PASSING CRITERIA:

Obtain 90 percent or better on the procedure. Tasks indicated by an asterisk (*) must receive at least 1 point or the evaluation is terminated. The procedure must be performed within the designated time or the performance receives a failing grade.

SCORING:

2 points—Task performed satisfactorily without prompting.
1 point—Task performed satisfactorily with self-initiated correction.
0 points—Task performed incorrectly or with prompting required.
NA—Task not applicable to the patient care situation

TASKS:	PEER	LAB	CLINICAL
* A. Wash hands	☐	☐	☐
B. Obtain and prepare equipment			
* 1. resuscitation bag and mask	☐	☐	☐
* 2. laryngoscope and blade, ET tubes	☐	☐	☐
* 3. suction equipment	☐	☐	☐
* 4. warm, dry towel	☐	☐	☐
* 5. turn on radiant warmer	☐	☐	☐
* 6. obtain and put on gloves	☐	☐	☐
C. Perform initial steps			
* 1. place patient on open warmer	☐	☐	☐
* 2. thoroughly dry patient	☐	☐	☐
* 3. remove wet towels	☐	☐	☐
* 4. position the patient	☐	☐	☐
* 5. suction the mouth, then nose	☐	☐	☐
* 6. intubate and suction trachea if thick meconium is present	☐	☐	☐
* 7. stimulate the patient	☐	☐	☐
D. Evaluate respirations			
* 1. if spontaneous, evaluate heart rate	☐	☐	☐
* 2. if absent, begin PPV after 15—30 seconds	☐	☐	☐
E. Evaluate heart rate (spontaneous respirations)			
* 1. greater than 100, evaluate color	☐	☐	☐
* 2. less than 100, begin PPV	☐	☐	☐
F. Evaluate heart rate (following PPV)			
* 1. less than 60, continue PPV, start chest compressions	☐	☐	☐
* 2. 60–80 and not increasing, continue PPV start compressions if heart rate less than 80	☐	☐	☐
* 3. 60–100 and increasing, continue PPV	☐	☐	☐
* 4. greater than 100, discontinue PPV when spontaneous ventilations return	☐	☐	☐
* 5. administer medications of heart rate is less than 80 after 30 seconds of PPV with 100% oxygen and chest compressions	☐	☐	☐
G. Evaluate color			
* 1. if blue, provide oxygen	☐	☐	☐

TASKS:	PEER	LAB	CLINICAL
* 2. if pink, or acrocyanosis, observe and monitor	☐	☐	☐
* H. Intubate patient if indicated	☐	☐	☐
* I. Continue to assess respirations, heart rate, and color	☐	☐	☐
* J. Assign a 1-minute and 5-minute Apgar score at appropriate times	☐	☐	☐
* K. Transport to NICU when stable	☐	☐	☐
* L. Record all actions and observations in patient chart	☐	☐	☐

SCORE:

Peer: _____ points out of _____ (60) _____ %

Lab: _____ points out of _____ (60) _____ %

Clinical: _____ points out of _____ (60) _____ %

TIME: _____ out of possible 20 minutes.

STUDENT SIGNATURES   INSTRUCTOR SIGNATURES

PEER: _____   LAB: _____

STUDENT: _____   CLINICAL: _____

NEONATAL PHYSICAL ASSESSMENT

OBJECTIVE

The student will be able to perform a neonatal assessment in a laboratory and clinical setting. This will be done following aseptic guidelines and in a competent manner as determined by lab and clinical instructors.

TASK A: Wash Hands. Before performing the assessment, the student should perform a thorough hand washing.

TASK B: Visual Inspection. Before touching the patient you should perform a visual inspection. Once the neonate has been handled, he or she may cry and become fussy, making it difficult to complete some aspects of the assessment.

Begin with a general, overall visual assessment of the patient. The size of the neonate will help in the determination of gestational age. Look for any obvious abnormalities or defects. Observe the skin color. Look for signs of cyanosis, meconium staining, or jaundice.

Note the posture that the patient is assuming in bed. An overall look at the body proportions should now be done.

Inspect and compare the size of the head to the rest of the body. The head may appear slightly large but overall should look appropriately sized. All of the limbs should be appropriately sized, when compared to the rest of the body. Examine the nose for the presence of nasal flaring, a sign of respiratory distress.

Next, visually examine the chest. The chest expansion should be equal on both sides. Any retractions present should be noted. Evaluate the respiratory rate by counting the chest rises. Note whether respirations are regular. Watch the movement of extremities to determine whether the movements are symmetrical and appropriate. Finally, determine and note the amount of lanugo on the patient to use for the gestational age assessment.

Task C: Head-to-Toe Examination. This part of the exam should begin at the head and progress systematically to the feet. The examination of the head begins with a gentle palpation of the fontanelles. Note whether they are soft or tight and bulging. Examine the ears for assessment of gestational age. The nose is now examined for the determination of patency. Lightly press one nare closed, while observing the patient's respiratory effort. Continued ease in ventilation indicates a patent nasal passage. Repeat the procedure on the opposite nare.

Examine the mouth by running a clean finger along the roof of the mouth to check for a cleft palate. The mouth is also visually inspected for the presence of anything that could block the airway.

Physically palpate the neck to determine the presence of any tumors or cysts that could occlude the trachea. Next, examine the thorax. This is a good point to evaluate and note the patient's skin and breasts for the gestational age assessment. The chest is then auscultated with a stethoscope. All aspects of the lungs should be auscultated, noting aeration, bilateral equality, and presence of any adventitious sounds. Now, auscultate the heart for the presence of any murmurs. Determine the heart rate and the point of maximal intensity.

Moving on to the abdomen, gently palpate for the presence of cysts or tumors that may be pushing up on the diaphragm. A flat or sunken abdomen may indicate a diaphragmatic hernia.

The genitalia are next examined for the purpose of the gestational age assessment. The extremities are then examine. Palpate brachial and femoral pulses. Of special interest are the creases on the soles of the feet, used in the gestational age assessment, which are noted at this point.

TASK D: Determine Gestational Age. Following the examination, the student will determine approximate gestational age from the physical signs using the Ballard or Dubowitz scale.

TASK E: Return Patient. At the completion of the assessment, the patient is returned to the incubator or bassinet and positioned appropriately.

TASK F: Document Results. The final step is to record the results of the assessment in the patient chart. The student should note any abnormalities found and document all findings.

PERFORMANCE EVALUATION 12
PHYSICAL ASSESSMENT

Date: Lab _____   Clinical _____   Hospital _____

Lab: Pass _____ Fail _____   Clinical: Pass _____ Fail _____

Student name _____   Instructor name _____

Number of required observations: Lab _____   Clinical _____

Number of times observed: Lab _____   Clinical _____

Number of required practices: Lab _____   Clinical _____

Number of times practice: Lab _____   Clinical _____

PASSING CRITERIA:

Obtain 90 percent or better on the procedure. Tasks indicated by an asterisk (*) must receive at least 1 point or the evaluation is terminated. The procedure must be performed within the designated time or the performance receives a failing grade.

SCORING:

2 points—Task performed satisfactorily without prompting.
1 point—Task performed satisfactorily with self-initiated correction.
0 points—Task performed incorrectly or with prompting required.
NA—Task not applicable to the patient care situation

TASKS:	PEER	LAB	CLINICAL
* A. Wash hands	☐	☐	☐
B. Visually inspect the neonate			
1. overall appearance	☐	☐	☐
2. proportions and posture	☐	☐	☐
3. head	☐	☐	☐
4. chest	☐	☐	☐
5. extremities	☐	☐	☐
6. lanugo	☐	☐	☐
C. Head-to-toe assessment			
1. Head			
a. fontanelles	☐	☐	☐
* b. ears	☐	☐	☐
* c. nose	☐	☐	☐
d. mouth	☐	☐	☐
e. neck	☐	☐	☐
2. Thorax			
* a. skin	☐	☐	☐

TASKS:	PEER	LAB	CLINICAL
* b. breasts	☐	☐	☐
* c. lungs	☐	☐	☐
d. heart	☐	☐	☐
3. Abdomen	☐	☐	☐
* 4. Genitalia	☐	☐	☐
5. Extremities			
* a. sole creases	☐	☐	☐
b. pulses	☐	☐	☐
* D. Determine gestational age from preceding assessment	☐	☐	☐
* E. Return patient to bed and position	☐	☐	☐
* F. Record results and observations	☐	☐	☐

SCORE:

Peer: _____ points out of _____ (46) _____ %

Lab: _____ points out of _____ (46) _____ %

Clinical: _____ points out of _____ (46) _____ %

TIME: _____ out of possible 15 minutes.

STUDENT SIGNATURES

PEER: _____

STUDENT: _____

INSTRUCTOR SIGNATURES

LAB: _____

CLINICAL: _____

CHEST X-RAY INTERPRETATION

OBJECTIVE

The student will be able to systematically examine a chest x-ray and determine appropriateness of tube placements and the presence of disease states. This will be accomplished by the student examining radiographs provided by lab and clinical instructors.

TASK A: Systematic Examination. The student will perform a systematic examination of the chest radiograph according to the following outline.

    Systematic Approach to Reading a Chest X-ray
1. Confirm correct patient and date.
2. Correct orientation. Patient's left side should be on your right as you view the radiograph.
3. Check the quality of the radiograph.

4. Identify artifact.
5. Confirm proper patient position.
6. Determine whether the radiograph is inspiratory or expiratory.
7. Examine the diaphragm.
8. Examine the abdomen.
9. Inspect the cardiac silhouette.
10. Examine the area of the lung hilum.
11. Inspect the respiratory tract:
    a. Trachea
    b. Position of the endotracheal tube
    c. Mainstem bronchus
    d. Lung fields
    e. Pleural surface

TASK B: Determination of Lung Pathology. At this point, the student will describe any lung pathology present to the lab and clinical instructor. The student is referred to Section 1 of this manual for a review of radiologic pathology.

TASK C: Suggest Treatment. This task is accomplished by the student offering suggestions regarding the treatment of the lung disease and any changes in endotracheal tube or other catheter position.

TASK D: Documentation. The performance is completed by documenting the findings in the patient chart. This should include any lung pathology present and tube and catheter placements.

PERFORMANCE EVALUATION 13
CHEST X-RAY INTERPRETATION

Date: Lab _____   Clinical _____   Hospital _____

Lab: Pass _____ Fail _____   Clinical: Pass _____   Fail _____

Student name _____   Instructor name _____

Number of required observations: Lab _____   Clinical _____

Number of times observed: Lab _____   Clinical _____

Number of required practices: Lab _____   Clinical _____

Number of times practice: Lab _____   Clinical _____

PASSING CRITERIA:

Obtain 90 percent or better on the procedure. Tasks indicated by an asterisk (*) must receive at least 1 point or the evaluation is terminated. The procedure must be performed within the designated time or the performance receives a failing grade.

SCORING:

2 points—Task performed satisfactorily without prompting.
1 point—Task performed satisfactorily with self-initiated correction.
0 points—Task performed incorrectly or with prompting required.
NA—Task not applicable to the patient care situation

TASKS:	PEER	LAB	CLINICAL
A. Systematically examine the x-ray	☐	☐	☐
* 1. check the identification tag	☐	☐	☐
* 2. orient to right and left	☐	☐	☐
* 3. determine exposure	☐	☐	☐
* 4. identify artifact	☐	☐	☐
* 5. determine patient position	☐	☐	☐
* 6. determine if inspiratory or expiratory	☐	☐	☐
* 7. examine the diaphragm	☐	☐	☐
* 8. examine the abdomen	☐	☐	☐
* 9. determine the proper position of the UAC and/or UVC	☐	☐	☐
* 10. examine the cardiac silhouette	☐	☐	☐
* 11. examine the lung hilum	☐	☐	☐
* 12. examine the trachea	☐	☐	☐
* 13. determine the proper position of the endotracheal tube	☐	☐	☐
* 14. examine the bronchus and lung tissue	☐	☐	☐
* B. Determine possible lung pathology present	☐	☐	☐
* C. Suggest appropriate treatment or changes	☐	☐	☐
* D. Document appropriate findings in patient chart	☐	☐	☐

SCORE:

Peer: _____ points out of _____ (34) _____ %

Lab: _____ points out of _____ (34) _____ %

Clinical: _____ points out of _____ (34) _____ %

TIME: _____ out of possible 20 minutes.

STUDENT SIGNATURES

PEER: _____

STUDENT: _____

INSTRUCTOR SIGNATURES

LAB: _____

CLINICAL: _____

UMBILICAL ARTERY CATHETER SAMPLING

OBJECTIVE

The student will demonstrate the ability to properly obtain a blood sample for analysis from an umbilical artery catheter in a laboratory and clinical setting. This will be done following aseptic guidelines and in a competent manner as determined by lab and clinical instructors. *NOTE:* **Never** attempt to draw a UAC sample without appropriate training under the supervision of someone who is very familiar with the procedure.

TASK A: Obtain Equipment. Obtain the needed equipment. Collect two 3 cc syringes, a blood gas syringe, two sterile gauze pads, Betadine and alcohol swabs, a heparin flush solution, paper to note pertinent information, two floor exam gloves, and eye protection. Any time you will be handling blood, it is mandatory that you protect yourself by wearing gloves and eye protection.

TASK B: Wash Hands. Before performing this procedure, the student will perform a thorough hand washing. Observe universal precautions.

TASK C: Prepare Equipment. Remove the syringes from their protective containers. Using sterile technique, fill one of the 3 cc syringes with 2 to 2.5 cc of the heparin flush solution. *Make certain that you are using a heparin flush solution that is specifically made for neonates.*

If any preparation of the blood gas syringe is necessary, do it at this point. Now write down the patient and clinical data on the paper and place the exam gloves on both hands. Before drawing the sample, clean the stopcock connection with Betadine and then with alcohol. Place one of the sterile gauze pads under the stopcock, and place another nearby for use later.

TASK D: Perform Procedure. To draw the sample, remove the cap on the three-way stopcock port used for sampling. Be cautious that you are using the correct port and the correct stopcock. If there is more than one stopcock, use the one that is closest to the entry point of the catheter into the abdomen.

Place the empty 3 cc syringe on the stopcock port and turn the stopcock lever off to the IV solution. This opens the stopcock between the catheter and the syringe.

Slowly draw back 2 cc of blood from the UAC. This flushes the line of any IV fluid that might contaminate your sample. Next, turn the stopcock halfway between the syringe and the IV port. This does two things: First, it prevents the arterial blood from squirting out of the stopcock port when you remove the syringe; second, it prevents IV fluid from contaminating the sample. To be safe, it may be advisable to pinch the IV tubing between your fingers while withdrawing the sample because some stopcocks may allow a leakage of IV fluid into your sample.

Now carefully remove the syringe from the stopcock and lay it on the gauze pad that you set out at the beginning. Next, place your blood gas syringe on the stopcock port, turn the stopcock lever back off to the IV, and draw your sample out. Most blood gas analyzers only require between 0.1 to 0.3 cc of blood. Make certain how much your analyzer will need before drawing the sample.

Turn the stopcock lever off to the blood gas syringe, remove the syringe, and expel any air bubbles. Place a cap on the syringe. If more than 10 to 15 minutes will elapse before analysis, the sample should be placed on ice.

Next, take the 3 cc syringe with the withdrawn blood and place it on the stopcock port. Turn the stopcock lever off to the IV port and loosen any air bubbles that may be in the hub of the syringe with your finger.

Follow this by withdrawing a small amount of blood into the syringe. This should remove all air bubbles so you do not inject them into the patient. Now carefully and slowly reinject the blood into the patient. Be sure to watch for air bubbles. When you have reinjected the blood, turn the stopcock lever off to the sampling port, remove the syringe, and replace it with the 3 cc syringe containing the flush solution.

Again, turn the stopcock lever off to the IV port and inject just enough of the flush solution to clear the UAC line of blood.

After injecting the heparin solution, turn the stopcock off to the syringe, remove the syringe, and replace the stopcock cap.

If your blood gas sample is contaminated with IV solution, it will usually have a very acid pH, without a corresponding increase in PCO_2. The hematocrit will also be much lower than previous readings. The sample itself will sometimes look diluted and watery. If your sample is questionable, redraw it, paying close attention to pinching off the IV tube while the sample is drawn.

TASK E: Complete Procedure. Clean up the area by disposing the used materials in an appropriate container. Make certain all connections are secure.

TASK F: Documentation. Complete the procedure by charting the blood gas results in the patient chart.

PERFORMANCE EVALUATION 14
UMBILICAL ARTERY CATHETER SAMPLING

Date: Lab _____   Clinical _____   Hospital _____

Lab: Pass _____ Fail _____   Clinical: Pass _____   Fail _____

Student name _____   Instructor name _____

Number of required observations: Lab _____   Clinical _____

Number of times observed: Lab _____   Clinical _____

Number of required practices: Lab _____   Clinical _____

Number of times practice: Lab _____   Clinical _____

PASSING CRITERIA:

Obtain 90 percent or better on the procedure. Tasks indicated by an asterisk (*) must receive at least 1 point or the evaluation is terminated. The procedure must be performed within the designated time or the performance receives a failing grade.

SCORING:

2 points—Task performed satisfactorily without prompting.
1 point—Task performed satisfactorily with self-initiated correction.
0 points—Task performed incorrectly or with prompting required.
NA—Task not applicable to the patient care situation

TASKS:	PEER	LAB	CLINICAL
A. Obtain equipment			
* 1. two 3 cc syringes	☐	☐	☐
* 2. blood gas syringe	☐	☐	☐
* 3. two sterile gauze pads	☐	☐	☐
* 4. Betadine and alcohol swaps	☐	☐	☐
* 5. heparin flush solution	☐	☐	☐
* 6. data slip	☐	☐	☐
* 7. two floor exam gloves	☐	☐	☐
* 8. eye protection	☐	☐	☐
B. Wash hands	☐	☐	☐
C. Prepare equipment			
1. remove syringes from containers	☐	☐	☐
* 2. fill one 3 cc syringe with 2.0 to 2.5 cc of a heparin flush solution	☐	☐	☐
* 3. place gauze pads in proper places	☐	☐	☐
* 4. prepare blood gas syringe	☐	☐	☐
5. record appropriate data on slip	☐	☐	☐
* 6. place exam gloves on hands	☐	☐	☐
* 7. place eye protection	☐	☐	☐
D. Perform procedure			
1. Clean stopcock	☐	☐	☐
* 2. place empty 3 cc syringe on stopcock	☐	☐	☐
* 3. turn stopcock off to IV line	☐	☐	☐
* 4. slowly withdraw 2 cc of blood	☐	☐	☐
* 5. turn stopcock back halfway	☐	☐	☐
* 6. remove syringe and place on sterile gauze	☐	☐	☐
* 7. place blood gas syringe on stopcock	☐	☐	☐
* 8. turn stopcock off to IV line	☐	☐	☐
* 9. withdraw blood sample	☐	☐	☐
* 10. turn stopcock off to syringe and remove the syringe	☐	☐	☐

TASKS:	PEER	LAB	CLINICAL
* 11. cap the blood gas syringe	☐	☐	☐
* 12. replace 3 cc syringe containing blood on stopcock	☐	☐	☐
* 13. turn stopcock off to IV line	☐	☐	☐
* 14. tap base of syringe with finger	☐	☐	☐
* 15. withdraw small amount of blood to remove bubbles	☐	☐	☐
* 16. slowly reinject blood to patient	☐	☐	☐
* 17. turn stopcock off and remove syringe	☐	☐	☐
* 18. place syringe with heparin solution on stopcock	☐	☐	☐
* 19. turn stopcock off to IV line	☐	☐	☐
* 20. tap base of syringe with finger	☐	☐	☐
21. withdraw small amount of blood to remove bubbles.	☐	☐	☐
* 22. inject 1 to 1.5 cc of flush into line	☐	☐	☐
* 23. turn stopcock off to syringe and remove	☐	☐	☐
* 24. replace stopcock port covering	☐	☐	☐
E. Complete procedure: clean up used materials and dispose of properly. Make certain all connections are secure.	☐	☐	☐
* F. Document results in patient chart	☐	☐	☐

SCORE:

Peer: _____ points out of _____ (80) _____ %

Lab: _____ points out of _____ (80) _____ %

Clinical: _____ points out of _____ (80) _____ %

TIME: _____ out of possible 10 minutes.

STUDENT SIGNATURES

PEER: _____

STUDENT: _____

INSTRUCTOR SIGNATURES

LAB: _____

CLINICAL: _____

RADIAL ARTERY PUNCTURE

OBJECTIVE

The student will demonstrate proper technique in preparing the patient and obtaining a radial artery blood sample. This will be done following aseptic guidelines and in a competent manner as determined by lab and clinical instructors.

The most common artery to obtain a blood gas in a premature neonate is the radial artery. This is because there are fewer possible complications and it can be visualized with the aid of a high-intensity light.

Occasionally you may attempt a brachial artery puncture, but it is more hazardous and it is usually second choice. *Never* puncture the femoral artery except in extreme emergency cases when it is your last choice. The area surrounding the femoral artery could easily contain the entire blood volume of the neonate without showing any outward signs.

TASK A: Review Chart. Check the order to determine any special conditions to be met. Verify that the patient is receiving the desired FiO_2 and that no procedures have taken place that may affect the test results. You should wait at least 15 minutes after suctioning or ventilator changes

TASK B: Obtain and Prepare Equipment. You will need a heparinized blood gas syringe or butterfly tubing with a 23 to 25 gauge needle and a syringe for the sample, Betadine and alcohol swabs, sterile gauze pads, a data slip, exam gloves, and eye protection. It is also advisable to have an assistant. When performing an arterial puncture on a premature infant, you may wish to use a cool temperature transilluminator for help in locating the artery.

TASK C: Wash Hands. Next, thoroughly wash the hands.

TASK D: Confirm Patient. Before performing any procedure, confirm that you have the correct patient by looking at the name bracelet attached to a patient limb.

TASK E: Prepare the Wrist. Prepare the wrist by carefully scrubbing it with the alcohol and Betadine swab. It is important to use the Betadine solution because of the number of alcohol-resistant microorganisms that currently exist. Allow the area to air dry. While the site is drying, put on the exam gloves and eye protection.

TASK F: Locate the Artery. If using a transilluminator, position the light so that it is aimed upward, near enough to the bedside to allow the patient's arm to reach the light. Carefully place the wrist on top of the light; hyperextend the hand slightly to visualize the artery. Blood vessels will appear as dark lines; the artery should pulsate with the heart rate.

If you are not using a transilluminator, gently palpate the wrist to locate the artery. Once you have located it, wipe the puncture site again with alcohol.

TASK G: Perform Procedure. When you have located the radial artery in the wrist, secure the blood gas syringe and, with the needle bevel up, insert the needle into the skin and direct it toward the radial artery. Advance the needle slowly until blood begins to fill the syringe. When you enter the artery, you should get a flash of blood and the syringe barrel will continue to fill.

If you miss the artery on the first advance, slowly withdraw the needle, because it is possible that you went through the artery.

When the correct amount of blood has filled the syringe barrel, remove the needle from the patient's wrist and immediately cover the insertion site with the gauze pad and hold pressure. Upon removal, the needle tip should be plugged with a rubber plug or other device. If using a butterfly needle, once you have entered the artery, the tubing should fill with blood. Allow the first drop of blood to fall from the end of the tubing onto a gauze pad. Then have your assistant attach the syringe to the end of the tubing and gently aspirate the necessary amount of blood.

The purpose of the assistant is to hold the patient and prevent excess movement, which may make the puncture very difficult, and to either hold the puncture site or analyze the blood gas sample. The key to a successful arterial puncture is to do it slowly and carefully. Do not attempt to hit the artery by moving the needle side to side once it is inserted. If you miss on the first attempt, withdraw the needle to where the top of the bevel is visible at the skin and move the syringe to the side and redirect the needle into the wrist.

Have your assistant hold the site while you analyze the sample or arrange for it to be analyzed. Gentle pressure should be applied to the site until bleeding has stopped, at least 5 minutes. If the sample will not be analyzed within 10 to 15 minutes, it should be placed on ice. Examine the site for any signs of hematoma or continued bleeding. Blanching of the hand requires immediate notification of the physician.

TASK H: Document Procedure. Complete the procedure by documenting the results of the blood gas and noting any side effects or complications of the procedure.

TASK I: Monitoring. The appropriate timing and method of monitoring the equipment and the patient should be determined. This is based on any orders, written department standards, and patient condition.

PERFORMANCE EVALUATION 15
RADIAL ARTERY PUNCTURE

Date: Lab _____   Clinical _____   Hospital _____

Lab: Pass _____ Fail _____   Clinical: Pass _____   Fail _____

Student name _____   Instructor name _____

Number of required observations: Lab _____   Clinical _____

Number of times observed: Lab _____   Clinical _____

Number of required practices: Lab _____   Clinical _____

Number of times practice: Lab _____   Clinical _____

PASSING CRITERIA:

Obtain 90 percent or better on the procedure. Tasks indicated by an asterisk (*) must receive at least 1 point or the evaluation is terminated. The procedure must be performed within the designated time or the performance receives a failing grade.

SCORING:

2 points—Task performed satisfactorily without prompting.
1 point—Task performed satisfactorily with self-initiated correction.
0 points—Task performed incorrectly or with prompting required.
NA—Task not applicable to the patient care situation

TASKS:	PEER	LAB	CLINICAL
A. Review chart	☐	☐	☐
B. Obtain equipment			
* 1. high-intensity light	☐	☐	☐
* 2. ABG syringe with 23 to 25 gauge needle or butterfly and syringe	☐	☐	☐
* 3. Betadine and alcohol swab	☐	☐	☐
* 4. sterile gauze pad	☐	☐	☐
5. data slip	☐	☐	☐
* 6. floor exam gloves	☐	☐	☐
* 7. eye protection	☐	☐	☐
* 8. assistant	☐	☐	☐
* C. Wash hands	☐	☐	☐
D. Confirm Patient	☐	☐	☐
* E. Prepare the wrist			
* 1. scrub with Betadine swab	☐	☐	☐
* 2. wipe with alcohol swab	☐	☐	☐
* 3. allow to dray	☐	☐	☐
* 4. place gloves on hands	☐	☐	☐
* 5. place eye protection	☐	☐	☐
* F. Position the high-intensity light	☐	☐	☐
G. Perform procedure			
* 1. locate radial artery	☐	☐	☐
* 2. insert needle toward the artery	☐	☐	☐
3. slowly advance the needle until the artery is penetrated	☐	☐	☐
* 4. slowly withdraw the needle and reattempt to puncture the artery (if missed on first attempt)	☐	☐	☐
* 5. withdraw needle from skin when sample is obtained	☐	☐	☐
* 6. immediately cover the site with gauze pad and hold pressure for 5 to 10 minutes	☐	☐	☐
7. check for adverse effects	☐	☐	☐
* H. Document results	☐	☐	☐
* I. Monitor appropriately	☐	☐	☐

SCORE:

Peer: _____ points out of _____ (48) _____ %

Lab: _____ points out of _____ (48) _____ %

Clinical: _____ points out of _____ (48) _____ %

TIME: _____ out of possible 15 minutes.

STUDENT SIGNATURES   **INSTRUCTOR SIGNATURES**

PEER: _____   LAB: _____

STUDENT: _____   CLINICAL: _____

HEEL PUNCTURE

OBJECTIVE

The student will demonstrate proper technique in preparing the patient and obtaining a capillary blood sample from the heel of a neonatal patient. This will be done following aseptic guidelines and in a competent manner as determined by lab and clinical instructors.

TASK A: Warm sample site. This is an important step that should be done as consistently as possible to achieve reliable blood gas results. The importance of consistency cannot be stressed enough. If the temperature and heating time change with every heel puncture, the values will be unreliable. Each NICU usually has its own method of heating the lower leg. Two common methods will be described here.

The first method is the simplest but also more expensive. It involves the use of a small, commercially produced plastic packet, containing chemicals that when mixed produce heat. The packet is wrapped in a cloth and then secured to the lower leg and foot.

The second technique of heating the heel should be available in any nursery. Obtain a clean cloth diaper or other small, clean cloth. Hold it under warm (approximately 44 to 45⁻C) running water for about a minute until it is fully saturated. Do not allow the cloth to come in contact with the bottom of the sink where it can gather bacteria, but rather hold it under the faucet with your hands and let the water run through it. It is important that the cloth be approximately the same temperature each time you do a heel puncture.

When the diaper has reached the desired temperature, squeeze all of the water out and roll it up. Return to the bedside with the damp cloth and obtain a plastic disposable diaper. Wrap the foot and lower leg with the warned cloth, and cover it with the plastic diaper, plastic side out, and secure it with the sticky tabs. This helps insulate the cloth to keep the heat in and also keeps the patient from kicking the cloth off.

Once either warmer is applied, wait 5 to 7 minutes to allow the circulation in the foot to increase before attempting the puncture. The increased circulation is secondary to the vasodilation that accompanies the heating of the limb.

TASK B: Wash Hands. Before doing a heel puncture, thoroughly wash your hands.

TASK C: Obtain Equipment. While waiting for the heel to warm, gather the necessary equipment. You will need a small lancet, Betadine and alcohol swabs, a heparinized capillary tube, end caps, a metal ``flea,'' a magnet, sterile gauze, a data slip, exam gloves, and eye protection. It is also helpful to have an assistant.

TASK D: Put on Gloves and Eye Protection. Put the gloves and eye protection on at this time in preparation for the puncture.

TASK E: Prepare Equipment. Following 5 to 7 minutes of heating, return to the bedside and prepare all of the equipment for use. This is done by opening the swabs and cautiously opening the lancet, being careful to maintain its sterility. Place all of the equipment nearby so it can be reached easily as needed.

TASK F: Perform Procedure. Unwrap the heel and quickly wipe it with the Betadine swab followed by the alcohol swab. Ideally, the heel puncture should be made on the anterolateral and posterior edge of the heel as shown in Figure A–10. A puncture made outside of the described area increases the risk of lacerating the posterior tibial artery or penetrating the calcaneus bone of the heel.

The blade of the lance should be parallel rather than horizontal with the foot to avoid any chance of cutting vessels or ligaments. The heel is now punctured following the preceding guidelines.

The puncture should be done by holding the foot in one hand, and holding the lance in the other. Position the lance directly above the desired puncture site. Perform the puncture by quickly advancing the lance, penetrating the skin adequately, and pulling the tip back out. As the blood forms a drop on the surface of the puncture, gather the blood into the heparinized capillary tube.

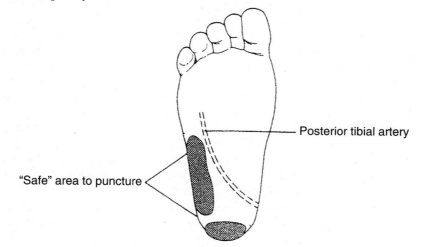

Figure A–10 *The heel is punctured in the outlined area.*

The blood should flow freely from the site with no squeezing. Blood enters the tube through a capillary action simply by placing one end into the blood droplet. Holding the opposite end slightly below the laceration will enhance blood flow into the capillary tube. Care should be taken not to allow air to enter the capillary tube.

The flow of blood from the laceration may be augmented by wiping the wound with the alcohol prep and removing any clotted blood. After gathering your samples, wipe the site again with alcohol and have your assistant apply gentle pressure with a gauze pad until bleeding stops.

All of the previously mentioned criteria can also be applied to a finger puncture in situations in which the heel cannot be punctured. The heel is the preferred site on premature infants.

TASK G: Cap the Tube. After placing the flea in the tube, both ends should be sealed with rubber caps.

TASK H: Mix Sample. Blood will clot quite easily in a capillary tube, so it is important to "flea" the sample unless it will be analyzed immediately. This is done by inserting a small steel pin into the tube and moving it back and forth in the sample with the magnet. Fleas, usually provided with the capillary tubes, help mix the blood with the heparin and reduce the risk of clotting. If the sample will not be analyzed within 10 to 15 minutes, it should be placed on ice.

TASK I: Document Results. Complete the procedure by documenting the blood gas results in the patient chart.

PERFORMANCE EVALUATION 16
HEEL PUNCTURE

Date: Lab _____   Clinical _____   Hospital _____

Lab: Pass _____ Fail _____   Clinical: Pass _____   Fail _____

Student name _____   Instructor name _____

Number of required observations: Lab _____   Clinical _____

Number of times observed: Lab _____   Clinical _____

Number of required practices: Lab _____   Clinical _____

Number of times practice: Lab _____   Clinical _____

PASSING CRITERIA:

Obtain 90 percent or better on the procedure. Tasks indicated by an asterisk (*) must receive at least 1 point or the evaluation is terminated. The procedure must be performed within the designated time or the performance receives a failing grade.

SCORING:

> 2 points—Task performed satisfactorily without prompting.
> 1 point—Task performed satisfactorily with self-initiated correction.
> 0 points—Task performed incorrectly or with prompting required.
> NA—Task not applicable to the patient care situation

TASKS:	PEER	LAB	CLINICAL
A. Wrap heel			
* 1. obtain heated cloth or chemical warmer	☐	☐	☐
* 2. select appropriate heel location	☐	☐	☐
* 3. wrap foot with cloth/warmer	☐	☐	☐
* 4. secure cloth/warmer	☐	☐	☐
* 5. allow heel to warm 5 to 7 minutes	☐	☐	☐
* B. wash hands	☐	☐	☐
C. Obtain equipment			
* 1. small-sized lance	☐	☐	☐
* 2. alcohol swab	☐	☐	☐
* 3. Betadine swab	☐	☐	☐
* 4. heparinized capillary tube	☐	☐	☐
* 5. metal flea and magnet	☐	☐	☐
* 6. sterile gauze	☐	☐	☐
7. rubber caps	☐	☐	☐
8. blood gas data slip	☐	☐	☐
* 9. floor exam gloves	☐	☐	☐
* 10. eye protection	☐	☐	☐
* D. Put on gloves and eye protection	☐	☐	☐
E. Prepare equipment			
* 1. open swabs	☐	☐	☐
* 2. open lance	☐	☐	☐
F. Perform procedure			
* 1. completely unwrap heel	☐	☐	☐
* 2. wipe heel with Betadine swap	☐	☐	☐
* 3. wipe heel with alcohol swab	☐	☐	☐
* 4. stick heel in appropriate location	☐	☐	☐
* 5. fill capillary tube with sample	☐	☐	☐
* 6. wipe site with alcohol swab after obtaining sample and hold pressure with gauze	☐	☐	☐
* G. Cap each end of the tube	☐	☐	☐
* H. Mix sample with flea	☐	☐	☐
* I. Document results in patient chart	☐	☐	☐

SCORE:

Peer: _____	points out of _____ (54) _____ %
Lab: _____	points out of _____ (54) _____ %
Clinical: _____	points out of _____ (54) _____ %

TIME: _____ out of possible 20 minutes.

STUDENT SIGNATURES	**INSTRUCTOR SIGNATURES**
PEER: _____	LAB: _____
STUDENT: _____	CLINICAL: _____

TRANSCUTANEOUS MONITOR

OBJECTIVE

Using a transcutaneous monitor (TCM), the student will demonstrate proper calibration and placement on patient in a laboratory and clinical setting. This will be done following aseptic guidelines and in a competent manner as determined by lab and clinical instructors.

TASK A: Obtain Monitor. First, obtain a clean transcutaneous monitor.

TASK B: Calibrate Monitor. Before placing on the patient, the monitor must be calibrated. The exact mechanism of calibration varies depending on the type of monitor used. Follow the manufacturer's instructions for proper calibration. Whatever method is used, the monitor must be calibrated to known levels of PO_2 and PCO_2. This is done by placing the sensor in a holding device and passing a flow of gas with a known concentration of oxygen and carbon dioxide to the sensor.

The PO_2 and PCO_2 measured during calibration is compared to the known PO_2 and PCO_2 of the calibration gas. The PO_2 and PCO_2 of the calibration gas is determined by multiplying the barometric pressure by the percentage of gas in the sample. For example, if the concentration of oxygen in the sample gas is 0.30 and the barometric pressure is 700 mm Hg, the monitor should read a PO_2 of 210 mm Hg (700 mm Hg × 0.30).

If the monitor is above or below the desired level, it is adjusted to read appropriately. Even if the calibration is totally automatic, the correct values must be verified by the practitioner.

Next, examine the membrane that covers the sensor. It should be free from tears or any other defect that may interfere with proper readings.

TASK C: Gather Equipment. Gather the equipment that you will need to attach the monitor, including alcohol swabs, doublesided adhesive discs, a contact medium, and a cotton ball.

TASK D: Select Appropriate Site. Now, turning your attention to the patient, select an appropriate site for placing the sensor. The site should ideally go on an area of the body that will not interfere with other monitors. Additionally, it should not be placed under the body or over bony areas such as the clavicles, sternum, scapulas, or hip. The area must be free from broken-down skin, burns, abrasions, or other excoriations. Avoid placing the sensor over the same site that it was just removed from.

TASK E: Wash Hands. Before attempting this skill, a thorough hand washing is done.

TASK F: Prepare Site. The next task is to prepare the site for the application of the sensor. Remove the alcohol swab and scrub the site. This removes skin oils and other substances that may interfere with proper bonding of the disc.

TASK G: Prepare Sensor. While the site is drying, apply the sticky disc to the sensor, pressing all around the sensor face to ensure adequate adhesion. Now remove all paper from the bottom of the disc and place a drop of contact medium on the surface of the electrode.

TASK H: Apply Sensor. You are now ready to apply the sensor to the skin. Place the sensor above the selected site and firmly press it onto the skin. The portion of the adhesive disc that is visible around the sensor should be gently pressed against the skin to remove air bubbles and ensure adhesion. The cotton ball may now be pressed onto the visible portion of the disc. This allows cotton fibers to adhere to the disc, thus preventing other objects from adhering.

With the sensor firmly on the patient, set the high and low alarm limits to the desired levels. If the monitor is equipped with a timer, set it at this time.

TASK I: Monitor the Readings. Transcutaneous readings should be monitored continuously and charted at least every 2 to 4 hours. While the monitor is on the patient, obtain blood gases as necessary to verify TCM readings and monitor the site for proper adhesion.

TASK J: Recalibrate Monitor. When the appropriate time limit is reached, remove the sensor. The sensor should be removed gently to prevent skin peeling or dermal stripping. When the sensor is removed, examine the site for any signs of burning or skin abrasion.

The monitor is then recalibrated and replaced on the skin following the previous steps. Site changes must be documented in the patient record.

PERFORMANCE EVALUATION 17
TRANSCUTANEOUS MONITOR

Date: Lab _____ Clinical _____ Hospital _____

Lab: Pass _____ Fail _____ Clinical: Pass _____ Fail _____

Student name _____ Instructor name _____

Number of required observations: Lab _____ Clinical _____

Number of times observed: Lab _____ Clinical _____

Number of required practices: Lab _____ Clinical _____

Number of times practice: Lab _____ Clinical _____

PASSING CRITERIA:

Obtain 90 percent or better on the procedure. Tasks indicated by an asterisk (*) must receive at least 1 point or the evaluation is terminated. The procedure must be performed within the designated time or the performance receives a failing grade.

SCORING:

2 points—Task performed satisfactorily without prompting.
1 point—Task performed satisfactorily with self-initiated correction.
0 points—Task performed incorrectly or with prompting required.
NA—Task not applicable to the patient care situation

TASKS:	PEER	LAB	CLINICAL
* A. Obtain monitor and clean as needed	☐	☐	☐
* B. Properly calibrate monitor			
1. determine proper calibration			
a. calculate PO_2 and PCO_2 values	☐	☐	☐
b. PO_2 and/or PCO_2 within limits	☐	☐	☐
c. condition of sensor membrane	☐	☐	☐
C. Gather equipment			
* 1. alcohol swabs	☐	☐	☐
* 2. double-sided sticky discs	☐	☐	☐
* 3. contact medium	☐	☐	☐
4. cotton ball	☐	☐	☐
* D. Select appropriate site on patient	☐	☐	☐
* E. Wash hands	☐	☐	☐
F. Properly prepare area			

	PEER	LAB	CLINICAL
* 1. scrub site with alcohol prep	☐	☐	☐
2. allow site to dry	☐	☐	☐

TASKS:

G. Properly prepare TCM sensor

	PEER	LAB	CLINICAL
* 1. apply sticky disc	☐	☐	☐
* 2. apply contact medium to sensor	☐	☐	☐

H. Apply sensor to the skin

	PEER	LAB	CLINICAL
* 1. firmly press sensor onto patient skin	☐	☐	☐
2. press cotton ball to visible portion of disc	☐	☐	☐
* 3. set high and low alarm limits	☐	☐	☐
* 4. set time limit as appropriate	☐	☐	☐

I. Monitor the TCM

	PEER	LAB	CLINICAL
* 1. obtain ABGs when indicated	☐	☐	☐
* 2. monitor for proper adhesion	☐	☐	☐
* 3. correlate TCM values with ABG values	☐	☐	☐

J. Remove TCM and recalibrate

	PEER	LAB	CLINICAL
* 1. remove after appropriate time	☐	☐	☐
* 2. check site for signs of burn or abrasions from removal	☐	☐	☐

SCORE:

Peer: _____ points out of _____ (46) _____ %

Lab: _____ points out of _____ (46) _____ %

Clinical: _____ points out of _____ (46) _____ %

TIME: _____ out of possible 20 minutes.

STUDENT SIGNATURES

PEER: _____

STUDENT: _____

INSTRUCTOR SIGNATURES

LAB: _____

CLINICAL: _____

PULSE OXIMETER

OBJECTIVE

The student will be able to correctly place a pulse oximeter on a patient and monitor for proper operation. This will be done following aseptic guidelines and in a competent manner as determined by lab and clinical instructors.

TASK A: Obtain Equipment. First, obtain a clean monitor and probe. A device to secure the probe to the patient should also be obtained at this time if a finger or limb probe will be used. A securing device is not necessary when using an ear probe.

TASK B: Wash Hands. Thoroughly wash your hands.

TASK C: Select Site. Now proceed to the patient bedside and select an appropriate site for the application of the monitor. The site should be clean, free of skin abrasions and excoriations, and allow adequate passage of light. On small infants, the probe is frequently placed on the wrist or the foot. On larger patients, a finger or toe is generally used. Cold extremities may indicate poor perfusion and may give inaccurate readings, and should be avoided if possible.

TASK D: Attach Probe. Apply the probe to the patient site with the wire from the probe coursing parallel to the limb. This action prevents bending the wire, possibly damaging it, and additionally averts accidental dislodging of the probe.

Secure the probe to the patient using an appropriate device. Position the probe so that the light transmitter and receiver are located directly opposite each other through the body. Sponge limb restraints with a Velcro fastener and Coban wraps are often used to secure the probe. The device should not only hold the probe securely but also block out extraneous light that may interfere with saturation readings. Avoid wrapping the probe too tightly, particularly on a small infant, because it can impede circulation or cause pressure injury.

If an ear probe will be used, attach the probe to the lobe of the selected ear. Set the high and low alarm limits to the desired levels.

TASK E: Monitor Readings. While the probe is in use, it should be regularly monitored for correlation with heart rate, proper positioning, and maintenance of desired oxygen saturation. This information should be charted at least every 2 to 4 hours.

TASK F: Change Site. The probe site should be changed on a regular basis, as determined by the department.

TASK G: Document Procedure. Document appropriate data in patient chart.

PERFORMANCE EVALUATION 18
PULSE OXIMETER

Date: Lab _____   Clinical _____   Hospital _____

Lab: Pass _____ Fail _____   Clinical: Pass _____   Fail _____

Student name _____   Instructor name _____

Number of required observations: Lab _____   Clinical _____

Number of times observed: Lab _____   Clinical _____

Number of required practices: Lab _____   Clinical _____

Number of times practice: Lab _____   Clinical _____

PASSING CRITERIA:

Obtain 90 percent or better on the procedure. Tasks indicated by an asterisk (*) must receive at least 1 point or the evaluation is terminated. The procedure must be performed within the designated time or the performance receives a failing grade.

SCORING:

2 points—Task performed satisfactorily without prompting.
1 point—Task performed satisfactorily with self-initiated correction.
0 points—Task performed incorrectly or with prompting required.
NA—Task not applicable to the patient care situation

TASKS:	PEER	LAB	CLINICAL
A. Obtain equipment			
* 1. monitor	☐	☐	☐
* 2. probe	☐	☐	☐
* 3. device to secure probe	☐	☐	☐
* B. Wash hands	☐	☐	☐
* C. Select proper site on patient	☐	☐	☐
D. Attach the oximeter probe to patient			
* 1. secure with Coban or restraint (if limb probe is used)	☐	☐	☐
* 2. alarm limits set	☐	☐	☐
E. Monitor the oximeter			
* 1. pulse and heart rate correlate	☐	☐	☐
* 2. continued proper positioning	☐	☐	☐
* 3. O_2 saturation maintained to desired levels	☐	☐	☐
* F. Change probe site per policy	☐	☐	☐
* G. Document appropriate data in patient chart	☐	☐	☐

SCORE:

Peer: _____   points out of _____ (24) _____ %

Lab: _____   points out of _____ (24) _____ %

Clinical: _____   points out of _____ (24) _____ %

TIME: _____ out of possible 10 minutes.

STUDENT SIGNATURES   **INSTRUCTOR SIGNATURES**

PEER: _____   LAB: _____

STUDENT: _____   CLINICAL: _____

VENTILATOR SETUP

OBJECTIVE

The student will be able to demonstrate the ability to set up a ventilator by attaching all necessary equipment and preparing the ventilator for placement on a patient. This will be done following aseptic guidelines and in a competent manner as determined by lab and clinical instructors. For this procedure, it is assumed that the ventilator has been appropriately cleaned beforehand.

TASK A: Obtain Equipment. First, you must obtain the necessary equipment. You will need a clean circuit, a clean humidifier, a temperature probe or thermometer, and a bacterial filter.

TASK B: Wash Hands. Next, it is necessary to wash your hands.

TASK C: Connect Equipment. You are now ready to attach the new circuit to the ventilator. Place the bacterial filter between the ventilator outlet and the humidifier inlet. This is a precautionary measure to filter the gas before it reaches the patient. Next, place the clean humidifier onto the heater assembly and connect the line from the ventilator to the inlet of the humidifier.

Remove the clean circuit from the protective wrapping and connect the inspiratory line to the outlet of the humidifier. Connect the expiratory line to the expiratory valve inlet. Connect the temperature probe or thermometer to the patient connection. Some newer circuits contain a heated wire; if so, the thermometer probes are connected at the humidifier outlet and the patient connection. Attach the appropriately sized pressure line to the patient connection.

TASK D: Set Parameters. Next, set initial parameters on the ventilator. If not dictated by department policy, initial parameters should be set as follows:

FiO_2—1.00
Rate—40 breaths per minute
PIP—20 mc H_2O
PEEP—3 cm H_2O
Flow—8 L/minute
Inspiratory time—0.5 second
Emergency pop-off pressure—25 cm H_2O
Mode—IMV

TASK E: Test Equipment. Test the ventilator by connecting the oxygen and air hoses to the wall outlet, occluding the patient connection in a sterile manner. Turn the ventilator to the IMV mode and ensure the PIP is being achieved. This confirms that there are no leaks in the circuit. Also test the ventilator alarms at this time to verify proper function.

TASK F: Cover Ventilator. The ventilator is now ready and should be covered with a plastic bag to keep it clean until use.

PERFORMANCE EVALUATION 19
VENTILATOR SETUP

Date: Lab _____   Clinical _____   Hospital _____

Lab: Pass _____   Fail _____   Clinical: Pass _____   Fail _____

Student name _____   Instructor name _____

Number of required observations: Lab _____   Clinical _____

Number of times observed: Lab _____   Clinical _____

Number of required practices: Lab _____   Clinical _____

Number of times practice: Lab _____   Clinical _____

PASSING CRITERIA:

Obtain 90 percent or better on the procedure. Tasks indicated by an asterisk (*) must receive at least 1 point or the evaluation is terminated. The procedure must be performed within the designated time or the performance receives a failing grade.

SCORING:

2 points—Task performed satisfactorily without prompting.
1 point—Task performed satisfactorily with self-initiated correction.
0 points—Task performed incorrectly or with prompting required.
NA—Task not applicable to the patient care situation

TASKS:	PEER	LAB	CLINICAL
A. Obtain equipment			
* 1. circuit	☐	☐	☐
* 2. humidifier equipment	☐	☐	☐
* 3. temperature probes	☐	☐	☐
4. bacterial filter	☐	☐	☐
* B. Wash hands	☐	☐	☐
C. Connect equipment to ventilator			
1. place bacterial filter between ventilator and humidifier inlet	☐	☐	☐
* 2. place humidifier on heating unit	☐	☐	☐
* 3. connect inspiratory line to humidifier outlet and expiratory line to exhalation valve	☐	☐	☐
* 4. connect temperature probes	☐	☐	☐

TASKS:	PEER	LAB	CLINICAL
* 5. connect pressure line to patient ``Y''	☐	☐	☐
* D. Set initial parameters	☐	☐	☐
E. Test equipment			
* 1. alarm function	☐	☐	☐
* 2. check for system leaks	☐	☐	☐
F. Cover with protective bag	☐	☐	☐

SCORE:

Peer: _____   points out of _____ (28) _____ %

Lab: _____   points out of _____ (28) _____ %

Clinical: _____   points out of _____ (28) _____ %

TIME: _____ out of possible 15 minutes.

STUDENT SIGNATURES   **INSTRUCTOR SIGNATURES**

PEER: _____   LAB: _____

STUDENT: _____   CLINICAL: _____

NEONATAL VENTILATOR CHECK

OBJECTIVE

The student will be able to demonstrate the ability to assess the current settings on a neonatal ventilator. The student will further demonstrate the ability to determine the appropriateness of settings by assessing patient status. This will be done following aseptic guidelines and in a competent manner as determined by lab and clinical instructors.

Ventilator monitoring is facilitated in most institutions by a ventilator flow sheet on which the ventilator checks are documented. Each flow sheet is unique to the institution and the student should become familiar with those in the NICUs in which he will be practicing.

This proficiency is designed to cover the basic components of the ventilator check; components are not presented in any particular order. Ventilator checks should be done at the frequency dictated by department standards, as well as after any changes are made, to ensure correct settings and proper function of the ventilator and associated monitors.

TASK A: Obtain Equipment. Begin the procedure by obtaining the required equipment. You will need a stethoscope, an oxygen analyzer, and proper equipment to suction the patient. If these items are already set up at the bedside, check them for proper function.

TASK B: Wash Hands. Before performing a ventilator check, a thorough hand washing is necessary.

TASK C: Assess Patient. After confirming that you have the correct patient, focus attention on the patient and perform a brief assessment. Assess the overall appearance of the patient, including skin color and body position, and note anything that looks abnormal or out of place. Watch the chest to evaluate the chest excursions. Check the heart rate and compare it to previous levels.

TASK D: Auscultate and Suction (As Needed). Before beginning the ventilator check, auscultate the lungs to evaluate aeration, the presence of adventitious sounds, and equality of breath sounds. Suction, if indicated. It is important to remove excess secretions from the airway to prevent false or fluctuating ventilator readings.

TASK E: Check and Record Ventilator Parameters. Now you may turn your attention to the ventilator and monitor. Whenever a ventilator monitor is being used, all pressures and rates should be read from it and not the ventilator. Before performing a ventilator check, drain any condensed water from the ventilator tubing. As each of the following parameters is checked, it should be recorded in the appropriate place on the ventilator flow sheet.

First, verify the mode of ventilation. This will usually be either IMV or CPAP. Next, count both the spontaneous and ventilator respiratory rates. This is followed by a check of the peak inspiratory pressure (PIP), and the positive end expiratory pressure (PEEP), inspiratory time (IT), or duration of positive pressure (DPP); I:E ratio, peak flow, analyzed FiO_2, and circuit temperatures. When volume ventilation is being done, the set and delivered volumes and pressures, as well as compliance, should be monitored.

Examine the humidifier to ensure that it is functioning properly and that the water supply is adequate. Next, check the ventilator and monitor alarms to confirm they are set appropriately and activated. Examine the endotracheal tube to verify it is at the proper depth and that the securing method is adhering and holding the tube steady. Look for signs of skin excoriations around the mouth and tube that may need attention. Finally, check the readings on the ECM and pulse oximeter and record in the appropriate location.

TASK F: Additional Charting. In addition to charting the previously mentioned parameters, document the patient's breath sounds; volume, color, and consistency of any sputum that was removed during suctioning; and the results of any blood gases that have been done. If any parameter changes have been done they should also be documented along with the rationale for the changes.

TASK G: Report Observations. Report any changes in status, adverse reactions, or unusual findings to the physician and any other appropriate personnel.

PERFORMANCE EVALUATION 20
NEONATAL VENTILATOR CHECK

Date: Lab _____   Clinical _____   Hospital _____

Lab: Pass _____ Fail _____   Clinical: Pass _____   Fail _____

Student name _____   Instructor name _____

Number of required observations:	Lab _____	Clinical _____
Number of times observed:	Lab _____	Clinical _____
Number of required practices:	Lab _____	Clinical _____
Number of times practice:	Lab _____	Clinical _____

PASSING CRITERIA:

Obtain 90 percent or better on the procedure. Tasks indicated by an asterisk (*) must receive at least 1 point or the evaluation is terminated. The procedure must be performed within the designated time or the performance receives a failing grade.

SCORING:

2 points—Task performed satisfactorily without prompting.
1 point—Task performed satisfactorily with self-initiated correction.
0 points—Task performed incorrectly or with prompting required.
NA—Task not applicable to the patient care situation

TASKS:	PEER	LAB	CLINICAL
A. Obtain equipment			
* 1. stethoscope	☐	☐	☐
* 2. oxygen analyzer	☐	☐	☐
* 3. suction equipment	☐	☐	☐
* B. Wash hands	☐	☐	☐
C. Assess patient			
* 1. confirm correct patient	☐	☐	☐
* 2. appearance	☐	☐	☐
* 3. chest excursion	☐	☐	☐
* 4. check heart rate	☐	☐	☐
* D. Auscultate (and suction as needed)	☐	☐	☐
E. Check each of the following:			
* 1. mode of ventilation	☐	☐	☐
* 2. respiratory rate (patient and ventilator)	☐	☐	☐
* 3. peak inspiratory pressure	☐	☐	☐
* 4. PEEP	☐	☐	☐
* 5. inspiratory time or DPP	☐	☐	☐

TASKS:		PEER	LAB	CLINICAL
*	6. I:E ratio	☐	☐	☐
*	7. peak flow	☐	☐	☐
	8. set and delivered volumes (as appropriate)	☐	☐	☐
	9. set and delivered pressures (as appropriate)	☐	☐	☐
	10. compliance (as appropriate)	☐	☐	☐
*	11. analyzed FiO_2	☐	☐	☐
*	12. circuit temperatures	☐	☐	☐
*	13. humidifier and water level	☐	☐	☐
*	14. ventilator and monitor alarms	☐	☐	☐
*	15. endotracheal tube position	☐	☐	☐
*	16. TCM or pulse oximeter readings	☐	☐	☐
F.	Additional charting			
*	1. breath sounds	☐	☐	☐
*	2. sputum volume, color, consistency	☐	☐	☐
*	3. blood gas results	☐	☐	☐
*	4. any pertinent information or ventilator changes	☐	☐	☐
G.	Report observations			
*	1. changes in status	☐	☐	☐
*	2. adverse reactions	☐	☐	☐
*	3. unusual findings	☐	☐	☐

SCORE:

Peer: _____ points out of _____ (66) _____ %

Lab: _____ points out of _____ (66) _____ %

Clinical: _____ points out of _____ (66) _____ %

TIME: _____ out of possible 15 minutes.

STUDENT SIGNATURES   **INSTRUCTOR SIGNATURES**

PEER: _____   LAB: _____

STUDENT: _____   CLINICAL: _____

VENTILATOR PARAMETER CHANGES

OBJECTIVE

The student will be able to demonstrate competency in making appropriate ventilator parameter changes when given blood gas data. This will be done in a competent manner as determined by lab and clinical instructors.

It should be remembered that there is no magic formula that determines the correct ventilator change. The determination of vent changes is based on principles that may differ from patient to patient and comes from ample clinical experience with neonates. This evaluation is only meant to allow the student to demonstrate the basic understanding of the principles that govern parameter changes. Because this proficiency requires a demonstration of knowledge and understanding, rather than a demonstration of manual application, it relies heavily on the textbook as the guide to decision making. Whether the student's choices are deemed correct is entirely at the discretion of the instructor.

TASK A: Determine Blood Gas Status. The first step is to determine the patient's current blood gas status and acid-base balance by using blood gas results, pulse oximetry, and/or transcutaneous monitoring. These results and data will be provided by the lab or clinical instructor.

TASK B: Evaluate Current Ventilator Settings. Assuming a change in setting is indicated from the blood gas and acid-base status, the next step is to evaluate the current ventilator settings to determine what changes should be made. Special attention is paid to the current FiO_2 rate, volumes, and pressures. Determine whether the settings are low, medium, or high and whether they are in equilibrium. In other words, is the rate high but the PIP low or are they both high or both low?

TASK C: Determine Possible Changes. At this point, the student will discuss all of the possible changes that can be made to normalize the blood gas or acid-base balance. The emphasis here is on the ability to demonstrate understanding of the relationship between ventilator parameters and how each change will affect the patient.

TASK D: Select Appropriate Changes. Based on the previous information and on the current clinical status of the patient, the student will select the most appropriate parameter change and explain the rationale to the instructor. As a part of this task, the student will also discuss any possible complications that may accompany the selected parameter change.

TASK E: Make the Changes. At this point, the student will actually make the selected changes on the ventilator. This requires that the student be familiar with the ventilator in use. Although ventilator familiarity has not been previously mentioned, it is important that the student understands all aspects of the ventilator before assuming care of the patient.

TASK F: Follow-Up. It is important to follow up any ventilator changes with a blood gas analysis on unstable patients or with a transcutaneous monitor on stable patients. This is to ensure that the change(s) had the desired effect on the patient.

TASK G: Documentation. The final task in this proficiency is to document the change(s) in the patient record. Of equal importance is an explanation of why the changes were made, any side effects or complications, and follow-up blood gas or TCM readings.

PERFORMANCE EVALUATION 21
VENTILATOR PARAMETER CHANGES

Date: Lab _____   Clinical _____   Hospital _____

Lab: Pass _____ Fail _____   Clinical: Pass _____   Fail _____

Student name _____   Instructor name _____

Number of required observations: Lab _____   Clinical _____

Number of times observed: Lab _____   Clinical _____

Number of required practices: Lab _____   Clinical _____

Number of times practice: Lab _____   Clinical _____

PASSING CRITERIA:

Obtain 90 percent or better on the procedure. Tasks indicated by an asterisk (*) must receive at least 1 point or the evaluation is terminated. The procedure must be performed within the designated time or the performance receives a failing grade.

SCORING:

2 points—Task performed satisfactorily without prompting.
1 point—Task performed satisfactorily with self-initiated correction.
0 points—Task performed incorrectly or with prompting required.
NA—Task not applicable to the patient care situation

TASKS:

	PEER	LAB	CLINICAL
* A. Determine acid-base and oxygenation status from ABG and/or TCM	☐	☐	☐
* B. Evaluate current ventilator settings	☐	☐	☐
* C. Determine all possible ventilator changes to normalize ABG	☐	☐	☐
* D. Select appropriate ventilator changes: discuss potential complications	☐	☐	☐
* E. Make appropriate ventilator changes	☐	☐	☐
* F. Follow up the changes on TCM and/or ABG	☐	☐	☐
* G. Document changes in patient chart	☐	☐	☐

SCORE:

Peer: _____   points out of _____ (16) _____ %

Lab: _____   points out of _____ (16) _____ %

Clinical: _____   points out of _____ (16) _____ %

TIME: _____ out of possible 20 minutes.

STUDENT SIGNATURES

PEER: _____

STUDENT: _____

INSTRUCTOR SIGNATURES

LAB: _____

CLINICAL: _____

VENTILATOR CIRCUIT CHANGE

OBJECTIVE

The student will be able to demonstrate the ability to remove a dirty ventilator circuit and replace it with a clean circuit without compromising patient status. This will be done in a competent manner as determined by lab and clinical instructors.

Once a patient is attached to the ventilator, the circuit may need to be changed occasionally. This is a skill that most respiratory care practitioners need to possess because they are often responsible for changing the ventilator circuits.

TASK A: Obtain Equipment. Obtain the necessary equipment. You will need a new or clean patient circle, a new humidifier, sterile water, and a stethoscope. If a resuscitation bag is not present at the bedside, obtain one for this procedure. The bag should be set to the appropriate FiO_2 and checked for proper function. Exam gloves and eye protection should be obtained and put on at is time.

TASK B: Wash Hands. Before changing a dirty circuit, always wash your hands thoroughly. Observe universal precautions.

TASK C: Prepare New Circuit. Proceed to the patient bedside with the necessary equipment. The first step in changing the circuit is to replace the existing humidifier with the new one. This is done by (1) bypassing the humidifier by removing the inlet and outlet circuit tubing and connecting them together or (2) removing the humidifier from the heater with the tubing intact. Be sure to turn the heater off before removing the humidifier. In either case, place the new humidifier onto the heating unit and attach the appropriate sterile water source.

Remove the new patient circuit from its protective covering, being careful to maintain sterility. Connect the clean inspiratory tubing to the outlet of the humidifier and place the expiratory tube near the expiratory valve where it can be reached easily. The patient connection, with all tubes firmly attached, is placed near the patient's head where it can be easily accessed.

The inspiratory line that connects the ventilator flow outlet to the humidifier is attached at one end to the humidifier inlet, with the opposite end placed near the ventilator flow outlet. The pressure tubing is placed near the point of connection to the monitor, where it can be easily accessed.

Task D: Change Circuit. With the equipment in place, the circuit is now ready to be changed. Have someone bag the patient while changing the circuit. It is easy to get confused with all the tubing and make a wrong connection, possibly compromising the patient. Bagging the patient allows you to be cautious and make the correct connections.

With the patient bagged, disconnect the used inspiratory line from the ventilator flow outlet and attach the new inspiratory line to the flow outlet. Now detach the used expiratory tubing from the expiratory inlet and replace it with the new expiratory tubing. Finally, disconnect the used pressure tubing from the pressure manometer port and replace it with the new tubing.

TASK E: Verify Circuit Function. Occlude the patient connection and verify that the desired pressure is being achieved in the new circuit.

TASK F: Attach Patient. Attach the patient connection to the endotracheal tube and check to verify the patient is being ventilated. This is done by auscultating the chest and watching the chest rise.

TASK G: Conclude Procedure. Turn the humidifier heater back on at this point and ensure its proper function. Next, properly dispose of the dirty circuit.

TASK H: Complete Ventilator Check. It is important to do a complete ventilator check following the circuit change to ensure there have been no changes in the parameters.

TASK I: Document Procedure. The final task is to document the procedure in the patient record. The documentation should include breath sounds and vital signs following the change, as well as patient toleration of procedure.

PERFORMANCE EVALUATION 22
VENTILATOR CIRCUIT CHANGE

Date: Lab _____   Clinical _____   Hospital _____

Lab: Pass _____ Fail _____   Clinical: Pass _____   Fail _____

Student name _____   Instructor name _____

Number of required observations: Lab _____   Clinical _____

Number of times observed: Lab _____   Clinical _____

Number of required practices: Lab _____   Clinical _____

Number of times practice: Lab _____   Clinical _____

PASSING CRITERIA:

Obtain 90 percent or better on the procedure. Tasks indicated by an asterisk (*) must receive at least 1 point or the evaluation is terminated. The procedure must be performed within the designated time or the performance receives a failing grade.

SCORING:

2 points—Task performed satisfactorily without prompting.
1 point—Task performed satisfactorily with self-initiated correction.
0 points—Task performed incorrectly or with prompting required.
NA—Task not applicable to the patient care situation

TASKS:	PEER	LAB	CLINICAL
A. Obtain equipment			
* 1. patient circuit	☐	☐	☐
* 2. humidifier equipment	☐	☐	☐
* 3. sterile water	☐	☐	☐
* 4. stethoscope	☐	☐	☐
* 5. resuscitation bag and mask (if not at bedside)	☐	☐	☐
* 6. put on exam gloves and eye protection	☐	☐	☐
B. Wash hands	☐	☐	☐
C. Prepare new circuit			
* 1. bypass or remove old humidifier	☐	☐	☐
* 2. turn off heater	☐	☐	☐
* 3. place new humidifier on heater	☐	☐	☐
* 4. remove new circuit from bag	☐	☐	☐
* 5. connect inspiratory line to humidifier outlet	☐	☐	☐
6. place expiratory line near expiratory valve	☐	☐	☐
7. place patient connection near patient head			
8. attach ventilator-humidifier connecting tube to humidifier inlet, opposite end placed near ventilator patient flow outlet	☐	☐	☐
9. place pressure tubing near pressure monitor	☐	☐	☐
D. Change circuit			
* 1. assistant manually ventilates patient	☐	☐	☐
* 2. disconnect ventilator-humidifier tubing from ventilator and replace with new tubing	☐	☐	☐
* 3. disconnect expiratory tubing from expiratory valve; replace with expiratory tube from new circuit	☐	☐	☐
* 4. disconnect pressure tubing from pressure monitor; connect new tubing	☐	☐	☐
* E. Occlude patient connection and verify pressure	☐	☐	☐
* F. Attach new circuit to patient: verify patient ventilation			
* 1. auscultate	☐	☐	☐

TASKS:	PEER	LAB	CLINICAL
* 2. chest excursion	☐	☐	☐
G. Conclude procedure			
* 1. turn on humidifier	☐	☐	☐
* 2. properly dispose of dirty circuit	☐	☐	☐
* H. Perform a complete ventilator check	☐	☐	☐
* I. Document procedure in patient chart	☐	☐	☐

SCORE:

Peer: _____ points out of _____ (54) _____ %

Lab: _____ points out of _____ (54) _____ %

Clinical: _____ points out of _____ (54) _____ %

TIME: _____ out of possible 15 minutes.

STUDENT SIGNATURES   **INSTRUCTOR SIGNATURES**

PEER: _____   LAB: _____

STUDENT: _____   CLINICAL: _____

SMALL-PARTICLE AEROSOL GENERATOR (SPAG)

OBJECTIVE

The student will be able to demonstrate proficiency in correctly assembling and filling a small-particle aerosol generator. This will be done in a competent manner as determined by lab and clinical instructors.

The small-particle aerosol generator is produced by ICN Pharmaceuticals, Inc. and is designed to deliver the antiviral drug ribavirin for the treatment of RSV.

TASK A: Review Chart. Before starting the procedure, the patient record should be reviewed. First, confirm the order for the treatment. The length of administration should be noted. Check the chart for any contraindications to administering the therapy. Confirm the documentation of RSV. Note the overall patient condition by reviewing vital signs, nursing notes, and physician notes.

TASK B: Precautions. Discuss the precautions that should be taken when delivering ribavirin therapy with a SPAG unit. Because of the teratogenic risks associated with the use of ribavirin, the student must demonstrate understanding of appropriate precautions when using this therapy. When a tent or hood is used, an outer hood or cover can be placed over the primary hood or tent. A vacuum tube is then placed in the space between the outer and inner covers. The idea behind this procedure is that any excess ribavirin delivered to the inner hood or tent will escape to the space between the two covers. It is then evacuated through the vacuum tube to the outside or through filters that remove the ribavirin. Other measures include the wearing of gowns, gloves, goggles, and masks by all who enter the room. Surgical masks do not filter the ribavirin, making the use of special, small-particulate filter masks necessary. It is recommended that pregnant or nursing females avoid exposure to ribavirin entirely. Except when immediate care is required, nebulizer flow should be turned off 10 to 15 minutes before opening the hood. However, the drying chamber flow should remain on to ensure adequate oxygenation and CO_2 removal. It is also recommended that ribarivin only be delivered in isolation rooms that are under negative pressure, have adequate air exchange, and vent to the outside.

TASK C: Obtain Equipment. The SPAG unit is self-contained, but the student should ensure that the following are present for proper function: drying chamber, nebulizer reservoir, and all connecting tubes.

TASK D: Wash Hands. Before starting the assembly of equipment, hands should be washed thoroughly.

TASK E: Assemble Equipment. The first step is to reconstitute the ribavirin into the nebulizer reservoir. This is done by mixing one vial (6 g) of the lyophilized ribavirin with sterile water for injection or inhalation, using sterile technique, and shaking the vial until the drug is completely dissolved. This mixture is then added to the nebulizer reservoir, again using sterile technique, and sterile water is added for a final volume of 300 ml. The next step is to assemble the nebulizer by inserting the stem into the nebulizer cap and placing the cap onto the reservoir. Next, the reservoir assembly is placed into the nebulizer housing and snapped into place. The drying chamber is then inserted through the wall of the SPAG housing and pressed firmly onto the O ring of the nebulizer output. Now, attach the appropriate gas flow tubes to the drying chamber and the nebulizer.

TASK F: Precautions. Before starting the SPAG, all present in the room, with the exception of the patient, should put on a gown, gloves, eye protection, and an appropriate mask. Ensure that the door to the room is closed.

TASK G: Evaluate Patient. Before starting the treatment, the patient should be thoroughly evaluated. The evaluation should include vital signs, breath sounds, oxygenation status, and any other evaluation deemed necessary according to hospital and departmental policy.

TASK H: Attach to Patient. After selecting the appropriate administration device, connect a hose from the drying chamber outflow opening to the opening of the administration device. Connect the source gas to the front of the SPAG housing and adjust the pressure to 26 psi, using the regulator gauge on the front of the SPAG. Now, open the flow to the nebulizer to full open and readjust the regulator to 26 psi, if needed. Adjust the nebulizer flow to 3.5 to

6.5 L/min. Now, open the flow to the drying chamber completely and readjust the regulator pressure to 26 psi, if needed. The flow rate is then adjusted to allow a combined flow with the nebulizer output of 15 L/min if delivered to a tent or headbox or 12 L/min if delivered to a mask. Visually ensure that the nebulizer is functioning.

TASK I: Conclude Procedure. After ensuring proper setup and function, exit the room, remove all protective gear and clothing, and place items in appropriate receptacles. Thoroughly wash hands.

TASK J: Monitoring. The appropriate timing and method of monitoring the equipment and the patient should be determined. This is based on any orders, written department standards, and patient condition.

TASK K: Document Procedure. The final task is to document the procedure in the patient record. This should include patient data, as well as medication dosage and precautions taken.

PERFORMANCE EVALUATION 23
SMALL-PARTICLE AEROSOL GENERATOR (SPAG)

Date: Lab _____   Clinical _____   Hospital _____

Lab: Pass _____ Fail _____   Clinical: Pass _____   Fail _____

Student name _____   Instructor name _____

Number of required observations: Lab _____   Clinical _____

Number of times observed: Lab _____   Clinical _____

Number of required practices: Lab _____   Clinical _____

Number of times practice: Lab _____   Clinical _____

PASSING CRITERIA:

Obtain 90 percent or better on the procedure. Tasks indicated by an asterisk (*) must receive at least 1 point or the evaluation is terminated. The procedure must be performed within the designated time or the performance receives a failing grade.

SCORING:

2 points—Task performed satisfactorily without prompting.
1 point—Task performed satisfactorily with self-initiated correction.
0 points—Task performed incorrectly or with prompting required.
NA—Task not applicable to the patient care situation

TASKS:	PEER	LAB	CLINICAL
A. Review chart			
* 1. check order	☐	☐	☐
* 2. contraindications	☐	☐	☐
* 3. documentation of RSV	☐	☐	☐
4. patient condition	☐	☐	☐
B. Precautions			
* 1. double hood	☐	☐	☐
* 2. vacuum device	☐	☐	☐
* 3. gown, gloves, goggles, mask	☐	☐	☐
* 4. turn off nebulizer before opening the hood	☐	☐	☐
* 5. isolation	☐	☐	☐
* 6. negative pressure room	☐	☐	☐
* 7. vent to outside	☐	☐	☐
C. Obtain equipment			
* 1. drying chamber	☐	☐	☐
* 2. nebulizer reservoir	☐	☐	☐
* 3. tubing	☐	☐	☐
* D. Wash hands	☐	☐	☐
E. Assemble equipment			
* 1. reconstitute the ribivarin	☐	☐	☐
* 2. add to reservoir to 300 ml	☐	☐	☐
* 3. place cap on nebulizer reservoir	☐	☐	☐
* 4. place nebulizer in housing	☐	☐	☐
* 5. insert drying chamber	☐	☐	☐
* 6. connect tubing	☐	☐	☐
F. Take precautions			
* 1. wear gown, gloves, goggles, mask	☐	☐	☐
* 2. close room door	☐	☐	☐
G. Evaluate patient			
* 1. vital signs, breath sounds, oxygenation status	☐	☐	☐
2. other evaluation as necessary	☐	☐	☐
H. Attach to patient			
* 1. connect SPAG to delivery device	☐	☐	☐
* 2. connect source gas	☐	☐	☐
* 3. adjust pressure to 26 psi	☐	☐	☐
* 4. adjust nebulizer flow	☐	☐	☐
* 5. adjust drying chamber flow	☐	☐	☐
* I. Conclude procedure: appropriate disposal of gear	☐	☐	☐
* J. Monitor appropriately	☐	☐	☐
* K. Document procedure in chart	☐	☐	☐

SCORE:

Peer: _____ points out of _____ (66) _____ %

Lab: _____ points out of _____ (66) _____ %

Clinical: _____ points out of _____ (66) _____ %

TIME: _____ out of possible 25 minutes.

STUDENT SIGNATURES   **INSTRUCTOR SIGNATURES**

PEER: _____   LAB: _____

STUDENT: _____   CLINICAL: _____

ADDITIONAL PERFORMANCE EVALUATIONS

The following blank performance evaluation is provided to allow the lab or clinical instructor or the student to make custom evaluations according to special procedures that may not be included in the preceding evaluations. Photocopies can be made as necessary.

METERED DOSE INHALER

OBJECTIVE

The student will be able to correctly assemble the necessary equipment and administer medication via a metered dose inhaler in a laboratory and clinical setting. This will be done following aseptic guidelines and in a competent manner as determined by lab and clinical instructors.

TASK A: Review the Chart. Before proceeding, the patient chart should be reviewed. The student should first check the order to ensure that the prescribed medication and dosage are appropriate and being followed. Evaluate the presence of any contraindications to the therapy and the patient's current condition, as noted in the progress and nursing notes. This will help the student prepare for interaction with the patient and any potential changes that may be warranted in the therapy.

The patient's response to previous therapy should be reviewed for possible adverse side effects or other problems encountered. These notes should serve as a follow-up and reminder of the report received on the patient. During the chart review, the student will note any orders or indications for patient isolation techniques.

TASK B: Obtain the Equipment. You will need the proper medication inhaler, a valved holding chamber with a mouthpiece or appropriate size mask, and a stethoscope for evaluation of breath sounds.

For patients old enough to perform the maneuver, generally those older than 5 years of age, peak flow measurements should be done before and after bronchodilator administration to evaluate the effectiveness of the therapy. You will therefore require a peak flow meter for these patients.

Finally, because of the possibility of contact with secretions, the student should obtain a pair of exam gloves.

TASK C: Wash Hands, Observe Universal Precautions. After gathering the necessary equipment, the student should perform a thorough hand washing, after which gloves should be worn.

TASK D: Confirm Patient. Before administration of any drug to a patient, confirm that you have the correct patient by looking at the name bracelet attached to a patient limb.

TASK E: Assess Patient. Before administering the therapy, the student should auscultate the patient's lungs and evaluate breath sounds. Careful auscultation is necessary to provide a baseline for comparison following therapy. The student should also check the pulse rate, respiratory rate and effort, and peak flow.

TASK F: Position Patient. To achieve the best expansion of the lung bases, the patient should be elevated to an upright position for the treatment. For patients who are unable to be elevated, the therapy may be modified as needed.

TASK G: Administer Therapy. Assemble the equipment by attaching the inhaler to the inlet of the valved holding chamber. Shake well.

Place the mouthpiece in the patient's mouth or the mask over the mouth and nose. Press the inhaler to actuate and release one puff of medication into the chamber. Allow the patient to breath in and out for 3 to 4 breaths, until the chamber is cleared of medication. An older child may be instructed to hold each breath for a few seconds before exhaling.

Repeat until the ordered number of medication puffs have been administered.

TASK H: Monitor the Patient. During the treatment, the patient is monitored for pulse rate, respiratory rate and pattern, and any adverse side effects.

TASK I: Conclude the Procedure. After the appropriate dose of medication has been administered, disassemble the device. If inhaled steroids have been given, the patient's mouth should be rinsed with water to help prevent yeast infection.

Now ask the patient to cough. Any secretions should be placed in a tissue or other appropriate receptacle. Repeat the patient assessment, including breath sounds, heart rate, respiratory rate and effort, and peak flow. Return the patient to the previous or other desired position.

TASK J: Record in the Patient Chart: Chart the appropriate information in the patient record. These data should include before and after breath sounds, heart rate, peak flows, and respiratory effort, as well as a description of patient toleration, sputum production, and any adverse effects.

Task K: Hand Washing. Wash hands again.

PERFORMANCE EVALUATION 24
METERED DOSE INHALER

Date: Lab _____   Clinical _____   Hospital _____

Lab: Pass _____ Fail _____   Clinical: Pass _____   Fail _____

Student name _____   Instructor name _____

Number of required observations: Lab _____   Clinical _____

Number of times observed: Lab _____   Clinical _____

Number of required practices: Lab _____   Clinical _____

Number of times practice: Lab _____   Clinical _____

PASSING CRITERIA:

Obtain 90 percent or better on the procedure. Tasks indicated by an asterisk (*) must receive at least 1 point or the evaluation is terminated. The procedure must be performed within the designated time or the performance receives a failing grade.

SCORING:

2 points—Task performed satisfactorily without prompting.
1 point—Task performed satisfactorily with self-initiated correction.
0 points—Task performed incorrectly or with prompting required.
NA—Task not applicable to the patient care situation

TASKS:	PEER	LAB	CLINICAL
A. Review chart			
1. check order	☐	☐	☐
2. contraindications	☐	☐	☐
3. patient condition	☐	☐	☐
4. past response to therapy	☐	☐	☐
5. orders or indications for isolation	☐	☐	☐
B. Obtain equipment			
1. medication inhaler	☐	☐	☐
2. valved holding chamber	☐	☐	☐
3. stethoscope	☐	☐	☐
4. peak flowmeter	☐	☐	☐
5. exam gloves	☐	☐	☐

TASKS:	PEER	LAB	CLINICAL
C. Wash hands; put on gloves	☐	☐	☐
D. Confirm identity of patient	☐	☐	☐
E. Assess patient			
1. breath sounds	☐	☐	☐
2. pulse rate	☐	☐	☐
3. respiratory rate and effort	☐	☐	☐
4. peak flow	☐	☐	☐
F. Position patient	☐	☐	☐
G. Administer therapy			
1. assemble inhaler and holding chamber	☐	☐	☐
2. apply to patient	☐	☐	☐
3. actuate canister	☐	☐	☐
4. allow patient to breathe until chamber is cleared	☐	☐	☐
5. instruct patient on proper technique	☐	☐	☐
6. repeat until ordered dose is given	☐	☐	☐
H. Monitor patient			
1. pulse rate	☐	☐	☐
2. respiratory rate and pattern	☐	☐	☐
3. adverse side effects	☐	☐	☐
I. Conclude procedure			
1. disassemble MDI from holding chamber	☐	☐	☐
2. have patient rinse mouth	☐	☐	☐
3. have patient cough	☐	☐	☐
4. reassess patient			
a. breath sounds	☐	☐	☐
b. pulse rate	☐	☐	☐
c. respiratory rate and effort	☐	☐	☐
d. peak flow	☐	☐	☐
5. Return patient to desired position	☐	☐	☐
J. Record results and observations	☐	☐	☐

SCORE:

Peer: _____ points out of _____ (66) _____ %

Lab: _____ points out of _____ (66) _____ %

Clinical: _____ points out of _____ (66) _____ %

TIME: _____ out of possible 25 minutes.

STUDENT SIGNATURES   INSTRUCTOR SIGNATURES

PEER: _____   LAB: _____

STUDENT: _____   CLINICAL: _____

PERFORMANCE EVALUATION FOR

_____

Date: Lab _____   Clinical _____   Hospital _____

Lab: Pass _____ Fail _____   Clinical: Pass _____   Fail _____

Student name _____   Instructor name _____

Number of required observations: Lab _____   Clinical _____

Number of times observed: Lab _____   Clinical _____

Number of required practices: Lab _____   Clinical _____

Number of times practice: Lab _____   Clinical _____

PASSING CRITERIA:

Obtain 90 percent or better on the procedure. Tasks indicated by an asterisk (*) must receive at least 1 point or the evaluation is terminated. The procedure must be performed within the designated time or the performance receives a failing grade.

SCORING:

2 points—Task performed satisfactorily without prompting.
1 point—Task performed satisfactorily with self-initiated correction.
0 points—Task performed incorrectly or with prompting required.
NA—Task not applicable to the patient care situation

TASKS:

	PEER	LAB	CLINICAL
_____	☐	☐	☐
_____	☐	☐	☐
_____	☐	☐	☐
_____	☐	☐	☐
_____	☐	☐	☐
_____	☐	☐	☐
_____	☐	☐	☐
_____	☐	☐	☐
_____	☐	☐	☐
_____	☐	☐	☐
_____	☐	☐	☐
_____	☐	☐	☐
_____	☐	☐	☐
_____	☐	☐	☐
_____	☐	☐	☐
_____	☐	☐	☐
_____	☐	☐	☐
_____	☐	☐	☐
_____	☐	☐	☐

TASKS:	**PEER**	**LAB**	**CLINICAL** (fill in title)
_____	☐	☐	☐
_____	☐	☐	☐
_____	☐	☐	☐
_____	☐	☐	☐
_____	☐	☐	☐
_____	☐	☐	☐
_____	☐	☐	☐
_____	☐	☐	☐
_____	☐	☐	☐
_____	☐	☐	☐
_____	☐	☐	☐
_____	☐	☐	☐
_____	☐	☐	☐
_____	☐	☐	☐
_____	☐	☐	☐
_____	☐	☐	☐
_____	☐	☐	☐
_____	☐	☐	☐
_____	☐	☐	☐
_____	☐	☐	☐
_____	☐	☐	☐
_____	☐	☐	☐
_____	☐	☐	☐
_____	☐	☐	☐
_____	☐	☐	☐
_____	☐	☐	☐
_____	☐	☐	☐
_____	☐	☐	☐
_____	☐	☐	☐
_____	☐	☐	☐
_____	☐	☐	☐
_____	☐	☐	☐
_____	☐	☐	☐

SCORE:

Peer: _____ points out of _____ (66) _____ %

Lab: _____ points out of _____ (66) _____ %

Clinical: _____ points out of _____ (66) _____ %

TIME: _____ out of possible 25 minutes.

STUDENT SIGNATURES

PEER: _____

STUDENT: _____

INSTRUCTOR SIGNATURES

LAB: _____

CLINICAL: _____

Bibliography and Suggested Readings

American Association for Respiratory Care. Clinical practice guideline for postural drainage therapy. *Respir Care.* 1991;36:1418–1426.

American Association for Respiratory Care. Clinical practice guideline for arterial blood gas analysis. *Respir Care.* 1992;37:913–917.

American Association for Respiratory Care. Clinical practice guideline for nasotracheal suctioning. *Respir Care.* 1992;37:898–901.

American Association for Respiratory Care. Clinical practice guideline for endotracheal suctioning of mechanically ventilated adults and children with artificial airways. *Respir Care.* 1993;38:500–504.

American Association for Respiratory Care. Clinical practice guideline for capillary blood gas sampling for neonatal and pediatric patients. *Respir Care.* 1994;39:1180–1183.

American Association for Respiratory Care. Clinical practice guideline for selection of an aerosol delivery device for neonatal and pediatric patients. *Respir Care.* 1995;40:1325–1335.

American Association for Respiratory Care. Clinical practice guidelines for selection of an oxygen delivery device for neonatal and pediatric patients. *Respir Care.* 1996;41:637–646.

National Heart, Lung, and Blood Institute. *Facts about Controlling Asthma.* NIH publication 97-2339, 1997.

APPENDIX B

SPECIALITY EXAMINATION STUDY GUIDE

GENERAL TEST-TAKING STRATEGIES

As you probably already know, there is no such thing as a perfect test. Every test you have ever taken will include areas that you feel are clear and fair and other areas that seem vague and unfair. Because it is impossible to prepare for exactly what will be on the Perinatal/ Pediatric Respiratory Care Specialty Examination, the best preparation is to understand some general strategies in test-taking. By following these strategies, the practitioner will be better prepared for any examination. Before examining each strategy, it must be understood that it *is* possible to learn how to take tests.

EFFECTIVE PREPARATION

The first step in effective preparation is to *begin early*. In fact, it is never too early to begin studying for the examination. If you have not already started, start today. Before you actually begin studying, you must know *what* to study. This study guide has been designed to do exactly that, to point out what to study in order to prepare for the Perinatal/Pediatric Specialty Examination.

The next important step is to *study regularly*. Just like exercise, studying is most effective when you do it on a regular basis. A successful test-taker is one who does no "cram" at the last minute. It is important to deliberately structure your time. Schedule a certain starting and stopping time. Set aside a certain time of day when you will study. Plan to study in an environment that is free from distractions. The amount of time is not as important as the environment. You can accomplish more in 15 minutes in a quiet, comfortable environment than studying for one hour in an environment with frequent disruptions and noise.

Ideally, the studying should be done in the same location and at the same time each day. Start with the most difficult areas first. It is the tendency of most people to work on the easy areas first and putting off the harder areas for later. Resist that temptation and work on the harder areas first.

If you are going to be studying for an hour or more, be sure to take a five- to ten-minute break at regular intervals. Do not study until you are exhausted and then take a break. Breaks every 30 minutes or so will help to keep you fresh. During the breaks, stand up and move around, do some relaxation exercises and massage your neck and other tense areas. Never try to study when you are tired or sleepy.

If you begin your studying early on, you will eventually reach the point where you feel you understand the material. When you reach this point, continue to study! It is beneficial to be *overprepared* when taking an examination. However, this is true only to a certain point. As a general rule, study for an additional 25% of the time you have spent thus far.

Another important strategy in examination preparation is to review tests that are similar to the one you will be taking. The sample test provided in this study guide will be an excellent review for the type of questions you will encounter. Understanding these types of questions and practicing the thought processes involved will be a tremendous help in your preparation. It is recommended that you become very acquainted with the test format by thoroughly reading the portion of this book dealing with the NBRC type questions. When reviewing and taking the sample examinations, duplicate the testing environment as much as possible. Take the sample examination using the same rules and regulations set down in the NBRC guidelines. Duplicate and use the supplied answer sheet. Mark your answers by filling in the bubble by the correct response with a pencil. Follow the time limit constraints. Get used to sitting and taking the practice examination in a two-hour session. Do not use a calculator or notes, because you will not have these available during the actual examination. By duplicating the conditions during practice examinations, your comfort level will increase before taking the actual examination, and your chances of successfully passing will increase.

Next, *organize* your studying. It is best to start by getting an overview of the material. For this examination, it may be best to break the test into general areas such as the three content areas, or even break it into smaller areas. As you review the chosen area, make note of the general ideas and themes. If you are studying from a textbook, highlight the main concepts and ideas. Writing notes will help reinforce the concepts in your memory.

The last step in examination preparation is to *review* your notes and material on a regular basis. Reviewing helps you to recall those areas previously studied and greatly enhances retention of the material.

ENVIRONMENTAL VARIABLES

Most everyone suffers from some degree of anxiety when taking an examination. Although stress cannot always be eliminated altogether, there are several things that can be done to lower the level of stress.

First, following the examination preparation steps outlined above will reduce the stress caused by entering the examination unprepared. One of the biggest stress producers is the feeling of being unprepared for what is on the examination. Proper preparation will greatly reduce this stress.

Stress is also reduced by entering the examination well rested and healthy. For this reason, it is unwise to cram the night before. Save the night before the test to relax and get to bed early. Arise early enough to arrive at the testing center at least 30 minutes before the examination is scheduled to start. A hurried morning, or an unexpected delay in transit only serve to increase anxiety. The more calm, cool, and collected you are when you begin the examination, the better you will do. Do not take a tranquilizer or other drug, which may interfere with your judgment or make you drowsy. Wear comfortable clothing, particularly in layers. This way you can adjust your own comfort level in the room by removing or adding a layer of clothing. Anything you can do to increase your comfort level will enhance your chances of success.

Although it is oftentimes impossible to avoid sickness, it is never too early to begin a regime of regular exercise. Physical well-being can tremendously enhance the ability to perform well on the examination. Some light exercise just before the examination will help to relax and loosen up tense muscles. Perhaps a brisk walk around the testing center would be possible before entering to take the examination.

During the examination, stop regularly to stretch your muscles, take a few deep breaths, close your eyes, and relax for just a few moments. This will help you fresh and avoid the fatigue that often accompanies long stretches of intense concentration.

USE OF YOUR TIME DURING THE EXAMINATION

For the Perinatal/Pediatric Respiratory Care Specialty Examination, you will be given two hours to complete 100 questions. In order to complete the examination within the allotted time period, it will be necessary to allocate your time wisely.

When the examination begins, the proctor will announce the starting time and the finishing time. You should bring an accurate watch that you can use to follow your progress through the examination. For this examination, if every question were allotted the same amount of time, you would have one minute and twelve seconds for each question. However, you will find that some questions can be answered much quicker and some will take longer to answer. The key is not to spend too much time on any one question. If you are spending too much time on a question, or you do not know the answer, circle it and return to it later. By circling the answer and coming back, there may be a question further into the examination that stimulates your thought process and will allow you to answer the previous question. If you elect to do this, take care when placing your responses on the answer sheet so as not to get succeeding answers in the wrong place. Periodically check the time and assess how well you are using the time. For example, by 30 minutes into the examination, you should be near question number 25, at one hour question number 50, and so on.

It may prove helpful to write any equations down before beginning the examination in the front of the booklet. This technique frees your mind from the stress of trying to recall the information when fatigue has set in and makes recall more difficult.

When you have reached the end of the examination, return to those questions you had circled and spend the remaining time answering them.

ANSWERING QUESTIONS WHEN YOU DO NOT KNOW THE ANSWER

The question always arises what to do with those questions in which the answer is not known. Is it best to leave it unanswered, or to simply guess? The answer to that question is that it is always better to guess than to leave the question unanswered. The Perinatal/Pediatric Specialty Examination is graded on how many correct answers are achieved out of 100 possible. Therefore, every unanswered question is counted as a missed question and counts against the candidate. Instead of randomly choosing an answer, there is a strategy for guessing that will improve your chance of getting the correct answer.

First, it cannot be emphasized strongly enough to thoroughly understand the question before attempting to answer the question. Look for words, such as not, never, always, will, which may change the nature of the question. Do not read anything into the question. Let us use the following question as an example.

TABLE B–1   Preparation for the Examination

A. Content
   1. Start early
   2. Know what to study
   3. Study regularly
     a. schedule a start and stop time
     b. plan a consistent time
     c. have a regular study area
   4. Study the most difficult areas first
   5. Take breaks at regular intervals
   6. Be overprepared rather than underprepared
   7. Review tests that are similar to the target test
     a. duplicate the expected testing conditions
   8. Organize your study
     a. start with an overview
     b. divide material into content areas
     c. make copious notes
   9. Review notes and materials regularly
B. Environmental Variables
   1. Decrease stress
     a. be prepared
     b. be rested
     c. relax
   2. Arrive early
     a. do relaxation exercises
     b. have proper materials
     c. wear comfortable, layered clothing

---

1. A neonate is being ventilated at a peak inspiratory pressure of 30 cm H_2O, with a PEEP of 5 cm H_2O at a rate of 40 breaths per minute and an FiO_2 of 0.40. The transcutaneous oxygen monitor is reading a PaO_2 of 45 mm Hg. Which of the following would you recommend?
   A. Increase the PIP to 35 cm H_2O
   B. Increase the PEEP to 7 cm H_2O
   C. Increase the temperature of the incubator
   D. Increase the FiO_2 to 0.50

If the candidate were to read into the question, any of the choices could be viable answers. For example, if the patient has RDS, we could justify increasing the PIP. However, the question does not tell us about breath sounds or chest excursion or even that the patient has RDS. Again, if the patient is being exposed to cold stress, it may be appropriate to increase the temperature of the incubator. The question does not tell us that the patient is cold and therefore we cannot justify increasing the temperature. These are examples of reading into the question more information than is given.

Once you feel you understand the question, examine each choice carefully. What you will try to do is to eliminate as many of the choices as possible to improve your odds of choosing the correct answer. For example, if you are given four choices, there is a 25% chance that you will guess correctly. If you can rule out one of the choices, the odds increase to 33%. If you can rule out two of the choices, the odds become 50%.

If none of the choices can be eliminated, go with your first impression. Although this is a poor method of answering a question, often one of the choices will "feel" right. Once the choice is made, do not second guess and continue changing the answer. This is true of the test in general. Once an answer has been chosen, do not change it unless you are certain the wrong choice was made.

In summary, read the question carefully until you understand what is wanted. Answer only what is asked, do not answer what you *think* should have been asked. Do not jump to any conclusions after reading the question and watch for key words in the question that may change the meaning of the question.

NBRC RULES FOR THE EXAMINATION

Before discussing the examination rules, it is important to point out that the NBRC has a study guide that is available to anyone who requests it. The study guide includes all administrative policies and rules for the examination as well as a section that details the examination matrix among test-taking hints. This booklet is available by request at the address that follows:

The National Board for Respiratory Care, Inc.
8310 Nieman Road
Lenexa, Kansas 66214
(913) 599-4200

In order to be better prepared for the examination, it is helpful to understand the basic rules that have been established for this examination. The following summarizes those rules that have been instituted by the NBRC.

1. Take several sharpened pencils (No. 2 only) with you to the examination, because it is possible that pencils will not be available at the test center. Pens, colored pencils, and felt-tip pens cannot be used.
2. Although the official time is kept by the test supervisor, it is advisable to bring a watch to help pace yourself.
3. Nothing (including calculators) may be taken into the examination room, except your admission papers and personal items (i.e., coat, pencils, etc.).
4. Nothing may be taken from the examination room.
5. You cannot ask any questions regarding the examination content during the test.
6. You will be provided a form on which you may comment on questions you believe to be misleading or inaccurate.

7. You may leave the examination room during the examination but only once you have the supervisor's permission to leave. Any time you miss while out of the room is part of the two-hour period and you are not given additional time.

8. There are several reasons in which a candidate may be dismissed from the test, including:
   - unauthorized admission
   - creating a disturbance or being abusive
   - giving or receiving help
   - attempting to remove test materials
   - taking the test for someone else

THE TEST MATRIX AND NBRC TYPE QUESTIONS

The test matrix is a description of the content of the examination and the number and type of question for each content area. In brief, the test is broken down into three main content areas: 1) Clinical Data; 2) Equipment/Quality Control; and 3) Therapeutic Procedures.

The NBRC uses three types of questions on the examination. The first and most basic type of question is the simple multiple choice question. The following is an example of this type of question:

1. Which of the following arteries exits directly from the aortic arch?
   A. Brachial
   B. Right internal carotid
   C. Left subclavian
   D. Pulmonary
   ANSWER: C

In this type of question, there is only one *best* response. Some questions of this type may have four possible answers; however, only one will be the *best* response.

A second variety of question found on the examination is the multiple true-false questions. An example of this type of question is as follows:

1. Which of the following test(s) is/are done to assess the status of the fetus?
   I. Silverman-Anderson
   II. Cordocentesis
   III. APGAR
   IV. "Shake Test"
      A. I, II and III
      B. I and II only
      C. II, III and IV
      D. II and IV only
   ANSWER: D

This type of question is best answered by evaluating each choice after thoroughly reading the question. Place a "T" or "F" by those which are true or false according to the question. The correct combination of choices can then be determined and the correct answer selected. Again, if all responses cannot be answered either "T" or "F," by answering the responses you are sure of, you can increase your chances of answering the question correctly by eliminating answers that contain false information.

The third type of question used on the examination is a situational set. In this type of question, the candidate is given a short patient care scenario followed by one or more questions. An example of this type of question is as follows:

1. A 32-week neonate is delivered and rushed to the resuscitation room. One minute following delivery you note that respiratory effort is weak, the heart rate is 85, the limbs are flaccid, the patient is cyanotic over its entire body, and it only grimaces when the nose is suctioned. This patient's Apgar score is:
   A. 1
   B. 3
   C. 5
   D. 7
ANSWER: B

2. With a heart rate of 85, this patient will require which of the following?
   A. Manual Ventilation
   B. Epinephrine
   C. Chest Compressions
   D. Arterial Blood Gas
ANSWER: A

The Perinatal/Pediatric Specialty Examination uses three levels of difficulty in the questions. The content areas and number of questions are outlined in Table B–2.

The easiest level is the *recall* question. In this type of question, the candidate is asked to identify and recall specific information. As an example, the question may ask where the pulse is palpated on a infant during a resuscitation. There are a total of 19 questions of this type: 6 in the clinical data area, 4 in the equipment/quality control data area and 9 in the therapeutic procedures area.

The next level of difficulty are the *application* questions. In this type of question, candidates must be able to relate their knowledge to changing conditions and situations. For example, the question may describe a patient whose arterial oxygen saturation is dropping. The candidate must then determine what the appropriate response would be. In the examination, there are a total of 61 questions of this variety: 18 in the clinical data area; 12 in the equipment/quality control area; and 31 in the therapeutic procedures area.

The most difficult of the three question types is the *analysis* type of question. These questions build on the first two types and require the candidate to analyze the given information and arrive at the correct solution. An example of this type of question would be to give the candidate current ventilator settings and the results of an arterial blood gas analysis.

TABLE B–2 Examination Content and Questions

Content Area	Recall	Application	Analysis
Clinical Data	6	18	6
Equipment/Quality Control	4	12	4
Therapeutic Procedures	9	31	10
Total	19	61	20

The candidate must then determine appropriate changes that need to be made on the ventilator. In the examination, there are a total of 20 questions of this type; 6 in the clinical data area; 4 in the equipment/quality control area; and 10 in the therapeutic procedures area.

PERINATAL/PEDIATRIC PRACTICE EXAMINATION

This practice examination is included to help prepare for the Perinatal/Pediatric Specialty Examination. It is recommended that this examination be taken under similar circumstances to the actual examination. The practitioner should allow two hours to take this examination. Please use the answer key on the following pages to answer the questions.

ANSWER KEY FOR PRACTICE EXAMINATION

QUESTION NUMBER	ANSWER			
	A	B	C	D
1.	○	○	○	○
2.	○	○	○	○
3.	○	○	○	○
4.	○	○	○	○
5.	○	○	○	○
6.	○	○	○	○
7.	○	○	○	○
8.	○	○	○	○
9.	○	○	○	○
10.	○	○	○	○
11.	○	○	○	○
12.	○	○	○	○
13.	○	○	○	○
14.	○	○	○	○
15.	○	○	○	○
16.	○	○	○	○
17.	○	○	○	○
18.	○	○	○	○
19.	○	○	○	○
20.	○	○	○	○
21.	○	○	○	○
22.	○	○	○	○
23.	○	○	○	○
24.	○	○	○	○
25.	○	○	○	○
26.	○	○	○	○
27.	○	○	○	○
28.	○	○	○	○
29.	○	○	○	○
30.	○	○	○	○
31.	○	○	○	○
32.	○	○	○	○
33.	○	○	○	○
34.	○	○	○	○
35.	○	○	○	○
36.	○	○	○	○
37.	○	○	○	○
38.	○	○	○	○
39.	○	○	○	○
40.	○	○	○	○

QUESTION NUMBER	ANSWER			
	A	B	C	D
41.	○	○	○	○
42.	○	○	○	○
43.	○	○	○	○
44.	○	○	○	○
45.	○	○	○	○
46.	○	○	○	○
47.	○	○	○	○
48.	○	○	○	○
49.	○	○	○	○
50.	○	○	○	○
51.	○	○	○	○
52.	○	○	○	○
53.	○	○	○	○
54.	○	○	○	○
55.	○	○	○	○
56.	○	○	○	○
57.	○	○	○	○
58.	○	○	○	○
59.	○	○	○	○
60.	○	○	○	○
61.	○	○	○	○
62.	○	○	○	○
63.	○	○	○	○
64.	○	○	○	○
65.	○	○	○	○
66.	○	○	○	○
67.	○	○	○	○
68.	○	○	○	○
69.	○	○	○	○
70.	○	○	○	○
71.	○	○	○	○
72.	○	○	○	○
73.	○	○	○	○
74.	○	○	○	○
75.	○	○	○	○
76.	○	○	○	○
77.	○	○	○	○
78.	○	○	○	○
79.	○	○	○	○
80.	○	○	○	○
81.	○	○	○	○
82.	○	○	○	○

QUESTION NUMBER	ANSWER			
	A	B	C	D
83.	○	○	○	○
84.	○	○	○	○
85.	○	○	○	○
86.	○	○	○	○
87.	○	○	○	○
88.	○	○	○	○
89.	○	○	○	○
90.	○	○	○	○
91.	○	○	○	○
92.	○	○	○	○
93.	○	○	○	○
94.	○	○	○	○
95.	○	○	○	○
96.	○	○	○	○
97.	○	○	○	○
98.	○	○	○	○
99.	○	○	○	○
100.	○	○	○	○

1. An 8-year-old patient is placed on a volume cycled ventilator. The following information is available:

Height	50 inches
Weight	60 pounds

   Which of the following is an appropriate tidal volume for this patient?
   A. 330 ml
   B. 450 ml
   C. 520 ml
   D. 600 ml

2. While performing an initial assessment on a newborn infant, the respiratory care practitioner notices that the entire body is blanched and pale with a rapid heart rate. This is most consistent with which of the following?
   A. Respiratory distress syndrome
   B. Hypovolemic anemia
   C. Congenital heart defect
   D. Acrocyanosis

3. A history given by a young woman presenting to the physician's office for her first prenatal examination reveals the following information:

Age:	23 years
Marital Status:	Unwed
Living Conditions:	Lives in low-income housing
Ethnicity:	Native American

   Which of the above factors would NOT be considered a high-risk factor?
   A. Age
   B. Marital Status
   C. Living Conditions
   D. Ethnicity

4. All of the following are indications for the administration of a bronchodilator EXCEPT
   A. Decreasing $PaCO_2$
   B. Decreased chest expansion
   C. Wheezes
   D. Increasing ventilator pressures

5. A 1300 g neonate is being ventilated at a peak pressure of 32 cm H_2O, a PEEP of 6 cm H_2O, an FiO_2 of 0.70, and a rate of 65 breaths per minute. During a ventilator check, the respiratory care practitioner notes that the heart sounds have shifted slightly to the left. A chest radiograph is obtained and upon viewing, it appears as though there is a "bat-wing" in the patient's thorax. Which of the following is the most probable diagnosis?
   A. Pneumonia
   B. Pneumomediastinum

    C. Pneumopericardium
    D. Pulmonary interstitial emphysema

6. Following 1 week of mechanical ventilation for treatment of diffuse trauma, a pediatric patient's lung compliance begins a worsening trend. The chest radiograph shows diffuse atelectasis throughout the lung fields. Current ventilator parameters are

Rate	18/minute
Vt	450 ml
FiO_2	0.56
Compliance	28 ml/cm H_2O

Which of the following is the most appropriate recommendation?
    A. Initiate chest physiotherapy.
    B. Initiate aerosolized bronchodilators.
    C. Initiate PEEP.
    D. Initiate antibiotic therapy.

7. A 12-year-old patient has been hospitalized for 4 weeks for the treatment of a head injury. The patient received a tracheostomy 24 hours previously. The following information is available:

Visual examination	Retractions
Auscultation	Coarse rhonchi

Which of the following would be most appropriate at this time?
    A. Suction the patient's airway.
    B. Initiate chest physiotherapy.
    C. Initiate mucolytic aerosol therapy.
    D. Increase the inspired humidity.

8. A premature neonate is being manually ventilated at a rate of 120 breaths/minute, a peak pressure of 35 cm H_2O, PEEP of 5 cm H_2O, and FiO_2 of 1.0. The following arterial blood gas is obtained.

pH	7.18
$PaCO_2$	65 torr
HCO_3	17 mEq/Liter
PaO_2	45 torr

Breath sounds are equal with good chest excursion and a loud ductal murmur is heard on auscultation. Which of the following is the BEST recommendation?
    A. Increase the FiO_2
    B. Increase the peak pressure.
    C. Increase the PEEP.
    D. Give bicarbonate.

9. A newborn is being mechanically ventilated on a time cycled, pressure limited ventilator. The ventilatory parameters are as follows.

Rate	40/minute
Peak pressure	32 cm H_2O
PEEP	5 cm H_2O
Inspiratory time	0.4 second

Which of the following is the I:E ratio?

A. 1:1.5

B. 1:2.25

C. 1:2.75

D. 1:3.5

10. A transcutaneous PO_2 monitor is being used on a 32-week the neonate. The respiratory care practitioner notes that the $TcPO_2$ is consistently lower than the actual PaO_2 and the monitor does not trend with PaO_2. Which of the following may be the cause/s of this inconsistency?

I. Inappropriate electrode temperature.

II. Patient has a compromised hemodynamic status

III. There is excessive pressure on the electrode.

IV. Excessive perfusion at the probe site.

A. I, II, IV only

B. II and III only

C. I, II, III, and IV

D. I, II, III only

11. Which of the following is the minimal liter flow used with an oxyhood to reduce the possibility of CO_2 retention?

A. 4 L/minute

B. 7 L/minute

C. 10 L/minute

D. 15 L/minute

12. Following 30 seconds of positive pressure ventilation using an FiO_2 of 1.0, the heart rate of a neonate being resuscitated is noted to be 18 beats in a 15-second period. Which of the following is the next step in the resuscitation?

A. Continue ventilation and monitor the heart rate.

B. Administer epinephrine 1:10,000 via instillation into the endotracheal tube.

C. Begin external cardiac compressions.

D. Initiate ECG monitoring.

13. Which of the following drugs would produce anesthesia for performing a bronchoscopy?

A. Morphine

B. Chloral Hydrate

C. Pancuronium

D. Fentanyl

14. While auscultating the chest of a 36-week neonate, the respiratory care practitioner hears an abnormal sound following the first heart sound, ending before the second sound is heard. This is BEST described as a:
    I. Systolic murmur
    II. Diastolic murmur
    III. End-systolic gallop
    IV. Primary murmur
       A. IV only
       B. I or III only
       C. II or IV only
       D. I only

15. An infant is being mechanically ventilated on a pressure limited, time cycled ventilator. The following information is available.

Rate	40/minute
Peak pressure	25 cm H_2O
PEEP	4 cm H_2O
I:time	1 second

    A recent chest radiograph shows signs of air trapping and the patient's ventilation is worsening. Which of the following is the BEST recommendation?
    A. Increase the rate of ventilation.
    B. Increase the peak pressure.
    C. Decrease the PEEP.
    D. Decrease the respiratory time.

16. One minute following delivery, a neonate is assessed to have a weak respiratory effort, heart rate of 135, acrocyanosis, and some flexion of the extremities. The baby cries and coughs when a suction catheter is inserted into the nares. Which of the following BEST reflects this patient's Apgar score?
    A. 9
    B. 7
    C. 5
    D. 3

17. While visually inspecting a 41-week neonate, the respiratory care practitioner notices that although the patient's body is pink, the hands and feet are blue in appearance. This phenomenon is known as:
    A. Acrocyanosis
    B. Peripheral cyanosis
    C. Poor perfusion to the extremities
    D. Patent ductus arteriosus

18. Palpation of the brachail pulses in a 2-day-old neonate shows them to be strong and equal while the femoral pulses appear to be of a decreased force. The most likely cause of this is:

A. Coarctation of the aorta
B. Patent ductus arteriosus
C. Ventricular septal defect
D. Diaphragmatic hernia

19. Which of the following would be considered a normal systolic blood pressure for a 1000 g neonate?
    A. 75 mm Hg
    B. 68 mm Hg
    C. 50 mm Hg
    D. 35 mm Hg

20. A neonate being ventilated on a pressure limited, time cycled ventilator has the following arterial blood gas values:

pH	7.29
$PaCO_2$	52 torr
PaO_2	75 torr
HCO_3	23 mEq/liter

    Which of the following would be the most appropriate changes?
    I. Increase the peak pressure.
    II. Decrease the ventilator rate.
    III. Increase the PEEP.
    IV. Increase the FiO_2.
        A. I, II, and IV
        B. I only
        C. I and II only
        D. I, II, III

21. A 35-week neonate is brought from the delivery room to the NICU for resuscitation. The respiratory care practitioner notes that the patient is in extreme respiratory distress with unequal chest excursion and a scaphoid abdomen. The most likely diagnosis:
    A. Respiratory Distress Syndrome
    B. Diaphragmatic hernia
    C. Pneumothorax
    D. Pulmonary Edema

22. A 3-week-old term infant is admitted to the pediatric unit for the treatment of croup. The suction regulator is still in the room from the previous pediatric patient with the regulator set at –75 mm Hg of pressure. The respiratory care practitioner should:
    A. Leave the regular at the present setting.
    B. Increase the pressure to –90 mm Hg.
    C. Decrease the pressure to –40 mm Hg.
    D. Recommend changing the regulator.

23. The presence of which of the following would indicate the least likelihood of a neonate developing Respiratory Distress Syndrome?
    A. PI
    B. PG
    C. PC
    D. L/S ratio of 1:1

24. Which of the following are required when attempting an intubation on a newborn?
    I. Laryngoscope and blade
    II. Pediatric bronchoscope
    III. Resuscitation bag and mask
    IV. Suction equipment
        A. I, II, and III only
        B. I, III, and IV only
        C. II, III, and IV only
        D. I, II, III, and IV

25. Ribavirin is indicated for which of the following infections?
    A. Respiratory syncytial virus
    B. Gram-positive bacteria
    C. Gram-negative bacteria
    D. Toxoplasmosis

26. While weaning a neonatal patient from mechanical ventilation, the patient becomes tachycardic with an increasing $PaCO_2$. The most appropriate recommendation for this patient is:
    A. Continue weaning the patient.
    B. Obtain a stat chest radiograph.
    C. Reinstitute mechanical ventilation.
    D. Extubate the patient.

27. Which of the following is used to evaluate the degree of respiratory distress in a newborn?
    A. Apgar Score
    B. Glasgow Score
    C. Silverman-Anderson Index
    D. Ballard Score

28. A 980 g, 29-week-gestation neonate is being manually ventilated following delivery. Chest excursion is poor despite high peak pressures. What is most likely to be seen on the chest radiograph of this patient?
    A. Distal air trapping
    B. Reticulogranular pattern
    C. Bilateral emphysematous opacities
    D. Streaky infiltrates

29. The respiratory care practitioner would recommend chest physiotherapy for all of the following reasons EXCEPT
    A. Treatment of atelactasis
    B. Pleural effusion
    C. Lung abscess
    D. Mobilization of secretions

30. A 6-year-old patient is being ventilated by a volume cycled ventilator. The following information is available

Vt	300 ml
Peak pressure	28 cm H_2O
PEEP	5 cm H_2O
Circuit Compliance	2 ml/cm H_2O

    Which of the following is the corrected tidal volume?
    A. 267 ml
    B. 250 ml
    C. 234 ml
    D. 175 ml

31. Following delivery of 35-week twins, twin B is requiring bag-mask ventilation with peak pressures of 35 cm H_2O, an FiO_2 of 0.7, and a rate of 55 breaths/min. Initial blood gas results are as follows:

pH	7.32
$PaCO_2$	46 torr
HCO_3	22 mEq/liter
PaO_2	65 torr

    Which of the following is the most appropriate initial action?
    A. Increase the peak pressure.
    B. Continue with the same therapy.
    C. Intubate the patient.
    D. Recommend the administration of surfactant.

32. Each of the following are hazards of oxygen use EXCEPT
    A. Explosion hazard
    B. Retinopathy of prematurity
    C. Oxygen toxicity
    D. Cerebral vasoconstriction

33. While testing a flow inflating resuscitation bag, the respiratory care practitioner notes that no pressure is generated when the patient connection is occluded and the bag is compressed. All of the following are possible problems EXCEPT
    A. The flow is too low.
    B. The valve seat is not tightened.
    C. There is a leak in the system.
    D. The pop-off valve is set at too low a pressure.

34. While suctioning a 38-week mechanically ventilated infant, the patient's heart rate drops to 85 beats/min. Which of the following is/are the most probable cause/s of this drop in heart rate?
    I. Excessive suctioning pressures
    II. Hypoxia
    III. Hypothermia from excessive exposure
    IV. Vagal stimulation
       A. I, II, and III
       B. I and III only
       C. II and IV only
       D. I, II, III, and IV

35. The cessation of a respiratory effort in the fetus or newborn following an uncorrected hypoxemic episode in which there is no further attempt to breathe is called:
    A. Asphyxia
    B. Hypercapnia
    C. Primary Apnea
    D. Secondary Apnea

36. A respiratory care practitioner is administering oxygen to a 40-week neonate by attaching oxygen tubing from a flowmeter to the incubator. The practitioner is unable to achieve an FiO_2 greater than 0.40. The most probable reason for not attaining the desired FiO_2 is:
    A. It is difficult to achieve an FiO_2 greater than 0.40 in any incubator.
    B. The practitioner is using an older incubator and must lift the arm with the attached red flag.
    C. The oxygen flow must be greater than 60 L/minute.
    D. The flowmeter is defective.

37. The respiratory care practitioner is asked to recommend a parasympatholytic drug for inhalation. Which of the following is the BEST recommendation?
    A. Albuterol sulfate
    B. Ipratropium bromide
    C. Cromolyn sodium
    D. Terbutaline sulfate

38. A respiratory care practitioner notes that the rate of the neonatal ventilator slows when the inspiratory time is increased. Which of the following is the probable cause?
    A. The rate timer is malfunctioning.
    B. The ventilator rate is limited by the I:E ratio.
    C. The ventilator utilizes an expiratory timer.
    D. The inspiratory flow rate is excessive.

39. While ventilating a neonate on an Infant Star ventilator, an audible alarm is triggered and AO2 is displayed. Which of the following is/are the most common cause/s of this alarm?
    I. Electrical failure
    II. A loss of gas pressure
    III. A blocked expiratory tube
    IV. A nonfunctioning expiratory valve
        A. I and II only
        B. I, II, and III only
        C. III and IV only
        D. IV only

40. While using a time cycled, pressure limited ventilator, the respiratory care practitioner is unable to achieve a peak pressure above 25 cm H_2O. Which of the following is the most likely cause?
    A. The inspiratory pop-off valve is activating.
    B. The oxygen pressure is below 30 psi.
    C. The ventilator is malfunctioning.
    D. The ventilator tubing is too compliant.

41. A neonatal patient with Bronchopulmonary Dysplasia is receiving oxygen via a cannula. The patient has had 3 episodes of epistaxis in the last 24 hours. Which of the following is the most likely cause?
    A. The prongs are too large.
    B. The FiO_2 is excessively high.
    C. The flow rate is excessive.
    D. The ambient humidity is low.

42. While using a sidestream type of end-tidal CO_2 monitor on a 10-year-old near-drowning patient being mechanically ventilated, the respiratory care practitioner notes that the analyzer fluctuates severely and oftentimes reads zero over a period of time. Which of the following is the most probable cause of this problem?
    A. The patient's condition is worsening.
    B. There is water in the sample tubing.
    C. The ventilator is being inappropriately managed.
    D. The analyzer is out of calibration.

43. While performing chest physiotherapy on a 31-week neonate, the respiratory care practitioner observes that the patient requires an increase in the FiO_2 0.30 above the starting level. The most appropriate response would be to:
    A. Discontinue the treatment.
    B. Attempt the treatment at a later time.
    C. Stop the treatment and suction the airway.
    D. Do nothing, this is a normal reaction to CPT.

44. Before extubation of a pediatric patient with a cuffed endotracheal tube, which of the following are important considerations?
    I. Withhold continuous feedings.
    II. Deflate the cuff.
    III. Hyperoxygenate the patient.
    IV. Thoroughly suction the tube.
        A. II, III, and IV
        B. I, II, and III
        C. III and IV only
        D. I, I, III, and IV

45. Which of the following sized endotracheal tubes would be appropriate for a 1400 g neonate?
    A. 2.0
    B. 2.5
    C. 3.0
    D. 3.5

46. While working on a 28-week neonate in a radiant warmer, the respiratory care practitioner notes that the low temperature alarm activates. The radiant heater is on and the patient's temperature is normal when measured rectally. Which of the following is the most likely cause of the alarm?
    A. The radiant warmer is malfunctioning.
    B. The environmental humidity is excessive.
    C. The desired set temperature is set too low.
    D. The temperature probe has fallen off the patient.

47. The parent of a newborn receiving home apnea monitoring notifies the respiratory care practitioner that the monitor has multiple false alarms. Which of the following would be the most appropriate initial action?
    A. Check for loose, misapplied, or broken electrodes.
    B. Recommend the patient receive a different monitor.
    C. Advise the patient to turn off the alarm.
    D. Suggest the parent ignore the alarm.

48. The respiratory care practitioner is asked to obtain an arterial blood gas on a 4-day-old infant with a history of a patent ductus arteriosus. Which of the following would BEST reflect pre-ductal blood flow?
    A. Right radial artery
    B. Left radial artery
    C. Umbilical artery
    D. Heel puncture capillary sample

49. The following arterial blood gas is obtained after placing a 39-week newborn in an oxygen hood at an FiO_2 of 0.35 at a flow of 5 L/min. The patient has a history of TTN, with subnormal $PaCO_2$ levels.

pH	7.32
$PaCO_2$	48 torr
$PaCO_2$	68 torr
HCO_3	24 mEq/liter

    Which of the following is the most appropriate initial action?
    A. Increase the FiO_2.
    B. Increase the flow to 8-10 L/min.
    C. Initiate chest physiotherapy.
    D. Place a larger oxyhood on the patient.

50. The "classic method" of measuring lung compliance and airway resistance on a neonate utilizes which of the following to estimate pleural pressure?
    A. Pneumotachograph
    B. Transthoracic catheter
    C. Mouth pressure
    D. Esophageal balloon

51. A 1200 g neonate on mechanical ventilation is being monitored with a pulse oximeter and transcutaneous monitor. Because the patient is unstable, many ventilator changes are being made. Which of the following recommendations would further enhance the ability to properly treat this patient?
    A. Close monitoring of the mean airway pressure
    B. Frequent chest radiographs
    C. The insertion of an umbilical artery catheter
    D. The addition of an end tidal CO_2 monitor

52. A 2-day-old neonate is being mechanically ventilated on an FiO_2 of 1.0, peak pressure of 32 cm H_2O and PEEP of 5 cm H_2O. A pulse oximeter is located on the right wrist and is consistently reading an SPO_2 of 98%. The following UAC blood gas results are obtained.

pH	7.28
$PaCO_2$	52 torr
PaO_2	43 torr
HCO_3	22 mEq/liter
SPO_2	;78%

    These results are consistent with which of the following?
    A. Ventricular septal defect
    B. Coarctation of the aorta
    C. Atrial septal defect
    D. Patent ductus arteriosus

53. While examining the chest radiographs of a 5-day-old mechanically ventilated neonate, the respiratory care practitioner notes an elevated diaphragm on the right side accompanied by a mediastinal shift toward the right lung. There is a decrease in the spaces between the ribs on the right side, and a slight hyperinflation of the left lung. The most likely diagnosis is:
    A. Respiratory Distress Syndrome
    B. Tension Pneumothorax
    C. Atelectasis
    D. Hyperinflation

54. A 10-year-old patient is admitted to the ICU with a history of head injury following an automobile accident. The physician asks that the patient's $PaCO_2$ be maintained at a level of 25 torr and that it be closely monitored. Which of the following is the BEST recommendation?
    A. Insertion of an arterial line
    B. Use of a trancutaneous monitor
    C. Frequent blood gas analysis
    D. Capnography

55. A 4-day-old newborn being monitored with a pulse oximeter and transcutaneous PCO_2 monitor is noted to have a drop in SPO_2 of 5–7% and a rise in the $PaCO_2$ of 3–4 torr when asleep. Which of the following is the most appropriate recommendation?
    A. Perform a sleep study.
    B. Initiate oxygen therapy.
    C. Initiate nasal CPAP at night.
    D. Monitor for accessory muscle activity.

56. While examining a 34-week neonate, the respiratory care practitioner notices moderate nasal flaring, intercostal retractions, and expiratory grunting. Which of the following is the most likely diagnosis?
    A. Choanal Atresia
    B. Respiratory Distress Syndrome
    C. Bronchopulmonary Dysplasia
    D. Neonatal Pneumonia

57. Assuming an atmospheric PO_2 of 160 torr at sea level with a barometric pressure of 760 mm Hg, which of the following would be the PO_2 at 6000 feet altitude?
    A. 129 torr
    B. 134 torr
    C. 145 torr
    D. 150 torr

58. An 8-year-old patient is being mechanically ventilated on a volume cycled ventilator. The following information is available.

Rate	18
FiO_2	0.65
Vt	450 ml
PB	725 mm Hg
PaO_2	85 torr
$PaCO_2$	43 torr
PH_2O	47 torr

Which of the following is the A-a DO_2?
A. 104 torr
B. 240 torr
C. 302 torr
D. 450 torr

59. All of the following are symptoms of Respiratory Distress Syndrome EXCEPT
   A. Nasal flaring
   B. Expiratory grunting
   C. Retractions
   D. Subcutaneous emphysema

60. A 5-year-old patient with asthma is admitted to the hospital for treatment. The patient is ordered on chest physiotherapy QID. Which of the following is the goal of the therapy on this patient?
   A. Improve oxygenation
   B. Monitoring the patient
   C. Mobilization of secretions
   D. Reversal of bronchospasm

61. Type 1, or early fetal heart decelerations, are the result of which of the following?
   I. Maternal hypotension
   II. Compression of the fetal head
   III. Placental insufficiency
   IV. Umbilical cord compression
      A. I and III only
      B. II and IV only
      C. II only
      D. III only

62. A 3-year-old patient is admitted to the emergency room with shortness of breath. The respiratory care practitioner notes the patient has retractions, diffuse bilateral wheezing, and an increased respiratory rate. The physician orders a medication nebulizer with cromolyn sodium and normal saline. Which of the following is the most appropriate action?
   A. Carry out the procedure as ordered.
   B. Recommend bronchoscopy.

C. Recommend a sympathomimetic drug be substituted for the cromolyn sodium.
D. Recommend the cromolyn sodium be given without saline.

63. A 4-year-old patient is ordered on low flow oxygen with humidity to relieve nasal dryness. Which of the following combinations would BEST fulfill the physician's order?
A. Oxygen cannula with a bubble humidifier.
B. Oxygen mask with a wick humidifier.
C. Oxyhood with a cascade humidifier.
D. Non-rebreathing mask with a bubble humidifier.

64. A respiratory care practitioner treating a newborn patient notes that the patient has worsening cyanosis despite increasing FiO_2. Physical examination shows the patient to be tachypneic with intercostal retractions. The patient has an audible systolic ejection click and a loud second heart sound. The chest x-ray shows a prominent main pulmonary artery with moderate cardiomegaly. Which of the following tests will BEST help determine the diagnosis?
A. Hyperoxia-hyperventilation test
B. A-a DO_2
C. Oxygen index
D. Pre- and post-ductal PaO_2 study

65. A 33-week newborn is initiated on mechanical ventilation with a time cycled, pressure limited ventilator. The following information is available.

Rate	55/minute
Peak Pressure	28 cm H_2O
PEEP	3 cm H_2O
FiO_2	0.55
Inspiratory Time	.50 second
Flow rate	8 L/min

Arterial blood gas results on the above settings are

pH	.28
$PaCO_2$	52 torr
PaO_2	65 torr
HCO_3	25 mEq/liter

On examination, the breath sounds are diminished with poor chest excursion. Which of the following would be the most appropriate action at this point?
A. Increase the peak pressure.
B. Increase the rate.
C. Increase the flow rate.
D. Order a stat chest x-ray.

66. The attending neonatologist asks for the pulse rate of a 28-week neonate following its delivery. The BEST location to assess this is:
A. The brachial artery

B. The femoral artery
C. The radial artery
D. The carotid artery

67. While using a venti-mask on a 10-year-old asthmatic patient, the respiratory care practitioner is unable to achieve the desired FiO_2. Which of the following is the most likely cause?
    A. The patient's tidal volume is too small.
    B. The mask is too large.
    C. The oxygen tubing is kinked.
    D. The oxygen flow is too low.

68. Which of the following is the BEST initial rate for mechanical ventilator of a newborn when no settings are specified?
    A. 100/minute
    B. 80/minute
    C. 60/minute
    D. 40/minute

69. While weaning a pediatric patient from mechanical ventilation, the respiratory care practitioner initiates pressure support ventilation. Which of the following methods BEST describes the proper level of pressure support?
    A. Increase pressure support until the patient's respiratory rate declines.
    B. Initiate pressure support at a level of 20 cm H_2O.
    C. Initiate pressure support until the patient is achieving the desired tidal volume.
    D. Initiate pressure support at the level of the peak pressure achieved during mechanical ventilation.

70. Following delivery via cesarean section, a newborn is brought to the resuscitation room. Following drying, positioning, and suctioning, the initial assessment determines the heart rate to be 85 with a weak respiratory effort. Which of the following is the next step in the resuscitation?
    A. Assess the patient's color.
    B. Bag and mask ventilation with 100% oxygen.
    C. Immediate intubation followed by manual ventilation.
    D. Administer 3 ml of 1:10,000 epinephrine IM.

71. A 4-week-old infant shows signs of increasing respiratory distress. Which of the following would be the BEST method of determining acid base balance?
    A. Radial artery puncture
    B. Capillary blood gas
    C. Transcutaneous $PaCO_2$ monitor
    D. Pulse oximeter

72. An infant with BPD has been hospitalized for 3 months. The patient currently has a tracheostomy, with stable oxygen requirements and ventilator parameters. Which of the following should be present before allowing the infant to receive home care?
    A. Normal chest x-ray
    B. Clear breath sounds
    C. Minimal secretions
    D. Adequate nutritional intake

73. Following an episode of reflux, a 38-week neonate shows signs of increasing respiratory distress and decreasing oxygen saturation as monitored on a pulse oximeter. Which of the following would be the BEST recommendation?
    A. Initiate chest physiotherapy.
    B. Obtain a chest radiograph.
    C. Change the feeding frequency.
    D. Check the patient's temperature.

74. The respiratory care practitioner assigned to the emergency room is asked to assess a 2-year-old female with a dry, nonproductive cough. The chart indicates that the patient has had no previous hospitalizations. Which of the following would be most helpful in assessing the cause of the cough?
    A. Interviewing the parents
    B. Pulmonary function studies
    C. Chest radiograph
    D. Blood cultures

75. A 6-hour-old neonate with RDS is being mechanically ventilated with a time cycled, pressure limited ventilator. The infant is noted to have increasing $PaCO_2$ levels. Which of the following would BEST be used to assess for a change in lung compliance?
    I. Breath sounds
    II. Pulse oximeter
    III. Transcutaneous monitor
    IV. Chest excursion
    A. I only
    B. I, II, and III
    C. II and III only
    D. I and IV only

76. A 3-week-old newborn being weaned from mechanical ventilation is receiving IV morphine 0.2 mg/kg q4 hours for agitation. The respiratory care practitioner should monitor the patient for all of the following EXCEPT
    A. Bradycardia
    B. Respiratory depression
    C. Hypotension
    D. Seizures

77. At flows of 6 to 15 L/minute, a non-rebreathing mask can deliver an FiO_2 of
    A. 0.7 to 1.0
    B. 0.5 to 0.7
    C. 0.4 to 0.5
    D. 0.3 to 0.4

78. While observing a 39-week neonate, the respiratory care practitioner notices that the left arm does not move while the other extremities are actively moving. Which of the following is the most probable cause of this lack of movement?
    A. Muscle wasting.
    B. Congenital abnormality.
    C. Possible fracture.
    D. This is a normal occurrence.

79. A term newborn with TTN is being administered oxygen via an oxyhood. The following information is available.

FiO_2	0.23
PaO_2	65 torr
$PaCO_2$	41 torr

    Which of the following would be the BEST recommendation?
    A. Decrease the FiO_2 to room air.
    B. Continue with the present levels of oxygen.
    C. Increase the FiO_2 to 0.30.
    D. Initiate the patient on a nasal cannula.

80. The respiratory care practitioner receives an order to initiate mechanical ventilation at a rate of 45 breaths per minute at an I:E ratio of 1:2. Which of the following inspiratory times would achieve the specified ratio?
    A. 0.54 second
    B. 0.48 second
    C. 0.44 second
    D. 0.40 second

81. While monitoring an intubated 11-year-old patient with epiglottitis, the respiratory care practitioner notes that the aerosol stops exiting the Brigg's adapter each time the patient inhales. Which of the following is the BEST recommendation?
    A. Increase the flow rate.
    B. Increase the FiO_2.
    C. Increase the humidity output.
    D. Change to an ultrasonic nebulizer.

82. An infant has chest physiotherapy ordered q4 hours while the feedings are ordered q3 hours. Which of the following is the BEST recommendation?
    A. Continue the therapy as ordered.
    B. Change the chest physiotherapy to q3 hours.

C. Change the feedings to q4 hours.

D. Discontinue the chest physiotherapy.

83. Following intubation and the initiation of mechanical ventilation on a 30-week neonate, the respiratory care practitioner receives an order to initiate chest physiotherapy. Which of the following would be appropriate methods of performing the therapy?

I. Hands

II. Vibrator

III. Resuscitation mask

IV. Percussor

   A. I, II, and IV only

   B. II and IV only

   C. II, III, and IV only

   D. I, II, III, and IV

84. A 6-year-old male patient is admitted to the emergency room with a history of headache and nausea. Pulse oximetry shows an SPO_2 of 95% on a nasal cannula at 3L/min. Initial arterial blood gas results are as follows:

pH	7.30
$PaCO_2$	48 torr
PaO_2	54 torr
HCO_3	22 mEq/liter
SPO_2	86% (per co-oximeter)

Which of the following is the most probable cause of the difference between the pulse oximeter and the co-oximeter reading?

A. Elevated level carboxyhemoglobin

B. Poor perfusion at the site of the probe

C. Co-oximeter out of calibration

D. Contaminated arterial blood sample

85. A 13-year-old postoperative patient is being mechanically ventilated on a volume cycled ventilator. The patient weighs 34 kg. The following information is available.

Rate	12/minute
Vt	500 ml
FiO_2	0.38

It is determined that the patient's ventilation needs to be augmented. Which of the following would be the most appropriate ventilator change?

A. Increase the rate.

B. Increase the tidal volume.

C. Increase both rate and tidal volume.

D. Increase the FiO_2.

86. Following 1 minute of external cardiac massage on a 800 g neonate, the heart rate remains below 80 beats/minute. The decision is made to instill epinephrine into the endotracheal tube. The correct dosage for this patient would be:
    A. 0.1 to 0.3 ml
    B. 1 ml given in two 0.5 ml boluses
    C. 8 mEq/liter
    D. 0.08 to 0.24 ml

87. Before performing a radial puncture, the respiratory care practitioner should perform which of the following tests?
    A. Shunt
    B. Alveolar/air
    C. Allen's
    D. Perfusion

88. The respiratory care practitioner notes a sudden change in the clinical status of a mechanically ventilated newborn. Auscultation reveals a shift of the heart sounds to the left. A stat chest radiograph is obtained and shows hyperlucency on the right with a left shift of the trachea. These findings are consistent with:
    A. Diaphragmatic hernia
    B. Right side pneumothorax
    C. Left side atelectasis
    D. Right side pneumonia

89. A 5-year-old patient is admitted to the emergency room with a history of upper respiratory infection for the past 2 days and a tight, inspiratory and expiratory stridor. The most appropriate aerosolized drug for this patient is
    A. Terbutaline sulfate
    B. Racemic epinephrine
    C. Albuterol
    D. Ipratropium bromide

90. A 5-year-old patient is receiving a continuously analyzed FiO_2 of 0.35 via a high flow wick humidifier attached to an air/oxygen blender. One hour later, the analyzed FiO_2 shows 0.27. Which of the following is a possible cause of the analyzer drift?
    A. The barometric pressure has decreased.
    B. The wick water reservoir has run dry.
    C. The analyzer is being affected by the humidity.
    D. The analyzer battery has run down.

91. Following 3 weeks of mechanical ventilation, a neonatal patient has been gradually weaned from ventilatory support. Current ventilator settings are

Rate	8/minute
Peak pressure	18 cm H_2O
PEEP	4 cm H_2O

Which of the following is the BEST recommendation?
A. Extubate the patient.
B. Continue weaning the patient.
C. Change to pressure support ventilation.
D. Place the patient on CPAP.

92. Which of the following types of tracheostomy tube is the most appropriate for home ventilator care?
A. Uncuffed tube.
B. Cuffed, fenestrated tube.
C. Foam cuff tube.
D. Cuffed, non-fenestrated tube.

93. While interviewing the parents of a mechanically ventilated infant, it is determined that the parents are currently undergoing a divorce. With regard to the possibility of home care, which of the following suggestions is the most appropriate?
A. The patient should be placed in a foster home until the divorce is final.
B. The patient is not a candidate for home care until the home environment is stable.
C. The patient should be placed with the parents of the mother or father.
D. The patient should be sent home to help bring the family back together.

94. A respiratory care practitioner working for a home care company is asked to teach a 16-year-old mother in the use of an apnea monitor for her newborn infant. Which of the following instructions should be recommended by the practitioner?
   I. Always lay the infant on its stomach.
   II. Contact the home care company in the event of frequent false alarms.
   III. Check for loose, misapplied, or broken electrodes.
   IV. Emphasize the importance of not becoming complacent.
      A. I, II, and III only
      B. II and III only
      C. II, III, and IV only
      D. I, II, III, and IV

95. A liquid oxygen tank is being used for home oxygen therapy. The following information is available.

Full weight	70 pounds
Current weight	45 pounds
Liter flow	2 L/min

Which of the following is the hours of oxygen left in the tank?
A. 7695 hours
B. 3250 hours
C. 450 hours
D. 128 hours

96. An arterial blood gas analysis would be indicated in all of the following circumstances EXCEPT
   A. A worsening of the clinical course
   B. Increasing retractions
   C. The appearance of jaundice
   D. The appearance of cyanosis

97. Which of the following is used to administer the drug ribavirin?
   A. Large volume nebulizer
   B. Ultrasonic nebulizer
   C. Small volume nebulizer
   D. Small particle aerosol generator

98. A 9-year-old patient admitted with status asthmaticus is being ventilated with a volume cycled ventilator. The respiratory care practitioner notices that the high pressure alarm triggers repeatedly, the patient is agitated and SPO_2 is dropping to below 90%. Which of the following should the practitioner do FIRST?
   A. Order a stat chest x-ray
   B. Auscultate breath sounds.
   C. Obtain an arterial blood gas sample.
   D. Recommend sedation for the patient.

99. Mean airway pressure increases with increases in which of the following?
   I. Peak inspiratory pressure
   II. Positive end expiratory pressure
   III. Total cycle time
   IV. Respiratory rate
   A. I and II only
   B. I, II, and III
   C. I, II, and IV
   D. II, III, and IV

100. Which of the following is the drug of choice for a neonate diagnosed with transposition of the great vessels?
   A. Sodium bicarbonate
   B. Dopamine
   C. Oxygen administered at a concentration of 1.0
   D. Prostaglandin E

ANSWERS TO PRACTICE EXAMINATION

Following each answer, a rationale is given pertaining to the answer followed by a reference in the textbook where the information can be found. On those answers without a reference, the rationale serves as the reference to the answer.

1. **Answer A.** Rationale: Pediatric patients should be ventilated at a tidal volume of 10 to 15 ml/kg of body weight. This patient weighs approximately 27.2 kg (60 pounds × .454 kg/pound = 27.24); therefore, the appropriate range of tidal volumes would be 272 ml to 408 ml.
   Reference: Chapter 15

2. **Answer B.** Rationale: The fact that the infant is pale and blanched indicates a lack of red blood cells. The most probable cause of those listed is hypovolemic anemia secondary to a loss of blood.
   Reference: Chapters 3, 4, and 10

3. **Answer A.** Rationale: The fact that the young woman is unwed, lives in low-income housing, and is included in a minority group, are all included as high-risk factors. Her age of 23 is not considered adolescence, which is often seen as being less than 18 years of age.
   Reference: Chapter 2

4. **Answer A.** Rationale: A decreasing $PaCO_2$ is indicative of excessive ventilation. Bronchospasm in which a bronchodilator is indicated, is manifest by worsening ventilation and would be seen as an increasing $PaCO_2$.
   Reference: Chapter 6

5. **Answer B.** Rationale: The high pressure of the ventilator along with the shift of the heart to the left indicate the possibility of an air leak. The chest radiograph confirms the presence of free air in the thorax. The "bat-wing" is the thymus gland, which is outlined by the free air in the mediastinum.
   Reference: Chapter 13

6. **Answer C.** Rationale: Worsening compliance and increasing atelectasis on chest x-ray indicate a loss of surface tension, probably secondary to the onset of ARDS. The initiation of PEEP will prevent the collapse of the alveoli, improving both compliance and atelectasis.
   Reference: Chapter 15.

7. **Answer A.** Rationale: The presence of retractions and coarse rhonchi indicate that secretions are narrowing the airway, increasing the resistance to breathing and creating the rhonchi.
   Reference: Chapter 6

8. **Answer D.** Rationale: On patients who have a large right-to-left ductal shunt, as indicated by the poor oxygenation on 100% oxygen and a loud ductal murmur, ventilation alone will not improve oxygenation or ventilation. The administration of bicarbonate is indicated in this scenario in an attempt to increase the pH, which, in turn, will reduce the pulmonary vasoconstriction and improve pulmonary blood flow, reducing the right-to-left shunt.
   Reference: Chapter 4

9. **Answer C.** Rationale: The I:E ratio is calculated by dividing 60 seconds by the rate to determine the total ventilatory cycle time. (60/40 = 1.5 seconds) The inspiratory time is then subtracted from the total time to calculate the expiratory time. (1.5 seconds –0.4 seconds = 1.1 seconds expiratory time) The final step is to divide the expiratory time

by the inspiratory time to calculate the I:E ratio. (1.1/0.4 = 2.75) The I:E ratio is therefore 1:2.75 in this scenario.
Reference: Chapter 15

10. **Answer D.** Rationale: Of the four choices, only an inappropriate temperature, compromised hemodynamic status and excessive electrode pressure would cause the described differences. Excessive perfusion would most likely cause the electrode to read more accurately.
Reference: Chapter 9

11. **Answer B.** Rationale: A liter flow of at least 7 liters per minute is necessary to wash out expired CO_2 and prevent the possibility of CO_2 retention.
Reference: Chapter 7

12. **Answer C.** Rationale: Following 15 to 30 seconds of positive pressure ventilation, if the heart rate is still below 80 beats/minute (this patient's heart rate is 72 beats/min), external cardiac compressions should be started.
Reference: Chapter 4

13. **Answer D.** Rationale: Of the four mentioned drugs, only fentanyl citrate can produce anesthesia.
Reference: Chapter 8

14. **Answer D.** Rationale: A sound heard following the first heart sound, which ends before the onset of the second sound, is a systolic murmur.
Reference: Chapter 5

15. **Answer D.** Rationale: At a rate of 40, the total cycle time is 1.5 seconds (60/40 = 1.5) At an inspiratory time of 1 second, the patient is not being allowed enough time (0.5 second) to expire. Decreasing the inspiratory time will increase the I:E ratio and allow for proper exhalation, reducing the air trapping and improving ventilation.
Reference: Chapter 15

16. **Answer B.** Rationale: The Apgar score for this patient is determined as follows:
Respiratory Effort: Weak, 1 point.
Heart Rate: 135, 2 points.
Color: Acrocyanosis, 1 point.
Muscle tone: Some flexion, 1 point.
Reflex Irritability: Coughs and cries to stimulation, 2 points.
Reference: Chapter 4

17. **Answer A.** Rationale: The blue appearance of the hands and feet when the body is pink is known as acrocyanosis and is commonly seen within the first 24 hours following delivery.
Reference: Chapter 5

18. **Answer A.** Rationale: The presence of a decreased femoral pulse in the presence of normal brachial pulses indicates a blockage in the aorta, which is reducing the force of the femoral pulse. The most likely cause of blockage is coarctation of the aorta.
Reference: Chapters 5 and 11

19. **Answer C.** Rationale: The range of systolic blood pressure for a 1000 g neonate is 39 59 mm Hg.
Reference: Chapter 5

20. **Answer B.** Rationale: The blood gas results indicate a need to increase ventilation. Of the given choices, only increasing the peak pressure will increase ventilation.
    Reference: Chapter 15
21. **Answer B.** Rationale: Although the respiratory distress and unequal chest excursion may be observed in the presence of a pneumothorax, the presence of a scaphoid (flat or sunken) abdomen indicates a lack of abdominal contents and, therefore, a diaphragmatic hernia is suspected.
    Reference: Chapter 5
22. **Answer A.** Rationale: For neonatal patients, a pressure range of –50 to –80 mm Hg is appropriate for suctioning.
    Reference: Chapter 6
23. **Answer B.** Rationale: The lipid, phosphatidylglycerol (PG), is not present in the amniotic fluid until mature surfactant is being produced around 35 to 36 weeks.
    Reference: Chapter 1
24. **Answer B.** Rationale: The only piece of mentioned equipment not required for an intubation is the bronchoscope. The bronchoscope would only be used under special circumstances when a normal intubation is not possible.
    Reference: Chapter 4
25. **Answer A.** Rationale: Ribavirin is indicated for the treatment of respiratory syncytial virus infections.
    Reference: Chapter 8
26. **Answer C.** Rationale: The patient is showing signs of a failure to wean. The patient should be reinstituted on mechanical ventilation and rested until a later time.
    Reference: Chapter 15
27. **Answer C.** Rationale: The Silverman-Anderson index is utilized to assess the degree of respiratory distress in a newborn.
    Reference: Chapter 5
28. **Answer B.** Rationale: The early gestational age along with the presence of poor lung compliance are indications of respiratory distress syndrome. The chest radiograph of this syndrome is described as a reticulogranular pattern.
    Reference: Chapter 13
29. **Answer B.** Rationale: Chest physiotherapy is used to treat processes that are occurring internally to the lungs. Pleural effusion occurs external to the lung and is not a process that would be improved by CPT.
    Reference: Chapter 6
30. **Answer C.** Rationale: Corrected tidal volume is calculated by subtracting the PEEP from the peak pressure (38 – 5 = 33). The result is then multiplied by the circuit compliance to arrive at the tubing loss (33 × 2 = 66 ml tubing loss). The tubing loss is then subtracted from the delivered total volume to arrive at the corrected tidal volume (300 – 66 = 235 ml).
    Reference: Chapter 15
31. **Answer C.** Rationale: Although the arterial blood gases are not at a dangerous level, the patient is requiring high levels of ventilory support to maintain the blood gases.

Before continuing with the care of the patient, the airway must be secured and maintained with an endotracheal tube.
Reference: Chapter 4

32. **Answer A.** Rationale: Although oxygen does enhance combustion, it is not an explosive gas. Explosion is therefore not a hazard.
Reference: Chapter 6

33. **Answer B.** Rationale: Flow inflation bags do not have valves to direct the flow of gas as do self-inflating resuscitation bags.
Reference: Chapter 4

34. **Answer C.** Rationale: The most common causes of bradycardia during suctioning are hypoxemia and stimulation of the vagal nerve.
Reference: Chapter 6

35. **Answer D.** Rationale: Secondary apnea follows primary apnea and results in a cessation of the breathing effort by the fetus or newborn. Secondary apnea can only be treated by mechanical ventilation.
Reference: Chapter 4

36. **Answer B.** Rationale: Older incubators were often equipped with an FiO_2 limiting device. To achieve FiO_2 of greater than 0.4, the operator must lift an arm on the front of the incubator, which, in turn, allows more oxygen to flow to the incubator environment.
Reference: Chapter 6

37. **Answer B.** Rationale: Of the listed respiratory drugs, only ipratropium bromide is in the category of parasympatholytic.
Reference: Chapter 8

38. **Answer C.** Rationale: When an expiratory timer is utilized on a ventilator, the expiratory time remains fixed as inspiratory time is changed. Therefore, as the inspiratory time is increased, the total breath time is increased, slowing the rate.
Reference: Chapter 15

39. **Answer C.** Rationale: The AO2 alarm indicates the ventilator has detected a peak pressure of 10 cm H_2O higher than the set level. This indicates a blocked expiratory tube or nonfunctioning expiratory valve.
Reference: Chapter 16

40. **Answer A.** Rationale: If the inspiratory pop-off emergency valve is set below the desired level of peak pressure, the operator will not be able to achieve a peak pressure above the level determined by the pop-off valve.
Reference: Chapter 15

41. **Answer C.** Rationale: When using a nasal cannula on neonatal patients, flow above 4 L/minute may lead to mucosal drying with subsequent epistaxis.
Reference: Chapter 6

42. **Answer B.** Rationale: In a sidestream analyzer, the sample is taken from the patient connection through a small diameter tube to the analyzer. Water, which can easily occlude the tube, can partially or totally block the tube and cause the analyzer to fluctuate or read zero if there is total blockage.
Reference: Chapter 9

43. **Answer A.** Rationale: Any patient who requires an increase of greater than 0.25 increase in the FiO_2 during CPT should be discontinued from the treatment. In this instance, the risk to the patient is greater than the benefit of the treatment.
    Reference: Chapter 6

44. **Answer D.** Rationale: All of the mentioned items are important considerations before performing extubation.
    Reference: Chapter 15

45. **Answer C.** Rationale: A size 3.0 endotracheal tube is used on patients weighing from 1000 to 2000 g.
    Reference: Chapter 4

46. **Answer D.** Rationale: The radiant warmer utilizes a negative feedback system to maintain the patient's temperature. When the probe is off the patient, it reads ambient temperature, which may be cooler than the desired set temperature. The radiant heater is then activated in an attempt to heat the patient. The low temperature alarm is activated when the probe fails to sense an increase in the temperature.
    Reference: Chapter 7

47. **Answer A.** Rationale: The most common source of false alarms on apnea monitors are loose, misapplied, or broken electrodes.
    Reference: Chapter 19

48. **Answer A.** Rationale: In the patient with normal cardiovascular anatomy, the right subclavian artery, which supplies the right radial artery, is the only mentioned artery that receives pre-ductal arterial blood flow from the aorta.
    Reference: Chapters 9 and 11

49. **Answer B.** Rationale: Flow rates of less than 7 liters per minute to an oxyhood may result in CO_2 retention by not flushing the expired CO_2 from the hood.
    Reference: Chapter 6

50. **Answer D.** Rationale: The "classic method" of determining lung compliance and airway resistance utilizes an esophageal balloon to estimate pleural pressure. Although also used, a pneumotachograph is used to measure flows and volumes, not pleural pressure.
    Reference: Chapter 5

51. **Answer C.** Rationale: Although pulse oximeters and transcutaneous monitors are valuable adjuncts in the care of unstable neonates, they cannot replace the need for arterial blood gas analysis. Because this patient is unstable with frequent ventilator changes, the presence of an umbilical artery catheter will greatly facilitate obtaining blood gases to follow the patient's progress. The catheter additionally provides a direct route for administration of drugs and fluids.
    Reference: Chapter 4

52. **Answer D.** Rationale: The high SPO_2 reading from the pulse oximeter is the result of pre-ductal blood perfusing the right arm while the blood from the umbilical artery reflects post-ductal blood flow. The difference between the two saturations indicates the shunt is in the ductus arteriosus, not in the heart itself.
    Reference: Chapter 11

53. **Answer C.** Rationale: Atelectasis will often cause the diaphragm to rise on the affected

side. It is often accompanied by a mediastinal shift toward the atelectatic area, a decrease in the rib interspaces, and hyperinflation of the opposite lung.
Reference: Chapter 13

54. **Answer D.** Rationale: In the absence of lung or heart disease, end-tidal CO_2 monitoring is a reliable, noninvasive method of monitoring arterial PCO_2 levels. Although transcutaneous monitors can also be used, they are not as reliable and accurate as capnography.
Reference: Chapters 6 and 12

55. **Answer A.** Rationale: The combination of a decrease in SPO_2 and a rise in the $PaCO_2$ while asleep indicates a possible sleep apnea. A sleep study would be useful in ruling out or confirming sleep apnea as a cause.
Reference: Chapter 10

56. **Answer B.** Rationale: Nasal flaring, grunting, and retractions are the three cardinal signs of Respiratory Distress Syndrome.
Reference: Chapter 5

57. **Answer A.** Rationale: For each increase in altitude of 1000 feet, the PO_2 decreases slightly more than 5 torr. Therefore, an increase of 6000 feet would result in a decrease in PO_2 of approximately 31 torr from sea level.
Reference: Chapter 18

58. **Answer C.** Rationale: The calculation of the A-a gradient is done by first determining the inspired PO_2. This is done by first subtracting the PH_2O from the barometric pressure and multiplying the resulting pressure by the FiO_2.
$(725 - 47) \times 0.65 = 678 \times 0.65 = 440.7$ or 441 P_1O_2.
The next step is to multiply the $PaCO_2$ by 1.25 (assuming the respiratory quotient is 0.8) and subtracting the result from the inspired PO_2.
$(43 \times 1.25 = 54; 441 - 54 = 387)$
The final step is to subtract the PaO_2 from the P_1O_2 to calculate the A-a gradient.
$387 - 85 =$ A-a gradient of 302 torr
Reference: Chapter 17

59. **Answer D.** Rationale: Subcutaneous emphysema is a symptom of an airleak syndrome. The airleak may result from the treatment of respiratory distress, but is not a symptom of the disease.
Reference: Chapter 10

60. **Answer C.** Rationale: An acute asthma attack is usually accompanied by the secretion of thick mucus, which can clog the airways and worsen air movement. The goal of chest physiotherapy therefore is to mobilize the secretions so that they can be removed.
Reference: Chapter 6

61. **Answer C.** Rationale: Early fetal heart decelerations are secondary to a vagal response, caused by compression of the fetal head during a contraction.
Reference: Chapter 2

62. **Answer C.** Rationale: The patient in this scenario is showing signs of acute airway bronchospasm, indicated by retractions, wheezing, and an increased respiratory rate. Cromolyn sodium is used to prevent bronchospasm and has no effect to reverse bron-

chospasm; therefore, a sympathomimetic drug is more appropriate therapy at this point.
Reference: Chapters 8 and 12

63. **Answer A.** Rationale: Low flow oxygen on a 4-year-old patient is best delivered via a nasal cannula humidified with a bubble humidifier.
Reference: Chapter 6

64. **Answer A.** Rationale: All of the described symptoms are indicative of persistent pulmonary hypertension of the newborn. The hyperoxia-hyperventilation test is used to either confirm or disprove the diagnosis.
Reference: Chapter 10

65. **Answer A.** Rationale: The fact that the chest excursion is poor, with diminished breath sounds indicates the lungs are not being expanded properly on inspiration. With an adequate PaO_2 and an elevated $PaCO_2$, the proper action is to increase the peak pressure in order to expand the lungs and improved ventilation.
Reference: Chapter 15

66. **Answer A.** Rationale: Palpation of the pulse rate is done at the brachial artery. The artery is easily accessible and easy to palpate.
Reference: Chapter 4

67. **Answer D.** Rationale: The two most common causes of a malfunctioning venturi mask are: 1) too low an oxygen flow, which results in a diminished air entrainment ratio; and 2) occlusion of the entrainment port.
Reference: Chapter 6

68. **Answer D.** Rationale: The initial rate of ventilation should be 40 breaths per minute either during resuscitation or when no parameters are specified.
Reference: Chapter 15

69. **Answer C.** Rationale: The level of pressure support is determined by augmenting the pressure support level until the patient reaches a desired tidal volume.
Reference: Chapter 15

70. **Answer B.** Rationale: Following the initial steps of the resuscitation, a weak inspiratory effort with a heart rate of 85 necessitates immediate bag and mask ventilation with an FiO_2 of 1.0. The patient's heart rate is then reassessed and further steps are initiated accordingly.
Reference: Chapter 4

71. **Answer B.** Rationale: To assess the acid base balance of an infant, a capillary blood gas is less traumatic to the patient and is comparable to arterial values when determining $PaCO_2$ and pH. The transcutaneous monitor does not measure pH and is therefore not sufficient to measure acid base balance. The pulse oximeter only measures oxygen saturation, which does not coincide with acid base balance.
Reference: Chapter 9

72. **Answer D.** Rationale: Besides having a stable airway, stable oxygen, and ventilator parameters, the patient should have nutritional intake adequate to maintain growth and development.
Reference: Chapter 19

73. **Answer B.** Rationale: Increasing respiratory distress and decreasing oxygen satura-

tions following an episode of reflux all indicate a possible aspiration of stomach contents. The chest radiograph would be helpful in checking for changes that may indicate aspiration.
Reference: Chapter 13

74. **Answer A.** Rationale: Any evaluation of a noncritical patient should always begin with a thorough history of the illness. In this case, it is unlikely that the patient could appropriately answer questions; therefore, the parents should be interviewed. The outcome of the interview will help determine what further diagnostic studies should be done.
Reference: Chapter 5

75. **Answer D.** Rationale: When using a pressure limited ventilator, changes in compliance are often first detected by a worsening or improvement of breath sounds and chest excursion, secondary to the tidal volume diminishing or increasing.
Reference: Chapter 15

76. **Answer D.** Rationale: Seizures are not associated with the use of morphine.
Reference: Chapter 8

77. **Answer A.** Rationale: At oxygen flows of 6 to 15 L/minute, a properly fitting nonrebreathing mask can deliver a range of FiO_2 between 0.7 and 1.0.
Reference: Chapter 6

78. **Answer C.** Rationale: A normal newborn will move all extremities symmetrically. Lack of movement in one extremity indicates a bone fracture, or possibly paralysis secondary to birth trauma.
Reference: Chapter 5

79. **Answer D.** Rationale: Due to the low level of FiO_2 and the adequate PaO_2, a nasal cannula would allow better patient access while maintaining the proper level of FiO_2.
Reference: Chapter 6

80. **Answer C.** Rationale: The appropriate inspiratory time is determined by first dividing the breath rate into 60 seconds to calculate the total cycle time ($60/45 = 1.33$ seconds). The next step is to add the two numbers of the desired I:E ratio together ($1:2 = 3$). The final step is to divide the total cycle time by the sum of the I:E ratio to calculate the inspiratory time ($1.33/3 = 0.44$ second).
Reference: Chapter 15

81. **Answer A.** Rationale: the loss of aerosol during inhalation indicates the patient's inspiratory flow demands are greater than that being provided by the nebulizer. The proper action is to increase flow to the patient.
Reference: Chapter 12

82. **Answer B.** Rationale: Because chest physiotherapy should always be done previous to a feeding, and due to the fact that feedings are vital to patient growth and development, the best recommendation in this scenario is to change the chest physiotherapy to match the feeding schedule.
Reference: Chapter 12

83. **Answer C.** Rationale: For this small of a patient, the use of the hands would be inappropriate to perform chest physiotherapy.
Reference: Chapter 6

84. **Answer A.** Rationale: An elevated carboxyhemoglobin can cause the pulse oximeter to interpret a higher oxyhemoglobin than is actually present. The pulse oximeter cannot distinguish between carboxyhemoglobin and oxyhemoglobin; therefore, it assumes that if the hemoglobin is not desaturated, it must be oxyhemoglobin. The history of headache and nausea are symptoms of an elevated carboxyhemoglobin and further reinforce the diagnosis.
    Reference: Chapter 9
85. **Answer A.** Rationale: At 34 kg of body weight, this patient's highest tidal volume is 510 ml (34×15 ml). Because the patient's tidal volume is already at the maximal level, the most appropriate change would be to increase the respiratory rate.
    Reference: Chapter 15
86. **Answer D.** Rationale: During a resuscitation, epinephrine is given in a dosage of .1 to .3 ml/kg of body weight. For this patient weighing 800 g, or 0.8 kg, the correct dosage is 0.08 to 0.24 ml.
    Reference: Chapter 4
87. **Answer C.** Rationale: The Allen's test, which checks for collateral circulation through the ulnar artery, should always be done before puncturing the radial artery.
    Reference: Chapter 9
88. **Answer B.** Rationale: The sudden change in clinical status with a shift of the heart sounds are initial clues of a pneumothorax. This is verified by the chest radiograph showing a hyperlucency on the right with a left shift of the trachea indicating a tension pneumothorax on the right side.
    Reference: Chapter 10
89. **Answer B.** Rationale: The history and examination findings of upper respiratory infection and stridor indicate the diagnosis of croup. The aerosolized drug of choice for croup is racemic epinephrine.
    Reference: Chapter 8
90. **Answer C.** Rationale: Whenever the FiO_2 is being measured continuously, the analyzer should be placed prior to the humidifier to avoid erroneous readings.
    Reference: Chapter 6
91. **Answer A.** Rationale: The current parameters are all at levels at which extubation is possible. Due to the small diameter of the endotracheal tube used on neonates, it is not recommended that they breathe on CPAP before extubation due to the resistance of the tube.
    Reference: Chapter 15
92. **Answer A.** Rationale: An uncuffed tracheostomy tube is preferred for use in the home care setting, to avoid laryngeal and tracheal damage. The patient is also able to vocalize as a small amount of gas is allowed to leak past the tube.
    Reference: Chapter 19
93. **Answer B.** Rationale: The effects of home care on the family are numerous. The presence of a sick infant in the home causes major disruptions of family life. The relationships among all family members often need to be gradually redefined. The family may have problems dealing with the health care and financial obligations, adding more

stress to the situation. In addition to the above-mentioned stressors, divorce will only worsen the situation and heap more stress on the parents.
Reference: Chapter 19

94. **Answer C.** Rationale: To avoid the chance that the mother may shut off the monitor in the event of frequent false alarms, she should be instructed to contact the home care company. The health care provider can then assess the situation and correct the false alarms. Because many false alarms are caused by lose, misapplied, or broken electrodes, the mother should be instructed basic troubleshooting in this area. Finally, there is a high degree of noncompliance in teenage parents; therefore, strict compliance to protocol should be reinforced.
Reference: Chapter 19

95. **Answer D.** Rationale: Calculating the amount of time left in a liquid track is done by multiplying the weight of the cylinder by 342 (the number of liters per pound of weight). This number is then divided by the liter flow to arrive at the number of minutes remaining. Dividing the total minutes by 60 calculates the hours remaining ($45 \times 342 = 15,390$ liters; $15,390/2$ L/min = 7695 minutes. $7695/60 = 128.25$ hours remaining)
Reference: Chapter 19

96. **Answer C.** Rationale: An arterial blood gas would not aid in the diagnosis or treatment of jaundice, whereas an arterial blood gas would help the practitioner diagnose and treat the other three.
Reference: Chapter 9

97. **Answer D.** Rationale: Due to the large volume of drug to administer, the length of time and the fact that it must be administered dry, ribavarin can only be delivered via a small particle aerosol generator (SPAG).
Reference: Chapter 8

98. **Answer B.** Rationale: With a history of status asthmaticus, this patient is at risk of developing barotrauma secondary to air trapping. This patient, with a sudden increase in peak pressure, agitation, and a dropping saturation could have a pneumothorax that could be quickly assessed by auscultation. A less dangerous situation would be the presence of secretions in the airway, preventing adequate gas exchange and increasing resistance. Again, auscultation is the quickest method of determining the necessity to suction.
Reference: Chapter 10

99. **Answer C.** Rationale: All of the items mentioned will increase mean airway pressure if they are increased, except for the total cycle time. Increases in the total cycle time actually reduce the respiratory rate, thus decreasing the mean airway pressure.
Reference: Chapter 14

100. **Answer D.** Rationale: In transposition of the great vessels, the only communication between the pulmonary blood flow and the systemic blood flow is through the ductus arteriosus. Prostaglandin E keeps the ductus patent, thus allowing mixing of oxygenated blood. This is one instance where administration of oxygen is not indicated because it promotes closure of the ductus.
Reference: Chapter 8

APPENDIX C

SELECTED AVERAGE LABORATORY VALUES

AVERAGE BLOOD CHEMISTRY VALUES FOR TERM INFANTS

ION	BIRTH	24 HOURS	48 HOURS
Sodium, mmol/L	147	145	149
Potassium, mmol/L	7.8	6.3	5.9
Calcium, mg/dl	9.3	7.8	7.9
Chloride, mmol/L	103	103	103
Glucose, mg/dl	73	63	59

AVERAGE BLOOD CHEMISTRY VALUES FOR LOW BIRTH WEIGHT INFANTS

ION	<1000 G	1001–1500 g	1501–2000 g
Sodium, mmol/L	138	133	135
Potassium, mmol/L	6.4	6.0	5.4
Chloride, mmol/L	100	101	105

AVERAGE HEMATOLOGIC VALUES

	BIRTH	1 MONTH	5 YEARS	10 YEARS
Hematocrit	54	40	40	40
Hemoglobin gm/dl	14–24	11–17	12.5–15	13–15.5
Platelets	140–300,000/mm3	200–470,000/mm3	150–450,000/mm3	13–15.5
Red blood count	4.8–7.1 million/mm3		4.2–6.2 million/mm3	13–15.5
White blood count	9000–30,000/mm3	5000–19,500/mm3	5000–10,000/mm3	13–15.5
Neutrophils	61%	35%	60%	13–15.5
Lymphocytes	31%	56%	30%	13–15.5
Total bilirubin	<2 mg/dl	<1 mg/dl	<1 mg/dl	13–15.5

CHARTS OF AVERAGE VITAL SIGNS

AVERAGE NEONATAL BLOOD PRESSURE

WEIGHT	SYSTOLIC (mm Hg)	DIASTOLIC (mm Hg)
750 g	34–54	14–34
1000 g	39–59	16–36
1500 g	40–61	19–39
3000 g	51–72	27–46

NORMAL PEDIATRIC VITAL SIGNS

AGE	PULSE RATE MALES	FEMALES
0–12 months	132–138	123–129
5 years	78–85	78–85
10 years	66–71	68–70
15 years	60–63	64–67

RESPIRATORY RATE

AGE	MALES	FEMALES
0–12 months	30–32	29–31
5 years	22	21
10 years	19	19
15 years	18	18

BLOOD PRESSURE

AGE	SYSTOLIC	DIASTOLIC
0–12 months	80 +/– 16	46 +/– 16
5 years	94 +/– 14	55 +/– 9
10 years	107 +/– 16	57 +/– 9
15 years	118 +/– 19	60 +/– 10

APPENDIX E

CONVERSION CHART: POUNDS AND OUNCES TO GRAMS

POUNDS

OUNCES	0	1	2	3	4	5	6	7	8	9	10	11
0	0	454	907	1361	1814	2268	2272	3175	3629	4082	4536	4990
1	28	482	936	1389	1843	2296	2750	3203	3657	4111	4564	5018
2	57	510	964	1417	1871	2325	2778	3232	3685	4139	4593	5046
3	85	539	992	1446	1899	2353	2807	3260	3714	4167	4621	5075
4	113	567	1021	1474	1928	2381	2835	3289	3742	4196	4649	5103
5	142	595	1049	1503	1956	2410	2863	3317	3770	4224	4678	5131
6	6	170	624	1077	1531	1984	2438	2892	3345	3799	4552	4706
7	198	652	1106	1559	2013	2466	2920	3374	3827	4281	4734	5188
8	227	680	1134	1588	2041	2495	2948	3402	3856	4309	4763	5216
9	255	709	1162	1616	2070	2523	2977	3430	3884	4337	4791	5245
10	283	737	1191	1644	2098	2551	3005	2459	3912	4366	4819	5273
11	312	765	1219	1673	2126	2580	3033	3487	3941	4394	4848	5301
12	340	794	1247	1701	2155	2608	3062	3515	3969	4423	4876	5330
13	369	822	1276	1729	2183	2637	3090	3544	3997	4451	4904	5358
14	397	850	1304	1758	2211	2665	3118	3572	4026	4479	4933	5386
15	425	879	1332	1786	2240	2693	3147	3600	4054	4508	4961	5415

Pounds = weight in grams/454
Grams = weight in pounds $\times$ 454

APPENDIX F

CONVERSION CHART: FAHRENHEIT TO CELSIUS

°F	°C	°F	°C
95.0	35.0	99.6	37.6
95.2	35.1	99.8	37.7
95.4	35.2	100.0	37.8
95.6	35.3	100.2	37.9
95.8	35.4	100.4	38.0
96.0	35.6	100.6	38.1
96.2	35.7	100.8	38.2
96.4	35.8	101.0	38.3
96.6	35.9	101.2	38.4
96.8	36.0	101.4	38.6
97.0	36.1	101.6	38.7
97.2	36.2	101.8	38.8
97.4	36.3	102.0	38.9
97.6	36.4	102.2	39.0
97.8	36.6	102.4	39.1
98.0	36.7	102.6	39.2
98.2	36.8	102.8	39.3
98.4	36.9	103.0	39.4
98.6	37.0	103.2	39.6
98.9	37.1	103.4	39.7
99.0	37.2	103.6	39.8
99.2	37.3	103.8	39.9
99.4	37.4	104.0	40.0

$°C = [(°F - 32) \times 5]/9$

$°F = [(°C \times 9)/5 + 32]$

APPENDIX G

CONVERSION CHART: FRENCH TO MILLIMETERS AND INCHES

FRENCH SIZE	DIAMETER (mm)	DIAMETER (INCHES)
1	1/2	0.013
2	2/3	0.026
3	1	0.039
4	1 1/3	0.052
5	1 2/3	0.065
6	2	0.078
7	2 1/3	0.091
8	2 2/3	0.104
9	3	0.118
10	3 1/3	0.131
11	3 2/3	0.144
12	4	0.157
13	4 1/3	0.170
14	4 2/3	0.183
15	5	0.196
16	5 1/3	0.209
17	5 2/3	0.233
18	6	0.236
19	6 1/3	0.249
20	6 2/3	0.262

APPENDIX H

CONVERSION CHART: INCHES TO CENTIMETERS

INCHES	CENTIMETERS
$^1/_4$	0.635
$^1/_2$	0.026
1	2.54
2	5.08
3	7.62
4	10.16
5	12.70
10	25.40
11	27.94
12	30.48
13	33.02
14	35.56
15	38.10
16	40.64
17	43.18
18	45.72
19	48.26
20	50.80
21	53.34
22	55.88
23	58.42
24	60.96

Inches = centimeters/2.54
Centimeters = inches $\times$ 2.54

789

PHYSICAL GROWTH CHART

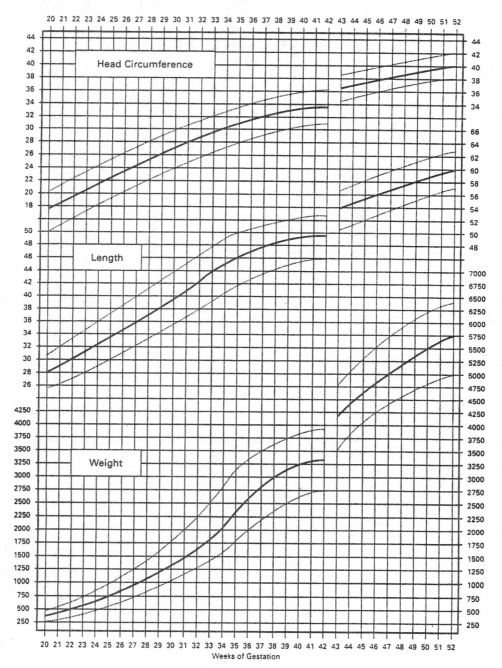

Weeks of Gestation

GLOSSARY

abruptio placentae   The abnormal separation of the normally implanted placenta from the uterus in a pregnancy of 20 weeks or more occurring before the delivery of the fetus.

acrocyanosis   A condition in the newborn characterized by a cyanotic discoloration of the hands and feet. Also known as peripheral acrocyanosis of the newborn.

active transport   The movement of molecules across a cell membrane through means of a chemical activity allowing the passage of large molecules, which would normally be unable to pass.

afterload   The resistance against which the left ventricle must eject its blood volume during systole. Afterload is created by the volume of blood already in the vascular system and the resistance of the vessel walls.

air bronchogram   The visualization of the air-filled bronchus on a chest radiograph. Normally not seen, it is visible when consolidated or atelectatic lung tissue behind the bronchus creates a white background on the radiograph against which the air-filled bronchus can be visualized. Additionally, it may indicate a dilation of the bronchus secondary to distal consolidation or atelectasis.

air leak syndrome

alae nasi   The external border located at the opening to the nasal passages. Being cartilaginous, it normally maintains the patency of the nasal openings during spontaneous ventilation.

almitrine   An experimental respiratory stimulant that is being investigated for possible treatment of neonatal apnea.

alpha-fetoprotein (AFP)   A protein normally synthesized by the liver, yolk sac, and GI tract of the fetus. Elevated levels of AFP in the amniotic fluid help in the diagnosis of neural tube defects such as spina bifida.

amniocentesis   A procedure in which a small amount of amniotic fluid is removed from the uterus. The needle used to extract the fluid is guided by ultrasound to locate a suitable pocket of fluid. The amniotic fluid is then analyzed for numerous fetal genetic defects and for fetal maturity.

amnion   The membrane that covers the fetal side of the placenta, the outer covering of the umbilical cord, and the entire internal surface of the uterus.

amplitude

anaerobic   Pertaining to the absence of oxygen.

analog   A continuous electrical signal often converted into a digital form, which is then displayed.

anemometer   A instrument designed to measure the force or speed of a gas flow.

anencephaly   A genetically transmitted defect in which the brain and spinal cord are absent, the cranium remains open, and the vertebral canal remains a groove.

anticipatory grief   Grief brought on by the anticipation of a traumatic event, such as the death of a loved one.

asphyxia   Severe hypoxia, which leads to hypoxemia, hypercapnia, acidosis, and eventual death if not corrected.

autosomal-recessive trait   A pattern of inheritance in which the transmission of a recessive gene results in a carrier state if the person is heterozygous for the trait, and in an infected state if the person is homozygous for the trait.

azidothymidine (AZT)   A thymidine-based antiviral drug that inhibits the replication of retroviruses. Used in the treatment of HIV infections.

azoospermia   A lack of spermatozoa in the semen.

balloon septostomy (Rashkind procedure)   The enlargement of an opening in the cardiac septum between the right and left atria. It is done under anesthesia by passing a deflated balloon attached to a cardiac catheter through the foramen ovale into the left atrium. The balloon is then inflated and pulled through the foramen ovale to enlarge its opening.

baroreceptor   A cluster of pressure-sensitive nerve endings found in the alls of the atria, the vena cava, the aortic arch, and the carotid sinus. Stretching of the nerves results in stimulation of central reflex mechanisms leading to vasodilation or constriction.

beta-lactam   A group of antibiotics (penicillins and cephalosporins) that inhibit bacterial cell wall synthesis.

blastocyst   The form of fetal embryologic development that follows development of the morula. It is a spherical mass of cells having a central, fluid-filled cavity called the blastocoele and surrounded by two layers of the cells: the triphoblast, which becomes the placenta, and the embryoblast, which becomes the embryo.

blastoderm   The layer of cells forming the wall of the blastocyst. It gives rise to the primary germ layers, the endoderm, mesoderm, and ectoderm.

blastomere   One of the two cells that develops in the first division of the fertilized ovum. The blastomere divides and subdivides to become the morula.

bonding   The attachment process that occurs between an infant and parents beginning with the planning of the baby. Bonding is initially stronger in the mother until delivery, when the father begins a strong bonding process.

Bourdon gauge   A gauge that uses a curled copper tube, closed at one end. As pressure in the gauge increases, the copper tube straightens slightly and, by a series of gears, causes a needle to move on the face of the gauge, reflecting either pressure or flow.

breech   Abnormal fetal delivery in which the fetus emerges feet, knees, or buttocks first.

bronchiolitis obliterans   A pulmonary disease marked by progressive inflammation and obliteration of the distal airways.

brown fat   A type of fat found in newborns. Due to its unique thermogenic activity, brown fat is a unique source of heat energy for the newborn.

calcaneus   The heel bone.

caput succedaneum   A localized pitting edema found in the scalp of a newborn that may overlie the sutures of the skull. It is the result of pressure from the cervix on the fetal head. Usually not dangerous, it disappears within the first few days of life.

barconic acid (H_2CO_3)   The compound formed by the reaction of carbon dioxide (CO_2)

and water (H_2O) or by the reaction of hydrogen ions (H^+) and bicarbonate (HCO_3). The reaction is enhanced by the presence of the enzyme carbonic anhydrase.

chemoreceptor   A sensory nerve stimulated by chemical stimuli such as CO_2 and H^+ ion concentration. Chemoreceptors located in the carotid artery detect changes in $PaCO_2$ and signal the central respiratory center to increase or decrease ventilation.

choana   The funnel-shaped opening between the posterior nares and the nasopharynx.

choanal atresia   A congenital anomaly in which a membranous or bony occlusion blocks the choana. Choanal atresia is caused by the failure of the nasopharyngeal septum to rupture during embryologic development.

chorioamnionitis   An inflammatory reaction in the amnion caused by infectious organisms in the amniotic fluid.

chorionic villi   The tiny vascular fibrils on the surface of the placenta that infiltrate the endometrium of the uterus. They form the point at which maternal and fetal blood exchange nutrients and blood gases.

choroid plexus   Tangled masses of tiny blood vessels found in the third, lateral, and fourth brain ventricles.

cognitive   That which pertains to the mental processes of comprehension, judgment, memory, and reasoning.

color flow mapping   The use of color images with ultrasound, which enables the technician to observe the direction of blood flow. Often used to visualize blood flow through the ductus arteriosus or other heart defect.

compliance   The measurement of the distensibility of the lung, measured by the lung volume produced per unit of pressure change.

compressible volume   That part of the tidal volume that does not reach the patient because it remains in expanded ventilator tubing.

compression factor   The amount of tidal volume that may be trapped in the ventilator tubing in relation to the amount of pressure applied to the tubing. Normally, it is calculated in milliliters per cm H_2O pressure.

conductive (conduction)   The transfer of heat from a warmer object in direct contact with a cooler object.

convective   The transfer of heat from a warm object to cooler air circulating over or around the object.

costophrenic angle   The angle at the bottom of the lung where the diaphragm and the chest wall meet as seen on a chest radiograph.

cotyledon   One of the visible segments on the maternal surface of the placenta containing the fetal vessels, chorionic villi, and the intervillous space.

CPAP

crackle   Formerly called "rales," crackles are described as fine bubbling sounds heard on auscultation of the lungs caused by air entering fluid-filled alveolus and distal airways.

Crigler-Najjar syndrome   A congenital, familial, autosomal abnormality in which glucuronyl transferase is deficient or absent. Characterized by nonhemolytic jaundice, an accumulation of unconjugated bilirubin, and severe disorders of the central nervous system.

cryotherapy   A treatment that uses cold as a destructive medium, usually liquid nitrogen.

cushingoid Having the characteristics of Cushing's disease: fat pads on the upper back and face, striae on the limbs and trunk, and excess hair on the face.

Dalton's law A law of physics stating that the sum of the pressure exerted by a mixture of gases is equal to the total of the partial pressures exerted by each gas if they were separated. $P_B = P_1 + P_2 + P_3...$

decerebrate As relating to posture, the extension and internal rotation of the arms and the extension of the legs with the feet in forced plantar flexion.

decorticate As relating to posture, the rigid flexion of the upper extremities at the wrists and elbows. The legs may also be in a flexed position.

decubitus A recumbent or horizontal position. For example, a lateral decubitus that is lying on one side.

DeLee suction A suction device in which the clinician supplies the suction to the catheter. Any debris is collected in a small collection tube, protecting the clinician from inhaling materials.

demand flow The ability of a ventrilator to provide flow to the patient in addition to the set flow rate. The additional flow is triggered by a mechanism that senses the negative pressure being created by the patient.

densities Relating to the shades of gray seen on a radiograph. Substances that absorb x-rays result in a white density. Substances that absorb little or no x-rays result in a dark density.

diaphragmatic papers An electrode that stimulates the diaphragm to contract. The electrode is maintained by an electronic controller on which the operator determines the rate and strength of contraction.

dichotomy A division or separation into two or more parts.

dilatation The widening of the cervix during labor measured during vaginal examination, expressed in cm or finger breadth. Full dilatation of the cervix is 10 cm.

disseminated Widespread or scattered.

disseminated intravascular coagulation (DIC) A grave coagulopathy that results from the overstimulation of the body's clotting and anticlotting processes in response to disease or injury.

doll's eyes A normal response in newborn infants is for the eyes to remain stationary as the head is rotated from side to side. This reflex is abnormal in adults. *See also* Oculocephalic.

Doppler The change in frequency when a sound is emitted by an object moving toward or away from an observer. In Doppler scanning, ultrasonic waves are reflected from a moving structure such as the heart to yield information on the structure.

doxapram hydrochloride A respiratory stimulant used to improve respiratory function. Often used for chronic pulmonary disease with associated hypercapnia.

DPPC (Dipalmitoyl phosphatidylcholine) The major phospholipid compound found in pulmonary surfactant. *See also* Phosphatidylcholine.

driving pressure The gradient between two pressures that causes a gas or substance to move from the area of higher pressure to the area of lower pressure. The larger the difference between the two pressures, the higher the driving pressure.

ductus arteriosus   The vascular channel that connects the pulmonary artery to the descending aorta in fetal circulation.

ductus venosus   The vascular channel in the fetal circulation that passes through the liver and connects the umbilical vein to the inferior vena cava.

duration of positive pressure   The time in which positive pressure is being applied to the airways. It is measured from the time the pressure elevates above baseline until it returns to baseline.

dyscrasia   An abnormal blood or bone marrow condition, such as aplastic anemia or Rh incompatibility.

dystocia   A pathologic or difficult labor.

ectoderm   The outermost of the three primary germ layers found in the developing embryo. The ectoderm gives rise to the nervous system, eyes, ears, epidermis, and mucous membranes.

effacement   The shortening of the vaginal part of the cervix and the thinning of its walls during labor. Effacement is expressed as a percentage of full effacement, which is 100%.

elasticity   The ability of a tissue to return to its original shape and size following a deforming stress being placed on it.

electromyography   A procedure to test and record the intrinsic ele3ctric activity in a skeletal muscle. This is done by applying electrodes to the skin and observing the electrical activity on an oscilloscope.

emesis   To expel the contents of the stomach through the esophagus and out the mouth.

empathy   The ability to recognize and share the emotions and feelings of another and to understand the meaning of that person's behavior.

encephalocele   A protrusion of the brain through a congenital defect in the skull.

endoderm   The innermost of the germ layers found in the developing embryo. From the endoderm arise the epithelium of the respiratory tract, the GI tract, the urinary tract, pharynx, tonsils, and thyroid gland.

engagement   The fixation of the presenting part of the fetus in the maternal pelvis. Engagement occurs when the presenting part is level with the ischial spines of the maternal pelvis.

enteral   Pertaining to the intestines, often associated with feedings or medications.

enzyme-linked immunosorbent assay (ELISA)   A laboratory test used to detect specific antigens or antibodies, using enzyme-labeled immunoreactants and a solid-phase binding support such as a test tube. It is commonly used in the diagnosis of the AIDS infection.

epistaxis   Bleeding from the nose due to a variety of causes.

erythroblastosis fetalis   A type of hemolytic anemia that occurs in newborns as a result of maternal-fetal blood group incompatibility involving the Rh factor and the ABO blood groups.

estriol   A naturally occurring human estrogen found in high concentrations in urine. Its level in the maternal urine may be used to ascertain the proper function of the placenta.

evaporative   As relates to the loss of heat through the changing of water to vapor on the surface of the skin.

extravasation   A passage of blood, serum, or lymph into the interstitial spaces of the tissue.

extrinsic   Developing or having its origin outside the body.

facilitated diffusion   The movement of ions or molecules through the cell membrane by the interaction with a carrier protein that aids in their passage. This is probably done by binding chemically with the ion or molecule and shuttling it through the membrane.

fertilization   The union of male and female gametes to form a zygote from which the embryo develops.

fetoscopy   A procedure in which a fetus may be directly observed in utero using a fetoscope introduced into the uterus through the abdominal wall. Samples of fluid or tissue may be produced for laboratory assessment.

fluidic   Pertaining to a valve that utilizes the coanda effect to direct the movement of a flow of gas.

Fontan procedure   A surgical treatment of hypoplastic left-heart syndrome in which the main pulmonary artery and the right atrium are connected.

fontanelle   The space on a new2born's cranium between the cranial bones, covered by a tough membrane.

foramen ovale   An opening in the septum separating the atria of the heart found in fetal circulation.

functional residual capacity (FRC)   The volume of gas remaining in the lungs following a normal exhalation.

fundus   As relating to the uterus, the end opposite the cervix.

galactosemia   An inherited, autosomal recessive disorder of galactose metabolism, characterized by a deficiency of the enzyme galactose-l-phosphate uridyl transferase. Hepatosplenomegaly, cataracts, and mental retardation often develop.

gastroschisis   A congenital defect characterized by an incomplete closure of the abdominal wall with protrusion of the viscera.

germinal matrix   An area of profuse vascularization in the developing fetal brain located adjacent to the walls of the ventricles.

glucagon   A hormone produced by the alpha cells found in the islets of Langerhans that stimulates the conversion of glycogen to glucose by the liver.

guaic   A wood resin used on a reagent strip to test for the presence of blood in the stool or urine.

hilum   The depression where the blood vessels, nerves, and bronchus enters the lungs.

human placental lactogen (HPL)   A placental hormone that may be deficient in certain abnormalities of pregnancy.

hydrocephaly   A pathologic condition characterized by an abnormal accumulation of cerebrospinal fluid within the cranial vault, resulting in dilation of the ventricles.

hydrolysis   The chemical alteration or decomposition of a compound with water.

hydrophobic   The property of repelling water molecules.

hydrops fetalis   The massive accumulation of fluid in the fetus or newborn often in association with erythroblastosis fetalis. Effusions of the pericardial, pleural, and peritoneal spaces also occur.

hydroscopic   The property of taking on water molecules.

hyperalimentation   The administration of a nutritionally adequate hypertonic solution consisting of glucose, protein hydrolysates, minerals, and vitamins through an indwelling catheter usually in the superior vena cava. Also called total parenteral nutrition, or TPN.

hyperlucency   As pertaining to a radiograph, that area which is very dark, indicating an accumulation of air or gas.

hyperosmolar   Pertaining to an increased concentration of osmotically active components such as electrolytes and proteins.

hyperpnea   A deep, labored, or rapid respiration.

hypoplasia   The incomplete or underdevelopment of an organ or tissue.

hypopnea   Shallow or slow respirations.

hypotonia   Having a smaller concentration of solute-to-solution ratio than that found in intravascular or interstitial fluids.

hypoxic-ischemic encephalopathy   A serious injury to the infant brain in which death of brain cells occurs secondary to hypoxemia or diminished cerebral blood perfusion accompanying systemic hypotension.

immunoglobulin   Any one of five distinct antibodies present in the serum and external secretions of the body.

inotropic   That which pertains to the strength or force of muscular contractions.

intervillous space   The space located between the chorionic villi of the placenta. The intervillous space acts as a reservioir for maternal arterial blood, which exchanges nutrients and waste with the fetal blood.

intrinsic   Originating within the body.

intussusception   The prolapse of one segment of bowel into the lumen of another segment.

kernicterus   An abnormal toxic level of bilirubin that accumulates in the tissues of the central nervous system, sometimes causing severe degenerative disorders.

Kling gauze   A brand name of wrapping gauze that comes in variable widths and lengths. Normally used to wrap around limbs and extremities.

lanugo   Soft, downy hair that covers the normal fetus from approximately the fifth gestational month until term, at which point it is nearly gone.

lavage   The process of instilling a sterile solution into an organ, including the trachea, in order to wash or to loosen secretions.

lethargy   The state of being indifferent, apathetic, or sluggish.

leukopenia   An abnormal process in which the number of white blood cells is diminished, usually indicated by a white cell count of less than 5000 cells per cubic millimeter.

leukotrienes   A class of biologically active compounds that occur naturally in leukocytes. Leukotrienes produce inflammatory and allergic reactions.

light-emitting diode (LED)   A small electron tube that emits light when charged with an electrical current.

linear drive   As pertaining to a piston-driven ventilator, the piston travels in a straight line front to back creating a square wave now pattern.

logarithm   The exponent that indicates the power to which a number must be raised to produce a given number. For example, in the formula $B^2 = X$, 2 is the logarithm of X.

Lucey Driscol syndrome   A syndrome possibly passed as an autosomal recessive trait characterized by inhibited uridine disphosphate glucuronosyl transferase and leading to rapidly progressive jaundice and kernicterus.

lymphadenophy   Used to denote any disorder of the lymph nodes or vessels.

mainstream nebulizer   A nebulizer designed to be used inline with the flow of inspired gas. In a mainstream nebulizer, the aerosol is created inline with the flow of gas, which then carries the aerosol to the patient.

MAS/KV   Abbreviation for milliampere seconds/kilovolt. Used to determine the necessary energy for exposing a radiograph.

meconium   A thick, dark green, sticky material that collects in the intestines of the fetus and becomes the material expelled during the first bowel movements. It is composed of intestinal secretions, amniotic fluid, and intrauterine debris.

meningomyelocele   A saclike protrusion of either the cerebral or spinal meninges through a congenital defect in the skull or in the vertebral column, which forms a cyst filled with cerebrospinal fluid.

mesoderm   The middle of the three germ layers found in the developing embryo. The mesoderm forms the bones, connective tissues, muscles, blood, vascular, and lymphatic tissues.

metered dose inhaler (MDI)   A small canister containing a prescribed drug that releases a specific dose of aerosolized drug when activated.

methacholine   A cholinergic drug that is aerosolized and delivered by inhalation to confirm the diagnosis of asthma.

micrognathia   Also called Pierre-Robin syndrome, a congenital underdevelopment of the mandible that may cause upper airway obstruction from the tongue falling back into the oropharynx.

microprocessor   A type of miniature device that contains the arithmetic, logic, and control circuitry necessary to interpret and execute program instructions.

morula   The clump of blastomeres formed by the dividing fertilized ovum.

mumur   As relating to heart sounds, a low-pitched fluttering or humming heard just before, during, or after the normal heart sounds.

muscarinic   Pertaining to that which stimulates the receptors of the postganglionic parasympathetic receptors.

necrotizing enterocolitis   An acute inflammation of the bowel that occurs primarily in preterm or neonates of low birthweight. Bacterial invasion of the intestinal wall may lead to perforation and peritonitis.

necrotizing tracheobronchitis   A localized area of tissue damage and death in the trachea and bronchi caused by the continual contact of pulsed gas delivered during high-frequency jet ventilation.

neutropenia   An abnormality resulting in a decrease in the number of blood neutrophils often associated with leukemia and infection.

nosocomial   Relating to the hospital. A nosocomial infection is one acquired during hospitalization.

obtundation   The use of a drug to soothe or deaden pain in order to reduce patient anxiety and discomfort. Often done by reducing the consciousness level of the patient.

occult   Being hidden from view or difficult to observe.

oculocephalic (reflex)   A reflex used to test the integrity of the brainstem. The head is quickly moved from side to side. Failure of the eyes to lag properly or to assume the midline position indicates a lesion on the ipsilateral side at the level of the brainstem.

oculovestibular (response)   This test is elicited by irrigating the external auditory canal with ice water. The normal response is a conjugate movement of the eyes toward the side of stimulation. Absence of the response indicates impairment of the pontine centers. Also called the caloric test.

oligohydramnios   An abnormally small amount of or the absence of amniotic fluid.

omphalocele   A congenital herniation of the intraabdominal viscera through the abdominal wall near the umbilicus.

optimism   A belief or disposition that everything will work out for the best.

ora serrata   The zigzag margin found in the retina of the eye.

ototoxic   Referring to a substance having a harmful effect on the eighth cranial nerve or on the organs of hearing and balance.

ovum   The female germ cell extruded from the ovary at ovulation.

oxidation   A reaction in which either the oxygen content of a compound is increased or the positive valence of a compound or radical is increased because of a loss of electrons.

pallor   The absence of normal color in the skin or an unnatural paleness to the skin.

paradoxical   Any situation or occurrence in which the outcome is the opposite of what is expected.

parenteral   Pertaining to the uptake of substances or medications by any route other than the digestive tract.

periventricular leukomalacia   The neuropathologic consequence of a generalized reduction in cerebral blood flow in the premature infant resulting in necrosis of the periventricular white matter.

persistent fetal circulation   A condition in which blood flow continues following the fetal pattern after delivery. The shunts involved include the ductus arteriosus and the foramen ovale.

pessimism   The tendency to always view the grim side of every situation.

petechiae   Small purple or red spots on the skin resulting from minute hemorrhages within the dermal or submucosal layers.

pharmacokinetics   The study of all aspects of drug use on the body to include routes of absorption and excretion, duration and action, and biotransformation.

pheochromocytoma   A chronic hypertension caused by a vascular tumor of the adrenal medulla or sympathetic paraganglia. It is characterized by hypersecretion of epinephrine and norepinephrine.

phosphatidylcholine (PC)   The major component of mature surfactant. It is the compound that is most active in lowering alveolar surface tensions. Its concentration is measured following amniocentesis to determine lung maturity. *See also* DPPC.

phosphatidylglycerol (PG)   One of the minor acidic phospholipids found in surfactant. Its presence in amniotic fluid signals the maturity of the fetal lungs.

phosphatidylinositol (PI)   One of the minor acidic phospholipids found in surfactant. PI is important in the stabilization of PC in the surfactant layer that lines the alveoli.

phospholipid　One of a class of compounds containing phosphoric acid, fatty acids, and a nitrogenous base. Phospholipids are found in many living cells.

pinna　The cartilaginous portion of the external ear.

placenta previa　An abnormal implantation of the placenta near to or covering the cervical opening.

pleural effusion　An abnormal accumulation of fluid between the lung and the pleural lining. The fluid is either a transudate, which is a relatively protein-free fluid extruded from a tissue, or an exudate, which is a fluid high in protein that has escaped from the blood vasculature.

pneumocardiogram　A test in which the respirations and electrocardiogram of an infant are monitored over a period of time in an attempt to discover apnea or candidates for SIDS.

pneumotachograph　An instrument that measures the velocity of expired gas flows.

polyhydramnios　A condition of excessive amounts of amniotic fluid, usually more than 2000 ml.

posthemorrhagic hydrocephalus　The abnormal accumulation of cerebrospinal fluid in the ventricles caused by blockage and obstruction that results from residual adhesions from the initial disease process.

preeclampsia　An abnormal condition occurring during pregnancy in which the maternal blood pressure elevates after week 24 of gestation. Hypertension is accompanied by proteinuria and edema. The etiology remains unknown.

primary apnea　A cessation of breathing with accompanying bradycardia that follows the onset of asphyxia in the fetus.

prolapse　The failing or sliding of an organ from its normal position.

pseudocholinesterase　A nonspecific cholinesterase that hydrolyses noncholine esters as w4ell as acetylcholine.

pseudocysts　A space or cavity containing a gas or liquid that does not have a lining membrane.

PSIG　Abbreviation for pounds per square inch, gauge. PSIG is used to identify the pressure in a gas cylinder as measured by an attached regulator gauge.

psychosocial　Pertaining to a combination of psychologic and social factors.

pulmonary hypoplasia　An abnormal underdevelopment of the pulmonary tree, often caused by a space-occupying lesion such as diaphragmatic hernia, which does not allow the lung to develop normally.

purulent　Producing or containing pus.

radiant　The transfer of heat from a warm object to a cooler object not in direct contact by the emission of heat rays.

radiopaque　A substance or object that does not allow the passage of x-rays. The result is a white area on the exposed film. Often used to assess the location of catheters and tubes in the body.

rebound effect　The sudden contraction, swelling, or edema that follows the effects of a bronchodilatory or vasodilatory drug.

reconcentration　The concept that a nebulized drug becomes higher in concentration as the fluid level diminishes. This is caused by a combination of evaporation of the diluent and the baffling of larger aerosol particles, which fall back into the solution and eventually make the drug concentration higher.

reduction   The addition of hydrogen to a substance, the removal of oxygen from a substance, or a decrease in the valence of the electronegative part of a compound.

reflux   An abnormal backward flow of fluid as in stomach fluids flowing up the esophagus.

regionalization   The organization of health care delivery within a geographic region that ensures availability of all hospital services to the population residing within the region and avoiding costly duplication.

resistance   The opposition to flow offered by the walls of the airways or of the blood vessels. Resistance is increased as the diameter of the vessel or airway is decreased.

reticulocytosis   An increase in the number of reticulocytes in the blood.

reticulogranular   A cloudy or hazy appearance of the lung fields seen on a chest radiograph of a patient with respiratory distress.

rhonchi   Abnormal breath sounds heard during auscultation caused by the airway being obstructed with secretions, muscular spasm, or external pressure. The sounds are described as a snore or rumbling, are more pronounced during exhalation, and usually clear with coughing.

roentgenograph   An exposed x-ray film.

rugae   Ridges or folds of skin found in the stomach and on the mature male scrotum.

scaphoid   A sunken anterior abdominal wall.

secondary apnea   A cessation of breathing accompanied by bradycardia and hypotension that follows extended asphyxia in the fetus or newborn. Spontaneous respirations will not occur again unless the infant is mechanically ventilated and the asphyxia reversed.

sensitivity   Pertaining to mechanical ventilation, the capacity to detect a patient-initiated breath by the spontaneous creation of negative pressure in the airway, allowing the ventilator to synchronize the mechanically assisted breaths.

septum primum   An embryologic structure in the developing heart, which eventually becomes the atrial and ventricular septum.

servo-controlled   A device that utilizes a feedback loop for control. An example is a home thermostat, which measures the temperature and triggers the furnace when the temperature drops below the set level. As the temperature rises above the set level, the thermostat stops the furnace.

sieve   A filter or mesh screen that only allows the passage of particles smaller than the openings in the filter or mesh.

simple diffusion   The movement of fluids or particles from an area of higher concentration to an area of lower concentration through a semipermeable membrane following brownian movement.

sine wave   A pressure or flow pattern that assimilates natural breathing patterns. The inspiratory and expiratory patterns appear as a semicircle above and below the line of no flow or no pressure.

sinus venosus   The embryologic structure in the fetal heart that eventually becomes the inferior and superior vena cava and a portion of the right atrium.

socialization   The process by which an individual learns to live within the expectations and standards of society.

sodium-potassium exchange resin (Kayexalate) A resin-containing solution administered via enema in which sodium ions are released from the solution and replaced by potassium ions in the intestines. Used to treat hyperkalemia.

solenoid A coil of wire in the form of a cylinder. When electrical current flows through the wire, a magnetic field is developed drawing a movable core into the coil.

spacer A device placed between the discharge port of a metered dose inhaler and the patient's mouth. Used to allow better distribution of the nebulized particles in the patient's tracheobronchial tree.

spectrophotometric infrared analysis The measurement of different species of hemoglobin in a blood sample by determining the amount of infrared light absorbed.

sphingomyelin A type of sphingolipid found in steady quantities in amniotic fluid. Compared with the concentration of lecithin, it is a part of the determination of lung maturation during the L/S ratio test.

static attraction The attraction of two tissues or objects that is maintained by a thin fluid layer between the two tissues or objects. An example is the attraction between the visceral and parietal pleura of the lungs and thorax.

stations The level of the biparietal plane of the fetal head in relation to the level of the ischial spines on the maternal pelvis measured in negative cm above the spines and positive cm below the spines.

stratum corneum The outermost layer of the skin composed of dead cells converted to keratin.

supine Lying on the back.

surfactant A combination of lipoproteins found in mature alveoli that reduce the surface tension of the pulmonary fluids.

systolic ejection clicks An extra heart sound heard during mid- to late systole having a click-like quality. A frequent cause of ejection clicks is prolapse of the mitral valve.

teratogen Any substance or agent that interferes with normal fetal development and causes one or more developmental abnormalities in the fetus.

third-party reimbursement The reimbursement for care in which an entity other than the receiver or the giver of care is responsible for payment. Usually assigned to an insurance company.

thoracic gas volume The volume of gas in the thorax as measured by a body plethysmograph. Thoracic gas volumes include gas that may or may not be in free communication with the airways.

Thorpe tube A method of measuring gas flows by using a free-floating ball inside a calibrated cylinder. The flow of gas causes the ball to rise in the cylinder, allowing the clinician to read flow from the height of the ball.

thrombocytopenia An abnormal reduction in the number of blood platelets. It is often a result of destruction of erythroid tissue in bone marrow or an immune response to a drug.

thromboxanes Following an injury to a vessel, thromboxanes are formed by the enzymes of plattelets and, when combined with ADP, act on nearby platelets to activate them also. The stickiness of these additional platelets causes them to adhere to the original platelets.

thrombus An aggregation of platelets, fibrin, clotting factors, and cellular elements of the blood that attaches to the interior wall of a vessel.

thymus   The primary central gland of the lymphatic system located in the mediastinum and extending superiorly into the neck to the lower edge of the thyroid gland.

thyrotoxicosis   A disorder characterized by an enlarged thyroid gland, exophthalmos, and hyperthyroidism of unknown origin. Also called Graves' disease.

time constant   The amount of time necessary to allow expiration from the respiratory system. One time constant is calculated by multiplying the compliance by the resistance. Ninety-five percent of the tidal volume is exhaled following three time constants.

titrate   The addition or administration of definite amounts of a solution or drug until a given endpoint or sign is achieved.

tocodynamometer   An instrument used to measure the force of uterine contractions.

tocolysis   Uterine relaxation resulting in a postponement of labor.

tonic posturing   An abnormal sign of brain dysfunction in which some or all skeletal muscles remain in a contracted state.

transducer   A device activated by some sort of received energy, which is then converted to a signal suitable for transmission over an electrical circuit.

transient   Pertaining to a temporary condition.

transillumination   The use of a high-intensity light passing through body tissues for the purpose of examining a structure interposed between the observer and the light source.

transthoracic oscillation   A novel modality of mechanical ventilation in which a chest shell is placed over the thorax and negative pressure is applied to the internal space of the shell at an extremely high rate.

Trendelenburg   A position in which the head is lower than the body and legs. Often used during chest physiotherapy to aid in bronchial drainage.

trophoblast   The layer of tissue that forms the wall of the blastocyst in the early stages of embryologic development.

truncus arteriosus   The embryologic structure of the developing heart, which becomes the aorta and pulmonary artery.

turfism   The claiming of a geographic or territorial region as belonging to an individual or organization.

turgor   The normal resiliency of the skin, which is a result of the outward pressure of the cells and interstitial fluid.

ultrafiltration   The act of filtering large molecules from small molecules by creating a pressure gradient across a filter containing small pores.

unstressed volume   The volume of gas in the lungs when the thorax is at its resting level.

updraft nebulizer   An aerosol-creating device in which the aerosol must exit the nebulizer in order to enter the inspiratory stream of gas going to the patient. Also called a sidestream nebulizer.

uteroplacental   Pertaining to the function, anatomy, and physiology of the uterus and placenta.

vaso-obliteration   The destruction of the retinal vasculature in the first stages of retinopathy of prematurity. In response to hyperoxia and other factors, the vessels may permanently constrict and become necrotic.

venoarterial   Removal of the blood from a large vein and returning the blood to an artery.

When used with ECLS, the blood is often removed from the right atrium and returned to the aorta.

venovenous   Removal of the blood from a vein and returning the blood to a vein.

ventricular-peritoneal shunt   A surgically created passageway in which the cerebrospinal fluid is diverted through a plastic tube to the abdominal cavity where it is absorbed. Used to drain excess amounts of fluid from the brain in hydrocephalus.

ventriculostomy   A surgically created opening opening that allows cerebrospinal fluid to drain from the ventricles of the brain to the cistera magna. Also known as the Torkildsen procedure.

vernix   An off-white, cheese-like substance that covers the skin of the fetus and newborn. It is composed of sebaceous gland secretions, lanugo, and epithelial cells. It aids in thermoregulation and in the delivery of the fetus by facilitating the passage through the birth canal.

viscosity   The thickness, density, and stickiness of a fluid. A viscous fluid is thicker and denser than a nonviscous fluid.

volume-assured pressure support

volume-controlled ventilation

volume support (VS)

Western blot   A laboratory test used to detect the presence of antibodies to specific antigens. It is thought to be more reliable than the ELISA test and is often used to verify the results of the ELISA test.

wheeze   A form of rhonchus that has the sound of a high-pitched whistle or a musical quality. Often heard over areas of airway constriction or obstruction.

INDEX